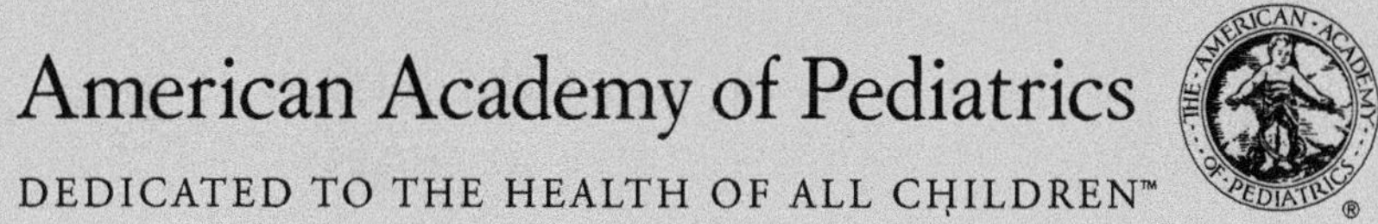

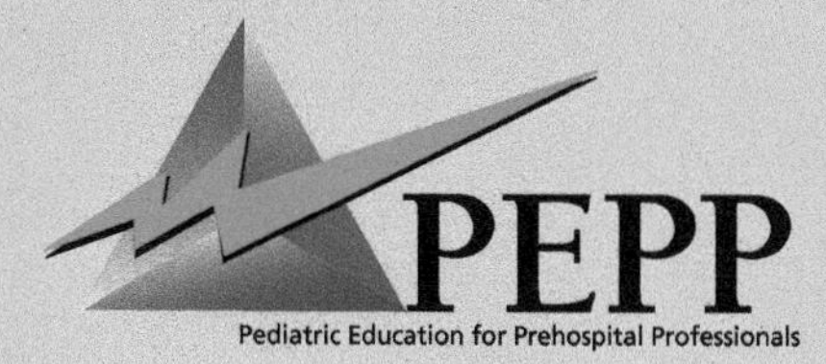

Pediatric Education
for Prehospital Professionals

REVISED THIRD EDITION

Editors

Susan Fuchs, MD, FAAP, FACEP

Bruce L. Klein, MD, FAAP

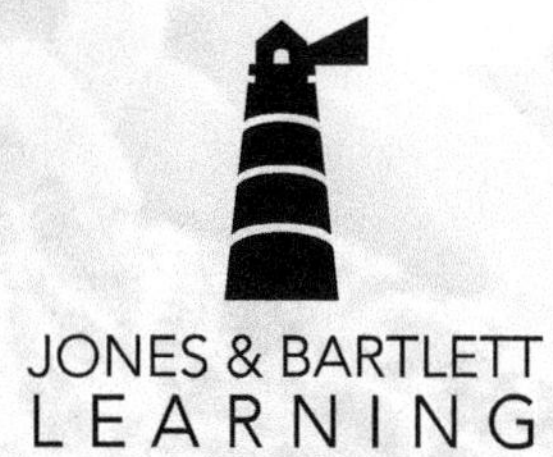

JONES & BARTLETT
LEARNING

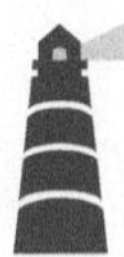

World Headquarters
Jones & Bartlett Learning
5 Wall Street
Burlington, MA 01803
978-443-5000
info@jblearning.com
www.jblearning.com

American Academy of Pediatrics
DEDICATED TO THE HEALTH OF ALL CHILDREN™

Thaddeus Anderson, Manager, AAP Maintenance of Competency and Simulation
Melissa Marx, Manager, AAP Life Support Programs
Michael Greenier, MPH, Life Support Simulation and Course Specialist
Caitlin E. Hahne, AAP Life Support Programs Assistant
Gina Pantone, AAP Division Coordinator
Wendy Simon, MA, CAE, Director, AAP Life Support Programs
American Academy of Pediatrics
141 Northwest Point Boulevard
Post Office Box 927
Elk Grove Village, IL 60009-0927
www.PEPPSite.com
www.aap.org

Jones & Bartlett Learning books and products are available through most bookstores and online booksellers. To contact Jones & Bartlett Learning directly, call 800-832-0034, fax 978-443-8000, or visit our website, www.jblearning.com.

Substantial discounts on bulk quantities of Jones & Bartlett Learning publications are available to corporations, professional associations, and other qualified organizations. For details and specific discount information, contact the special sales department at Jones & Bartlett Learning via the above contact information or send an email to specialsales@jblearning.com.

This material is made available as part of the professional education programs of the American Academy of Pediatrics. No endorsement of any product or service should be inferred or is intended. The Academy has made every effort to ensure that contributors to the *Pediatric Education for Prehospital Professionals (PEPP), Revised Third Edition* materials are knowledgeable authorities in their fields. Readers are nevertheless advised that the statements and opinions are provided as guidelines and should not be construed as official Academy policy. The recommendations in this publication or the accompanying resources do not indicate an exclusive course of treatment. Variations taking into account individual circumstances, nature of medical oversight, and local protocols may be appropriate. The Academy and the publisher disclaim any liability or responsibility for the consequences of any actions taken in reliance on these statements or opinions.

There may be images in this book that feature models; these models do not necessarily endorse, represent, or participate in the activities represented in the images. Any screenshots in this product are for educational and instructive purposes only. Any individuals and scenarios featured in the case studies throughout this product may be real or fictitious, but are used for instructional purposes only.

Products are included for informational purposes only. Inclusion in this publication does not imply endorsement by the American Academy of Pediatrics.

Production Credits
Chief Executive Officer: Ty Field
President: James Homer
EVP, Chief Product Officer: Ed Moura
Executive Publisher: Kimberly Brophy
Executive Acquisitions Editor: Christine Emerton
Editor: Alison Lozeau
Production Manager: Jenny L. Corriveau
Associate Production Editor: Nora Menzi
Vice President of Marketing: Alisha Weisman
Vice President of Sales, Public Safety Group: Matthew Maniscalco
Director of Sales, Public Safety Group: Patricia Einstein
VP, Manufacturing and Inventory Control: Therese Connell
Composition: diacriTech
Cover Design: Kristin E. Parker
Director of Photo Research and Permissions: Amy Wrynn
Cover Image: © Bruce Ayres/Getty Images
Printing and Binding: RR Donnelley
Cover Printing: RR Donnelley

To order this product, use ISBN: 978-1-284-13303-5

The Library of Congress has cataloged the first printing as follows:
Pediatric Education for Prehospital Professionals / American Academy of Pediatrics. — 3rd ed.
p. ; cm.
PEPP
Includes bibliographical references and index.
ISBN 978-1-4496-0763-0 — ISBN 978-1-4496-7043-6
I. American Academy of Pediatrics. II. Pediatric Education for Prehospital Professionals (Program) III. Title: PEPP.
[DNLM: 1. Emergencies. 2. Child. 3. Emergency Medical Services—methods. 4. Pediatrics. WS 205]

618.92'0025—dc23

2012017921

6048

Printed in the United States of America
23 22 21 20 13 12 11 10

Brief Contents

Contents

PEPP Steering Committee

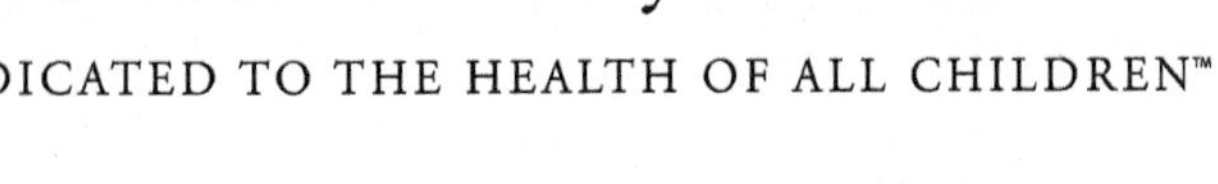

Deena Brecher, MSN, RN, APN, ACNS-BC, CEN, CPEN
Representative – Emergency Nurses Association
Cincinnati, OH

Thomas Breyer, FF/NRP
Representative – International Association of Fire Fighters
Washington, DC

Kathleen M. Brown, MD, FAAP, FACEP
Representative – American College of Emergency Physicians
The George Washington University School of Medicine
Children's National Medical Center
Washington, DC

James M. Callahan, MD, FAAP, FACEP
Representative – National Association of EMS Physicians
The Children's Hospital of Philadelphia
Philadelphia, PA

Susan Fuchs, MD, FAAP, FACEP
Co-Editor, *PEPP Revised Third Edition*
Representative – AAP Committee on Pediatric Emergency Medicine
Feinberg School of Medicine
Northwestern University
Associate Director, Division of Emergency Medicine
Ann and Robert H. Lurie Children's Hospital of Chicago
Chicago, IL

Brandon Kelley
Representative – National Association of State EMS Officials
Cheyenne, WY

Bruce L. Klein, MD, FAAP
Co-Chair, PEPP Steering Committee
Co-Editor, *PEPP Revised Third Edition*
Representative – AAP Section on Transport Medicine
Johns Hopkins Children's Center
Baltimore, MD

Katherine Remick, MD, FAAP
Representative – National Association of Emergency Medical Technicians
Austin, TX

Stephen G. Simon, MS, EMT-P, EFO
Representative – International Association of Fire Chiefs
Roanoke, VA

Keith Widmeier, BA, NRP, CCEMT-P, EMSI
Representative – National Association of EMS Educators
Cincinnati, OH

Cynthia Wright-Johnson, MSN, RNC
Representative - National Association of State EMS Officials
Baltimore, MD

Acknowledgments

Editors: Susan Fuchs, MD, FAAP, FACEP, and Bruce L. Klein, MD, FAAP

Authors

The American Academy of Pediatrics and Editors acknowledge with appreciation the contributions of the following individuals in the development of this resource.

Andrew Bartkus, RN, MSN, JD, CEN, CCRN, CFRN, NREMT-P, FP-C
Albuquerque, NM

Angela M. Bowen, RN, BSN, CPEN, NREMT-P
East Tennessee Children's Hospital
Knoxville, TN

Kelly Buddenhagen, NREMT-P
Ellijay, GA

Glen W. Clegg
Zephyrhills, FL

Twink Dalton, RN, MS, CNS, NREMT-P
Longmont, CO

Fidel O. Garcia, Paramedic
Grand Junction, CO

Carol Gupton, BS, NREMT-P
Omaha, NE

Bryan Hess, NREMT-P
Gunnison, CO

Gail Larkin, BS, NREMT-P
Long Island City, NY

Jennifer McCarthy, MAS, MICP
Crawford, NJ

Shannon Watson, NREMT-P
St. Louis, MO

Elizabeth M. Wertz Evans, RN, BSN, MPM, FACMPE, CPHQ, CPHIMS, FHIMSS
Cranberry Township, PA

Keith Widmeier, NREMT-P, BA
Somerset, KY

Contributors

The American Academy of Pediatrics and Editors acknowledge with appreciation the contributions of the following individuals in the development of the Procedures.

Bruce L. Klein, MD, FAAP
Johns Hopkins Children's Center
Baltimore, MD

Kristen Nelson McMillan, MD, FAAP
Johns Hopkins University School of Medicine
Baltimore, MD

Karen Schneider, MD, MPH, FAAP
Johns Hopkins University
Baltimore, MD

Physician Reviewers

The American Academy of Pediatrics and Editors acknowledge with appreciation the contributions of the following individuals in the development of this resource.

Terry Adirim, MD, MPH, FAAP
Director, Office of Special Health Affairs
Health Resources and Services Administration

Jeffrey R. Avner, MD, FAAP
Children's Hospital of Montefiore

Carol D. Berkowitz, MD, FAAP, FACEP
Harbor-UCLA Medical Center

Deena Brecher, MSN, RN, APN, ACNS-BC, CEN, CPEN
Representative – Emergency Nurses Association
Cincinnati, OH

Thomas Breyer, FF/NRP
Representative – International Association of Fire Fighters

Kathleen M. Brown, MD, FAAP, FACEP
Representative – American College of Emergency Physicians

Casey Buitenhuys, MD
Stanford University Hospital and Clinics

Marilyn J. Bull, MD, FAAP
Riley Hospital for Children at IU Health

James M. Callahan, MD, FAAP, FACEP
Representative – National Association of Emergency Medical Services Physicians

William A. Carey, MD, FAAP
Mayo Clinic

Meta L. Carroll, MD, FAAP
Northwestern University Feinberg School of Medicine

Christopher E. Colby, MD, FAAP
Mayo Clinic

Ronald Dieckmann, MD, MPH, FAAP, FACEP
University of California, San Francisco

Timothy Erickson, MD, FACEP, FAACT, FACMT
University of Illinois College of Medicine

George L. Foltin, MD, FAAP, FACEP
NYU School of Medicine

Susan Fuchs, MD, FAAP, FACEP
Co-Editor, *PEPP Revised Third Edition*
Representative – AAP Committee on Pediatric Emergency Medicine

Marianne Gausche-Hill, MD, FAAP, FACEP
Harbor-UCLA Medical Center

Phyllis L. Hendry, MD, FAAP, FACEP
University of Florida Health Science Center, Jacksonville

Stephen R. Karl, MD, FAAP, FACS
Avera McKenna Hospital and University Health Center

Brandon Kelley
Representative – National Association of State EMS Officials

Bruce L. Klein, MD, FAAP
Co-Chair, PEPP Steering Committee
Co-Editor, *PEPP Revised Third Edition*
Representative – AAP Section on Transport Medicine

Katherine Remick, MD, FAAP
Representative – National Association of Emergency Medical Technicians

Peter Di Rocco, MD
John A. Burns School of Medicine

Steven M. Selbst, MD, FAAP
Jefferson Medical College

Ghazala Q. Sharieff, MD, FACEP, FAAEM
University of California, San Diego

Stephen G. Simon, MS, EMT-P, EFO
Representative – International Association of Fire Chiefs

Paul E. Sirbaugh, DO, FAAP
Baylor College of Medicine/TCH

Michael G. Tunik, MD, FAAP
NYU School of Medicine

Keith Widmeier, BA, NRP, CCEMT-P, EMSI
Representative – National Association of EMS Educators

Cynthia Wright-Johnson, MSN, RNC
Representative - National Association of State EMS Officials

Board Reviewers

The editors would like to acknowledge the work of the American Academy of Pediatrics Board-appointed reviewer.

Carden Johnston, MD, FAAP, FRCP
University of Alabama at Birmingham School of Medicine

EMS Reviewers

Jason Ambrose, EMT-P, NCEE
Virginia Beach, VA

Gary R. Anderson, AEMT
Layton, UT

Steven K. Frye, BS, NREMT-P
College Park, MD

Kevin M. Gurney, BS, CCEMT-P, I/C
Waterville, ME

Peter D. Johnson, EMSI/NREMTP
Oxford, CT

Deb Kaye, BS, NREMT
Willmar, MN

Greg LaMay, BS, NREMT-P, NCEE
Tyler, TX

Judith Lynch, AA
Oakville, CT

Shannon McDaniel, EMS-I
Seymour, CT

Charlene Phelps, EMTI
Starksboro, VT

Katharine P. Rickey, BS, NRParamedic
Barnstead, NH

Superintendent Roland Webb, PCP
Delta, BC, Canada

Susan Siorek, RN, BSN, TNS
Maywood, IL

Pamela N. Taylor, EMT-P, PI
Westfield, IN

Photoshoot Acknowledgments

We would like to thank the following people and institutions for their collaboration on the photoshoots for this project. Their assistance was greatly appreciated.

Erica D'Errico
Schenectady, NY

Glen E. Ellman
Fort Worth Fire Department
Fort Worth, TX

Medical Advisor: Anthony Caliguire, Lieutenant REMT-P
Scotia Fire Department
Scotia, NY

Paul Felts
Ballston Lake, NY

PEPP History

The Pediatric Education for Prehospital Professionals (PEPP) Course is a tapestry of 25 years of collaboration, brainstorming, review, revision, and refinement by hundreds of physicians, nurses, paramedics, EMTs, and EMS educators dedicated to improving prehospital care of children. It is the most widely used and most extensively referenced course in pediatric prehospital care. The statistics paint an impressive picture: from 2000–2013, the American Academy of Pediatrics (AAP) registered 29,151 courses, and awarded PEPP certificates of completion to 320,794 students! The PEPP learning system is an honored cornerstone of EMS and pediatric life support education in the United States and worldwide.

The earliest history of the course dates back to 1990, to a period in American EMS when very little evidence-based information was available about safe and effective practices in prehospital care of infants and children. The original course was officially born in Dr. Ron Dieckmann's back office at San Francisco General Hospital, as a project of the California Pediatric Emergency and Critical Care Coalition, to address widening alarm over dangers and deficiencies in prehospital care of children being documented in medical journals and the lay media. The California EMS Authority funded the initial project through a federal block grant to a new committee formed by the Coalition named the California "PEP (Pediatric Education for Paramedics) Task Force."

After two years of fact-finding, deliberation and collaboration with representatives from the AAP, American College of Emergency Physicians (ACEP) and National Association of EMS Physicians (NAEMSP), the original California PEP Task Force published *Pediatric Education Guidelines for Paramedics* in 1993. The manuscript outlined desired educational goals, learning objectives, and components for a pediatric-specific curriculum for paramedics. The *Guidelines* were formally approved for all California paramedic training programs by the California EMS Commission and concurrently adopted and published by ACEP as the first national consensus document on prehospital pediatric care.

That same year, ACEP established a national committee on pediatric prehospital care, which became the "National PEP Task Force." Chaired by Dr. Dieckmann, the committee translated the California *Guidelines* into a practical "curriculum" for primary paramedic education in pediatrics. Then, in 1996, the Task Force released the first complete "PEP Course" with coordinated state-of-the art learning materials customized for prehospital providers. The course reflected the inspirational work of multiple state EMSC projects—especially the Washington Pediatric Prehospital Care Project, headed by Dena Brownstein in Seattle, and the California Pediatric Airway Project, directed by Dr. Marianne Gausche-Hill in Los Angeles. The new course was an interactive, highly visual, assessment-based "learning system" that included multiple linked components: a student manual, instructor manual, PowerPoint slide set, and an instructional video. Moreover, the learning system was developed and archived electronically and disseminated on a CD to allow rapid and inexpensive national distribution to site instructors, as well as easy modification with anticipated ongoing enhancements in prehospital clinical care.

1998 was a watershed moment in the course's history. That year, the AAP, the country's largest professional pediatric organization, identified prehospital care of children as a critical element of community pediatric services, and invested its vast clinical expertise and administrative and educational resources in the systematic dissemination of the course nationally and internationally. The AAP assumed financial and administrative ownership of the broadening PEP initiative, under the dedicated and visionary leadership of Linda Lipinsky, AAP Director of Life Support Programs. To oversee ongoing course development, improvements in teaching materials, and establishment of a sustainable national training network and fiscal infrastructure, the AAP appointed a permanent oversight group, the "National PEPP Steering Committee," with representatives from all organizations countrywide involved in pediatric prehospital care. The original committee included Bob Bailey, Pam Baker, Dr. Dena Brownstein, Dr. David Burchfield, Dr. Art Cooper, Dr. Susan Fuchs, Dr. Marianne Gausche-Hill, Tricia Kunz-Howard, Dr. Deborah Mulligan-Smith, Michael Pante, Gary Rainey, Steve Strawderman, Dr. Robert Wiebe, and Dr. George Woodward. Dr. Dieckmann served as first PEPP chairperson.

In the transition of the course to the AAP, a significant modification occurred in the scope and overall vision of the initiative: the earlier moniker "PEP" was changed to "PEPP" or "Pediatric Education for Prehospital Professionals." Every letter and word in the course's new name reflected strongly-held tenets of the Steering Committee: "Pediatric" to embody the full emphasis of the course on care of children; "Education" to reflect the goal for a broader cognitive and affective context for learning beyond conventional training; "Prehospital" to convey a special focus on the unique aspects of care delivery in the out-of-hospital environment; "Professionals" to promote commitment of both BLS *and* ALS personnel to effective pediatric care delivery.

At the beginning of the national rollout, the AAP entered into a key business partnership with Jones & Bartlett Learning, who had long experience in the arena of EMS educational publications. A major proponent in the production and dissemination of PEPP as a state-of-the art learning system was Jones & Bartlett's executive publisher, Kimberly Brophy, who became an invaluable ex-officio member of the PEPP Committee and vigorous advocate in the PEPP national effort.

A significant development in the early proceedings of the committee was the adoption of the Pediatric Assessment Triangle (PAT) as the centerpiece of the PEPP learning system. This paradigm was created by Drs. Dieckmann, Brownstein, and Gausche-Hill to introduce an integrative, visual, easily-remembered approach to assessment of infants and children.* Soon after introduction of the course, the PAT became the PEPP "brand" and the ongoing course logo. Then, in 2005, following the enthusiastic adoption of the PAT by PEPP learners, the PAT was established as the approved assessment model for all American pediatric life support courses in a national consensus meeting sponsored by the Federal EMSC Program. Since then, the PAT has become the recommended approach to assessment of children not only in PEPP, but also in APLS: The Pediatric Emergency Medicine Resource, the Emergency Nurse Pediatric Course (ENPC) for nurses, and in all pediatric life support programs countrywide. Studies in Los Angeles and elsewhere have confirmed that the PAT is a valuable tool when applied by nurses at triage and when used accurately by paramedics to drive prehospital pediatric care.

The inaugural fully-packaged PEPP course enjoyed meteoric success. The first edition of the 2000 "PEPP Manual" sold 91,233 copies—an astounding volume for a medical reference in any field. A year later, PEPP received its first major national accolade: the "EMSC National Heroes Award" from the Emergency Medical Services for Children Program, Maternal and Child Health Bureau, and National Highway Traffic Safety Administration, to recognize outstanding achievements in improving care of infants and children.

After the release of the first edition, the National PEPP Steering Committee pushed to extend its reach further into the prehospital provider communities. The second edition of the highly popular PEPP student manual was published in 2006 by Jones and Bartlett and sold 100,795 copies! The concepts and teaching methods outlined in the second edition were further embellished by the addition of the first online, interactive PEPP refresher course. This electronic program represented a further evolution of the learning system to accommodate providers who had previously completed the primary PEPP course and needed continuing refresher education. The online course offered a new option—learners could study pediatric concepts and perform self-assessment remotely, any time, at their convenience, with only a computer and web access.

After the release of the second edition, Dr. Brownstein who had helped usher the course through its first 15 years of history became the national chairperson. Thereafter, Dr. Susan Fuchs, a national leader in EMSC and original PEPP Committee member assumed the co-chairpersonship of the committee along with Michael Pante, a New Jersey paramedic, representative from the National Association of EMS Educators and also original PEPP Steering Committee member.

In 2008, a final piece of the original vision of the Steering Committee for an inclusive educational product for all prehospital provider levels was implemented when the AAP published the first PEPP student manual specifically for BLS providers. Since the course's introduction, the AAP has awarded 57,742 PEPP certificates of completion to BLS students.

In 2013, the AAP announced a partnership with the National Association of Emergency Medical Technicians (NAEMT). The AAP and NAEMTs agreement recognizes the value of collaborating with all providers in the continuum of pediatric emergency care.

The third edition of the student manual was released in 2014, amid a widening scope of influence of the course in multiple other countries in the Western world, who have adopted PEPP as the international standard of pediatric prehospital education. Following the release of the third edition manual, NAEMT adopted the third edition of the PEPP textbook for use within their Emergency Pediatric Care (EPC) course.

Historical summary prepared by Ron Dieckmann, MD, MPH
University of California, San Francisco

*Dieckmann RA, Brownstein D, Gausche-Hill M. The Pediatric Assessment Triangle: A Novel Approach to Pediatric Assessment. *Pediatric Emergency Care*, Vol 26, No 4, 2010: 312–315.

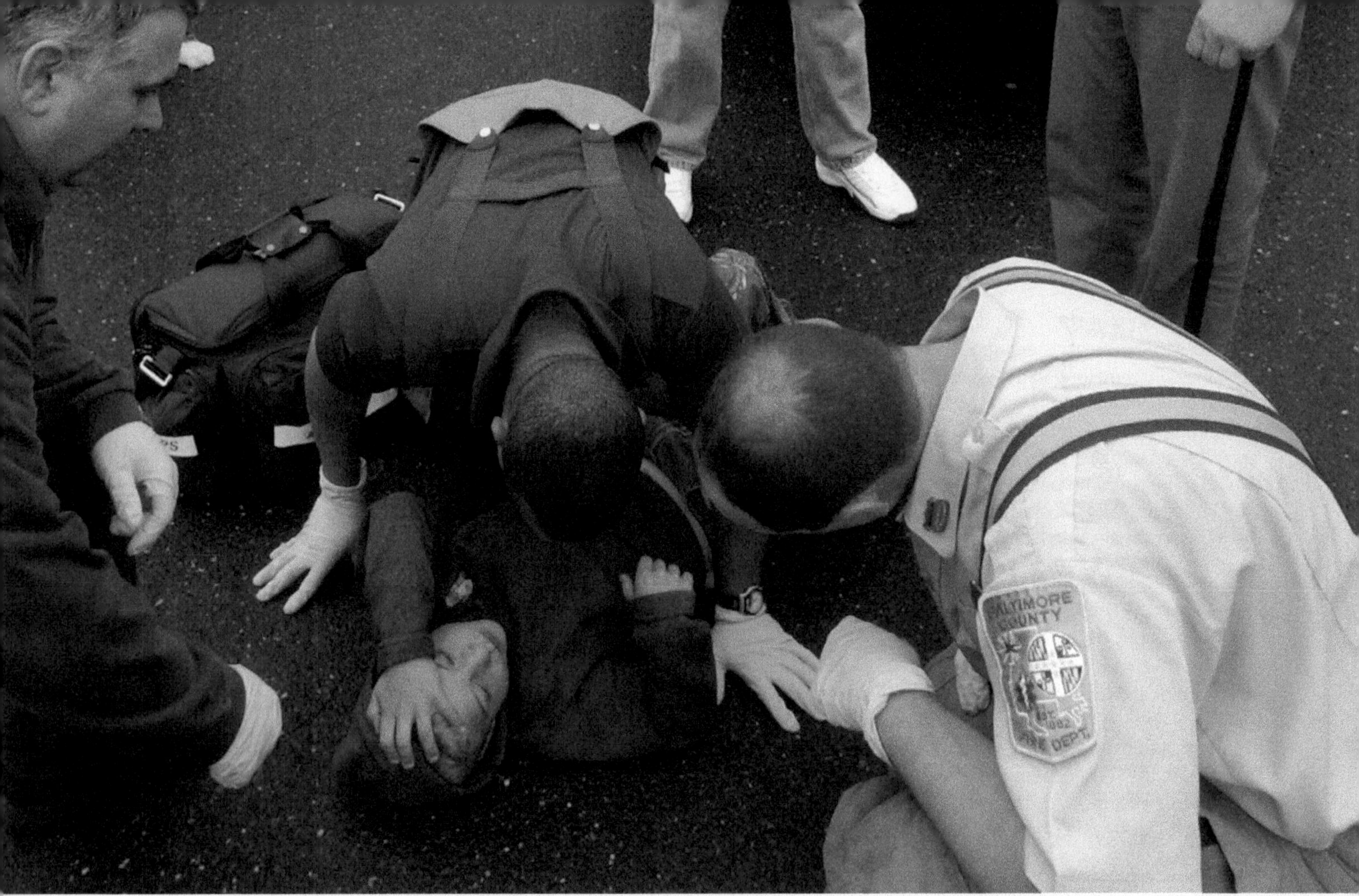

Learning Objectives

1. Describe *Pediatric Education for Prehospital Professionals (PEPP)* as a program that meets national education priorities in emergency care of children.
2. Discuss the special challenges for the prehospital professional in pediatric assessment.
3. Recognize the key features of prearrival preparation and the scene size-up.
4. Differentiate the three elements of the Pediatric Assessment Triangle (PAT) in the primary (initial) assessment.
5. Describe the important pediatric considerations for each step in the hands-on ABC sequence of the primary assessment.
6. Recognize clinical situations requiring pain assessment and management.
7. Discuss guidelines for when to stay on scene and treat, and when to immediately transport an ill or injured child, including appropriate mode of transport.
8. Outline the unique considerations in the additional assessment of a child, including history taking, secondary assessment, monitoring devices, and reassessment.

Pediatric Assessment

Chapter 1

Introduction

Caring for a critically ill or injured infant or child is one of the most stressful duties of the prehospital professional. Key history may be unreliable or unknown because the patient may be too young to have descriptive language, or the child may be afraid and unable to accurately recount the key events. The caregiver may be sobbing, frightened, and anxious for reassurance. Examination may be limited because of the child's small size and resistance to hands-on evaluation. **Vital signs** may be deceptive because of normal age-based variations, and the difficulty in obtaining them accurately. It is the job of the prehospital professional to bring comfort to the child, caregiver, or family, and to bring order to the chaos on scene. The prehospital professional must conduct an accurate assessment and deliver effective emergency treatment to the child.

The *Pediatric Education for Prehospital Professionals* (PEPP) course, developed by the American Academy of Pediatrics (AAP), provides the core cognitive knowledge and skills to prepare prehospital professionals for comprehensive assessment and management of critically ill and injured infants and children. PEPP materials are designed to meet the national Emergency Medical Services (EMS) education standards for all levels of emergency medical provider, as established by the United States Department of Transportation's National Highway Traffic Safety Administration (NHTSA). Therefore, some of the terminology previously used in PEPP (general, initial, and additional assessment) has been modified to reflect the national EMS core content.

Effective emergency care of children involves many professionals inside and outside of the hospital setting. Two of the most important concepts for comprehensive and high-quality out-of-hospital pediatric emergency care are teamwork and prevention. Teamwork involves professionals working together to develop and implement comprehensive clinical services, professional education, and appropriate administrative oversight specifically for children. Prevention involves professionals recognizing the limitations of an emergency care system oriented toward treatment after an illness or injury occurs, and working to change potentially dangerous conditions before an event of this type occurs. Of all community activities that can improve children's overall health and well-being, prevention of acute injury and illness is by far the most cost-effective. "Making a difference," as described in detail in Chapter 16, involves new roles for prehospital professionals in injury and illness prevention, in their professional day-to-day duties, and as part of their activities as community leaders and health advocates.

Accurate assessment of a child with a serious illness or injury requires special knowledge and skills. For patients of all ages, the prehospital professional's evaluation includes five steps: (1) scene size-up, (2) primary (initial) assessment using the **Pediatric Assessment Triangle (PAT)**, (3) history taking, (4) **secondary assessment** including physical examination and monitoring devices, and (5) **reassessment**. The primary and secondary assessments have well-defined components that follow the same sequence used for adult patients. However, all five steps in assessment have

Case Study 1

A 7-year-old unhelmeted boy rode his bicycle out of his driveway into the path of an oncoming car. According to witnesses, the car was moving about 30 mph (50 kph), the victim was struck and thrown approximately 15 ft (4.5 m), and he was unconscious for 1–2 minutes. On your arrival, he is crying and anxious but responds appropriately to questions. He is complaining that his stomach hurts. He has no abnormal airway sounds, grunting, flaring, or retracting. His skin is pale. The respiratory rate is 30 breaths/min, there are equal breath sounds with good air exchange, and the pulse oximetry reading is 98% on room air. His heart rate is 150 beats/min, and his blood pressure is 80/40 mm Hg. The radial pulse is absent, and the femoral pulse is weak. Capillary refill time is 4 seconds.

1. How badly injured is this child, and which physiologic process requires your emergent attention?
2. Should this child's pain be treated?

important pediatric modifications. In the emergency department (ED), physicians and nurses continue the assessment with an additional step, diagnostic testing, often with the benefit of ancillary tests.

Summary of Assessment Flowchart

This chapter introduces a flowchart that reflects the sequence of pediatric assessment taught by the PEPP course. The flowchart reinforces the interconnecting relationships of the different assessment components. Sometimes the assessment sequence must be stopped after the primary assessment to allow the prehospital professional to treat potentially life-threatening problems and initiate transport. For example, when a child has a critical injury, the secondary assessment must be deferred until after the child has been resuscitated and stabilized. Reassessment, however, is required in every case to monitor response to treatment, guide further interventions, and assist with transport and triage decisions. While monitoring devices such as a pulse oximeter or a bedside glucose check do provide diagnostic testing, further diagnostic testing is a hospital-based evaluation that often requires specialized tools, such as laboratory tests and radiologic procedures.

Scene Size-Up

↓

Primary Assessment
Using the PAT
Hands-on ABCDEs
Transport Decision: Stay or Go

↓

History Taking

↓

Secondary Assessment
Physical Exam
Monitoring Devices

↓

Reassessment

Scene Size-Up

On the way to the scene, prepare mentally to approach and treat an infant or child, and to interact with a distressed family. This means planning for a pediatric scene size-up, pediatric equipment and medication requirements, and age-appropriate assessment. All pediatric equipment and medications should be routinely checked, because they are less often used by most prehospital professionals and it is easy to become unfamiliar with their application. The information from dispatch on age and gender of the child, location of the scene, and chief complaint or mechanism of injury (or both) is the basis for prearrival preparation.

At the scene, begin the size-up by looking for possible safety threats to the child, caregiver, bystanders, or prehospital professionals. Examples of safety threats include spilled toxins, open containers of alcohol, drug paraphernalia, weapons, or

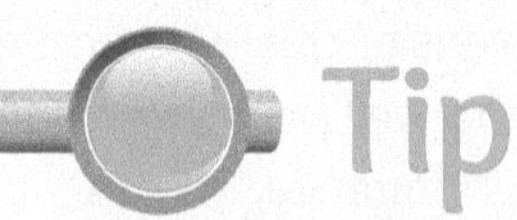

Tip

On the way to the scene, mentally rehearse your approach to the assessment and treatment of an infant or child, and the expected interaction with a caregiver or family. Dispatch information, when available, about the child's age can be helpful to mentally prepare for age-appropriate developmental considerations and for anticipating equipment and medication requirements for assessment and treatment.

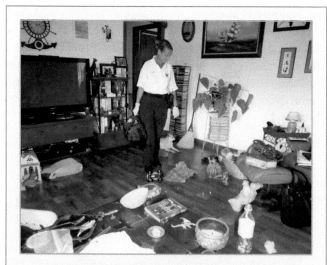

Figure 1-1 Environmental assessment.

fire. The child actually may be a safety threat if he or she has an infectious disease, such as varicella or meningococcemia.

Evaluating the setting includes an inspection of the physical environment and watching family-child or caregiver-child interactions (**Figure 1-1**). For example, documenting observations of dangerous scene conditions and inappropriate statements from caregivers greatly assists child protective services if the child is later determined to be a victim of inflicted injury. On the scene, be like a sponge; soak up as much useful information as possible to ensure scene safety.

Primary Assessment: The Pediatric Assessment Triangle

After the scene size-up, begin a primary assessment of the child. The primary assessment must have a developmentally appropriate approach. This assessment includes a visual and auditory "general impression" of the child, and uses the PAT as a standardized method to gather this information.

Scene Size-Up
↓
Primary Assessment
Using the PAT
Hands-on ABCDEs
Transport Decision: Stay or Go
↓
History Taking
↓
Secondary Assessment
Physical Exam
Monitoring Devices
↓
Reassessment

Rapid assessment is essential to determine level of acuity and urgency for treatment and transport. Ask yourself, "is the patient sick or not sick?" In the case of a child who is a victim of trauma with a known mechanism of injury, or of a child with a clear-cut complaint of pain in a specific anatomic location, the assessment may be straightforward. Still, careful evaluation is needed to identify less obvious, but potentially serious injuries or physiologic instability. For a child with an illness, the assessment may be much trickier. The prehospital professional must elicit information on the onset, duration, severity, and progression of symptoms, often from a child who cannot accurately provide such history. Moreover, illness complaints may be vague and less specific to an anatomic region. Whether the child has an injury or an illness, the PAT helps to identify physiologic instability, direct resuscitation priorities, and determine the timing of transport.

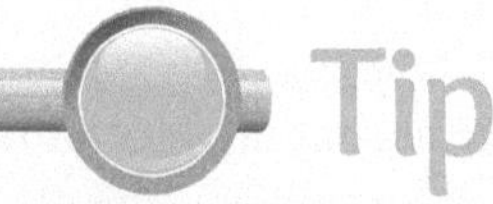

Use the PAT at the point of initial contact with every child, regardless of age or presenting complaint.

Developing a General Impression: The PAT

The PAT is an easy tool to use during the rapid, primary assessment of any child (**Figure 1-2**). It allows the prehospital professional to develop a first general impression of the patient's status with only visual and auditory clues. By using the PAT at the point of first contact with the patient,

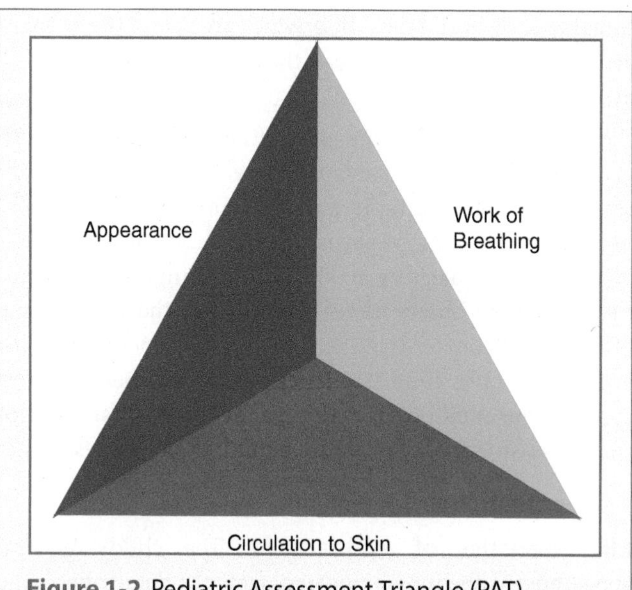

Figure 1-2 Pediatric Assessment Triangle (PAT).

the prehospital professional can immediately establish a level of severity, determine urgency for life support, and identify the general type of physiologic problem. Continued use of the PAT gives the prehospital professional a way to track response to therapy and determine timing of transport. It also allows for communication among medical professionals about the child's physiologic status and for accurate radio reporting.

There are three components of the PAT that together reflect the child's overall physiologic status: (1) appearance, (2) work of breathing, and (3) circulation to the skin. The PAT is based on listening and seeing, and does not require a stethoscope, blood pressure cuff, cardiac monitor, or pulse oximeter. The PAT does not require numbers. The PAT should be completed in less than 30 seconds and is designed to organize a time-honored process of "across the room assessment," an intuitive process that experienced pediatric providers do instinctively.

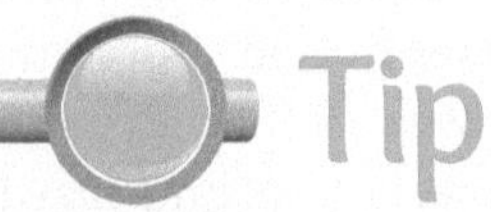

Tip

The elements of the PAT incorporate auditory and visual clues that should be obtained from "across the room," without appearing threatening to an already anxious child.

The PAT

Together, the physical characteristics of the PAT provide an accurate initial picture of the child's underlying cardiopulmonary status and level of consciousness. Although the PAT does not necessarily lead to a diagnosis, it identifies the general category of the physiologic problem and establishes urgency for treatment or transport. The PAT does not replace traditional vital signs and the ABCs, which are part of the primary assessment in the next phase of the physical evaluation.

The patient characteristics emphasized by the three arms of the PAT did not originate with PEPP. Experienced health care providers have always intuitively used these characteristics to obtain a rapid first "general impression" of ill or injured children. What is unique about the PAT is its systematic approach to making, integrating, and communicating these observations. The PAT is the cornerstone of the PEPP course. Use the PAT in every encounter with every child. Over time, it will become an indispensable and spontaneous method for making a rapid initial "sick or not sick" assessment of ill or injured children of all ages.

Appearance

Characteristics of Appearance. The child's general appearance is the most important factor in determining the severity of the illness or injury, the need for treatment, and the response to therapy. Appearance reflects the adequacy of ventilation, oxygenation, brain perfusion, body homeostasis, and central nervous system (CNS) function. There are many characteristics of appearance; the most important are summarized in the "tickles" (TICLS) mnemonic: tone, interactiveness, consolabilty, look/gaze, and speech/cry (**Table 1-1**).

Table 1-1 Characteristics of Appearance: The "Tickles" (TICLS) Mnemonic

Characteristic features to look for
• Tone Is she moving or vigorously resisting examination? Does she have good muscle tone? Or is she limp, listless, or flaccid?
• Interactiveness How alert is she? How readily does a person, object, or sound distract her or draw her attention? Will she reach for, grasp, and play with a toy or examination instrument, such as a penlight? Or is she uninterested in playing or interacting with the caregiver?
• Consolability Can she be consoled or comforted by the caregiver? Or is her crying or agitation unrelieved by gentle reassurance?
• Look/Gaze Does she fix her gaze on a face? Or is there a "nobody home," glassy-eyed stare?
• Speech/Cry Is her speech or cry strong and spontaneous? Or is it weak, muffled, or hoarse?

Adapted from Dieckmann RA, Brownstein D, Gausche-Hill M. The Pediatric Assessment Triangle: a novel approach to pediatric assessment. *Pediatr Emerg Care.* 2010:26;312–315.

Identifying abnormal appearance is a better way to detect subtle abnormalities in behavior than the conventional "alert, verbal, painful, unresponsive" (AVPU) scale or the Pediatric Glasgow Coma Scale (GCS) for neurologic evaluation. Most children with mild to moderate illness or injury are "alert" on the AVPU or "15" on the Pediatric GCS, although some may have an abnormal appearance

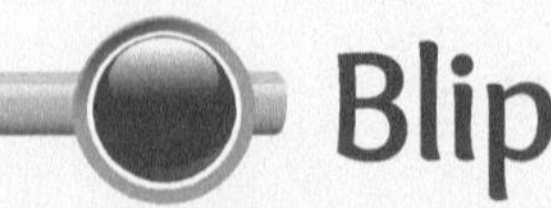

Blip

In assessing patients with mild to moderate illness or injury, numerical "scoring" methodologies and severity scales for levels of consciousness are rarely useful. These classical neurologic evaluation systems work best in patients with severe injury or illness and serious brain dysfunction.

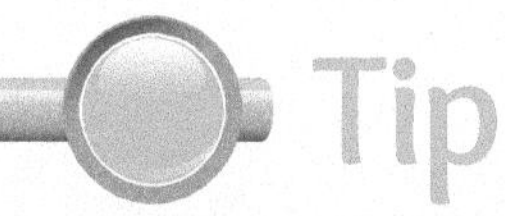

Never ignore the pale infant, the "nobody home stare," or the infant who does not respond appropriately to stimulation.

and a potentially serious underlying problem. Therefore, assessing a child's appearance is the most useful first thing to do in evaluating every pediatric patient.

Techniques to Assess Appearance. Assess the child's appearance from the doorway. This is Step 1 in the PAT. Techniques for assessment of a conscious child's appearance include observing from a distance; allowing the child to remain in the caregiver's lap or arms; using distraction tools, such as bright lights or toys, to measure the child's ability to interact; and kneeling down to be at eye level with the child. An immediate "hands-on" approach may cause agitation and crying, and may complicate the assessment. Unless a child is unconscious or obviously critically ill, get as much information as possible by observing the child before touching the child or taking vital signs.

One example of a child with a normal appearance is an infant who holds himself or herself upright in the mother's arms, makes good eye contact, and has good color (**Figure 1-3**). An example of an infant with a worrisome appearance is a toddler who makes poor eye contact with the caregiver or prehospital professional and is pale and listless (**Figure 1-4**).

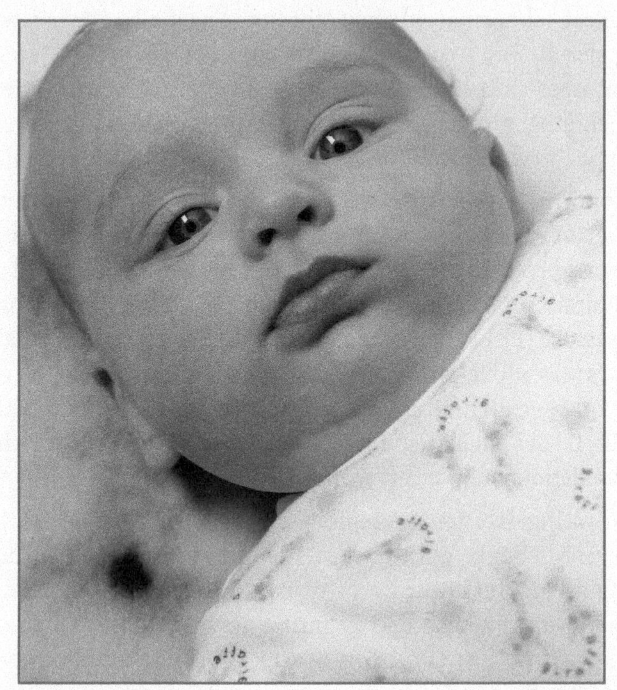

Figure 1-3 A child making good eye contact is normal and a sign of a good appearance.

An abnormal appearance may have many causes: inadequate oxygenation, ventilation, or brain perfusion; systemic abnormalities, such as poisoning, infection, or hypoglycemia; or acute or chronic brain injury. Regardless of the cause, a child with a grossly abnormal appearance is seriously ill or injured and needs immediate life support efforts to increase oxygenation, ventilation, and perfusion.

Although an alert, interactive child is usually not critically ill, there are some cases where a child may have life-threatening problems despite an initially normal appearance. Toxicologic or traumatic emergencies are good examples:

1. A child with acetaminophen, iron, or a cyclic antidepressant overdose may not show symptoms immediately after ingestion. Despite the child's normal appearance, he or she may develop deadly complications in the coming minutes or hours.
2. A child with blunt trauma and solid organ injury may be able to maintain adequate core perfusion, despite internal bleeding, by increasing cardiac output and systemic vascular resistance; therefore, he or she may appear normal during the primary assessment. However, when these compensatory mechanisms fail, the child may acutely "crash," with rapid progression to decompensated shock. Pallor may be the only finding on the PAT that suggests impending disaster.

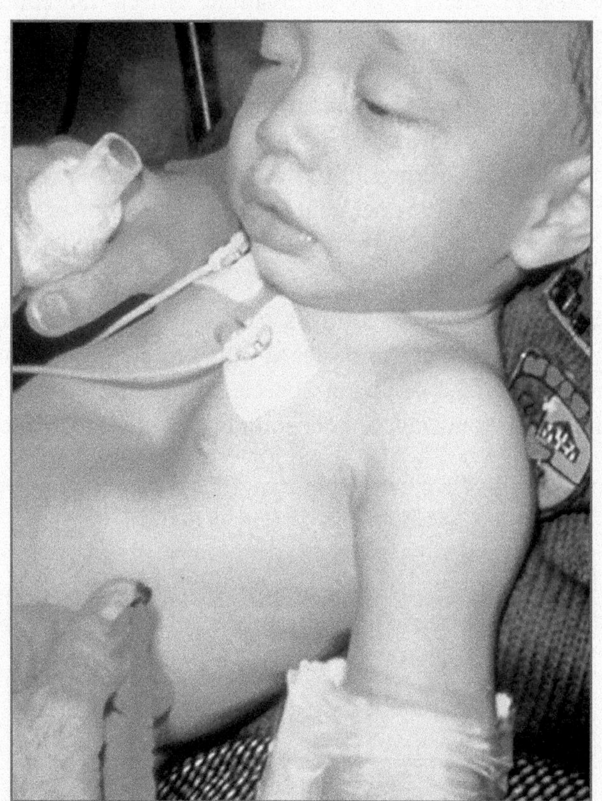

Figure 1-4 A limp, pale child unable to make eye contact or a child with retractions may be critically ill or injured.

A benign appearance should never justify a denial of transport. However, a normal appearance usually means that a transport with "lights and siren" is not necessary.

Age differences are associated with important developmental differences in psychomotor and social skills. "Normal" appearance and behavior vary by age group, as discussed in Chapter 2. Children of all ages engage their environment: newborns do this through energetic sucking and crying; older infants, by smiling or tracking a light; toddlers through physical exploration; and adolescents through speech. Knowledge of normal child development through the age groups should guide the assessment of appearance and result in more accurate treatment and transport decisions. Although appearance reflects the severity of illness or injury, it does not identify the cause. Appearance is the "screening" portion of the PAT. The other elements of the PAT (work of breathing and circulation to the skin) provide more specific information about the type of physiologic derangement, while giving additional clues about severity.

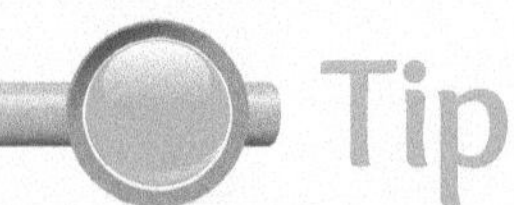

The child's general appearance is the single most important feature when assessing severity of illness or injury, need for treatment, and response to therapy.

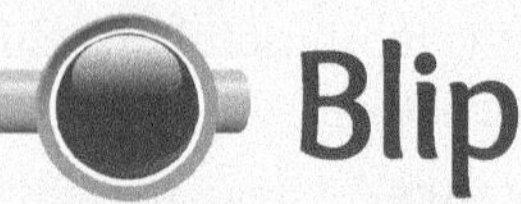

Although an alert, interactive child is usually not critically ill, there are some exceptions to the reliability of general appearance as an indicator of stable cardiopulmonary and neurologic function. The most common exceptions are ingestions with delayed physiologic effects and blunt injury with slow internal bleeding.

Work of Breathing

Characteristics of Work of Breathing. In children, work of breathing is a more accurate indicator of oxygenation and ventilation than respiratory rate or breath sounds on auscultation, the standard measures of breathing effectiveness in adults. Work of breathing reflects the child's attempt to compensate for abnormalities in oxygenation and ventilation, and it is a proxy for the effectiveness of gas exchange. This component of the PAT requires listening carefully for abnormal airway sounds and looking for signs of increased breathing effort. It is another "hands-off" evaluation method that does not require a stethoscope or pulse oximeter. **Table 1-2** summarizes the key characteristics of work of breathing.

Abnormal Airway Sounds. Examples of abnormal airway sounds that can be heard without a stethoscope are snoring, muffled or hoarse speech, stridor, grunting, and wheezing. Abnormal airway sounds provide information about the physiology and anatomic location of the breathing problem.

Table 1-2 Characteristics of Work of Breathing

Characteristic	Features to Look for
Abnormal airway sounds	Snoring, muffled or hoarse speech, stridor, grunting, wheezing
Abnormal positioning	Sniffing position, tripoding, refusing to lie down
Retractions	Supraclavicular, intercostal, or substernal retractions of the chest wall; head bobbing in infants
Flaring	Flaring of the nares on inspiration

Snoring, muffled or hoarse speech, and stridor suggest an upper airway obstruction. Snoring or gurgling occurs when the oropharynx is partially obstructed by the tongue and soft tissues. Muffled or hoarse speech reflects inflammation of the glottis or supraglottic structures. Stridor is a high-pitched sound heard on inspiration, or during inspiration and expiration, reflecting an obstruction at the level of the glottis or subglottic trachea. All of these sounds reflect abnormal airflow through partially obstructed upper airway structures. Obstruction of the upper airway passages can occur in a variety of illnesses and injuries, including croup, foreign body aspiration, and bacterial upper airway infections, or as a result of bleeding or edema.

Abnormal lower airway sounds that may be heard during the PAT include grunting and wheezing. Grunting is a sound produced by partial closure of the glottis on the end of expiration. Grunting is a form of auto positive end-expiratory pressure (PEEP), a way to distend lower respiratory tract air sacs (alveoli) to promote maximum gas exchange. Grunting involves exhaling against a partially closed glottis. This short, low-pitched sound is best heard at the end of the exhalation and is easily mistaken for whimpering.

Grunting is often present in children with moderate to severe hypoxia, and it reflects poor gas exchange because of obstruction in the lower airways and alveoli. Conditions that cause hypoxia and grunting are pneumonia, pulmonary contusion (bruising of the lungs), and pulmonary edema (fluid in air sacs).

Wheezing is the result of movement of air across partially blocked small airways. At first, wheezing usually occurs during exhalation and can be heard only by auscultation of the chest with a stethoscope. As the airway obstruction increases and breathing requires more work, wheezing is often present during inhalation and exhalation. With more obstruction, wheezing may be audible without a stethoscope. Finally, if respiratory failure develops, work of breathing may diminish and the wheezing may not be heard at all. The most common cause of wheezing in childhood is asthma, although wheezing may also be associated with bronchiolitis (a viral respiratory infection in infants) and lower airway foreign body aspiration.

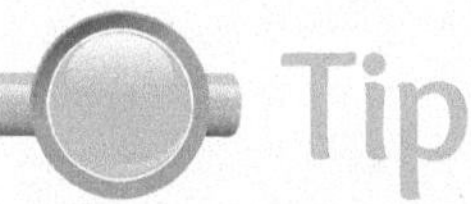

Tip

Abnormal airway sounds can provide excellent information about breathing effort, type of breathing problem, location of the breathing problem, and potential degree of hypoxia.

Visual Signs of Increased Work of Breathing. There are several useful visual signs of increased work of breathing. These signs reflect an increased breathing effort by the child to improve oxygenation and ventilation. The presence of certain physical features, such as abnormal positioning, retractions, and nasal flaring, reflect overall illness or injury severity. Abnormal positioning is usually evident from the doorway. There are several types of abnormal postures that can indicate the child is struggling to improve airflow. A child who is in the sniffing position is trying to align the axes of the airways to improve patency and increase airflow (**Figure 1-5**). This position is usually the result of severe upper airway obstruction. The child who refuses to lie down, or who leans forward on outstretched arms (tripoding), is creating optimal mechanical positioning to use accessory muscles of respiration (**Figure 1-6**). The sniffing position and tripoding are abnormal and indicate airway obstruction, increased work of breathing, and severe respiratory distress.

Retractions are physical signs of increased work of breathing. Retractions represent the recruitment of accessory muscles of respiration to provide more "muscle power" to move air into the lungs in the face of airway or lung disease or injury. To optimally observe retractions, expose the child's chest. Retractions are a more useful measure of work of breathing in children than in adults because a child's chest wall is less muscular, and the inward excursion of skin and soft tissue between the ribs is more apparent. Retractions may be in the supraclavicular area (above the clavicle), the intercostal area (between the ribs), or the substernal area (under the sternum), as illustrated in **Figure 1-7**. Another form of accessory muscle use seen only in infants is "head bobbing," which is the use of neck muscles to assist breathing during times of severe hypoxia.

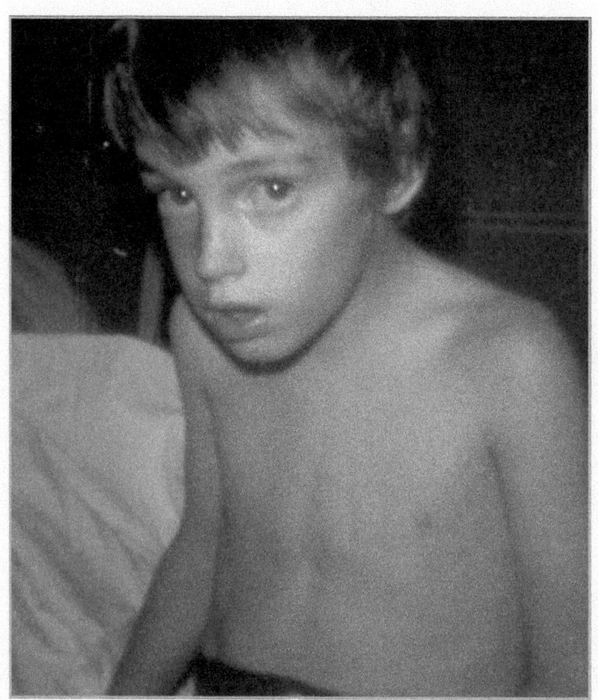

Figure 1-5 The sniffing position opens up the airways to improve patency.

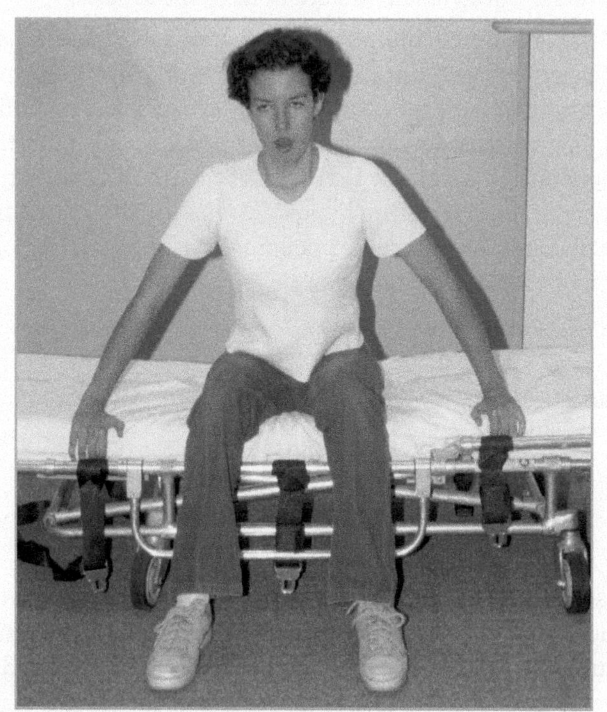

Figure 1-6 The abnormal tripod position indicates the patient's attempts to maximize accessory muscle use.

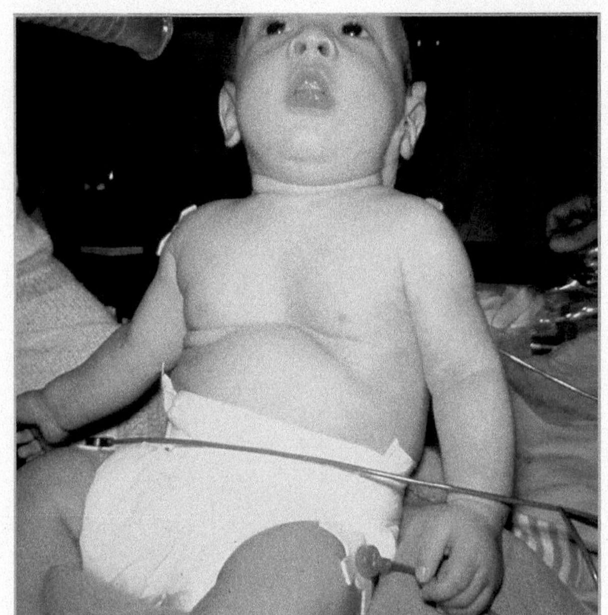

Figure 1-7 Retractions indicate increased work of breathing and may occur in the supraclavicular, intercostal, and substernal areas.

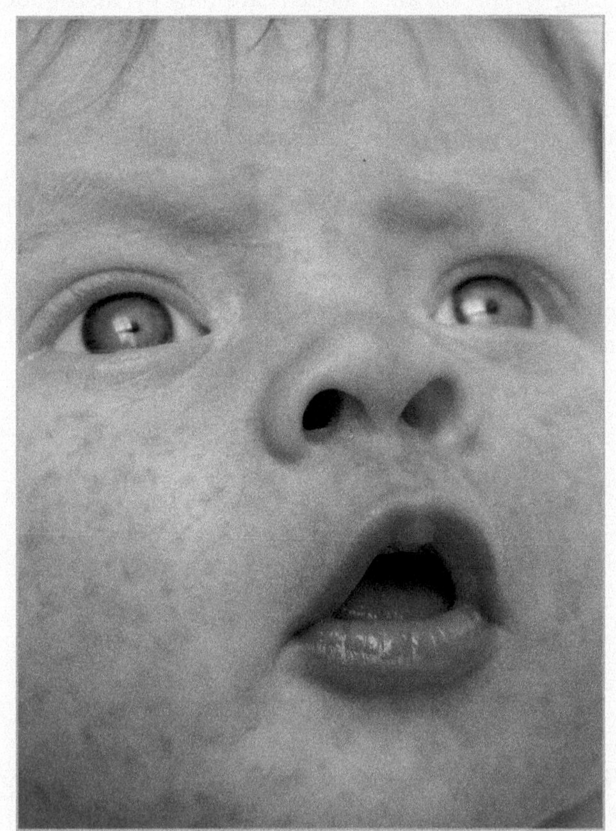

Figure 1-8 Nasal flaring indicates increased work of breathing and moderate to severe hypoxia.

The infant extends the neck as he or she inhales, and then allows the head to fall forward as he or she exhales.

Nasal flaring is another sign of accessory muscle use that reflects significant increased work of breathing (**Figure 1-8**). Nasal flaring is the exaggerated opening of the nostrils during labored inspiration and indicates moderate to severe hypoxia. It reflects the child's extra effort to breathe during hypoxic stress, usually caused by such conditions as croup, pneumonia, asthma, bronchiolitis, or pulmonary contusion.

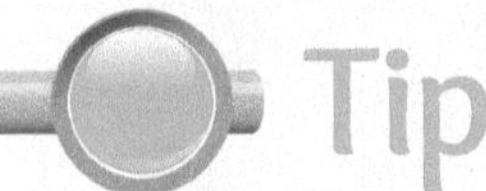

Tip

Head bobbing is a form of accessory muscle use specific to infants and is indicative of increased work of breathing.

Techniques to Assess Work of Breathing. Step 2 in the PAT is assessing work of breathing. Begin by listening carefully from a distance for abnormal airway sounds. Next, look for key physical signs. Note if the child has an abnormal posture, most notably the sniffing position or tripoding. Next, have the caregiver uncover the chest of the child for direct inspection, or have the child undress on the caregiver's lap. Look for intercostal, supraclavicular, and substernal retractions, and note if there is head bobbing in infants. After examining for retractions, inspect for nasal flaring. This stepwise process is critical for gathering accurate information. After an infant or child begins to cry, assessment of work of breathing becomes more difficult.

Children may have increased work of breathing because of abnormalities anywhere in their upper or lower airways, alveoli (air sacs), pleura (membrane surrounding the lungs and lining the walls of the pleural cavity), or chest wall. The type of abnormal airway sounds gives an important clue to the anatomic location of the illness or injury process, whereas the number and type of physical signs of increased work of breathing helps in determining the degree of physiologic stress.

Combining assessment of appearance and work of breathing can also help establish the severity of the child's illness or injury. A child with a normal appearance and increased work of breathing is in respiratory distress. An abnormal appearance and increased work of breathing suggests respiratory failure. An abnormal appearance and abnormally decreased work of breathing implies impending respiratory arrest.

Circulation to Skin

Characteristics of Circulation to Skin. The goal of rapid circulatory assessment is to determine the adequacy of cardiac output and core perfusion, or perfusion of the vital organs. The child's appearance is one indicator of brain perfusion, but abnormal appearance may be caused by other conditions unrelated to circulation, such as hypoxia, hypoglycemia, brain injury, or intoxication. For this reason, other signs of adequacy of perfusion must be added to the evaluation of appearance to assess the child's true circulatory status.

An important sign of core perfusion is circulation to the skin. When cardiac output is inadequate, the body shuts down circulation to nonessential anatomic areas, such as the skin and mucous membranes, to preserve blood supply to the most vital organs (brain, heart, and kidneys). Therefore, circulation to the skin reflects the overall status of core circulation. Pallor, mottling, and cyanosis are key visual indicators of reduced circulation to the skin and mucous membranes. **Table 1-3** summarizes these characteristics.

Pallor may be the first sign of poor skin or mucous membrane perfusion. Pallor may be the only visual sign apparent in a child with compensated shock, and indicates reflex peripheral vasoconstriction to shunt blood away from the skin to the core. Pallor may also be a sign of anemia or hypoxia. Mottling is another sign of inadequate skin perfusion, reflecting vasomotor instability (abnormal blood vessel tone) in the capillary beds of the skin. Mottled skin has patchy areas of vasoconstriction (pallor) mixed with areas of vasodilation (cyanosis or erythema). Mottling may also be a normal physiologic response in a child exposed to cold environmental temperatures.

Cyanosis is blue discoloration of the skin and mucous membranes. It is the most extreme visual indicator of poor perfusion or poor oxygenation. Do not confuse acrocyanosis (blue hands and feet in a newborn or infant less than 2 months of age) with true cyanosis. Acrocyanosis is a normal finding when a young infant is cold, and it reflects vasomotor instability rather than hypoxia or shock. True cyanosis is a late finding of respiratory failure or shock. A hypoxic child is likely to show other physical abnormalities long before turning blue. These abnormalities may include abnormal appearance with agitation or lethargy,

Table 1-3 Characteristics of Circulation to Skin

Characteristic	Features to Look for
Pallor	White or pale or mucous membrane coloration from inadequate blood flow
Mottling	Patchy skin discoloration caused by vasoconstriction or vasodilation
Cyanosis	Bluish discoloration of skin and mucous membranes

and increased work of breathing. A child in shock may also have pallor or mottling. Never wait for cyanosis to begin treatment with supplemental oxygen. However, the presence of cyanosis is always a critical sign that requires immediate intervention with breathing support.

Abnormal circulation to the skin, in combination with an abnormal appearance, suggests shock. However, the abnormalities in appearance in early phases of compensated shock may be subtle, and some children may remain alert. As perfusion worsens and compensatory mechanisms fail, appearance becomes abnormal, reflecting inadequate delivery of oxygen and glucose to the brain. Another clue to the presence of shock is effortless tachypnea, or tachypnea without signs of increased work of breathing. Effortless tachypnea is a reflex mechanism that allows the body to blow off carbon dioxide to compensate for the metabolic acidosis caused by poor peripheral perfusion (lactic acidosis). Hypocarbia (low blood CO_2 levels) generates a respiratory alkalosis and helps to restore normal pH (blood acid-base balance). Effortless tachypnea is different from the rapid and labored respirations that are present with illnesses and injuries associated with airway or lung pathology.

Techniques to Assess Circulation to Skin. Step 3 in the PAT is evaluating circulation to the skin. Be sure the child is exposed long enough for visual inspection, but not long enough to become cold. A cold child may have normal core perfusion, but abnormal circulation to the skin. Cold circulating air temperature is the most common reason for misinterpretation of skin signs, and an exposed young infant may become hypothermic quickly, even at normal ambient temperatures.

Inspect the skin and mucous membranes for pallor, mottling, and cyanosis. Look at the face, chest, abdomen, and extremities, and then inspect the lips for cyanosis. In dark-skinned children, circulation to the skin is sometimes more difficult to assess, and the lips, mucous membranes, and nail beds are the best places to look for pallor or cyanosis (**Figure 1-9**). Combining assessment of appearance and circulation to the skin can also help establish the severity of the child's illness or injury. A child with a normal appearance and poor circulation to the skin is possibly cold. An abnormal appearance and circulation to the skin suggests the child is in shock.

Using the PAT to Evaluate Severity and Illness or Injury. The PAT provides a general impression of the pediatric patient. The intent is to provide a standardized approach to the "general impression" and an immediate picture of the child's physiologic status. By combining the three components of the PAT, the prehospital professional should be able to answer three critical questions: (1) How severe is the child's illness or injury? (2) What is the most

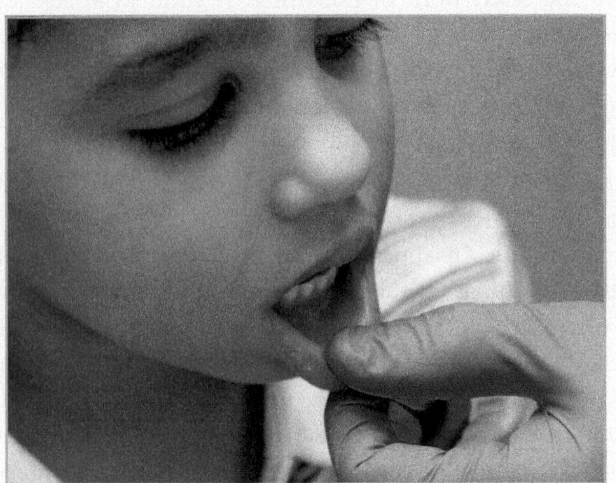

Figure 1-9 In dark-skinned children, circulation to the skin is sometimes more difficult to assess, and the lips, mucous membranes, and nail beds may be the best places to look for pallor or cyanosis.

likely physiologic abnormality? (3) What is the urgency for treatment? This information helps the prehospital professional select the most important actions: how fast to intervene, what type of general and specific treatment to give, and how rapidly to transport.

The three elements of the PAT work together and allow a rapid assessment of the child's overall physiologic stability. For example, if a child is interactive and pink, but has mild intercostal retractions, the prehospital professional can take time to approach the child in a developmentally appropriate manner to complete the primary assessment. However, if the child is limp, with unlabored rapid breathing and pale or mottled skin, shock is likely. In this case, the prehospital professional must move rapidly through the primary assessment and begin resuscitation. A child who has an abnormal appearance, but normal work of breathing and normal circulation to skin, probably has a primary brain dysfunction or a major metabolic or systemic problem, such as postictal state, subdural hemorrhage, concussion, intoxication, hypoglycemia, or sepsis.

The PAT has two important advantages. First, it allows the examiner to quickly obtain critical information about the child's physiologic status before touching or agitating the child. Second, the PAT helps set priorities for the rest of the hands-on primary assessment. The PAT takes only seconds, it helps to identify the need for lifesaving interventions, and it assists in the transition into the next phase of hands-on physical assessment.

The three components of the PAT (appearance, work of breathing, and circulation to the skin) can be assessed in any sequence, unlike the ordered ABCDEs of resuscitation discussed next.

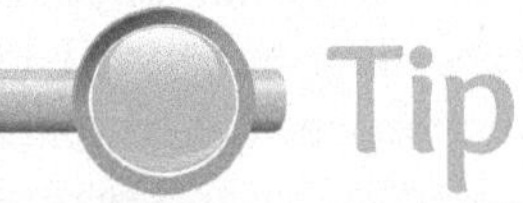

By combining the three components of the PAT, the prehospital professional can answer three critical questions: (1) How sick or injured is the child? (2) What is the most likely physiologic abnormality? (3) What is the urgency for treatment?

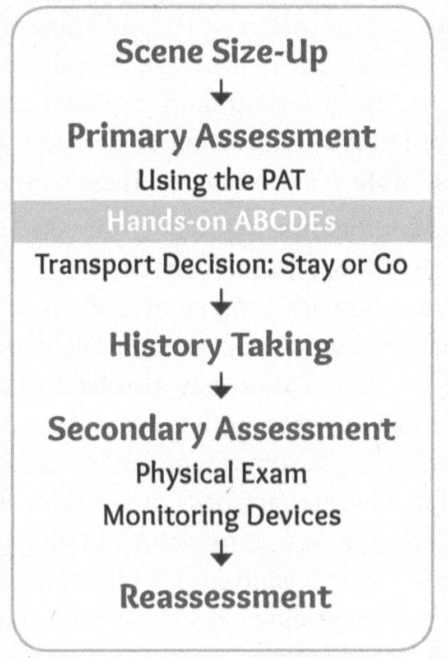

Primary Assessment: ABCDEs

Hands-on ABCDEs

The primary assessment continues to try to identify life-threatening conditions using an ordered hands-on physical evaluation of the ABCDEs. It provides a prioritized sequence of life-support interventions to reverse critical physiologic abnormalities. As in adults, there is a specific order for treating life-threatening problems as they are identified, before moving to the next step. The steps are also the same as with adults, but there are important pediatric differences in anatomy, physiology, and signs of distress. ABCDE assessment involves the following components:

1. Airway
2. Breathing
3. Circulation
4. Disability
5. Exposure

Airway

The PAT may identify the presence of an airway obstruction based on the presence of abnormal airway sounds. However, the loudness of the stridor or wheezing is not necessarily related to the amount of airway obstruction. For example, children with asthma in severe distress may have little or no wheezing. Similarly, children with an upper airway foreign body below the vocal cords may have minimal stridor. Abnormal positioning and retractions provide further information about the degree of obstruction, as does the quality of air entry on auscultation during the hands-on assessment.

If the airway is open, ensure that the chest rises with each breath. If a child has assumed a position that maximizes his or her ability to maintain a spontaneously open airway, allow the child to remain in that position of comfort. If gurgling is present, there may be mucus, blood, or a foreign body in the mouth or upper airway. Oropharyngeal suctioning of mucus or blood, or removal of a visible foreign body, very often restores patency. If the airway is totally obstructed, advanced life support (ALS) interventions are necessary.

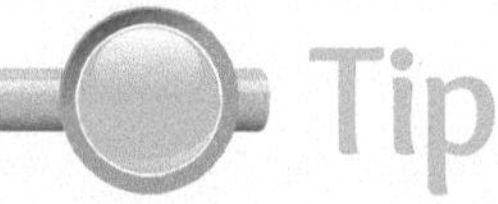

Tip

"Red flag" respiratory rates are less than 20 breaths/min for children younger than 6 years of age and less than 12 breaths/min for children younger than 18 years of age.

Breathing

Respiratory Rate. Verify the respiratory rate per minute by counting the number of chest rises in 30 seconds, then doubling that number. Interpret the respiratory rate carefully. Normal infants may show "periodic breathing" or variable respiratory rate with short (<20 second) periods of apnea. Therefore, counting for only 10–15 seconds may give a falsely low respiratory rate.

The significance of respiratory rates may be confusing. Rapid respiratory rates may simply reflect high fever, anxiety, pain, or excitement. Normal rates, however, may occur in a child who has been breathing rapidly with increased work of breathing for some time and is now becoming fatigued. Finally, interpretation requires knowledge of normal values for age (**Table 1-4**).

Serial assessment of respiratory rates may be especially useful, and the trend is sometimes more accurate than any single value. A sustained increase or decrease in respiratory rate is usually significant.

Pay close attention to extremes of respiratory rate. A very rapid respiratory rate (>60 breaths/min for any age), especially with abnormal appearance or marked retractions, indicates respiratory distress and possibly respiratory failure. An abnormally slow respiratory rate is always worrisome because it might mean respiratory failure. Red flags are respiratory rates less than 20 breaths/min for children younger than 6 years of age, and less than 12 breaths/min for older children. A normal respiratory rate alone never guarantees adequate oxygenation and ventilation. The respiratory rate must be interpreted along with appearance, work of breathing, and air movement.

Table 1-4 Normal Respiratory Rate for Age

Age	Respiratory Rate (breaths/min)
Infant	30–60
Toddler	24–40
Preschooler	22–34
School-age child	18–30
Adolescent	12–16

Auscultation. Listen with a stethoscope over the midclavicular and midaxillary lines during inhalation and exhalation to hear abnormal lung sounds, such as crackles and wheezing (**Figure 1-10**). Inspiratory crackles indicate disease in the alveoli (air sacs) themselves. Often crackles are not heard on auscultation, even when the child has a pathologic condition, such as pneumonia. The younger the child, the more difficult it is to appreciate abnormal sounds during auscultation. Expiratory wheezing indicates lower airway obstruction. Auscultation also helps evaluate

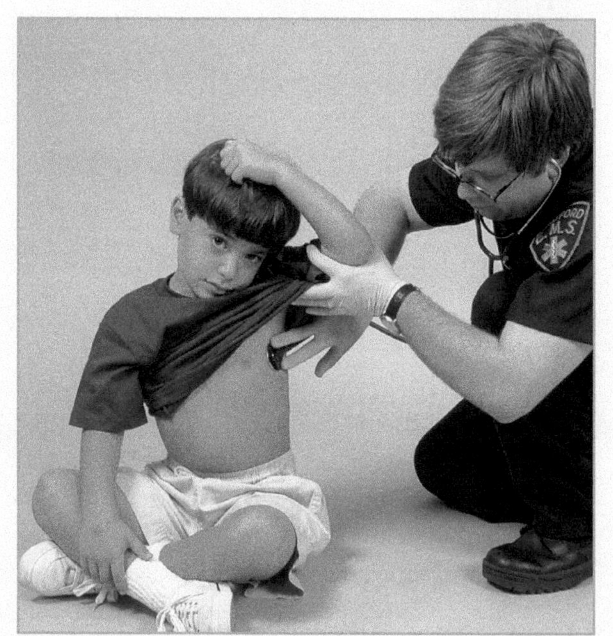

Figure 1-10 Listen for air movement over the midaxillary line.

the volume of air movement and effectiveness of work of breathing. A child with increased work of breathing and poor air movement may be in impending respiratory failure.

Table 1-5 lists abnormal breath sounds, their causes, and common examples of associated disease processes.

Circulation

The PAT provides important visual clues about circulation to the skin. Information obtained from the hands-on evaluation of heart rate, pulse quality, skin temperature, capillary refill time, and blood pressure provide further information on the adequacy of perfusion.

Table 1-5 Interpretation of Abnormal Breath Sounds

Sound	Cause	Examples
Stridor	Upper airway obstruction	Croup, foreign body aspiration, retropharyngeal abscess
Wheezing	Lower airway obstruction	Asthma, foreign body, bronchiolitis
Expiratory grunting	Inadequate oxygenation	Pulmonary contusion, pneumonia, drowning
Inspiratory crackles	Fluid, mucus, or blood in airway	Pneumonia, pulmonary contusion
Absent breath sounds despite increased work of breathing	Severe airway obstruction (upper or lower airway)	Physical barrier to transmission of breath sounds, foreign body, severe asthma, hemothorax, pneumothorax, pleural fluid, pneumonia, pneumothorax

Heart Rate. Methods used to assess adult circulatory status (heart rate and blood pressure) have important limitations in children. First, normal heart rate varies with age, as noted in **Table 1-6**. Second, tachycardia may be an early sign of hypoxia or poor perfusion, but it may also reflect less serious conditions, such as fever, anxiety, pain, and excitement. Like respiratory rate, interpret heart rate within the context of the overall history, PAT, and primary assessment. A trend of increasing or decreasing heart rate may be quite useful, and may suggest worsening hypoxia or shock, or improvement after treatment. When hypoxia or shock becomes critical, the heart rate falls, leading to frank bradycardia. Bradycardia indicates critical hypoxia or ischemia. With tachycardia greater than 180 beats/min, an electronic monitor is necessary to accurately determine heart rate.

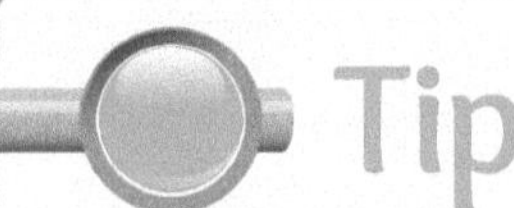

A rapid initial respiratory rate may simply reflect high fever, anxiety, pain, excitement, and not any real physiologic or anatomic problem. Noting a trend of an abnormal respiratory rate is more useful for indicating true pathology.

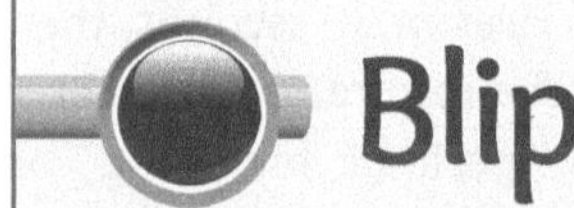

Be careful not to underestimate respiratory distress in a child with a pulse oximetry reading above 94%. This child may be using increased work of breathing and tachypnea to compensate for serious hypoxic stress.

Case Study 2

A 2-year-old boy was found face down in the family swimming pool. He was under water for no more than 1 minute but required cardiopulmonary resuscitation by the mother to get him breathing again. On arrival of EMS, the child is alert, pink, and clinging to his mother. Respirations appear regular and nonlabored at 26 breaths/min. When you examine him further, he screams and fights you. You are unable to obtain a blood pressure or heart rate, or assess lung sounds. The mother is sobbing and frightened.

1. How useful is the PAT in evaluating severity of illness and urgency for care?
2. In what ways is the PAT different than the ABCDEs in the primary assessment?

Pulse Quality. Feel the pulse to ascertain pulse quality. Normally, the brachial pulse is palpable medial to the biceps in the antecubital fossa (**Figure 1-11**). Note the quality as either weak or strong. If the brachial pulse is strong, the child is probably not hypotensive. If a peripheral pulse cannot be felt, attempt to find a central pulse. Check the femoral pulse in infants and young children, or the carotid pulse in an older child or adolescent. If there is no pulse, or the pulse is low (<60 beats/min) and the child is symptomatic with poor circulation, start cardiopulmonary resuscitation (CPR) (see Chapter 5 for more information).

Skin Temperature and Capillary Refill Time. Next, do a hands-on evaluation of circulation to the skin. Although children with normal circulation may have cool hands and feet, the skin should be warm above the wrists and ankles. With decreasing perfusion, the extremities become cooler proximally. Check capillary refill time in a fingertip, toe, or heel, or on the pads of the fingertips. Normal capillary refill time is less than 2 to 3 seconds. The value of measuring capillary refill time is controversial for several reasons: the peripheral perfusion baseline may vary from child to child; environmental factors, such as cold room temperature, may complicate interpretation; and it may be difficult for the prehospital professional to accurately count seconds under critical circumstances. The capillary refill time is just one element in the assessment of circulation. It must be evaluated in the context of the PAT and other perfusion characteristics, such as heart rate, pulse quality, and blood pressure.

Signs of circulation to the skin (skin temperature, capillary refill time, and pulse quality) are helpful tools to assess a child's circulatory status, especially when performed consecutively on a child who is not cold.

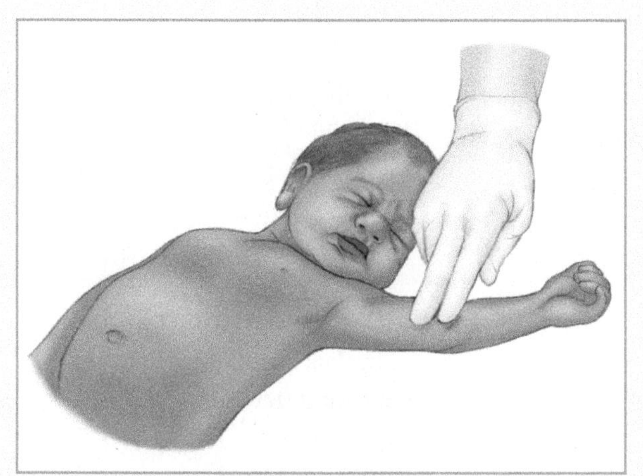

Figure 1-11 The anatomic position of the brachial pulse is medial to the biceps muscle.

Table 1-6 Normal Heart Rate for Age

Age	Heart Rate (beats/min)
Infant	100–160
Toddler	95–150
Preschooler	80–140
School-age child	70–120
Adolescent	60–100

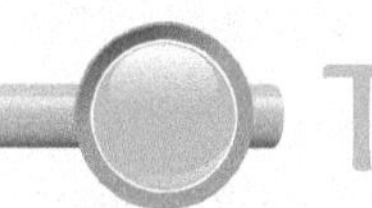

Interpret heart rate in the context of the overall history, PAT, and entire physical assessment.

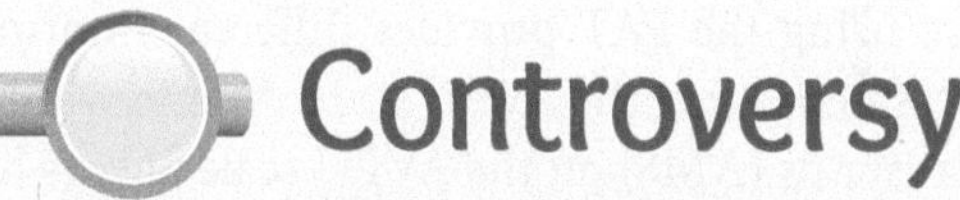

The value of capillary refill time is controversial. Peripheral perfusion may be variable in some children, and such environmental factors as ambient temperature may have a strong influence on capillary refill time.

Disability

Assessment of disability, or neurologic status, involves quick evaluation of the two main parts of the CNS: the cerebral cortex and the brainstem. First assess neurologic status, which is controlled by the cerebral cortex, by looking at appearance as part of the PAT; then assess the level of consciousness using the AVPU scale (**Table 1-7**). Evaluate the brainstem by checking the responses of each pupil to a direct beam of light. A normal pupil constricts after a light stimulus. Pupillary response may be abnormal in the presence of drugs, ongoing seizures, hypoxia, or impending brainstem herniation. Next, evaluate motor activity. Look for symmetric movement of the extremities, seizures, posturing, or flaccidity.

AVPU Scale. The AVPU scale is a standardized method of assessing the level of consciousness in all patients.

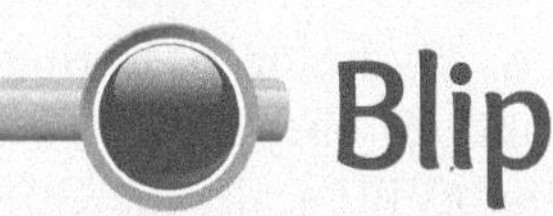

Neither the AVPU scale nor the Pediatric GCS allows assessment of restless or agitated behavioral states.

Table 1-7 AVPU Scale

Category	Stimulus	Response Type	Reaction
Alert	Normal environment	Appropriate	Normal interactiveness for age
Verbal	Simple command or sound stimulus	Appropriate or inappropriate	Responds to name; nonspecific or confused
Painful	Pain	Appropriate, inappropriate, or pathologic	Withdraws from pain or sound or motion without purpose or localization of pain; posturing
Unresponsive			No perceptible response to any stimulus

It helps categorize motor response based on simple responses to stimuli. The patient is either alert, responsive to verbal stimuli, responsive only to painful stimuli, or unresponsive.

Abnormal Appearance and the AVPU Scale. Assessment of appearance using the PAT provides different information than assessment using the AVPU scale. A child with an altered mental status (AMS) on the AVPU scale always has an abnormal appearance in the PAT, because such a child almost always has a serious or critical condition. However, a child with a mild to moderate illness or injury may be alert on the AVPU scale, but have an abnormal appearance in the PAT. Assessing appearance using the PAT may provide an earlier indication of the presence of serious illness and injury.

The accuracy of the AVPU scale is controversial and it has a few important limitations. Its ability to predict the extent of neurologic compromise has not been well tested in children. Its scope is limited in the evaluation of children with restless or agitated states. The scale only addresses decreased levels of responsiveness, a problem common to all of the current prehospital methods for disability assessment. However, it is easy to remember (there are no numbers to recall) and to use. The more complicated Pediatric GCS involves memorization and numerical scoring, tasks that may be hard to remember and apply in critical situations (see Chapter 7 for Pediatric GCS). Recent data suggest that the motor component of the GCS alone is the best predictor of neurologic outcome. The much simpler-to-administer motor component of the GCS may be adequate for mental status evaluation in the field. The motor categories of the GCS from lowest point value to highest are (1) no response, (2) extensor posturing, (3) flexor posturing, (4) withdrawing, (5) localizing, and (6) obeying instructions (as age-appropriate). Like the AVPU scale, the GCS does not address degrees of neurologic disability in children who are restless, agitated, or combative.

Exposure

Proper exposure of the child is necessary for completion of the primary physical assessment. The PAT requires that the caregiver remove part of the child's clothing to allow careful observation of the face, chest wall, and skin. Completing the ABCDE components of the primary assessment may require further exposure to fully evaluate physiologic function, anatomic abnormalities, and unsuspected injuries. Pay attention to the need for privacy, even for prepubescent children, when possible. Be careful to avoid heat loss, especially in infants, by covering the child up as soon as possible. Infants and younger children have a larger body surface to body weight ratio and are at a greater risk to rapidly lose body heat when left exposed. Cold stress in critically ill or injured patients can increase metabolic demands, worsen the effects of hypoxia and hypoglycemia, and adversely affect the response to resuscitative efforts.

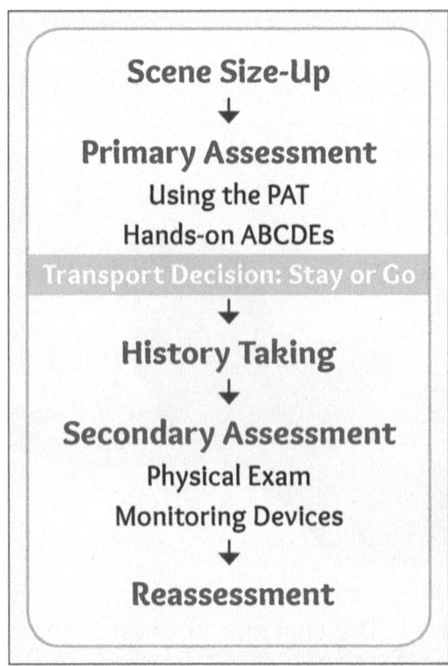

Primary Assessment: The Transport Decision: Stay or Go?

After completing the PAT and the hands-on ABCDEs, and beginning resuscitation as necessary, the prehospital professional must make a crucial decision: should they immediately transport the child to the ED, or should they continue with the additional assessment and treatment on scene? Should they transport the child, or is there a more appropriate mode of transport available (e.g., aeromedical services, pediatric specialty transport teams)? Should the child be transported to a local community hospital, for either treatment or stabilization, or does the child need to go directly to a trauma center or pediatric specialty hospital? This decision process is different for each child and for each EMS system.

Basic Life Support System

In a basic life support (BLS) system, field treatment options are limited. An early request for ALS backup or transport is appropriate if the scene is unsafe for the child, caregiver, or prehospital professional, or when a child has:

- A serious mechanism of injury
- A history compatible with serious illness
- A physiologic abnormality noted on primary assessment
- A potentially serious anatomic abnormality
- Significant pain

ALS

ALS System. In an ALS system with more extensive treatment options, the transport decision is often complex. Major factors to consider include:

- The type of clinical problem (injury versus illness)
- The expected benefits of ALS treatment in the field
- Local EMS system treatment and transport policies
- The ALS provider's comfort level
- Transport time

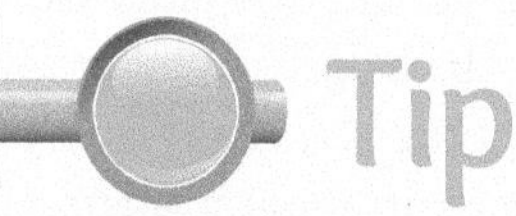

Deciding when to go and when to stay is different for each child and for each EMS system.

The Clinical Problem

If the 9-1-1 call is for trauma, and if the child has a serious mechanism of injury, a physiologic abnormality, or a potentially significant anatomic abnormality, or if the scene is unsafe, immediate transport is imperative. In these cases, stabilize the spine, manage the airway and breathing, stop external bleeding, and then transport. Attempt vascular access on the way to the ED. Examples of such patients include a child with an abnormal appearance after a closed head injury from a fall, or a child struck by a car who has a painful, deformed femur.

If the 9-1-1 call is for illness, the decision to stay or go is less clear cut and depends on the following factors: expected benefits of treatment, EMS system regulations, comfort level, and transport time.

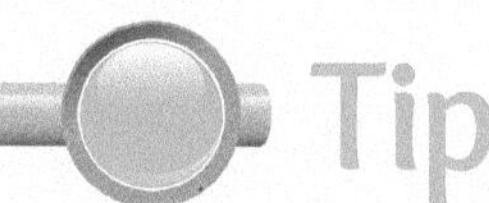

If the child is physiologically unstable, defer or omit history taking and physical examination.

Expected Benefits of Treatment

The time it takes to reach operative care in the hospital has a major effect on the outcomes of children with serious injuries. Therefore, rapid transport after initial stabilization of the cervical spine, airway, and breathing is extremely important. The time it takes to reach hospital care may also significantly affect the outcomes of children with certain medical illnesses. For example, a child in cardiogenic shock benefits most from rapid transport to definitive care, because the hospital is the best place for lifesaving treatments of this rare and complex condition.

However, some critically ill children benefit from ALS treatment on scene. For example, for a child who is seizing, early treatment with a benzodiazepine is the best hope to get the seizure under immediate control and avoid additional anticonvulsant administration and endotracheal intubation. Similarly, the risk of brain injury is decreased if glucose is administered to the unconscious diabetic child at the time that the prehospital professional recognizes hypoglycemia with a bedside test.

EMS System Regulations

The decision to stay or go often is defined by EMS system regulations about treatment and transport. For example, some systems allow prehospital professionals to treat a child in cardiopulmonary arrest with ALS interventions until either the resuscitation is successful or death is declared. Other systems require transport after initial resuscitation is underway, with the decision to discontinue efforts left to the ED staff.

Comfort Level

Whenever a prehospital professional believes that the illness or injury requires a higher level of care, it is best to initiate transport quickly. Moreover, whenever the prehospital professional feels uncomfortable with a critical intervention, it is best to transport and attempt the intervention on the way to the ED, rather than on scene. For example, a child with hypotensive (decompensated) hypovolemic shock usually deserves one attempt at vascular access on scene, then fluid administration on the way to the ED. The time spent on multiple intravenous attempts on scene might be better spent in transporting the child to definitive care, where the underlying cause of shock can be more appropriately addressed.

Transport Time

The time to the nearest ED is another key factor. A shorter transport time ordinarily supports a shorter scene time. For example, if a child has ingested a potentially lethal poison, immediate transport is prudent if the ED is close by, because of the complications related to delay of definitive care. However, if transport time is long, consider initiating treatment on scene.

Summary of Primary Assessment

The components of the pediatric primary assessment include the general impression, the ABCDEs, immediate resuscitation needs, and transport decision. The PAT is the basis for the general impression. It includes evaluation of the characteristics of appearance, work of breathing, and circulation to the skin, and uses clues obtained by looking and listening from across the room. The primary assessment includes a hands-on evaluation of pediatric-specific indicators of cardiopulmonary or neurologic abnormalities. Although vital signs can be useful in the primary assessment, they can also be misleading. They must be interpreted in the context of age and the overall general and primary assessments. Interventions may be necessary at any point in the ABCDE sequence. After the ABCDEs, another crucial decision is whether to stay on scene and begin treatment or transport immediately. The type of clinical problem, the expected benefits of earlier transport, the local EMS policies, the prehospital professional's comfort level, and the transport time are all important elements in the transport decision.

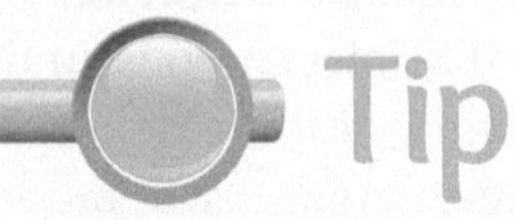

Always perform reassessment to track problems and monitor response to treatment.

History Taking

History taking has two objectives and should be performed on both medical and trauma patients:

1. To obtain a complete description of the main complaint.
2. To determine the mechanism of injury or circumstances of illness.

If the child seems to be physiologically unstable based on the primary assessment, the prehospital professional may decide to transport immediately and defer the history and secondary assessment. If the child is stable and the scene is safe, the prehospital professional should obtain a thorough history and complete the secondary assessment on the scene and before transport. As opposed to the primary assessment, which focuses on physiologic problems that may be immediately life-threatening, this secondary assessment focuses on anatomic abnormalities, which are rarely life-threatening.

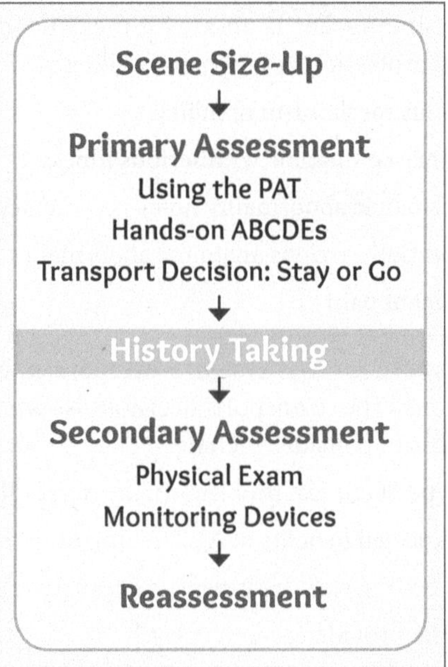

A history should be obtained from the caregiver of the pediatric patient, or from the caregiver and the older child or adolescent. In some cases, it may be helpful to interview the adolescent separate from the caregiver; many adolescents are hesitant to disclose information about drug use or sexual activity (as it relates to the current illness or injury) in front of their caregiver. The history provides important information that assists the prehospital professional in analyzing assessment findings. The SAMPLE mnemonic may be used to elicit information: Signs and Symptoms, Allergies, Medications, Past medical problems, Last food or liquid, and Events leading up to this illness or injury (**Table 1-8**).

Children with special health care needs often require additional history collection, but the type of history

Table 1-8 Pediatric SAMPLE Components

Component	Explanation
Signs and symptoms	Onset and nature of symptoms of pain or fever Age-appropriate signs of distress
Allergies	Known drug reactions or other allergies
Medications	Exact names and doses of ongoing drugs Timing and amount of last dose Timing and dose of analgesics or antipyretics
Past medical problems	History of pregnancy, labor, delivery Previous illness or injuries Immunizations
Last food or liquid	Timing of the child's last food or drink, including bottle or breastfeeding
Events leading to the injury or illness	Key events leading to the current incident Fever history

necessary is dependent on the underlying illness or condition. The use of an Emergency Information Form can be extremely helpful in obtaining critical information about these patients. More information about children with special health care needs can be found in Chapter 11.

If a child has an apparently minor condition (e.g., low-grade fever, feeding difficulties, fussiness, minor trauma), be careful not to overlook clues to possible serious underlying conditions. Ingestions, metabolic problems, and systemic infections may present with nonspecific findings in infants and toddlers. Consider child maltreatment when the physical findings are not logically related to the complaint leading to the call, or if the history is implausible or changes.

Secondary Assessment: Physical Examination

Often this portion of the assessment is not possible because of transport and treatment priorities. Sometimes it is unnecessary because the problem has been fully evaluated in earlier phases of the assessment, or the complaint and history are minor or well localized (e.g., minor laceration or twisted ankle).

If the child with traumatic injuries is stable on scene and does not need resuscitation after the primary assessment, or if he or she is on the way to the hospital but does not require ongoing treatment, perform a detailed secondary assessment.

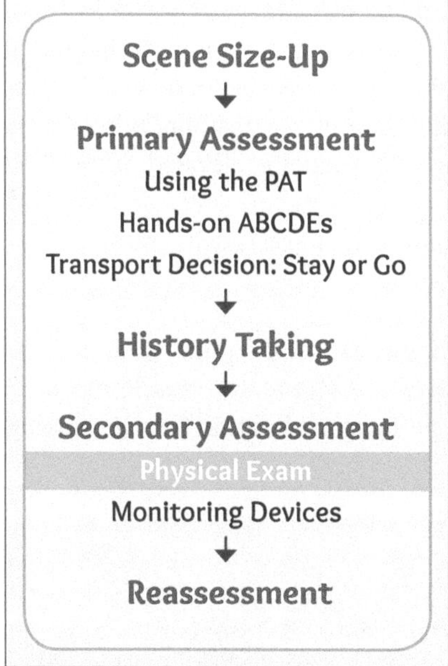

This physical evaluation must include all anatomic areas affected and builds on the findings of the primary assessment and history taking.

Use the toe-to-head sequence for the detailed secondary assessment of infants, toddlers, and preschoolers. This approach allows the prehospital professional to gain the child's trust and cooperation, and increases the accuracy of the physical findings. Ask for the assistance of the caregiver in the assessment. Note the following special anatomic characteristics of children when performing the secondary assessment.

General Observations

Observe the clothing for any unusual odors or for stains that might suggest a poison. If poisoning is suspected, remove soiled or dirty clothing and save it, and wash the child's skin with soap and water.

Skin

Observe the skin carefully for rashes and bruising patterns that may suggest maltreatment, as discussed in Chapter 13. Look for bite marks; straight line marks from cords or straps; pinch marks; or hand, belt, or buckle pattern bruises. Patterned injuries, or those with a geometric shape, are often indicative of abuse. Inspect for nonblanching petechial or purpuric lesions (which may indicate severe infections), and look for any new lesions that develop during transport.

Head

The younger the infant or child, the larger the head is in proportion to the rest of the body (**Figure 1-12**). This disproportionate size increases the risk for head injury with deceleration, such as in motor vehicle crashes. Look for bruising, swelling, and hematomas. Significant blood can be lost between the skull and scalp of a small infant.

Assessment of the anterior **fontanelle** in infants younger than 9–18 months old can provide helpful information (**Figure 1-13**). If possible, the fontanelle should be assessed with the infant in a sitting position. A bulging and **nonpulsatile fontanelle** suggests elevated intracranial pressure caused by **meningitis**, **encephalitis**, or **intracranial** bleeding. A sunken fontanelle suggests dehydration.

Eyes

A thorough evaluation of pupil size, reaction to light, and symmetry of **extraocular** muscle movements may be difficult to perform in infants. Gently rocking infants in the upright position often gets them to open their eyes. A colorful distracting object can then be used to help assess eye movements.

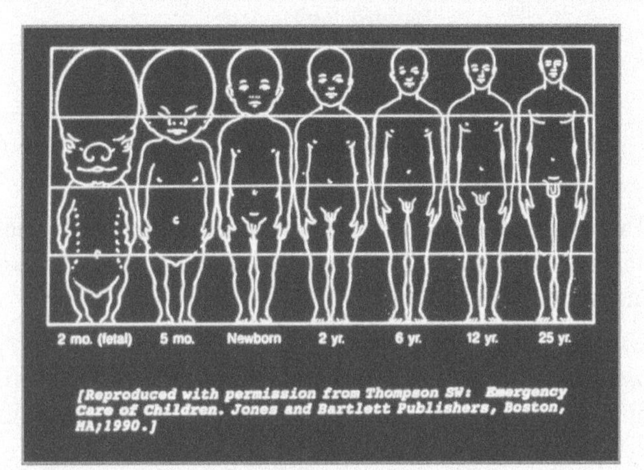

Figure 1-12 The relationship of the head to the body changes with advancing age.

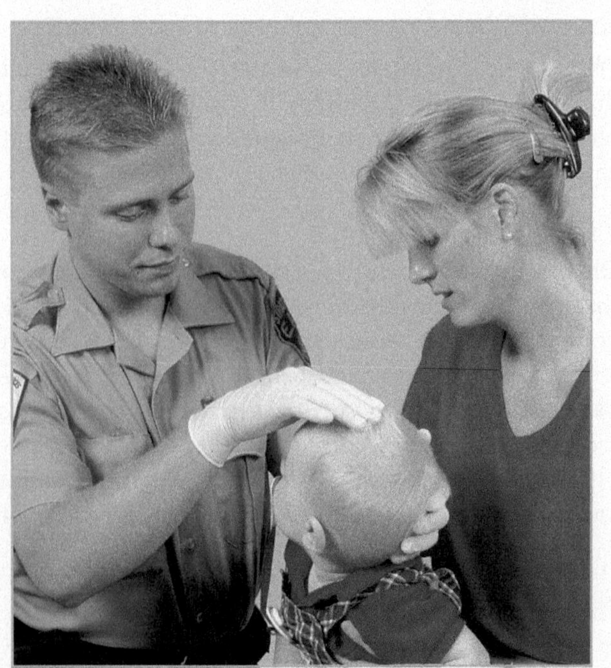

Figure 1-13 The anterior fontanelle of the infant is a window to the CNS.

Nose

Young infants preferentially breathe through their noses, so nasal congestion with mucus can cause marked respiratory distress. Gentle bulb or catheter suction of the nostrils may bring relief (**Figure 1-14**). Leaking blood (**rhinorrhea**) or cerebrospinal fluid (CSF) suggests a **basilar skull fracture**.

Ears

Look for any drainage from the ear canals (**otorrhea**). Leaking blood or CSF suggests a basilar skull fracture. Check for bruises behind the ear or **Battle sign**, another indicator of basilar skull fracture. The presence of **pus** may indicate an ear infection or perforation of the ear drum.

Mouth

In the trauma patient, look for active bleeding and loose teeth. Note the smell of the breath. Some ingestions are associated with identifiable odors, such as **hydrocarbons**. Acidosis, as in **diabetic ketoacidosis**, may impart a sweet or "fruity" smell to the breath.

Neck

Examine the **trachea** for **edema** or bruising. Listen with a stethoscope over the trachea at the midline (**Figure 1-15**). This is a quick and easy way to differentiate between very proximal airway obstruction (usually mucus in the nose) and true wheezing or stridor. The neck should also be assessed for a tracheal shift or jugular vein distention (JVD). These are classic signs of tension pneumothorax, but occur late in

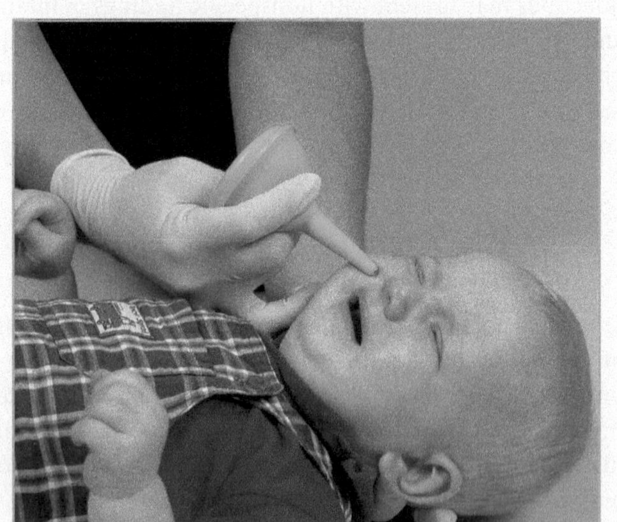

Figure 1-14 Gentle bulb suction may bring relief to the infant.

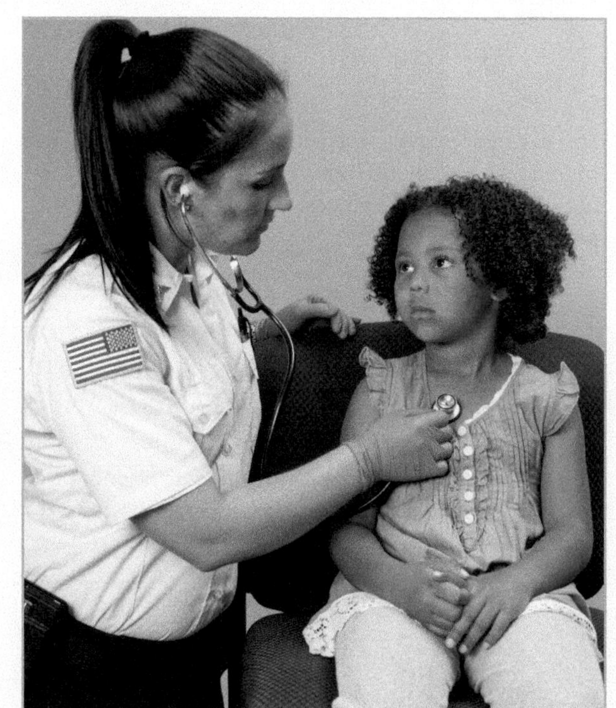

Figure 1-15 Listen at the trachea to distinguish the origin of abnormal airway sounds.

the physiologic process. JVD may not be present if there are other injuries present that have led to hypovolemia.

Chest

Reexamine the chest for penetrating injuries, lacerations, bruises, or rashes. If the child is injured, feel the clavicles and every rib for tenderness or deformity.

Back

Inspect the back for lacerations, penetrating injuries, bruises, or rashes.

Abdomen

Inspect the abdomen for any bruising, swelling, deformities, or rashes. In the trauma patient, redness or bruising under the site of protective straps, or "seat belt sign," may be apparent. Also, inspect the abdomen for distention. Gently palpate the abdomen and watch closely for guarding or tensing of the abdominal muscles, which may suggest infection, obstruction, or intra-abdominal injury. Note any tenderness or masses. If an infant or toddler has been crying for a prolonged period of time, or if a child's respiratory effort has been supported with a bag-valve-mask, this may also lead to abdominal distention because of air that has been pushed into the stomach.

Extremities

Assess for symmetry. Compare both sides for color, warmth, size of joints, and tenderness. Put each joint through a full range of motion while watching the eyes of the child for signs of pain; understandably, if there is obvious deformity of the extremity suggesting a fracture, this technique should not be used. If there is a suspected fracture present, assess for a pulse, capillary refill, motor function, and sensation distal to the injury.

Vital Signs

Although pulse and respirations have been assessed in the primary assessment, they may or may not have been formally counted and recorded because of circumstances of resuscitation or brevity of transportation. It is important to obtain and record these vital signs to make further assessment of the child's changing condition. When resuscitation is necessary, pulse and respirations should be monitored frequently but additional vital signs may be deferred until the child has stabilized or the transportation is completed.

Blood Pressure. Blood pressure determination and interpretation may be difficult in children because of the lack of patient cooperation, confusion about proper cuff size, and problems remembering normal values for age. **Figure 1-16A** illustrates the different sizes of blood pressure cuffs, and **Figure 1-16B** demonstrates the technique for getting a correct blood pressure in the arm or thigh. Always use a cuff with a width of two-thirds the length of the upper arm or thigh. For patients 3 years of age or younger, technical difficulties reduce the value of a blood pressure in the field. When shock is suspected in this age group based on other assessments (e.g., history, mechanism, PAT), consider attempting blood pressure once on scene, but do not delay treatment or transport. For patients older than 3 years of age, try one blood pressure measurement in the field, then move on to the rest of the assessment.

For children older than 1 year of age, an easy formula for determining the lower limit of acceptable blood pressure by age is as follows: minimal systolic blood pressure = 70 + (2 × age, in years). For example, a 2-year-old toddler with a systolic blood pressure of 65 mm Hg is hypotensive. **Table 1-9** shows approximate normal minimal systolic blood pressure values for different ages. High blood pressure is not a clinical problem for children in the field. Assume that a blood pressure is within normal limits if an infant or young child is agitated, is crying, has pink skin, and has easily palpable peripheral pulses. In a patient with this clinical profile, do not delay transport to obtain a blood pressure. Remember, a normal blood pressure measurement may be misleading. Although a low blood pressure definitely indicates hypotensive shock, a "normal" blood pressure frequently exists in children with compensated shock.

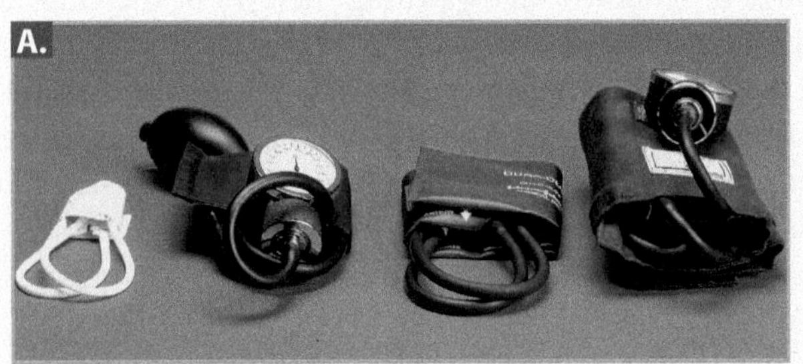

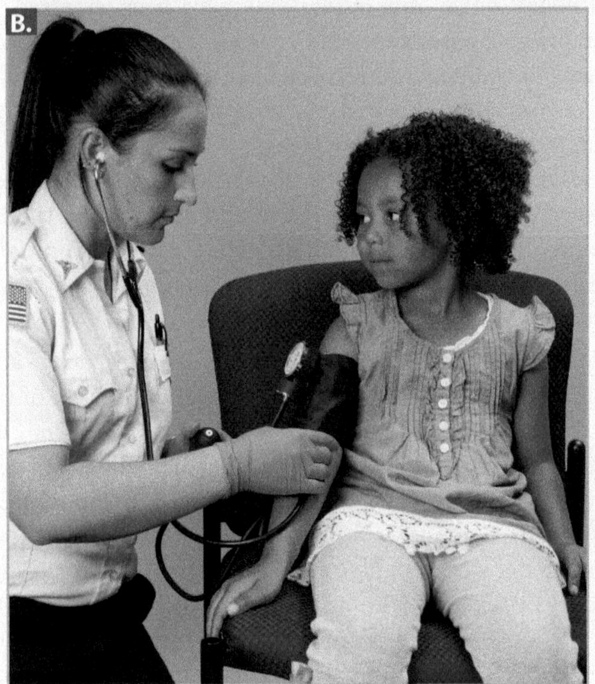

Figure 1-16 **A.** There are several different blood pressure (BP) cuff sizes: neonatal, infant, child, and adult. **B.** To obtain an accurate BP reading, use a cuff that is two-thirds the length of the child's upper arm.

Table 1-9 Minimum Blood Pressure by Age

Age	Minimal Systolic Blood Pressure (mm Hg)
Infant (birth to 12 mo)	>60
Toddler (1–3 yr)	>70
Preschooler	>75
School-age child	>80
Adolescent	>90

Note that a widening pulse pressure (systolic pressure minus diastolic pressure) may occur secondary to increased intracranial pressure and early septic shock; a narrowing pulse pressure may be seen early in hypovolemic shock.

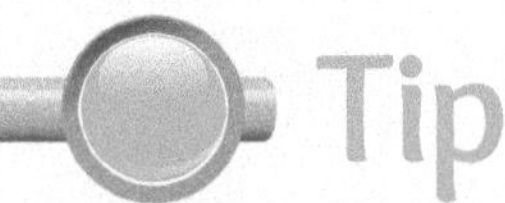

For patients younger than 3 years of age, the value of obtaining a blood pressure in the field may be outweighed by the technical difficulties of getting an accurate measurement.

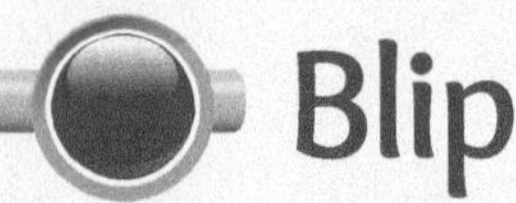

Do not depend on blood pressure readings to diagnose shock. A "normal" blood pressure frequently exists in compensated shock.

Assessment of Pain: A New Vital Sign

It is easy for the prehospital professional to ignore, underestimate, or misinterpret the signs and symptoms of pain in infants and young children. Children are much less likely to receive effective pain medications than adults. Studies have demonstrated reluctance by all levels of emergency care personnel to administer medications to children for control of pain and anxiety. The younger the child, the less likely the child will receive effective **analgesia** and **anxiolysis**. However, adult and pediatric experience has validated the effectiveness of analgesia in the prehospital setting to decrease pain, without causing respiratory depression or interference with the accuracy of physical assessment.

Pain is present with most types of injury and with many illnesses. Inadequate treatment of pain has many adverse effects on the child and family. Pain itself causes significant morbidity and misery for the child and family or caregivers, and interferes with the prehospital professional's accurate assessment of physiologic abnormalities. Children who do not receive appropriate analgesia are more likely to have exaggerated pain responses to subsequent painful procedures. Even neonates have demonstrable chronic changes in pain perception when they are subjected to painful procedures without the benefit of analgesia. Posttraumatic stress is also more common among children who experience pain during acute illness and injury and do not receive pharmacologic relief. Hence, just as with adults, it is essential to carefully assess pain in all children and to consider effective methods to provide relief from suffering when appropriate.

Local EMS protocols are now requiring that prehospital professionals assess and manage pain as a part of the secondary assessment. Indeed, evaluation of pain has become a new vital sign in all ages, including children. Appropriate pain management relieves distress of the child and family or caregivers, and facilitates communication, physical assessment, and ease of transport.

Assessment of pain must take into consideration the developmental age of the patient. The ability to recognize pain improves as the age of the child increases. For example, in a preverbal infant, crying and agitation unrelieved by being held by the caregiver may be caused by hunger, hypoxia, or pain. In infants, further assessment is essential to identify sources of pain before administration of analgesia. In contrast, verbal children older than 3 years of age are usually quite vocal about pain. Therefore, in older children, pain scales using pictures of facial expressions (Wong-Baker FACES Scale) or visual analogue scores (VAS) may be helpful in assessing the need for pharmacologic relief of pain. **Figure 1-17** illustrates the Wong-Baker FACES Scale. Although such "self-report" scales have not yet been extensively used in the prehospital environment, they have been validated in other settings to provide an immediate evaluation of intensity of pain, and to monitor response to treatment.

There is much overlap between the management of fear and anxiety and the management of pain in infants and young children. Many nonpharmacologic and pharmacologic methods relieve anxiety and reduce the perception of pain, as summarized in **Table 1-10**. Remaining calm and providing quiet professional reassurance to caregivers and child are the first important steps. A calm caregiver helps to make the child calm and more at ease. Distraction techniques may be extremely helpful in reducing pain. Many prehospital providers learn to use toys, "magic tricks," or engaging stories to provide distraction. Some EMS systems have developed a "toolbox" with distraction equipment to facilitate pain relief (**Figure 1-18**). Keeping the caregiver with the child and sometimes holding the child are also useful strategies.

In older children, visual imagery techniques can often be helpful. Ask the child where he or she would most prefer to be at the present time, then assist the child in closing his

Table 1-10 Methods of Prehospital Analgesia and Anxiolysis

Nonpharmacologic	Pharmacologic
Calm manner	Morphine
Caregiver assistance through presence or holding	Fentanyl Nitrous oxide
Distraction techniques with "toolbox" of toys	Benzodiazepines
Ice	12%–25% sucrose for neonates
Visual imagery	
Pacifier	
Music	
Splinting of fractures	

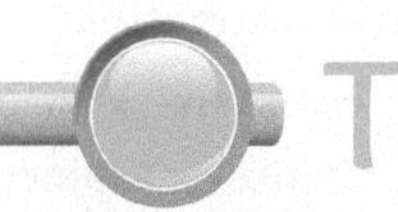

Tip

Pain is often considered an additional vital sign. Pain management can help relieve distress of the child and family, greatly facilitate communication and physical assessment, assist in timely provision of necessary interventions, and ease the transport process.

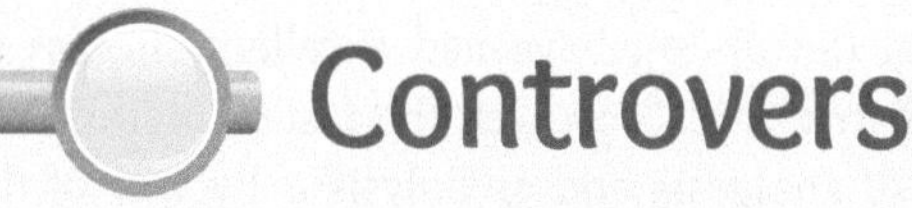

Controversy

Although "self-report" pain scales have not yet been extensively used for pediatric patients in the prehospital environment, they have been validated in other clinical settings. They can help provide an immediate evaluation of pain intensity, and they can aid in monitoring response to treatment.

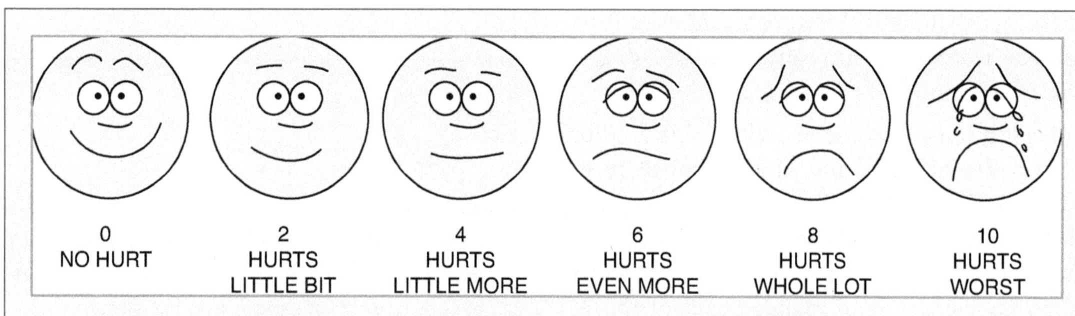

Figure 1-17 Wong-Baker FACES Pain Rating Scale for self-assessment of pain.

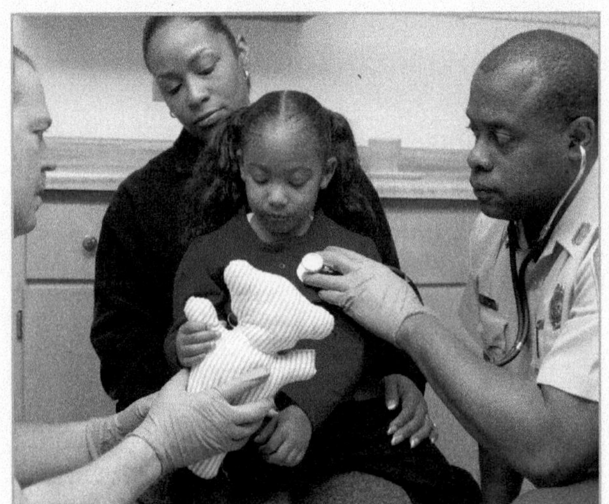

Figure 1-18 Use distraction techniques to help reduce the child's pain.

or her eyes and visualizing a more tranquil or enjoyable environment. Music is also a very effective distraction.

Pharmacologic methods for reducing pain are also a standard of prehospital care. Opiates, benzodiazepines, and nitrous oxide are available to prehospital professionals in many EMS systems. Intramuscular medications are less effective because children fear needles, and the injection site pain may last for days. Analgesic and anxiolytic drugs may be easily delivered through inhalation techniques, by the transmucosal (e.g., sublingual, intranasal, rectal) route, or by the transdermal route, although experience is still limited. Several techniques, such as inhaled nitrous oxide and rectal diazepam, have had excellent success in prehospital pediatric care. However, the fastest method for administration of analgesia and anxiolysis is by way of the intravenous route. Intravenous (IV) delivery provides the most effective and most controllable or titratable method. A downside is it does involve establishing vascular access, which like the intramuscular (IM) route is usually painful. Also, the child's response to pain and anxiolytic medication is sometimes unpredictable and must be carefully weighed against unwanted side effects. Medications to reduce pain also cause sedation and can result in respiratory depression, bradycardia, hypoxemia, hypotension, and even loss of protective airway reflexes. Occasionally, anxiolytic drugs cause a paradoxical worsening of agitation.

Assessment of pain has become a "vital sign," and management of pediatric pain and anxiety must be a routine part of field care in all EMS systems. This entails a thorough understanding of available nonpharmacologic techniques, medications, potential medication contraindications and complications, and management of those complications.

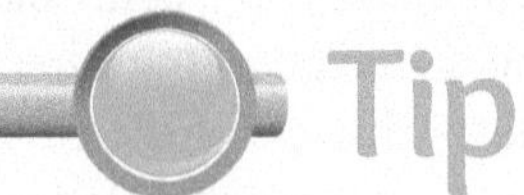

Analgesic and anxiolytic drugs may be easily delivered through inhalation, transmucosal (e.g., sublingual, intranasal, rectal) routes, or transdermal routes. Several techniques, such as inhaled nitrous oxide and rectal diazepam, have had excellent success in prehospital pediatric care.

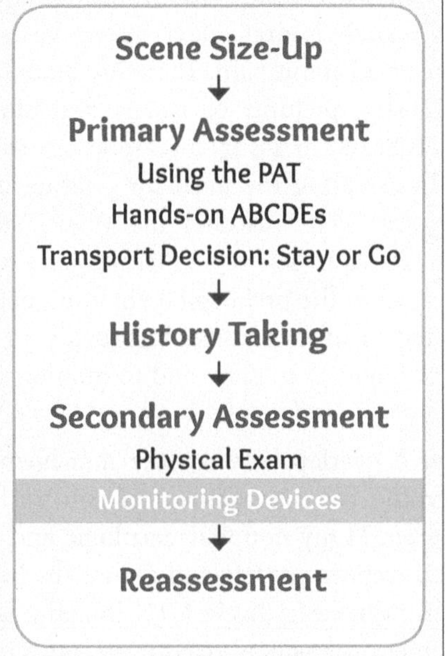

Secondary Assessment: Monitoring Devices

Pulse Oximetry

Oxygen Saturation. Pulse oximetry is an excellent tool to assess how well a child is breathing. **Figure 1-19** illustrates the technique of placing a pulse oximetry probe on a young child. In infants and younger children, the patient may tolerate the probe more readily if a wrap-around probe is used and it is placed around the toe or the foot. A pulse oximetry reading above 94% saturation on room air indicates good oxygenation. Be careful not to underestimate

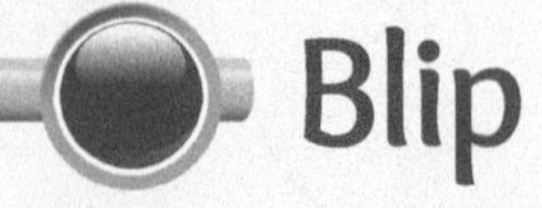

Be careful not to underestimate respiratory distress in a child with a pulse oximetry reading above 94%. This child may be using increased work of breathing and tachypnea to compensate for serious hypoxic stress.

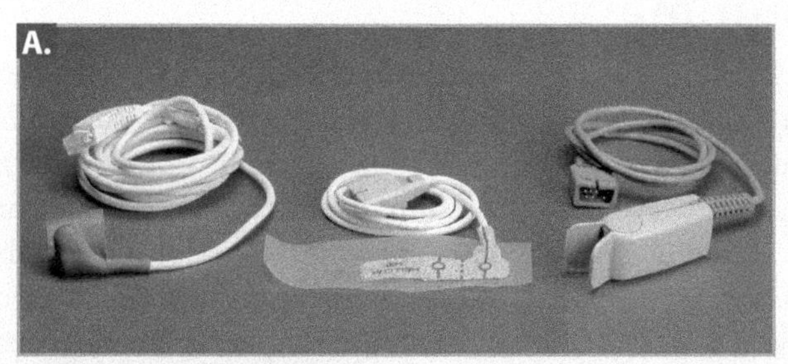

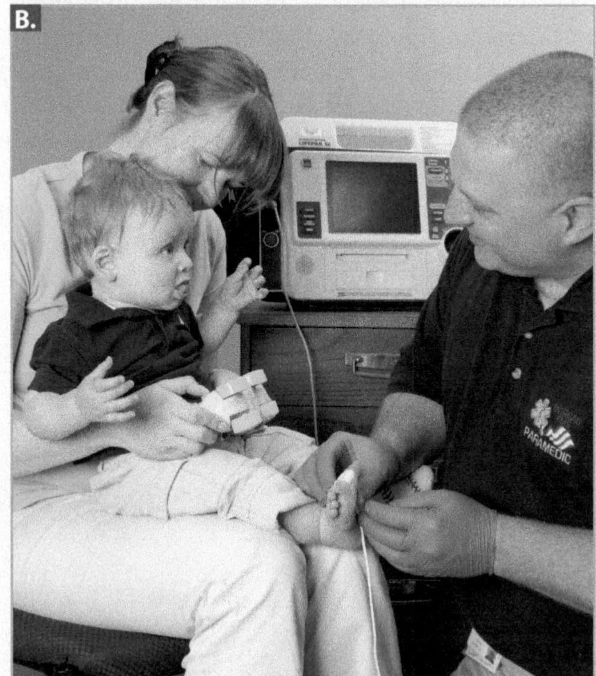

Figure 1-19 **A.** Various pulse oximeter probes wrap around or clip onto digits or earlobes. **B.** Pulse oximetry is an excellent tool for assessing the effectiveness of breathing.

respiratory distress in a child with a reading above 94%. Sometimes the child can compensate for hypoxia by significantly increasing work of breathing and respiratory rate, and pulse oximetry may not reflect the true severity or urgency of the respiratory problem. As with any other measurement, interpret pulse oximetry in the context of the "big picture," including work of breathing, appearance, and circulation.

Although pulse oximetry is quite helpful in identifying a child with moderate respiratory distress, it can also help identify the child in respiratory failure. When the pulse oximetry reading is below 90% saturation in a child on 100% oxygen by a nonrebreathing mask, this usually represents respiratory failure requiring **assisted ventilation**. However, sometimes a child in severe respiratory distress or early respiratory failure may maintain measured oxygen saturation by increasing work of breathing and respiratory rate. This child may not appear to be critically ill by pulse oximetry alone. Again, interpret pulse oximetry together with the rest of the assessment to accurately evaluate the degree of respiratory distress or failure.

Additional Monitoring Devices

The prehospital professional can perform some types of specific testing in the field, such as rapid glucose determinations, 12-lead ECG monitoring, capnography, and other specialty testing available in local EMS areas.

Diagnostic Testing

The diagnostic testing portion of the assessment frequently requires ancillary testing, such as laboratory and radiographic evaluations. Diagnostic testing is usually part of in-patient assessment in the ED, the hospital pediatric ward, or the pediatric intensive care unit.

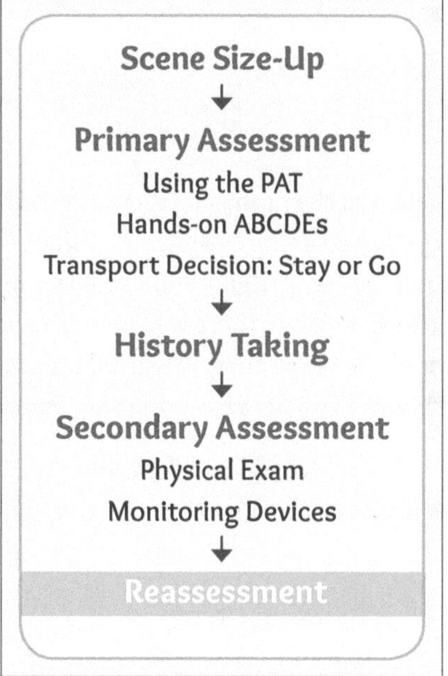

Reassessment

Perform reassessment of all patients to gauge the response to treatment and to track the progression of identified physiologic and anatomic problems. New problems may also be identified on reassessment. Data from the reassessment will guide ongoing treatment. The elements in the reassessment are:

1. The PAT
2. The ABCDEs with repeat vital signs
3. Assessment of positive anatomic findings
4. Review of the effectiveness and safety of treatment

The elements in the reassessment are also the basis for determination of an appropriate transport destination and for accurate, pediatric-specific radio or telephone communications with medical oversight or the ED.

Radio Reporting

Proper radio reporting promotes a seamless transfer of care from the prehospital to the ED setting, maximizing the ability of all clinicians to provide efficient and effective care. A good radio report transmits vital data completely and concisely, highlighting pediatric-specific information to allow the ED team to best prepare for the patient's arrival. If available, provide the ED a patient weight, as reported by the caregiver or as obtained by a length-based resuscitation tape. Recent studies have indicated, however, that estimates of weight determined by length-based tapes may underestimate a child's weight because of the increase in the prevalence of childhood obesity. For a step-by-step explanation, see **Field Reporting, Procedure 1**.

Summary

After the primary assessment, and beginning any necessary resuscitative efforts, the prehospital professional must determine the severity of the illness or injury and make a decision regarding mode and timing of transport. If additional evaluation is appropriate, perform a detailed history and secondary assessment either on scene or on the way to the ED. These additional phases of assessment are not indicated if there is an acute life-threatening or limb-threatening problem that requires the prehospital professional's ongoing attention. The secondary assessment is more for the detection of anatomic problems than for evaluation of physiologic abnormalities. Always perform reassessments to observe the patient's response to interventions, and to guide changes in treatment, transport, and triage. Diagnostic testing refers to laboratory and radiographic evaluation to determine causation, and mainly occurs after arrival in the ED and during hospitalization for admitted patients.

Case Study 3

You are called to the home of a 2-month-old boy who stopped breathing and turned blue according to his babysitter. He reportedly had a fever all day. The infant is lying supine; his skin is pale and mottled. When touched, the infant becomes extremely irritable and exhibits a high-pitched, screeching cry. When left alone, he appears lethargic and poorly responsive. There is no abnormal positioning, and no abnormal airway sounds, stridor, nasal flaring, or grunting. The respiratory rate is 60 breaths/min and unlabored. The heart rate is 200 beats/min. His peripheral pulses are weak and his extremities are cool to the touch. Capillary refill time is approximately 5 seconds.

1. Does this infant's appearance suggest a serious problem?
2. Is this infant in shock?

CASE STUDY ANSWERS

Case Study 1 — page 4

Beware of the pale child! Consider any child who has experienced significant trauma and is pale at the scene to have significant blood loss until proven otherwise. Children are able to compensate for blood loss and hypovolemia through catecholamine surges, which cause tachycardia and peripheral vasoconstriction. These reflexes inhibit the circulation to the skin and result in a pale patient. Although this child could have had a significant head injury based on mechanism of injury, his level of consciousness is reasonably normal; therefore, the initial issue needing emergent attention is hemorrhagic shock. Abdominal injuries with blunt trauma to the liver or spleen can result in significant internal bleeding without external signs of injury. Many children with internal bleeding do not always have abdominal tenderness. Indicators of suspected hemorrhagic shock are mild tachycardia, weak pulses, delayed capillary refill, and a borderline low blood pressure (80 mm Hg/palp). This child requires timely transport to a trauma center with pediatric capabilities. Delay vascular access until the child is en route to the hospital.

This child is also clearly in pain. However, weigh the benefits of pharmacologic therapy to relieve pain against the potential for circulatory collapse, delay in transport, and the need to effectively assess appearance. Use opiate analgesics, such as morphine, in patients with suspected compensated hemorrhagic shock cautiously because of morphine's vasodilatory effect.

Case Study 2 — page 14

The PAT is an accurate tool to evaluate severity of illness or injury, and to determine the urgency for providing lifesaving care. Upon arrival at the scene of this patient, it is quite reassuring to find the toddler alert, pink, and with nonlabored respirations. His vigorous responses make it difficult to perform the conventional ABCDE assessment. Since this child clearly has no serious immediate cardiorespiratory problems, is alert and awake, and fights your examination, history taking and secondary assessment can occur. However, the prehospital professional should transport every infant or child who has had a submersion injury to a hospital for observation of progression of symptoms. Still, the findings on the PAT allow the prehospital professional to slow the pace and get more information while on the scene. There is no need for immediate resuscitative interventions, and the prehospital professional can avoid the risk of "lights and siren" transport.

Anytime there is an unwitnessed submersion event, consider that a traumatic injury may be present. The usual mechanism of a toddler pool drowning involves falling less than 3 ft (1 m) into a body of water. In this scenario, it is unlikely that he has sustained a significant head or spinal injury. Furthermore, if he is moving his neck without apparent discomfort while in his mother's arms, but then vigorously screams and fights when you attempt to examine him, it is unlikely that spinal stabilization will be helpful (and may prove more harmful and distressing than not). Local protocols govern this decision. Although treatment and transport of this patient are not emergent, ongoing assessment during transport is necessary. Pulmonary complications of submersion, primarily hypoxia, may have a delayed presentation.

Case Study 3 — page 26

Any infant who has an acute life-threatening event, who reportedly stopped breathing or turned blue, deserves EMS transport, regardless of his or her appearance on your arrival. In this case, the need for urgent treatment and transport is obvious. One of the PAT indicators of shock in this infant is altered appearance. Although that finding could be due to causes other than poor brain perfusion (e.g., infection, trauma, toxins, hypoxia), the presence of effortless tachypnea and pale, mottled skin supports the diagnosis of shock. Alternating lethargy and irritability may progress to unresponsiveness as perfusion worsens.

The hands-on examination confirms the suspicion of shock. This patient's heart rate is rapid at 200 beats/min, with weak peripheral pulses, cool extremities, and delayed capillary refill. Even without a blood pressure, the abnormal appearance and skin findings suggest that he should be treated for hypotensive shock. Although the cause of shock is unknown, treatment of any type of hypotensive shock includes vascular access and 20-mL/kg boluses of crystalloid fluid. Make one attempt at vascular access on the scene and then rapidly transport this patient to definitive care. Reassess his response to therapy frequently en route.

SUGGESTED READINGS

Textbooks

American Academy of Orthopaedic Surgeons. *Emergency Care and Transportation of the Sick and Injured*. 10th ed. Burlington, MA: Jones & Bartlett Learning; 2011.

American Academy of Pediatrics and the American College of Emergency Physicians. *APLS: The Pediatric Emergency Medicine Resource*. 5th ed. Burlington, MA: Jones & Bartlett Learning; 2012.

Anne M, Agur A, Dalley A. *Grant's Atlas of Anatomy*. 11th ed. Philadelphia, PA: Lippincott Williams & Wilkins; 2004.

Bledsoe B, Porter R, Cherry R. *Essentials of Paramedic Care*. New Jersey: Prentice Hall; 2003.

Chameides L, Samson RA, Schexnayder SM, Hazinski MF. *PALS Provider Manual*. American Heart Association; 2011.

Zitelli B, Davis H. *Atlas of Pediatric Physical Diagnosis*. 4th ed. Philadelphia, PA: Mosby; 2002.

Articles

Gausche M. Out-of-hospital care of pediatric patients. *Pediatr Clin North Am*. 1999;46(6):1305–1327.

Green SM. Cheerio Laddie! Bidding farewell to the Glasgow Coma Score. *Ann Emerg Med*. 2011;58:427–430.

Thompson DO, Hurtado TR, Liao MM, Byyny RL, Gravitz C, Haukoos JS. Validation of the Simplified Motor Score in the out-of-hospital setting for the prediction of outcomes after traumatic brain injury. *Ann Emerg Med*. 2011;58:417–425.

Warren J. Guidelines for the inter- and intrahospital transport of critically ill patients. *Crit Care Med*. 2004;32(1):256–262.

Other Resources

Aehlert B. *Mosby's Comprehensive Pediatric Emergency Care*. Sudbury, MA: Elsevier; 2006.

American Academy of Pediatrics. Emergency information forms and emergency preparedness for children with special health care needs (policy statement). *Pediatrics*. 2010;125:829–837.

Nieman CT, Manacii CF, Super DM, Mancuso C, Fallon WF Jr. Use of Broselow tape may result in the under resuscitation of children. *Acad Emerg Med*. 2006;(10):1011–1019.

Proehl JA. Initial assessment and resuscitation. In: Hoyt KS, Selfridge-Thomas J, eds. *Emergency Nursing Core Curriculum*. 6th ed. St. Louis, MO: Saunders Elsevier; 2007:125.

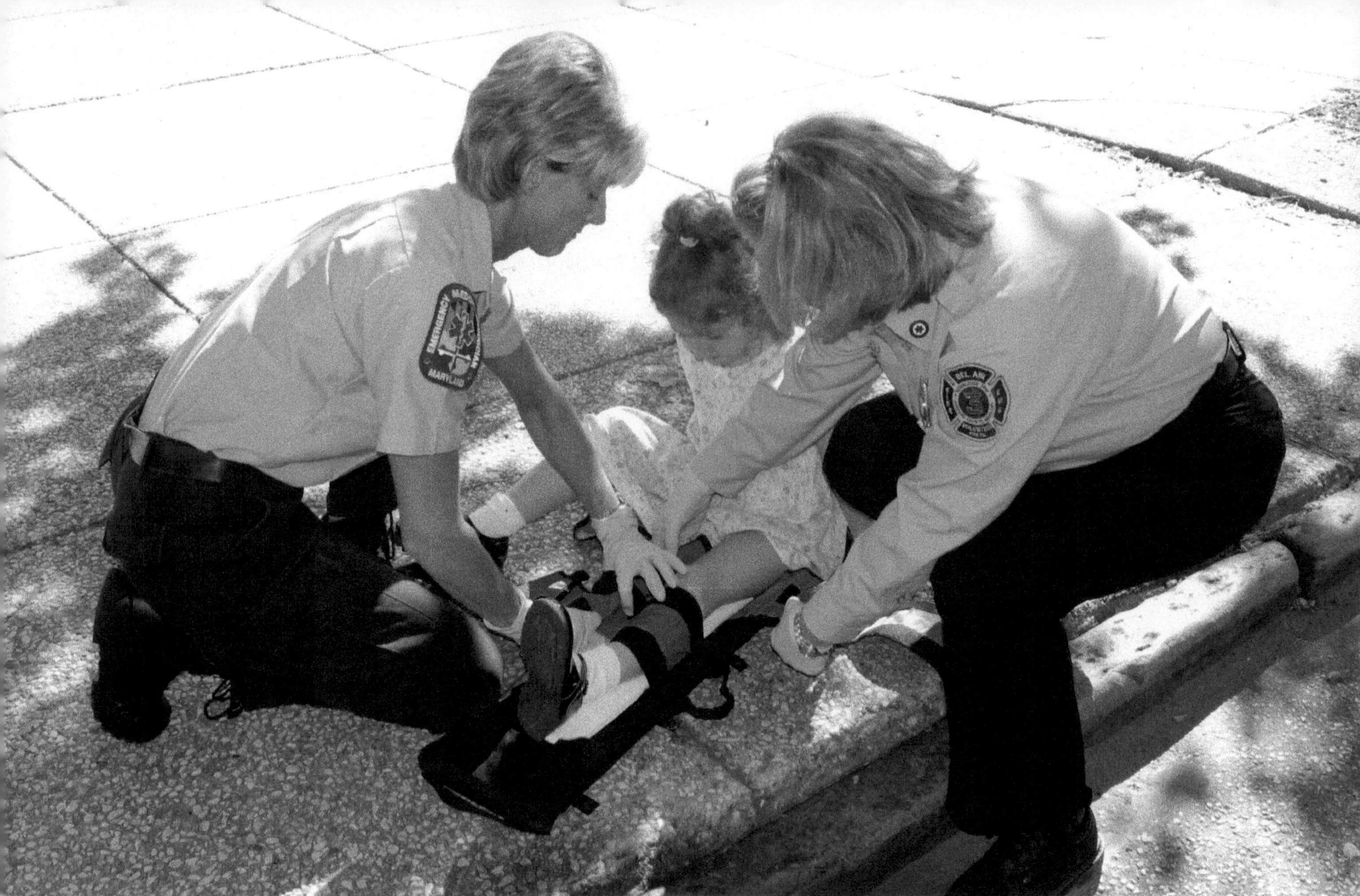

Learning Objectives

1. Discuss the communication challenges in handling emotional responses of a family with a child who is ill or injured.
2. List the expected changes in vital signs with advancing age.
3. Describe key growth and development characteristics for the following groups: infants, toddlers, preschoolers, school-aged children, adolescents, and children with special health care needs.
4. Explain unique anatomic and physiologic characteristics that influence assessment of children in each group.

Using a Developmental Approach

Chapter 2

Introduction

Infants and children constitute a small percentage of all patients seen in an emergency medical services (EMS) system. An even smaller percentage requires advanced life support (ALS). EMS providers must become comfortable with pediatric-specific information to promote success while interacting with this special patient population. Because of the unique anatomic, physiologic, and developmental differences in children, EMS providers must be well versed in normal developmental changes in infants and children. To successfully complete a pediatric patient assessment, the provider must be able to incorporate an understanding of how a child's physical growth and psychosocial development relate to his or her condition.

In addition to knowing the growth and developmental characteristics of the different age groups, the prehospital professional must be aware of special considerations when assessing a child with special health care needs (CSHCN). Sometimes the chronologic age of the CSHCN does not correspond with his or her developmental stage, and physical growth may not reflect emotional maturity.

Caring for a child also includes caring for the family. In addition to parents, caregivers, friends, and siblings may be present. Each person may have a different response to the child who is ill or injured, and the prehospital professional must be prepared to care for the entire "extended" family of friends and relatives. Communication skills are often as important as assessment and treatment skills in establishing an atmosphere of trust and comfort. Creating such an atmosphere requires that the prehospital provider have a confident and professional attitude toward children's care, and use age-appropriate pediatric skills. Communication skills become especially important in the event of a mass-casualty incident or natural disaster (see Chapter 9).

This chapter addresses age-specific growth characteristics and assessment techniques for physiologically stable children from infancy to adolescence, and for CSHCN. Chapter 1 addresses general assessment techniques for the acutely ill or injured child, and Chapter 11 expands the discussion on CSHCN.

Case Study 1

You receive a 9-1-1 call about a fussy infant. On your arrival, a frantic mother meets you at the door with her 4-week-old daughter in her arms. The infant is crying inconsolably. She has no retractions, but her skin is mottled on both the trunk and the extremities. Her arms and legs are cool. The mother tells you that the baby has been fussy all day, vomiting all her feedings, and the mother thinks her stomach looks big. She had a brief episode of limpness and pallor, and the mother gave her several rescue breaths before calling 9-1-1.

1. What are the steps to assess and treat this child, and how will you address the mother's concerns?
2. What are the worrisome findings in this infant?

Pediatric Calls and Response From Family and Providers

Every family responds differently when a child is ill (**Figure 2-1**). Having an ill child places immense pressure on the family unit. Common responses are reviewed in **Table 2-1**. Although some caregivers' responses may seem too emotional or illogical, listen to their concerns. Acting as an advocate for proper care allows the EMS provider to best approach the pediatric patient. Caregivers usually know the patient best and can provide vital information that allows the EMS interaction to be successful. Children, even infants, can quickly sense emotions in adults.

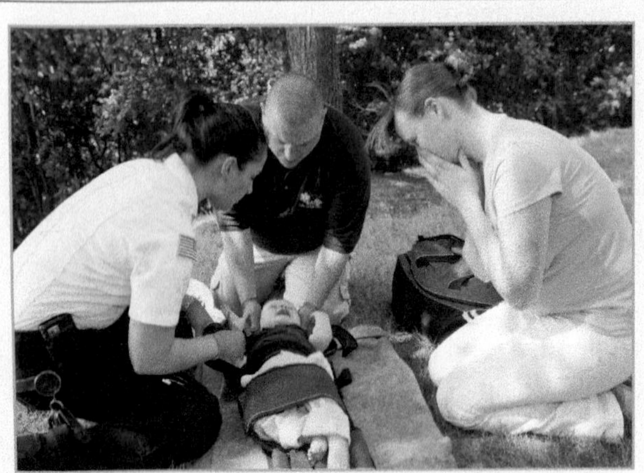

Figure 2-1 Every family responds differently to a child's illness or injury.

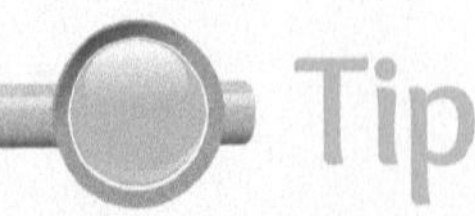

A family's response to a child's illness or injury is fluenced by the child's developmental level, previous erience with the medical system, coping strategies, e, availability of support systems, and nature of the ncy.

Just as a family may respond emotionally to a pediatric patient, so too may EMS providers. EMS providers may also experience any of the emotional responses as outlined in Table 2-1. Acting in a calm, professional manner gains trust from the family or caregivers and also helps the EMS crew to establish control of a potentially emotional situation. This approach also allows the providers to gain as much valuable information as possible from the family or caregivers, which ultimately helps triage the patient to the correct emergency department or include the most accurate differential diagnosis as part of the patient assessment.

The best way to reduce provider stress related to patient interactions is to remain current with pediatric treatment standards. Being familiar with the pediatric equipment location, currently stocked equipment, and medications also decreases stress while interacting with an ill child. Because of the limited number of pediatric calls, being well versed with the pediatric devices on an EMS unit becomes increasingly important.

Often providers feel guilt after interacting with a sick infant or child. It is common for providers to think about the pediatric situation after the call. Depending on the situation, a single patient interaction can cause reflection for days, weeks, or months. Any provider can experience difficult emotions after a stressful pediatric call. EMS providers should seek professional help from a licensed mental health professional when unresolved stress results from these interactions.

Communication With the Child and Family or Caregiver

To effectively approach infants and children, EMS providers should account for developmental information as it relates to the patient assessment at hand. Similar to interaction with adults, each pediatric patient is unique with a distinct

Table 2-1 Common Responses of Caregivers to Acute Illness or Injury in a Child

Response	Description
Disbelief	Caregivers may be struggling with the child's illness or injury. They may seem too calm or unconcerned.
Guilt	Caregivers may be horrified that they were unable to recognize the serious nature of their child's condition or that they were unable to prevent an injury. They may focus their attention on what should have been done, rather than on the child's immediate situation.
Anger	Caregivers may show their concern as anger, and they may direct their anger at the prehospital professional. Caregivers may become hostile when the prehospital professional makes efforts to stabilize their child. They may attempt to refuse transport.
Physical symptoms	Caregivers may have tachycardia, nausea, headache, chest pain, sweaty palms, dry mouth, or hyperventilation.

personality that can impact the EMS provider's ability to obtain pertinent assessment information. Calling 9-1-1 is often a stressful situation for the patient and family. Approaching the patient gently and at his or her eye level is important in initiating communication with the child. The best policy is to be honest with a child, because distrust can interfere with effectively finding important information about the situation at hand. Observing the patient's behavior can provide clues to age-specific actions.

In addition to communication with the pediatric patient, communication with the caregiver or family is also important. Children seek clues from their parents regarding safety. Infants and children are never a single-patient EMS call. The family and caregivers must be treated as potential patients in the situation, because their involvement can provide necessary information to properly handle the situation. Whenever possible, the pediatric patient and family or caregiver should be kept together. A successful pediatric patient interaction includes information gathering from family and primary caregivers. Effective communication is the cornerstone of effective out-of-hospital care.

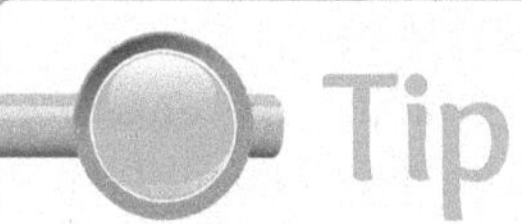

Communication skills are often as important as assessment and treatment skills.

Vital Signs Through the Ages

A common challenge in evaluating infants and children is determining when vital signs are normal based on the age of the patient. Respiratory rate, heart rate, blood pressure, and temperature all change with age. The presence or absence of fever, anxiety, or pain and the child's activity level also affect vital signs. In ill or injured children, the prehospital professional must distinguish the impact of these outside influences on vital signs from changes caused by pathologic processes. Chapter 1 presents key physical characteristics and assessment techniques that assist the prehospital professional in separating a "sick" child from a "not sick" child.

Respiratory Rate

Although normal values for vital signs vary with age, there are a variety of physiologic or anatomic bases for these changes. The normal range of respiratory rate slows with age because of an increase in the number of alveoli and increasing lung volume and lung compliance with physical growth. **Table 2-2** lists the normal respiratory rate for age.

Table 2-2 Normal Respiratory Rate for Age

Age	Respiratory Rate (breaths/min)
Infant (birth–12 mos)	30–60
Toddler (1–3 yr)	24–40
Preschooler	22–34
School-aged child	18–30
Adolescent	12–16

At times there is a problem with accurate counting of the rate, especially if the count is done in a 15-second interval. In infants, observe and count abdominal excursions for 30 seconds to obtain an accurate respiratory rate. As a child grows, breathing becomes less dependent on abdominal muscles and the diaphragm and more dependent on the chest muscles. Observing thoracic excursions for 15–30 seconds provides an accurate respiratory rate in an older child.

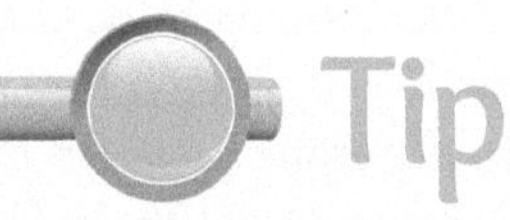

In infants, observe abdominal excursions and count rate for 30–60 seconds to obtain an accurate respiratory rate.

Heart Rate

The baseline heart rate of infants and children slows with age, reflecting increasing control of the heart rate by the vagus nerve. The vagus nerve transmits cholinergic impulses, which slow the beating of the heart. **Table 2-3** lists normal heart rates for age. In addition, by 2 years of age a circadian rhythm in heart rate is present, seen in a fall of 10–20 beats/min, while the child is asleep. One confusing factor in assessing a child's heart rate during different phases of the sleep–wake cycle, or during different phases of respiration, is that the child's rhythm is more irregular than an adult's. This sinus arrhythmia is more prominent in toddlers to school-aged children and is caused by immature vagus nerve control (**Figure 2-2**).

Table 2-3 Normal Heart Rates for Age

Age	Heart Rate (beats/min)
Infant (birth–12 mos)	100–160
Toddler (1–3 yr)	90–150
Preschooler	80–140
School-aged child	70–120
Adolescent	60–100

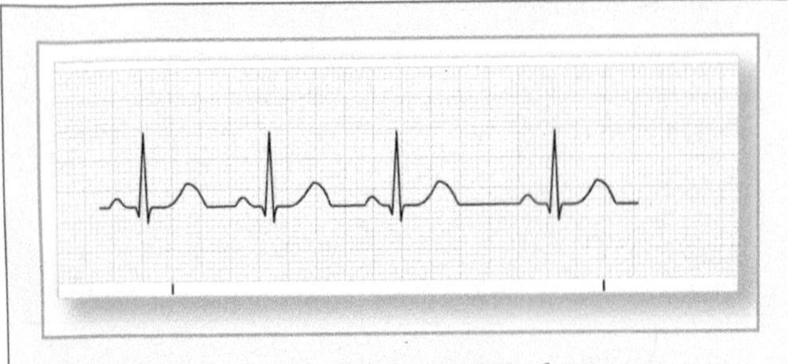

Figure 2-2 Electrocardiogram (ECG) of a sinus arrhythmia.

Blood Pressure

A child's blood pressure increases with age (**Table 2-4** lists normal systolic blood pressure values for age). The measured blood pressure is affected by equipment size. A cuff that is too small gives falsely elevated readings, whereas one that is too large gives readings that are too low. If diastolic pressure cannot be auscultated, obtain a systolic pressure by ating the pulse. This value is approximately 10 mm Hg than an auscultated pressure because of the relative itivity of palpation in appreciating initial pulsations uff is deflated.

Table 2-4 Normal Blood Pressure Values for Age

Age	Minimal Systolic Blood Pressure (mm Hg)
Infant (birth–12 mos)	>60
Toddler (1–3 yr)	>70
Preschooler	>75
School-aged child	>80
Adolescent	>90

Temperature

Body temperature also varies with age and site of measurement. Newborn temperatures are often higher than those of older children, averaging 37.5°C (99.5°F) during the first 6 months of life. After 3 years of age, the temperature falls to below 37.2°C (99°F), and finally to 36.7°C (98°F) by 11 years of age. There is also a circadian rhythm to body temperature that develops by 5 years of age. This results in a lower temperature at night and a higher temperature during the day. In infants, when a recorded temperature is important to the assessment, and the child is stable, ask the caregiver to obtain a rectal temperature. A rectal temperature is the accepted standard. A tympanic temperature may be acceptable in older children (>1 year) but may not be accurate based on the technique of the caregiver. Temperature may also be obtained with temporal artery thermometers. These devices use infrared technology to measure temperature in the superficial temporal artery. If obtained with good technique, these are quite accurate. An axillary temperature is approximately 1°C (2°F) lower than the rectal temperature. Normal body temperature decreases with increasing distance from the central circulation.

Growth Rates

Physical growth of infants and children includes body (somatic) growth and organ system growth. Skeletal and muscular growth has two spurts, the first from birth to 4 years of age and the second in adolescence (ages 9–14 for girls, ages 10–16 for boys). Brain, spinal cord, and nerve growth occurs maximally in the first few years of life and reaches adult proportions by 10 years of age.

The presence or absence of key secondary sex characteristics, especially pubic hair, marks a physiologic turning point for children. Genital growth begins about 8 years of age in girls and 9 years of age in boys, but there is significant variation. When children have visible pubic hair, they have usually attained adult physiology.

Anatomic Changes

Neck and Airway

The neck is short in infancy and elongates during childhood because of vertebral growth. As this occurs, anatomic landmarks also change in shape, size, and location. The epiglottis changes from a U-shape to the longer and thinner adult structure (**Figure 2-3**). It also moves in location from the level of the C1 vertebra to the C3 vertebra as the child's height increases. At birth, the larynx is only one-third the adult size. It becomes wider and longer until 3 years of age, and undergoes another growth spurt during puberty. At birth, the trachea is one-third the adult length, and increases 300% in circumference by puberty.

Chest and Lungs

At birth, the chest wall is round (anteroposterior, or AP, diameter equals lateral diameter). As the infant grows, it flattens out (lateral growth exceeds AP growth). Because an infant's chest wall is thin, heart and lung sounds are transmitted throughout the chest. Breath sounds are often audible on inspiration and expiration (bronchovesicular). In addition, secretions present anywhere in the respiratory tract are often heard throughout the chest. In an infant, respirations are mainly abdominal, because of the greater role of the diaphragm in breathing mechanics. By 6 years of age, breathing becomes more thoracic in origin, because of the development of chest wall musculature.

The lung tissue itself also changes with age. At birth, an infant has only 8% of the adult number of alveoli. The number of alveoli increases until 8 years of age, after which they increase in size but not number.

Heart

At birth, the right ventricle is the same size as the left ventricle, a function of the demands of fetal circulation. This accounts for a right axis deviation seen on electrocardiograms (ECGs) in infants. However, the left ventricle quickly grows in size and muscle mass, and greatly outsizes the right ventricle with age. The left ventricle reaches adult proportions of 2:1 by 1 year of age.

Abdomen

A newborn infant has a protuberant abdomen for numerous reasons. The liver is relatively large, the stomach is more horizontal, and the lungs expand downward with movement of the diaphragm. The stomach capacity increases from 30–90 mL at birth, to 210–360 mL by 1 year of age, and 500 mL by 2 years of age. It assumes a more vertical position during childhood and reaches an adult volume of 750–900 mL. The abdomen also

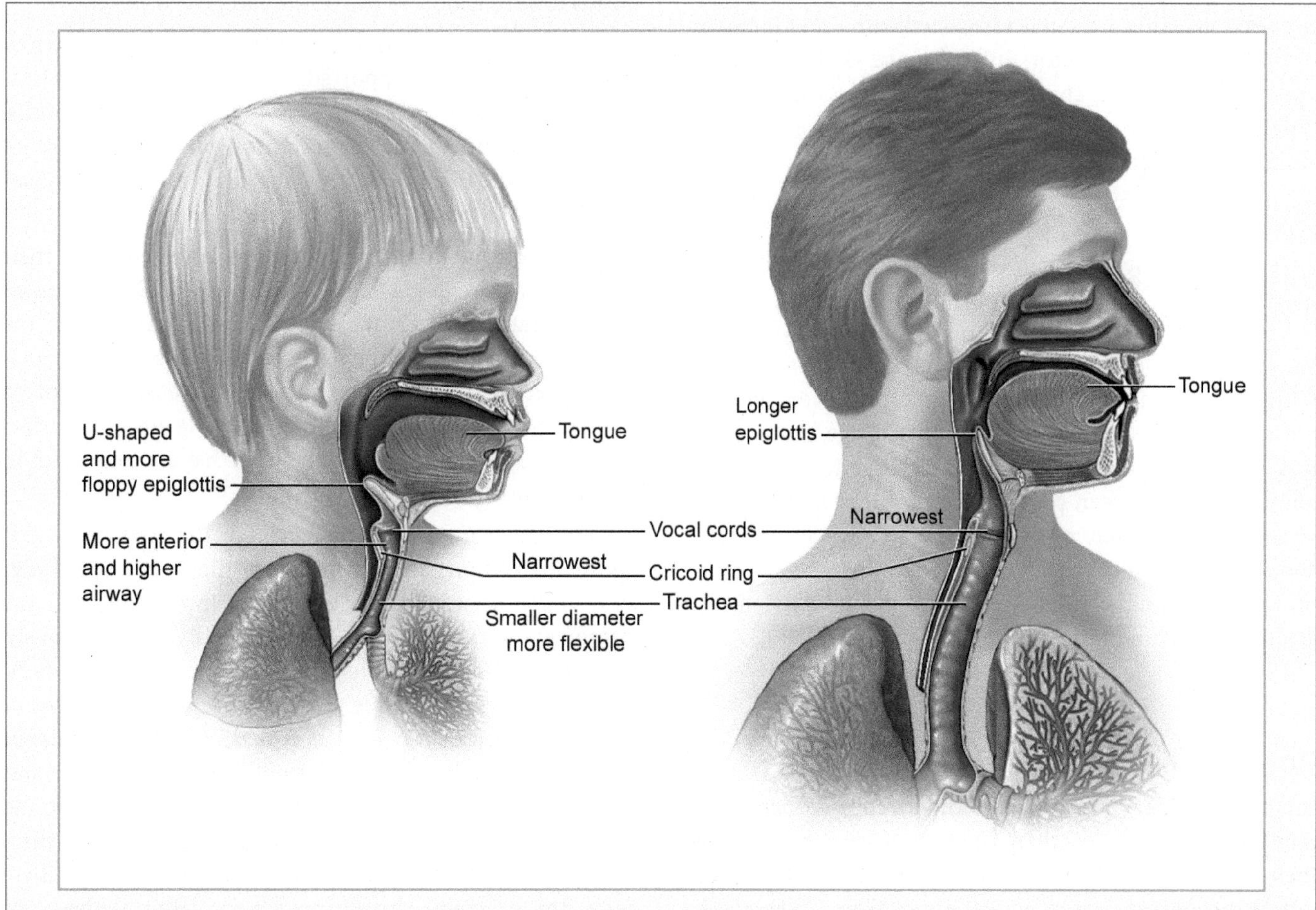

Figure 2-3 Differences between the child and adult airways.

seems protuberant in toddlers because of a normal lumbar lordosis (curvature) of the spine. The abdomen becomes more scaphoid (flat) in school-aged children.

Musculoskeletal System

In infants and young children, new longitudinal bone growth occurs in secondary centers of ossification at the end of the long bones, vertebral bodies, and the cranium (physeal plates). These cartilaginous growth plates are relatively weak and are vulnerable to fractures exclusive to childhood. Bone growth ends with the ossification of the growth cartilage and union of the epiphysis and diaphysis. Growth in children is asymmetric, with the lower extremities, especially the distal extremities (e.g., feet), growing before puberty and the trunk during puberty.

Muscle growth includes an increase in the size of muscle cells. There is a growth spurt in the number of muscle cells at 2 years of age, with a maximal increase during puberty. The proportion of muscle mass to body weight changes during childhood, going from 1:5 at birth to 1:3 in adolescence.

Nervous System

The growth of the nervous system occurs rapidly during infancy. It is 25% the adult size at birth, 50% by 1 year of age, 80% by 3 years of age, and 90% by 7 years of age. This includes growth of glial cells, dendrites, and synaptic connections. This growth is associated with rapid increase in fine motor, gross motor, and language skills of infants and toddlers. These changing competencies impact the type of assessment techniques appropriate for evaluating children of different ages.

Summary of Changes in Vital Signs and Anatomy Through Childhood

Vital signs are useful for assessment but are sometimes difficult to obtain and difficult to interpret. Not only do normal vital signs change significantly with age, but respiratory and heart rates are especially sensitive to adrenaline release because of fear, pain, anxiety, cold, or high activity level. Other anatomic changes in the airway, chest, heart, abdomen, musculoskeletal system, and nervous system occur throughout childhood and require adaptations in assessment techniques.

Infants

Developmental Characteristics

Infants are vulnerable and have a limited number of behaviors (**Figure 2-4**). Infants less than 2 months of age spend most of their time sleeping or eating. They are not yet able to tell the difference between parents and other caregivers or strangers. They need to be kept warm, dry, and fed. They experience the world through their bodies. Being held, cuddled, or rocked soothes the infant. Hearing is also well developed at birth, and calm and reassuring talk is often helpful.

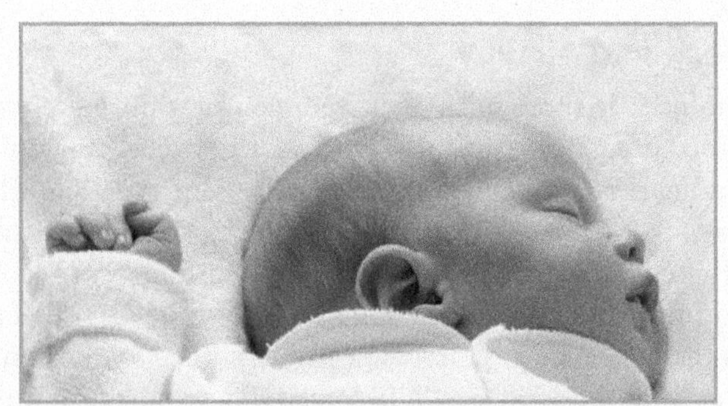

Figure 2-4 Infants are vulnerable creatures, with a limited number of behaviors.

Infants between 2 and 6 months of age are more active, which makes them easier to evaluate. They spend more time awake, they begin to make eye contact, and they recognize caregivers. Healthy infants in this age group have a strong suck, active extremity movement, and a vigorous cry. They may follow a bright light or toy with their eyes, or turn their heads toward a loud sound or the caregiver's voice.

Between the ages of 6 and 12 months, most infants learn to talk or babble, sit unsupported, reach for toys, move objects from one hand to another, and put things in their mouths. At approximately 1 year of age, most infants start to scoot or crawl, pull themselves to a standing position, "cruise" furniture, and possibly start to walk.

At 7–8 months, infants show a clear preference for their parents or caregivers, and by the age of 9–10 months demonstrate stranger anxiety, making separation of the child and caregiver for the purposes of assessment or transport especially problematic. They are most easily comforted by their parent or by a familiar adult. **Table 2-5** summarizes anatomic and physiologic differences that are important in the assessment and care of the infant.

The infant's capacity to interact with the environment is limited, and signs and symptoms of illness are not always easy to appreciate. Because of these factors, always take the caregiver's perception that "something is wrong" seriously. *An infant in the first 3 months of life who is reported to be fussier than usual, feeding poorly, or sleeping excessively, or who has a temperature greater than 38°C (100.4°F) must be seen by a physician.* It is important to find out if there has been a recent history of trauma, how the infant was acting before the event, and if the infant has been healthy since birth. Find out if the infant was born at term and if there were any problems during pregnancy, labor, delivery, or immediately after the birth.

Table 2-5 Anatomic and Physiologic Features of Infants

• Infants are nose breathers for the first several months of life. Obstruction of the nose from secretions, blood, or edema may cause respiratory distress.
• The muscles of the infant's chest wall are not yet developed, and the abdominal muscles are the main muscles used for breathing. "Belly breathing" is normal in infants and may become exaggerated as breathing becomes more rapid.
• Retractions are easily seen in the infant with respiratory distress.
• A faster metabolic rate increases the need for oxygen and nutrients.
• Because of immature temperature regulation and high body surface-to-mass ratio, infants are at risk for heat loss and hypothermia if left undressed.
• The head is large in proportion to the body (**Figure 2-5**) and may be a potential source of significant heat loss.

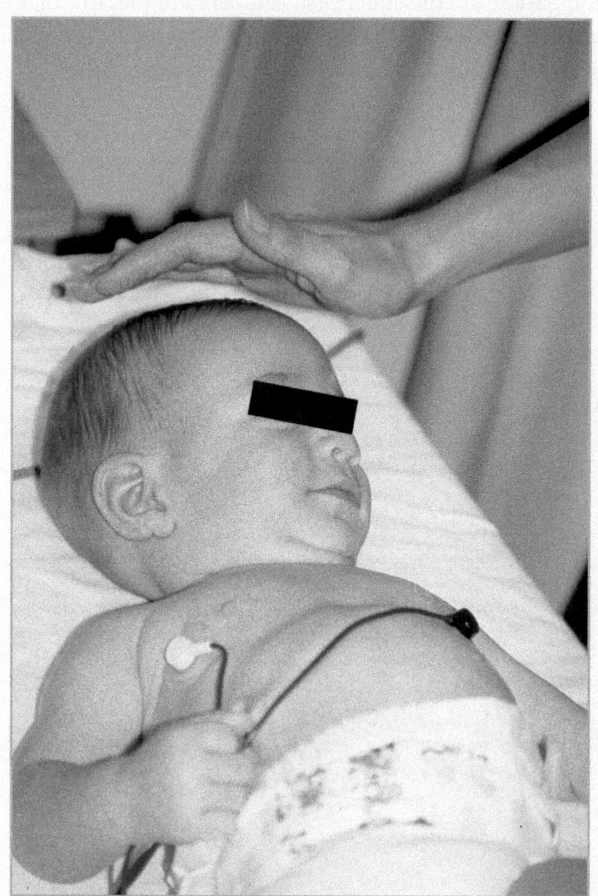

Figure 2-5 The infant's head is disproportionately large compared to older children and adults. The head may be a source of significant heat loss.

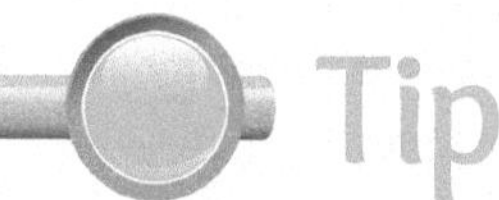

Tip

An infant less than 3 months of age who is reported to be fussier than usual, feeding poorly, or sleeping excessively, or who has a temperature greater than 38°C (100.4°F) must be seen by a physician.

In the first few months of life, excessive irritability or sleeping, fever, and poor feeding may be symptoms of a very serious illness, such as sepsis or congenital heart disease. Apnea is a common chief complaint in the infant. Periods of apnea may be a sign of infection, heart disease, seizure activity, head injury, or a metabolic problem, such as hypoglycemia. As the infant grows older and the behavioral repertoire expands, making the "sick" versus "not sick" decision becomes easier.

Common Conditions in Infants

- Viral syndromes (vomiting and diarrhea)
- Respiratory problems
- Fever
- Ear infections
- Sudden unexpected infant death (SUID)
- Child abuse

Assessment of the Infant

Conduct the assessment of the infant using the following principles:

- Obtain the name of the patient and use it while interacting with the patient.
- Obtain the normal disposition of the patient and compare it to the current behavior being displayed. Any acute change in disposition should be noted and relayed during the transfer-of-care report. Communicate with the infant using a confident but smiling face directed at the infant.
- Have the caregiver hold the infant while the EMS provider completes the assessment. Unless the infant requires a lifesaving intervention, the infant is better assessed in the arms of someone with whom he or she is familiar.
- Observe, auscultate, and palpate in this order to get the most information with the least amount of stress to the infant (**Figure 2-6**).
- Approach the infant slowly and calmly, because loud voices and quick movements may frighten him or her.
- Squat down or sit at "baby level."
- Observe the interaction of the infant with the caregiver. At 7–8 months, infants may begin to show stranger anxiety.

- A comfortable environment is important. An infant who is happily snuggled in a caregiver's arms may become fussy and cry when unwrapped and placed on cold sheets.
- If the infant begins to cry, a pacifier, blanket, or favorite toy may help to calm him or her. Avoid feeding the infant who is seriously ill or injured.
- Perform the assessment based on the infant's activity level. For example, if the infant is calm, get the respiratory rate and auscultate lung sounds at the beginning of the assessment.
- Make nonthreatening physical contact first, such as touching an extremity to assess warmth and capillary refill. Perform the most upsetting parts of the examination last.
- Use a warmed stethoscope and warm hands and handle the infant gently. Avoid doing anything potentially painful or distressing until near completion of the assessment. It is difficult to assess heart and lung sounds or to palpate the abdomen when the infant is crying.
- Consider offering the infant a toy as a distraction.
- In the older infant who may have stranger anxiety, have the caregiver remove the baby's clothing. Remove one item of clothing at a time, and then replace it, if possible, to avoid heat loss and hypothermia.

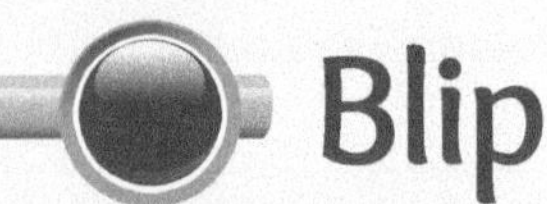

The older infant is fearful of separation and develops stranger anxiety. Approach slowly and assess the infant while he or she is being held by the caregiver.

Toddlers

Developmental Characteristics

Toddlers (ages 1–3 years) experience rapid changes in growth and development. By approximately 18 months of age, the toddlers are able to run, feed themselves, play with toys, and communicate with others. They begin making their own decisions and asserting their independence. The "terrible two" stage actually begins at about 1 year of age and often lasts into the third year. Toddlers are mobile and opinionated, and may be terrified of strangers. They are illogical by nature and are intensely curious but lack a sense of danger. Problem solving is concrete because toddlers cannot reason abstractly. Learning is done by trial and error, with little anticipation of consequences. Toddlers are playful, magical thinkers and are tremendously self-centered. They understand ownership and label things (e.g., toys) as "mine."

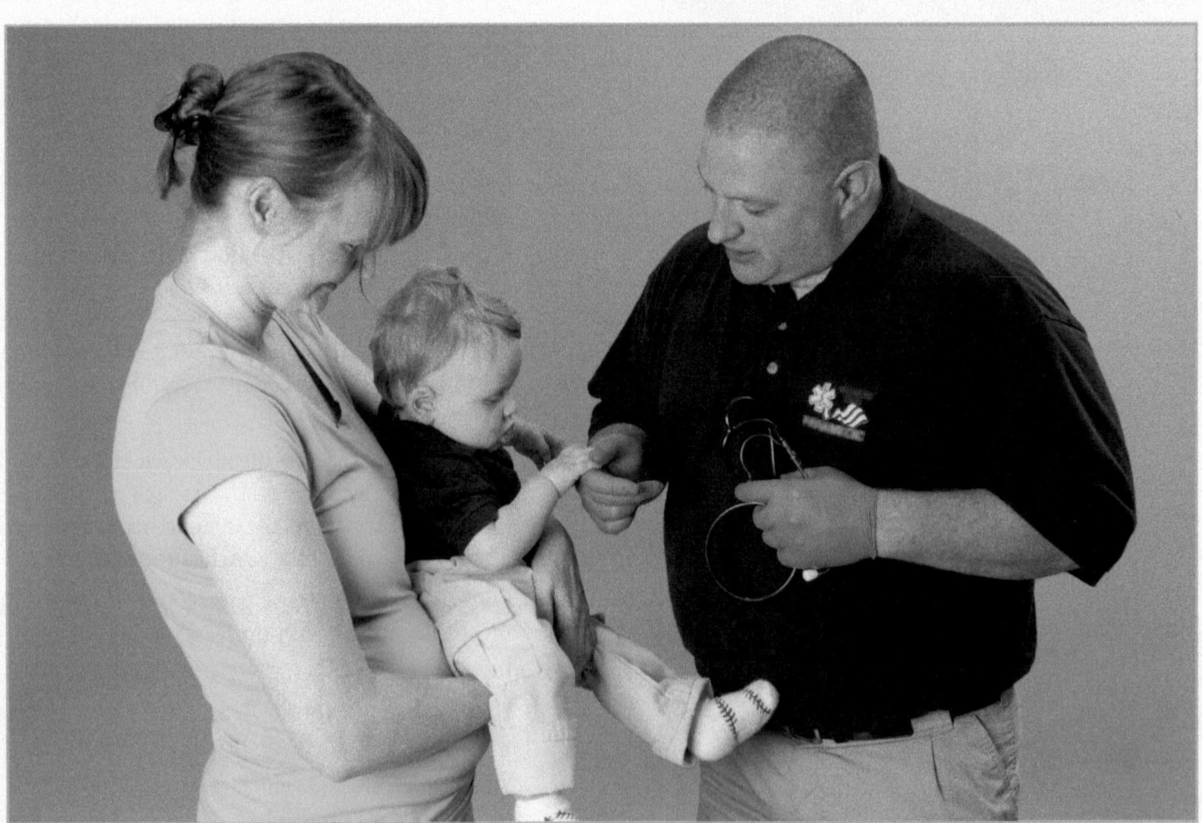

Figure 2-6 Approaching an infant: observe the infant in the caregiver's arms before palpating or auscultating.

Case Study 2

You respond to a call for a 2-year-old who is having respiratory difficulty. On your arrival, you hear a barking cough from the child's room. When you enter, the child is sitting up in bed and starts to cry, and hides behind his mother. With crying, his breathing becomes noisier, and he becomes more anxious. Even though he has pajamas on, you can see suprasternal retractions. His skin is pink. His mother states he was fine today, but suddenly woke up during the night "gasping for air."

1. Is this appropriate behavior for this child?
2. How can you assess this child without making him more upset?

Language capabilities vary widely. Some toddlers utter only single words, whereas others may speak in paragraphs. They often understand what is being said, even if they cannot respond with words. Older toddlers may remember earlier experiences with doctors or nurses, such as vaccinations or stitches, and be fearful about being examined.

The toddler's anatomy and physiology are much like the infant's, notably a large head and use of abdominal muscles to breathe. Thermoregulation is better, and limb muscles are more developed.

Common Ailments in Toddlers

- Viral syndromes (vomiting and diarrhea)
- Respiratory problems
- Febrile seizures
- Ear infections
- Child abuse
- Unintentional ingestions
- Open wounds

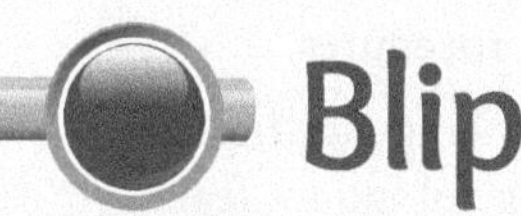

Blip

Do not separate the older infant or toddler from the caregiver.

Assessment of the Toddler

Conduct the assessment of the toddler using the following principles:

- Obtain the name of the patient and use it while interacting with the patient.
- Obtain the normal disposition of the patient and compare it to the current behavior being displayed. Any acute change in disposition should be noted and relayed during the transfer-of-care report.
- Approach the toddler slowly and keep physical contact to a minimum until he or she is familiar with you. Watch the toddler's activity level and behavior as you approach.
- Communicate with the toddler using a confident but friendly tone of voice.
- Sit or squat and use a quiet, soothing voice. Allow the toddler to remain on the caregiver's lap.
- Use play and distraction tools, such as a penlight or teddy bear, to help with the assessment (**Figure 2-7**). Introduce equipment slowly and encourage the toddler to hold it.
- Talk to the toddler, preferably about himself or herself. Admire his or her clothes; ask about pets or recent events. A toddler is the center of his or her universe.
- Give the toddler limited choices, such as "Do you want me to listen to your belly or your heart first?" This provides the toddler with a sense of control.
- Avoid questions that the toddler can answer with "no."
- Use simple, concrete terms. Provide a lot of reassurance and praise.
- Perform the most critical parts of the assessment first, working from toe to head, with the head and neck last.
- Ask for caregiver assistance with the assessment. The toddler is often less upset if the caregiver removes the toddler's clothes or administers oxygen.
- If necessary, ask the caregiver to gently palpate the toddler's extremity to test for pain.
- Do not expect toddlers to sit still and cooperate. Be flexible but thorough.
- In certain situations, the toddler may be extremely difficult to examine. If he or she is alert but resists the examination, determine the need for transport based on history. Use of lights and sirens during transport may increase the toddler's level of fear.

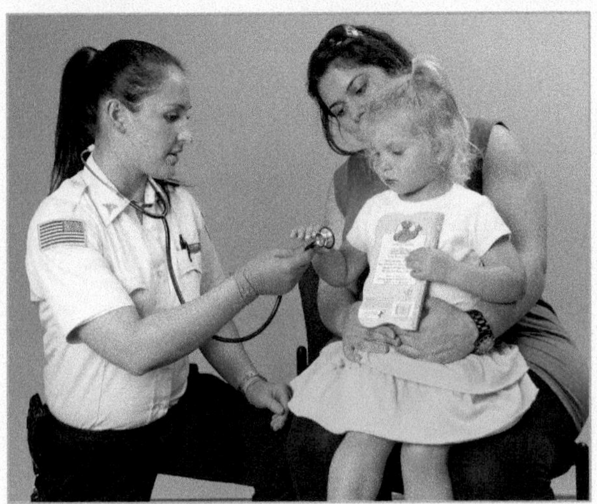

Figure 2-7 Approaching a toddler: offer a toy or distraction tool to help with the assessment.

Preschoolers

Developmental Characteristics

Preschoolers (ages 3–5 years) are creative and illogical thinkers (**Figure 2-8**). They are not always able to distinguish between fantasy and reality, and they have many misconceptions about illness, injury, and bodily functions. For example, a preschooler might think of a cut as "my insides leaking out." If you tell a preschooler you are going to take his or her pulse, they may ask, "Where are you going to take it and will I get it back?" Common fears for this age group include body mutilation, loss of control, death, darkness, and being left alone. Attention span is short. It is always best to maintain honesty about painful procedures. Information should be told as close to the procedure as possible to avoid miscommunication and increased anxiety. Preschool patients can be easily distracted by caregivers or friendly EMS providers. Positively rewarding these patients can help them maintain a good memory about interacting with EMS.

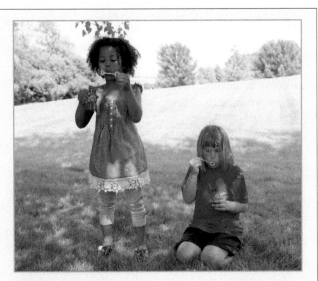

Figure 2-8 Preschoolers are creative and illogical thinkers.

Common Ailments in Preschoolers

- Unintentional ingestions
- Respiratory problems
- Febrile seizures
- Viral syndromes (vomiting and diarrhea)
- Open wounds
- Child abuse

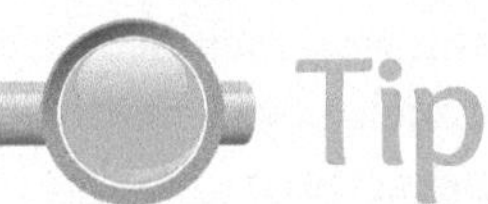

Tip

Preschoolers are creative thinkers who fear loss of control. Explain procedures in simple terms, allow them to handle equipment, and assess from toe to head.

Assessment of the Preschooler

Conduct the assessment of the preschooler using the following principles:

- Obtain the name of the patient, and use it while interacting with the patient.
- Obtain the normal disposition of the patient and compare it to the current behavior being displayed. Any acute change in disposition should be noted and relayed during the transfer-of-care report.
- Use simple terms to explain procedures.
- Choose words carefully, using language that is age-appropriate and that does not induce fear.
- Clarify any apparent misconceptions.
- Use dolls or puppets, if available, to explain what you are doing.
- When appropriate, allow the child to handle equipment (**Figure 2-9**). Allow the patient to help.
- Set limits on behavior—for example, "You can cry or scream, but don't bite or kick."
- Praise good behavior.
- Use games or distraction tools.
- Use dressings or bandages freely.
- Focus and carry out one thing at a time.

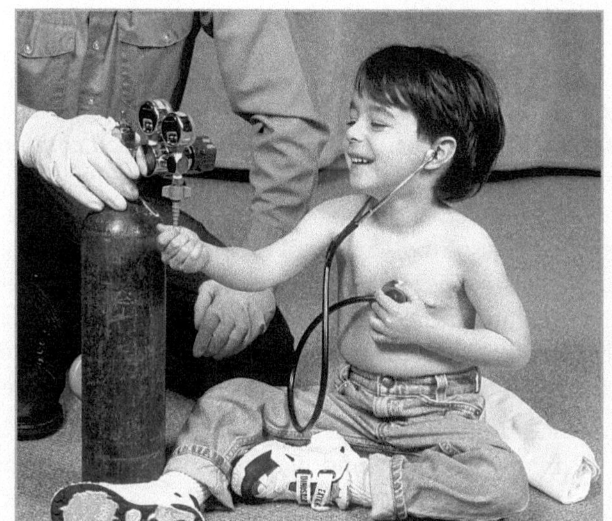

Figure 2-9 When approaching a preschooler, allow the child to handle the equipment.

School-Aged Children

Development Characteristics

School-aged children are talkative, analytical, and able to understand the concept of cause and effect (**Figure 2-10**). They feel a sense of accomplishment as they acquire new skills. Their knowledge of how bodies work may be sketchy, and they have limited ability to gauge the seriousness of a particular illness or injury. With careful choice of words, they can understand simple explanations about their bodies, and they like to be involved in their own care.

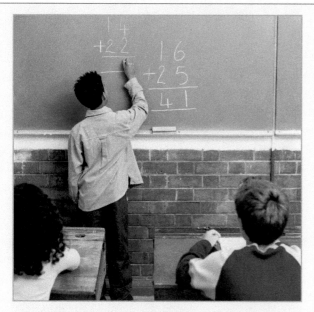

Figure 2-10 School-aged children are talkative, analytical, and able to understand the concept of cause and effect.

Common fears include separation from parents and friends, loss of control, pain, and physical disability. They are often afraid to talk about their feelings and may be unable to put their feelings into words. As they become more mobile and more independent, they begin to take more risks. They live in the present. Belonging and peer group support are important.

The anatomy and physiology of a child is similar to an adult's by about 8 years of age.

Common Conditions in School-Aged Children

- Poisonings/ingestion
- Respiratory problems
- Fractures (e.g., sports injuries)
- Open wounds
- Viral syndromes (vomiting and diarrhea)

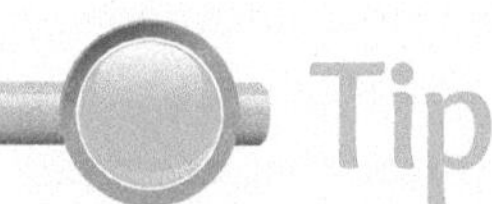

School-aged children fear separation from caregivers, loss of control, pain, and physical disability. Explain procedures and anticipate questions, provide privacy, and conduct assessment from head to toe.

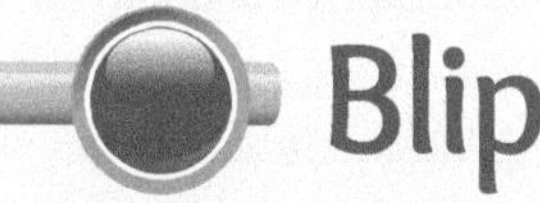

Offering choices that are not real violates the child's sense of trust. Tell the school-aged child what you are going to do, and do it!

Assessment of the School-Aged Child

Conduct the assessment of the school-aged child using the following principles:

- Obtain the name of the patient, and use it while interacting with the patient.
- Obtain the normal disposition of the patient and compare it to the current behavior being displayed. Any acute change in disposition should be noted and relayed during the transfer-of-care report.
- Speak directly to the child, and then include the caregiver. Be careful not to offer too much information.
- Anticipate the child's questions and fears, and discuss them immediately.

- Explain in simple terms what is wrong and how it will affect them. For example, when speaking to a 5-year-old, you may explain, "Your arm bone is broken, but the doctor will be able to fix it good as new. We'll give you some medicine in your arm to help stop it from hurting so much."
- Explain procedures immediately before doing them. Never lie to a child, telling the child that something will not hurt or that you are almost finished if this is not true. Remember that the child may not ask questions, even if he or she has real concerns.
- Ask the older school-aged child if he or she would like to have the caregiver present.
- Provide privacy. Children in this age group are modest. Expose the child for physical assessment as necessary and cover him or her up when done.
- If physical restraint is necessary to complete a procedure or to guarantee the safety of the child or crew, tell the child what is going to happen and then do it.
- Do not negotiate unless the child really has a choice. For example, it is okay to ask the child if he or she would like the intravenous (IV) line in the right or left hand but not to ask if it is okay to start an IV when it must be done.
- Let the child be involved in his or her own care. Children in this age group are afraid of being out of control (**Figure 2-11**).
- Reassure the child that being ill or injured is not a punishment.
- Praise the child for cooperating. Be careful not to be irritable if the child does not cooperate.
- The physical assessment can usually be done in the head-to-toe format.

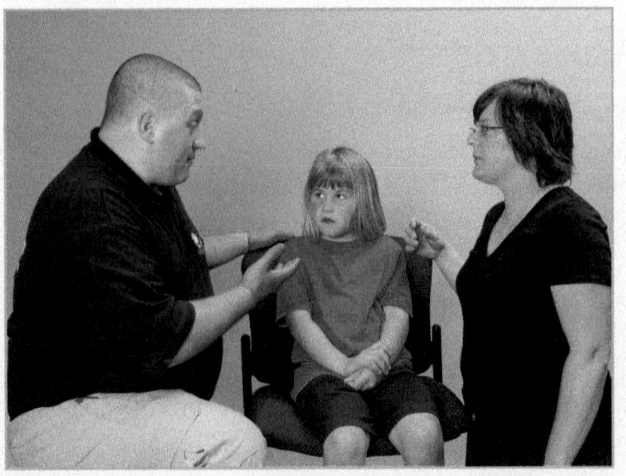

Figure 2-11 Approaching a school-aged child: let the child be involved in his or her own care.

Adolescents

Growth and Development Characteristics

Adolescents sometimes seem to share some characteristics of toddlers: they are very mobile but may lack common sense. However, adolescents are rational, understand cause and effect, and are able to express themselves with words. Adolescence is a time of experimentation and risk-taking behaviors (**Figure 2-12**). Adolescents often believe they are immune to danger, that they are "indestructible." They gradually shift from relying on family to relying on friends for psychological support and social development.

Adolescents struggle with independence, loss of control, body image, sexuality, and peer pressure. Anything that makes them different from their peers causes anxiety. Psychosomatic complaints are common in this age group. They may have mood swings or depression, and when ill or injured may act younger than their age, leaving a scared child in an adult body.

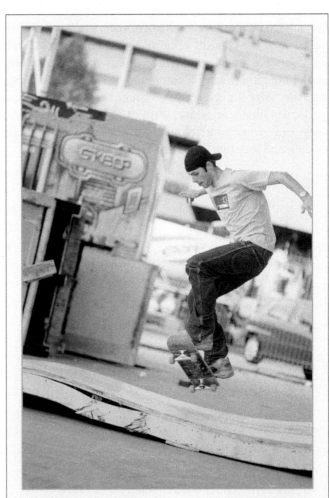

Figure 2-12 Adolescence is a time of experimentation and risk-taking behaviors.

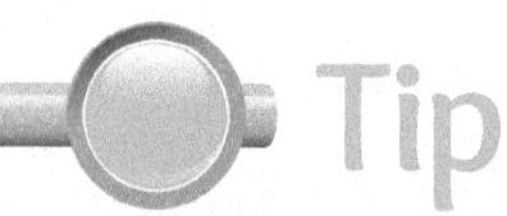

Adolescents struggle with independence, loss of control, body image, sexuality, and peer pressure. Provide concrete information, respect their privacy, and speak to them directly.

Common Conditions in Adolescents

- Poisonings/drug ingestion
- Respiratory problems
- Fractures (e.g., sports injuries)
- Open wounds

Assessment of the Adolescent

Conduct the assessment of the adolescent using the following principles:

- Obtain the name of the patient, and use it while interacting with the patient.
- Obtain the normal disposition of the patient and compare it to the current behavior being displayed. Any acute change in disposition should be noted and relayed during the transfer-of-care report.
- Provide accurate information about the illness or injury, normal body functions, and interventions. Explain what you are doing and why.
- Encourage the patient to ask questions and to be involved in his or her own care.
- Show respect. Speak directly to the adolescent. Do not turn to the caregiver for initial information (**Figure 2-13**).
- Respect the adolescent's modesty, privacy, and confidentiality unless it places him or her at risk.
- Be honest and nonjudgmental.
- Do not be misled by the adolescent's size or make assumptions about his or her comprehension of events. Adolescents may misinterpret the seriousness of the situation. They may also have many fears about permanent injury, disfigurement, or "being different" as a result of the illness or injury. Give adolescents accurate information and anticipate their questions or fears.
- Avoid becoming frustrated or angry if the adolescent does not talk or is uncooperative.
- Enlist the adolescent's friends to help persuade the adolescent to cooperate with the assessment or treatment, if he or she resists.

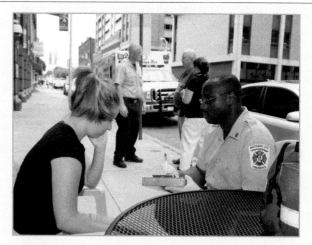

Figure 2-13 When approaching an adolescent, speak to him or her directly.

Children With Special Health Care Needs

Growth and Development Characteristics

When working with children with special health care needs (CSHCN), it is important to consider developmental age, rather than chronologic age. Information about the patient should be obtained from caregivers. If an EMS provider does not fully understand the child's medical or developmental history, it is better to be honest than to feign understanding and potentially place the patient at risk. CSHCN may have any type of chronic condition that affects health, normal growth, or development. This may include physical disability, developmental or learning disability, technologic dependency, or chronic illness. The developmental or learning disability may include mental impairment, difficulties in communication, sensory impairment, or limitations in physical activity. The child who is technology dependent may have a home ventilator, tracheostomy, gastric feeding tube, or long-term IV device. Specific categories of patients and methods of assessment and treatment are discussed in Chapter 11.

The number of children in the community with special needs is growing. Prehospital professionals must be familiar with the conditions and types of technology used in assessing and treating CSHCN. These children may require transport and care for exacerbation of their illness or for an unrelated illness or injury.

Unique aspects related to children with special needs include:

- Baseline vital signs may be outside the age-appropriate values.
- Weight may be significantly higher or lower than expected.

- Standard prehospital quick reference guides may be inaccurate.
- The child may have a limited ability to endure respiratory distress or shock.
- Be alert for a latex allergy.

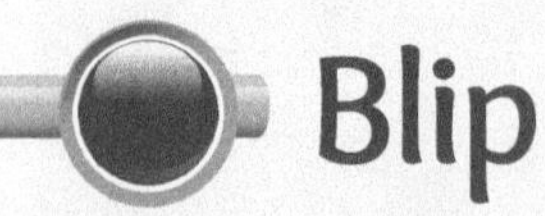

Do not assume that a child with a physical disability is cognitively impaired. Always ask the caregiver to clarify the child's normal level of functioning and interaction.

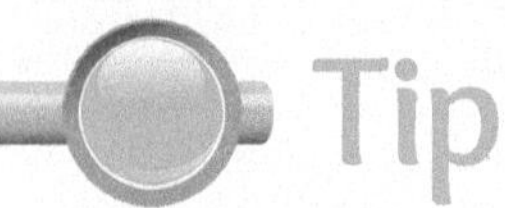

Even if a disabled child cannot talk or interact, show your respect by introducing yourself, explaining what you are doing, and providing verbal reassurance.

Assessment of a CSHCN

Conduct the assessment of the CSHCN using the following principles:

- Obtain the name of the patient, and use it while interacting with the patient.
- Obtain the normal disposition of the patient and compare it to the current behavior being displayed. Any acute change in disposition should be noted and relayed during the transfer-of-care report. Include the impressions of the caregiver in chart documentation. Ask the caregiver what he or she thinks of the child's condition, activity, and behaviors. Find out if the caregiver believes that the child is "not acting right."
- Get a careful history from the caregiver. The caregiver can provide detailed information about the child's medical history, medications, and current complaints. He or she is also aware of how best to approach the child, and of typical responses and behaviors.
- Approach the child with a developmental delay gently and using techniques appropriate to his or her developmental level, not chronologic age. Use language and techniques tailored to the child's cognitive level to communicate.
- Do not assume that the child with a physical disability is mentally impaired (**Figure 2-14**). Ask the caregiver about the child's level of function and interaction with others. To get at baseline functional level you might query, "What would Johnny be doing right now, if he were feeling well?"
- Use polite, professional behavior; acknowledge the caregivers' expertise; and take their concerns seriously. Families of chronically ill children usually have had extensive experience with the medical system. If most of their experiences have been good, they will very likely perceive the prehospital professional as an ally. However, if they have had bad experiences, they may feel a need to be very vigilant in protecting their child and be perceived as difficult or controlling.
- Keep in mind the amount of stress that the caregiver of a CSHCN may be experiencing and be sympathetic. It is often helpful to acknowledge their stress about the care being provided.

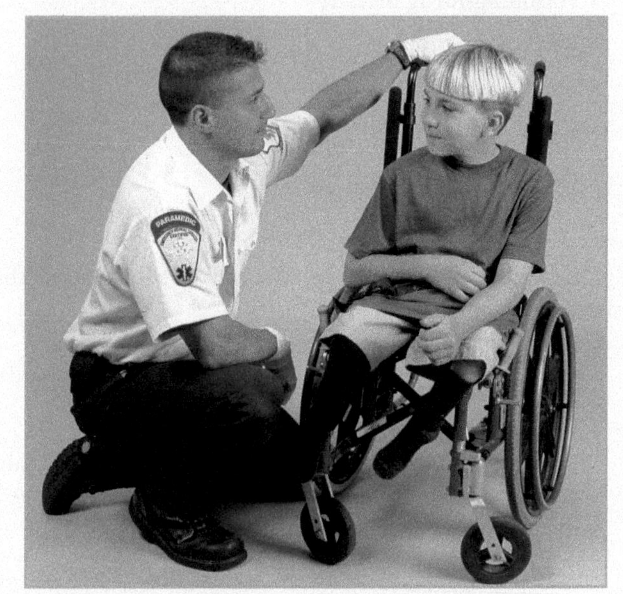

Figure 2-14 Approaching the CSHCN: obtain a thorough history and identify developmentally appropriate approaches that work best with the child.

Tips for the EMS Provider

Infant (0–12 months):

- Be diligent about keeping infants warm and dry to limit hypothermia.
- This is a particularly stressful time for parents adjusting to the eating, sleeping, and crying cycle; sometimes this is complicated by postpartum depression, which can be a risk factor for abuse.
- Persistent crying or irritability can be a symptom of serious illness.
- Although infants sleep a lot, they should rouse easily; inability to rouse a baby should be considered an emergency.
- Head control is limited until closer to 6 months, so when handling a baby, make sure to support the head and neck well.
- By 6 months, babies should make eye contact; lack of eye contact in a sick infant could be a sign

of significant illness, depressed mental status, or delayed development.

- By 6–12 months, infants are at risk for foreign body aspiration and poisoning because of exploration of the environment with their mouths.
- Reduce separation anxiety by keeping the child and parent together during evaluation and involving the parent in the treatment if appropriate.
- Crawling and walking can increase exposure to physical dangers and injuries.

Toddlers (12–36 months):

- Persistent crying or irritability can be a symptom of serious illness.
- Due to a lack of molars, there is an increased risk of choking, because children may not be able to grind up food before swallowing.
- Increased mobility increases exposure to physical dangers and injury.
- Distracting a child with a flashlight or toy may aid in physical examination.
- Allow a child to hold objects of importance to him or her (e.g., blanket).
- Try to make the interaction as positive as possible; painful procedures make for lasting impressions.

Preschool children (3–5 years):

- The rapid increase in language means they understand much of what is said if simple terms are used.
- Respect the patient's modesty and cover him or her up after the physical examination.
- Foreign body airway obstruction risk continues to be high.
- Offer choices to the patient if appropriate (e.g., "Should I listen to your front first or the back?").
- Do not waste time trying to use logic to convince preschoolers; they are concrete thinkers. Avoid frightening or misleading comments.
- Appealing to their magical thinking may allow you to do more (e.g., "This magic mist will help you breathe better [nebulizer].").
- Communicate about procedures as close to doing them as possible.
- Respect modesty.

School-aged children (6–12 years):

- Provide simple explanations for illness and treatments.
- Be honest about painful procedures.
- If possible, provide sense of control by giving choices.
- Respect the patient's modesty.
- Ask about school/sports/activities or interests to allow patients to warm up to you faster.

Adolescents (13–18 years):

- Explain things as clearly and honestly as you would to an adult.
- Give choices when appropriate.
- Respect modesty.
- Be honest about procedures that will cause discomfort.
- Address concerns and fears about the lasting effects of their injuries.
- Adolescence includes hormonal surges, emotions, and peer pressure; there is increased risk for substance abuse, self-endangerment, pregnancy, and dangerous sexual practices.

Summary

Understanding the developmental characteristics for each age group is essential for accurate assessment and treatment of the child in the out-of-hospital environment. Good field care requires good communication with the child and family. The family may include a large number of people, all of whom become "patients." CSHCN pose additional challenges in assessment, but their caregivers can be a great asset in guiding field evaluation and management.

Every call experience offers the ability for an EMS provider to learn something. With pediatric patients, the opportunities are larger than with adults. Postcall self-evaluation and call critique can offer providers an opportunity to identify ways to improve for the next pediatric patient interaction.

Case Study 3

You respond to the scene of a bike versus automobile crash. The rider is a 14-year-old boy, who is now walking around the scene. He was wearing a helmet and denies any loss of consciousness. His only complaints are that his wrist hurts, the front wheel of his bike is bent, and he will be late to meet his friends. He does not want to be examined, definitely does not want to go to the hospital, and starts to leave the scene as you approach him.

1. Is this teenager's reaction normal?
2. What techniques can help you adequately assess his injuries?

CASE STUDY ANSWERS

Case Study 1 — page 32

Even though the mother is frantic, it is important to get additional history: Was the infant full-term? Did she have any problems with delivery or after birth? Has she had feeding problems or vomiting in the past? Any fever or diarrhea?

Infants in the first few months of life have a limited range of behaviors, so anything out of the ordinary in the child's feeding, sleeping, or basic activity level is concerning for serious underlying illness or injury. Any infant who reportedly had an apneic episode that resulted in color change (pallor, cyanosis) or unresponsiveness may have had an apparent life-threatening event (ALTE). Causes of ALTE include sepsis, congenital heart disease, metabolic abnormalities, seizures, gastroesophageal reflux, and brain injury. These diagnoses are impossible to establish in the out-of-hospital setting and require emergency department evaluation.

Reassuring the mother is important, but this baby may be critically ill, and requires rapid assessment and transport. Although an infant's extremities may be mottled because of cold, mottling of the trunk is an extremely worrisome sign, reflecting poor perfusion. The possibility of hypovolemic shock is supported by the baby's cool extremities and history of vomiting. Furthermore, although infants can develop abdominal distention because of crying and swallowing air, abdominal distention in association with vomiting and signs of shock (abnormal appearance and abnormal circulation to skin) suggest serious pathology, such as intestinal obstruction.

Move the baby quickly into the ambulance, explaining what you are doing and why to the mother. If local protocol permits, allow the mother to ride with you to the hospital. Treatment of this infant includes administration of oxygen by a face mask and rapid transport to an emergency department. Prevention of heat loss by swaddling the baby and applying a hat is important, because hypothermia is a risk for a small infant. Consider vascular access en route, with a bolus of 20 mL/kg of crystalloid fluid.

Case Study 2 — page 39

Toddlers are often fearful of strangers, so enlisting the help of parents or caregivers makes patient assessment much easier. Allow the child to remain with the parent. Sit on the bed or crouch down to the child's eye level, and use a calm soothing voice. You can use distractions, such as a penlight, or ask about a stuffed animal on the bed, to gain the child's attention and to evaluate interactivity. Ask the parent to remove the child's pajamas and observe the work of breathing, including suprasternal, subcostal, or intercostal retractions, and respiratory rate. Although your main concern is the child's respiratory status, you may have to perform other portions of the hands-on examination, such as touching or tickling the child's toes before you get to the chest. When listening to breath sounds, warm the stethoscope beforehand, and explain what you are doing. If the child resists, you may be able to listen to a stuffed animal first, and allow the child to do the same, before resuming your examination.

Your assessment reveals the child's respiratory rate is 32 breaths/min and heart rate is 128 beats/min. You decide to give the child oxygen, but he refuses to keep the oxygen mask in place even with his mother's help, a response you recognize is typical of a toddler who is not seriously ill. For transport to the hospital, you secure the child on the stretcher, allowing his mother to accompany you in the ambulance, and direct blow-by oxygen in his direction.

Case Study 3 — page 45

This teenager is asserting his independence but is not legally able to give consent or refuse care, unless he is emancipated. He may not realize the risks of occult injury. Show respect, be honest and nonjudgmental, and speak directly to him. Explain why it is important to check him for potentially serious injuries, and offer him the privacy of the ambulance to conduct the examination. If he still refuses care, attempt to contact his parents or caregivers or enlist the assistance of police.

SUGGESTED READINGS

Textbooks

American Academy of Pediatrics, American College of Emergency Physicians. *APLS: The Pediatric Emergency Medicine Resource*. 5th ed. Burlington, MA: Jones & Bartlett Learning; 2012.

Behrman R, Kliegman R, Jenson H. *Nelson Textbook of Pediatrics*. 17th ed. Philadelphia, PA: Saunders; 2004.

Chameides L, Samson RA, Schexnayder SM, Hazinski MF. *PALS Provider Manual*. American Heart Association; 2011.

Marx JA, Hockberger RS, Walls RM. *Rosen's Emergency Medicine Concepts and Clinical Practice*. 7th ed. Philadelphia, PA: Mosby; 2009.

Tittinalli J. *Emergency Medicine: A Comprehensive Study Guide*. 7th ed. Columbus, OH: McGraw Hill; 2011.

Zitelli B, Davis H, McIntire S, Nowalk AJ. *Zitelli and Davis' Atlas of Pediatric Physical Diagnosis*. 6th ed. Philadelphia, PA: Elsevier; 2012.

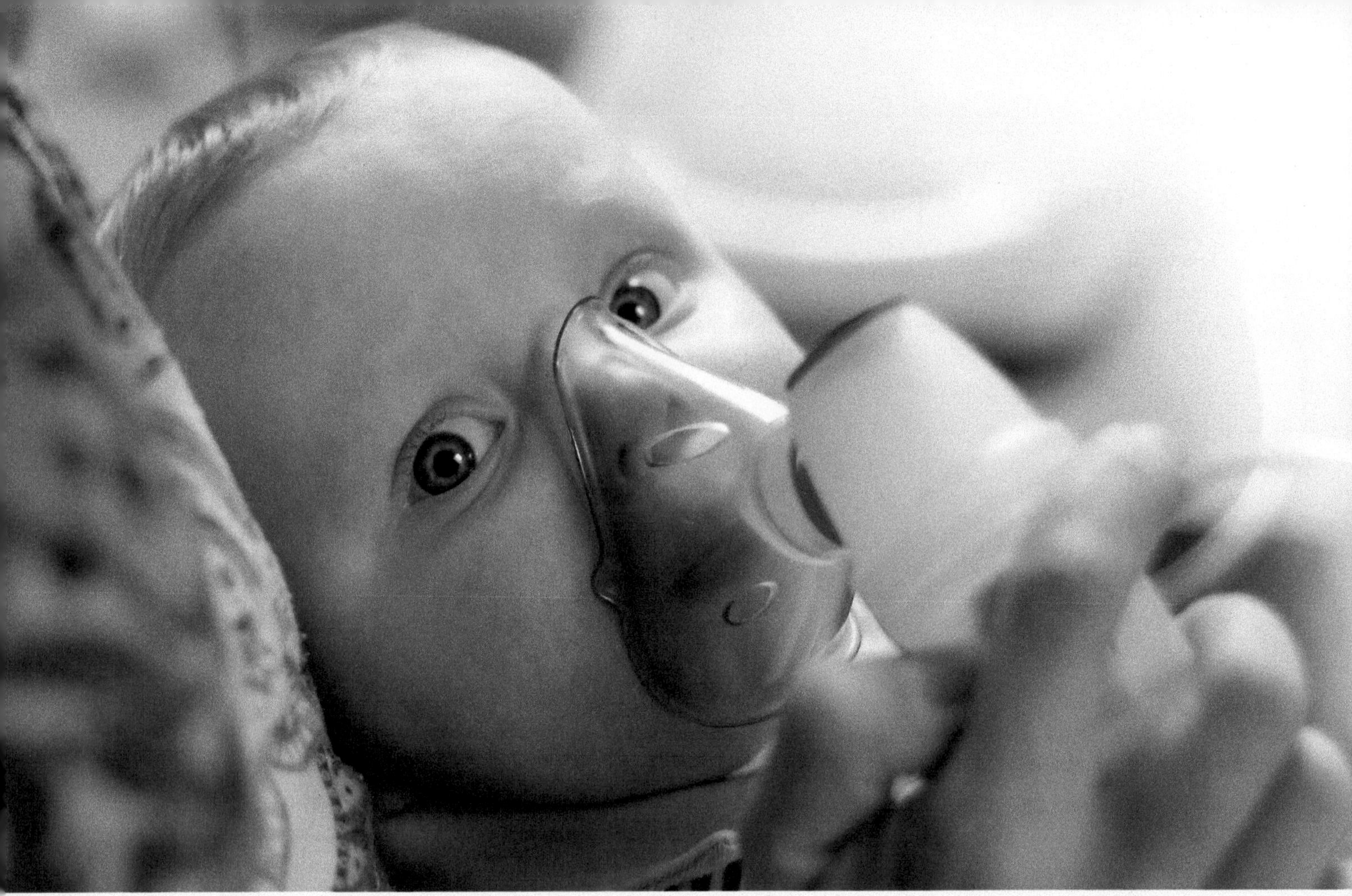

Learning Objectives

1. Describe how to assess airway and breathing, including interpreting information from the Pediatric Assessment Triangle and the ABCDEs.
2. Differentiate between respiratory distress, respiratory failure, and respiratory arrest based on history, physical examination, and physiologic monitoring.
3. Define the physiologic information provided by pulse oximetry and capnometry, recognize situations in which each should be used, and recognize appropriate management responses to abnormal measurements.
4. Outline a general treatment strategy, going from the least to the most invasive, for children with respiratory compromise.
5. Contrast the key signs, symptoms, and management of upper airway obstruction versus lower airway obstruction.
6. Discuss possible complications of assisted ventilation, and outline strategies to identify and correct these complications.

Respiratory Emergencies

Chapter 3

Introduction

Respiratory disease is the most frequent pediatric prehospital medical problem. Of all conditions causing respiratory disease in children, asthma is the most common. However, many other illnesses, foreign bodies, and trauma cause respiratory problems in children. Good assessment and early intervention for pediatric respiratory problems can avert serious illness and preventable death, and may shorten treatment time in the emergency department (ED).

Focusing on certain key physical signs and symptoms allows the prehospital professional to rapidly assess the effectiveness of gas exchange in the airways and lung alveoli. Using the Pediatric Assessment Triangle (PAT) is an important first step in determining the severity of disease, localizing the physiologic problem, and beginning treatment. Appearance reflects the overall state of ventilation and oxygenation. Increased work of breathing indicates either airway obstruction at some level or a problem in gas exchange at the alveolar level; it is often an early sign of hypoxia or hypercapnia. Fading respiratory effort is a sign of severe hypoxia or hypercapnia. Cyanosis of the skin or mucous membranes also indicates severe hypoxia.

In addition to the PAT, the primary assessment includes counting the respiratory rate; appropriately exposing all pediatric patients to ascertain work of breathing as part of the examination (this can be done in a nonthreatening manner by asking the parent or caregiver to lift the child's shirt or clothing to reveal retractions); performing hands-on chest auscultation; evaluating the heart rate; and obtaining pulse oximetry. This assessment not only provides a picture of respiratory function, but also helps prioritize general and specific treatments, and interventions and timing of transport.

Respiratory Distress and Failure

Respiratory distress, failure, and arrest are three points on a continuum of physiologic response to different types of hypoxic stress. Causes of hypoxic stress are variable and include asthma, bronchiolitis, croup, pneumonia, and chest wall injury. Although these three points in the continuum (respiratory distress, failure, and arrest) have different clinical characteristics in theory, in reality they are part of a spectrum that is not black or white. **Respiratory distress** is an abnormal physiologic condition identified by increased work of breathing. Increased respiratory rate; supraclavicular, suprasternal, intercostal, or subcostal retractions; use of accessory muscles; and nasal flaring are signs that alone or together indicate increased work of breathing. These physical signs represent the patient's attempt to make up for decreased gas exchange in the lungs and airways and to maintain oxygenation and ventilation. The brain is still getting enough oxygen, and the child's appearance is relatively normal.

Case Study 1

You are dispatched to the home of a 22-month-old boy who is having difficulty breathing. His mother says that for 2 days he has had a slight fever and has been "wheezing," especially when he cries or becomes more active. He suddenly awoke tonight acutely short of breath and now is making a very loud noise each time he breathes in. The child has no prior history of wheezing or respiratory illness.

The child is sitting on his mother's lap looking anxious, but makes eye contact and cries weakly when you approach. He makes loud, harsh noises with each inspiration. His color is pink, but he has marked supraclavicular and suprasternal retractions and nasal flaring. Respiratory rate is 42 breaths/min and the heart rate is 180 beats/min. The blood pressure is not obtained. His skin is warm, and he has strong pulses and normal capillary refill time. He has good air movement with loud, harsh breath sounds heard on each inspiration. Lower airway sounds are obscured by these loud inspiratory noises.

1. How sick is this child?
2. Are this child's findings more likely to be caused by upper airway or lower airway obstruction, and how will you manage him in the field?

Respiratory failure occurs when the infant or child exhausts his or her energy reserves or can no longer maintain oxygenation and ventilation. When the effects of the respiratory insult begin to overwhelm the child's ability to respond, he or she begins to decompensate. Respiratory failure may occur when chest wall muscles get tired after a long period of increased work of breathing (e.g., a child with severe asthma who is very tight and has been working hard to breathe for several hours); when the insult is severe and progressive (e.g., fulminant pneumonia); or when there is a failure of central respiratory drive (e.g., a child with a severe closed-head injury). An abnormal appearance (agitation or lethargy) or cyanosis in a child with an increased work of breathing indicates respiratory failure. An abnormally low respiratory rate and decreased respiratory effort, usually with bradycardia, also indicates respiratory failure. Respiratory failure must be treated immediately to restore good oxygenation and ventilation, and to prevent respiratory arrest.

Signs of failure are decreased level of consciousness, slow to agonal respirations, grunting, decreasing pulse oximetry, and bradycardia or inappropriate slowing of the heart rate.

Respiratory arrest means absence of effective breathing. If ventilation and oxygenation are not immediately supported, respiratory arrest rapidly progresses to full cardiopulmonary arrest. Most episodes of cardiac arrest in pediatric patients begin as respiratory arrest. Intervening at this point often prevents cardiac arrest. Early intervention in respiratory failure and arrest have a far better chance of producing neurologically intact survivors than treatment of cardiac arrest, which has an extremely low probability of survival.

Prearrival Preparation

Based on dispatch information and while en route to the scene, prepare mentally for management of respiratory distress and failure by reviewing the appropriate assessment techniques and treatment options for the child's age. This includes recalling an age-based approach to assessment as outlined in Chapter 1, equipment needs, and the likely treatment and transport options. Also, anticipate the determinants of whether to stay on scene and treat or to manage the airway and transport immediately to the ED.

Scene Size-Up

Be sure the scene is safe, and there are no obvious illness or injury threats. Assess the environment for foreign body risks, medications, noxious gases, fumes, chemicals, or smoke. Document scene conditions if environmental factors may be contributing to anticipated respiratory problems. If indicated, make sure to wear personal protective equipment (PPE), question how many patients are in the home or facility, determine if additional resources are needed, and attempt to determine mechanism of injury (MOI), nature of illness (NOI), and the need for cervical spine precautions or immobilization.

General Assessment: The PAT

Evaluating the Presenting Complaint

Find out the nature of the presenting complaint by asking several directed questions, as suggested in **Table 3-1**. After

Table 3-1 Key Questions About the Presenting Complaint

Key Question	Possible Medical Problem
Has your child ever had this kind of problem before?	Asthma, chronic lung disease
Is this the first time that your child has had trouble breathing?	Asthma, chronic lung disease
Is your child taking any medications?	Asthma, chronic lung disease, congenital heart disease
Has your child had a fever?	Pneumonia, bronchiolitis, croup
Did your child suddenly start coughing/choking/gagging?	Foreign body aspiration or ingestion
Has your child had an injury to his or her chest?	Pulmonary contusion, pneumothorax

the primary assessment, in patients with mild distress, there is time to get a more complete SAMPLE history (see Table 3-9) on scene as part of the focused history. If the child is in respiratory failure, do this later, while en route to the ED.

Assessment of Respiratory Status

Using the PAT

Begin the assessment with the PAT, as discussed in the chapter on patient assessment. Carefully evaluate appearance, work of breathing, and skin circulation. The PAT helps establish how sick the child is, the type of physiologic abnormality (respiratory distress or respiratory failure), the level of obstruction if present (upper or lower airway), and the urgency for treatment. Table 1-2 in Chapter 1 lists physical features in the child to help make these clinical distinctions by simple observation and listening.

Appearance

Appearance reflects the adequacy of oxygenation and ventilation in a child with difficulty breathing. If the child is compensating effectively for the respiratory insult, the appearance is fairly normal, and the TICLS mnemonic (see Table 1-1 in Chapter 1) shows an interactive child with good tone and color, and normal vocalizations, who looks or gazes at someone. If the child is not compensating, the appearance is abnormal, and the child has abnormal findings in the TICLS mnemonic because his or her brain is impaired from hypoxia or hypercapnia. Abnormal appearance is a spectrum of clinical states, so that the severity of respiratory failure determines how abnormal the child appears. Also, assessing appearance guides urgency of basic life support (BLS) versus advanced life support (ALS) treatment. Even if ALS procedures are required, start with BLS procedures while preparing to implement ALS procedures based on local protocol.

ALS

Example 1: A 3-year-old child who has stridor and retractions, but is running around the room and has a normal appearance, requires general noninvasive treatment and transport. The child is compensating effectively and is only in respiratory distress.

Example 2: An 8-year-old child who is agitated or inconsolable, with wheezing and increased work of breathing, has an abnormal appearance, and is probably hypoxic. The child is beginning to decompensate and is in early respiratory failure. In addition to general noninvasive treatment, this child requires immediate specific ALS treatment on scene with a **bronchodilator**, then rapid transport to an ED.

Example 3: A 3-year-old child who has been working hard to breathe for hours and is now sleepy or poorly responsive has an abnormal appearance. The altered mental status is the result of severe hypoxia or hypercapnia, reflecting late respiratory failure, and impending respiratory arrest. These patients require immediate **assisted ventilations** with airway adjuncts, such as **oropharyngeal airway (OPA)** or **nasopharyngeal airway (NPA)** using a bag-mask device on scene and possibly advanced airway procedures. This may include endotracheal intubation, supraglottic airways, or dual lumen airway.

Work of Breathing

To assess for adequate breathing, sometimes the patient needs to be appropriately exposed. Attempt to visualize the thorax in a nonthreatening manner while keeping the child warm. Look for signs of increased work of breathing:

1. Abnormal positioning (tripoding, "sniffing" position)
2. Abnormal airway sounds (e.g., snoring, stridor, wheezing, or grunting)
3. Retractions (or head bobbing in infants)
4. Nasal flaring

The significance of each of these findings is discussed in Chapter 1. These indicators of breathing effort help to identify the anatomic location of the problem (upper airway, lower airway, or lung alveoli), the severity of the physiologic dysfunction (respiratory distress, failure, or arrest), and the urgency for treatment (immediate resuscitation, general treatment only on scene with specific treatment en route, general and specific treatment on scene). In addition to abnormal airway sounds (stridor, wheezing, and grunting), retractions and the use of accessory muscles may help localize the site of airway problems. Use of the accessory muscles of the neck and suprasternal and supraclavicular retractions occurs more often with upper airway obstruction. Predominant subcostal and intercostal retractions and the use of abdominal muscles tend to localize an obstructive process to the lower airways. It is hard to recognize some of these signs when the child has on clothing; if needed, appropriately remove clothing to ascertain these other clinical signs.

Circulation to Skin

Finally, evaluate skin color. Cyanosis is an ominous sign, signaling profound hypoxia and the need for assisted ventilation. However, a child may have severe hypoxia without an obvious change in skin color. Pulse oximetry is very helpful; use it whenever available in a child with respiratory distress or respiratory failure.

Primary Assessment: The ABCDEs

After the PAT, perform the second portion of the primary assessment, the hands-on ABCDEs. There are three parts to the "B" or breathing evaluation:

1. Respiratory rate
2. Auscultation for air movement and abnormal breath sounds
3. Pulse oximetry

Respiratory Rate

In the noncritical patient, determine respiratory rate by sitting the child in the caregiver's lap and exposing the patient's chest. Count the rise and fall of the abdomen over 30 seconds, and then double that number. Normal respiratory rates vary in children of different ages (see Table 1-4 in Chapter 1). Always think about respiratory rates in the context of the PAT and the overall clinical assessment. Respiratory rate may be affected by level of activity, fever, anxiety, and metabolic state.

A respiratory rate of greater than 60 breaths/min is abnormal in a child of any age and should be a signal for careful evaluation for other signs of respiratory or circulatory problems. Even more dangerous is a rate that is too slow for age. A respiratory rate of less than 20 breaths/min in a sick child younger than 6 years of age, or a rate of less than 12 breaths/min in a sick child younger than 15 years of age may be a sign of respiratory failure, and immediate intervention is required.

Auscultation for Air Movement and Abnormal Breath Sounds

Assess air movement by placing the stethoscope and listening for the amount of air movement with each breath (**Figure 3-1**). Poor air movement may exist in children with respiratory problems for many reasons, as outlined in **Table 3-2**.

Table 3-2 Causes of Poor Air Movement in Children

Functional Problem	Possible Causes
Obstruction of airway	Asthma, bronchiolitis, croup, foreign body
Restriction of chest wall movement	Chest wall injury, severe **scoliosis** or kyphosis
Chest wall muscle fatigue	Prolonged increased work of breathing, muscular dystrophy
Decreased central respiratory drive	Head injury, intoxication
Chest injury	Rib fractures, pulmonary contusion, pneumothorax

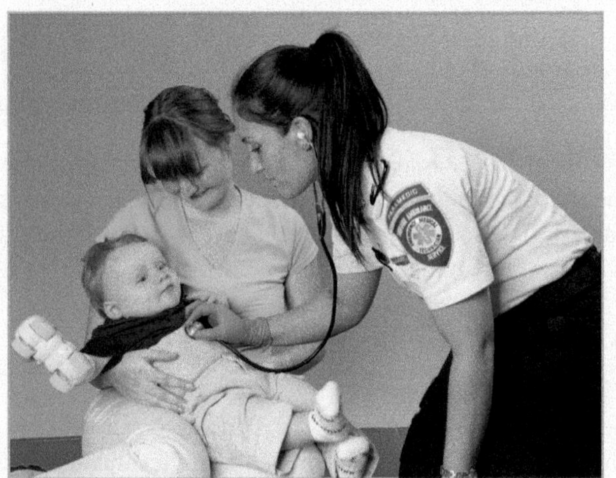

Figure 3-1 Assess air movement by placing the stethoscope and listening for the amount of movement with each breath.

Assessing air movement, or the volume of air exchanged with each breath, allows clinical estimation of **tidal volume**. Tidal volume is one of two factors that determine minute ventilation: the volume of air exchanged per minute. **Minute ventilation** is the basis for gas exchange in the lungs.

$$\text{Minute Ventilation} = \text{Tidal Volume} \times \text{Respiratory Rate}$$

This equation shows the connection between tidal volume and respiratory rate. A child may not have enough gas exchange if tidal volume is low, even with a normal or fast respiratory rate. Also, a normal or increased tidal volume does not mean there is enough gas exchange if the respiratory rate is too slow.

While listening for air movement, also listen for abnormal breath sounds. Table 1-5 in Chapter 1 summarizes the types and causes of abnormal breath sounds. Stridor, which is usually inspiratory in nature at least initially, is indicative of upper airway obstruction, whereas crackles and wheezes are associated with lower airway processes.

Pulse Oximetry

Pulse oximetry is a useful tool for detecting and measuring hypoxia. **Figure 3-2** illustrates possible sites for placement of the oximetry probe. **Pulse Oximetry, Procedure 9**, explains how to use a pulse oximeter. The pulse oximeter emits red light of two different wavelengths. These are absorbed differently by saturated and desaturated hemoglobin. The sensor on the pulse oximeter measures the transmission of the two wavelengths of red light, and a computer in the machine then determines the percentage of hemoglobin saturated with oxygen. When properly applied, *and if there is a good arterial tracing*, a reading of 95% or higher means normal blood oxygen saturation. *A value of 94% or less on room air is abnormal and is a signal to give supplemental oxygen.* A reading of less than 90%, with the patient on 100% oxygen, usually indicates respiratory failure in a previously healthy individual.

Patients with uncorrected cyanotic heart disease and some patients with chronic respiratory problems (e.g., cystic fibrosis) have a low oxygen saturation at baseline. In this type of patient, obtain the baseline value from the caregiver and attempt to provide enough oxygen to get the child to his or her baseline pulse oximetry level. Providing more oxygen than is needed to achieve the baseline pulse oximetry level may actually suppress ventilation by reducing the child's hypoxic drive to breathe. In normal children, hypercapnia or increased carbon dioxide pressure stimulates the drive to breathe, but in some children with chronic respiratory disease, hypercapnia is a constant state. In such cases, hypoxia becomes the stimulus to breathe. Overtreating hypoxia disturbs this regulatory function, and may paradoxically decrease drive to breathe and make the child worse. The preferred saturation rate is between 94% and 99%.

One must be careful not to overinterpret low oxygen saturation. Pulse oximetry is an adjunct to physical assessment. Falsely low readings are common with pulse oximetry. Movement by the child, cold extremities or a cold ambient temperature, and interference by light in the child's surroundings all may cause inaccurate pulse oximetry readings. Check probe placement, the quality of the tracing, and the child's clinical state before treating. Inaccurate readings or the inability to obtain a reading may also occur in children in shock with poor perfusion. However, give these children oxygen even if they do not have respiratory distress and regardless of pulse oximeter readings. It is also important not to underinterpret a normal pulse oximetry reading. *Sometimes an apparently normal oxygen saturation above 94% may be present in a child with significant respiratory distress, who is compensating by increased work of breathing.* Always use pulse oximetry in combination with physical assessment to ensure accurate interpretation of adequacy of breathing.

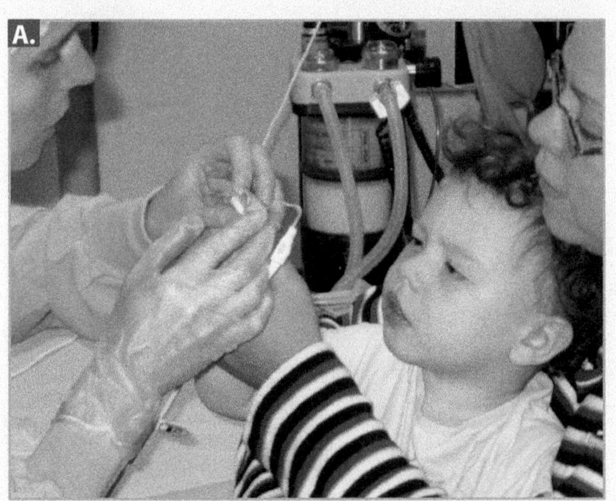

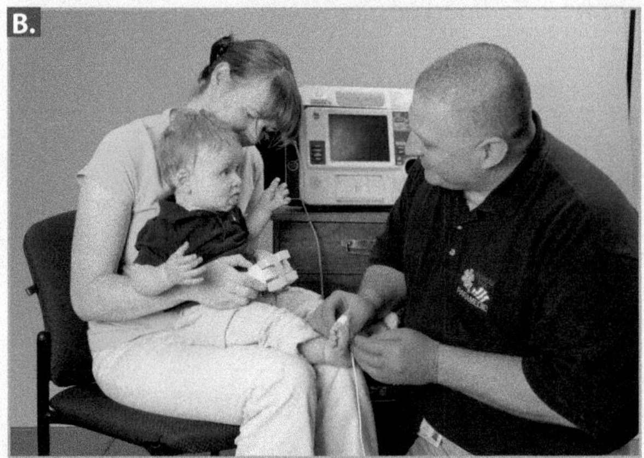

Figure 3-2 Possible sites for placement of the oximetry probe.

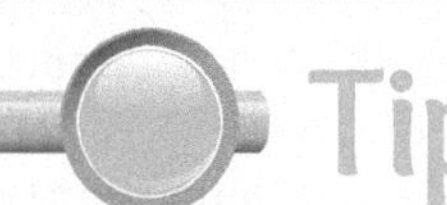

Remember, the pulse oximeter does not detect the adequacy of ventilation. A patient who is receiving supplemental oxygen may have a normal pulse oximeter reading but not have adequate ventilation. **Capnometry**, which quantitatively measures exhaled carbon dioxide, monitors carbon dioxide levels and adequacy of ventilation.

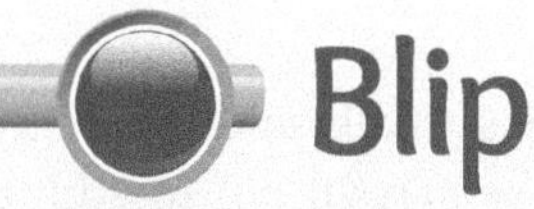

Be careful not to overinterpret low oxygen saturation. Match with the physical findings.

General Noninvasive Treatment

For every child in respiratory distress, begin general noninvasive treatment. *The general noninvasive treatment of every noncritical patient is the same—allow patient to assume a position of comfort and supply oxygen, if tolerated* (**Figure 3-3**). This is the only treatment for patients in respiratory distress without upper or lower airway obstruction. If the child is in respiratory failure or arrest, perform assisted ventilation immediately with airway adjuncts and consider advanced airways based on local protocols.

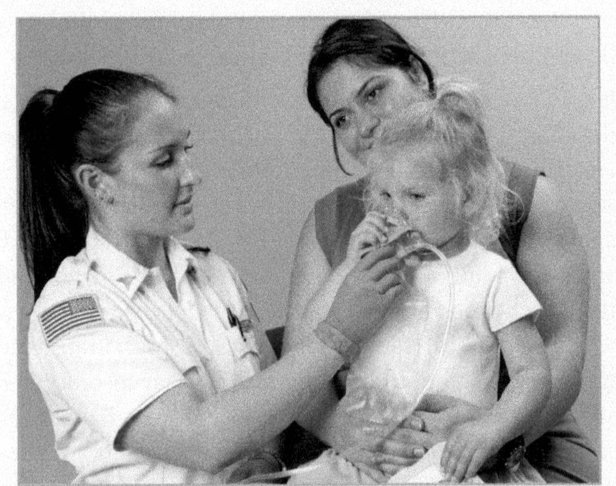

Figure 3-3 Always keep a child with respiratory distress in his or her position of comfort.

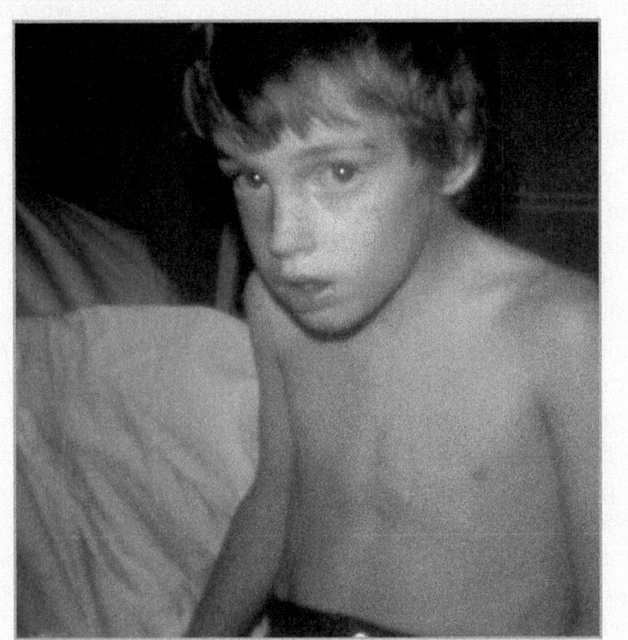

Figure 3-4 Sniffing position.

Positioning

A child in respiratory distress naturally moves into the position that provides the best air exchange, called the "position of comfort." For example, a child with severe upper airway obstruction may get into the "sniffing position" to straighten the airway and open the air passages (**Figure 3-4**). A child with severe lower airway obstruction may voluntarily take the "tripod" posture (sitting up and leaning forward on outstretched arms) to help accessory muscles (**Figure 3-5**). Infants and toddlers may be most comfortable in their caregiver's arms or lap. Do not move a child from his or her position of comfort. This might worsen the respiratory distress. In the ambulance, keep the dyspneic child safely restrained in an upright position, unless the child requires assisted ventilations or has other physiologic problems that require treatment in a supine position.

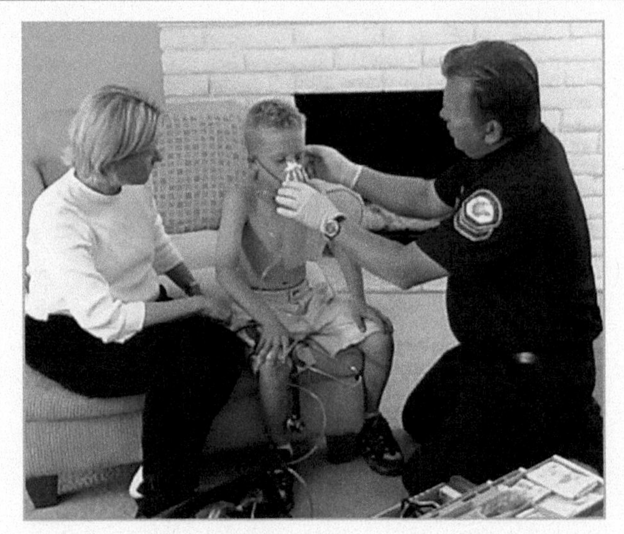

Figure 3-5 Tripod position.

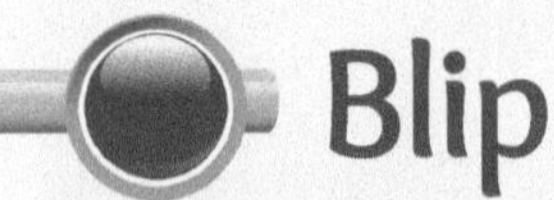

Blip

Do not move a child from his or her position of comfort.

Oxygen

Treatment with high-flow oxygen is usually safe. If the child has chronic respiratory illness, be careful not to administer too much oxygen. The prehospital professional must weigh the possible benefits of giving oxygen against the risks of agitating the child and worsening the respiratory distress. This is a special concern in a child with an unstable airway. Oxygen toxicity in newborns, especially premature newborns, is occasionally an issue in the prehospital setting. Newborns with respiratory distress, cyanosis, or other signs of respiratory disease require high-flow, 100%

oxygen. Newborns without signs of hypoxia no longer require 100% oxygen as explained in Chapter 10.

Most children accept oxygen therapy, especially if the prehospital professional is creative in the approach. This often means getting the help of the caregiver. If a child resists the use of a mask or nasal cannula, have the caregiver give blow-by oxygen from the end of the oxygen tubing or from tubing inserted into a cup (**Figure 3-6**).

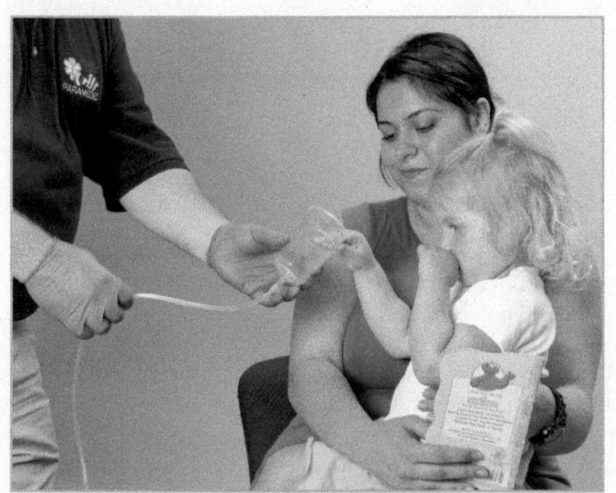

Figure 3-6 If the child resists application of a mask or nasal cannula, administer oxygen through a nonthreatening object, such as a cup.

Oxygen Delivery

Give oxygen to any child with clinical signs of cardiopulmonary distress or failure, or with a history suggesting possible abnormalities in gas exchange. The delivery method should provide the concentration of oxygen most appropriate for the child's condition, degree of cooperation, respiratory effort, and age. For a step-by-step explanation of this procedure, see **Oxygen Delivery, Procedure 3**.

Summary of General and Initial Respiratory Assessment and General Noninvasive Treatment

The PAT is a good tool for determining the effectiveness of gas exchange, based on observation of appearance and work of breathing. If the PAT suggests respiratory distress, begin general noninvasive treatment with oxygen and keep the child in his or her position of comfort. The PAT also identifies the critical child in respiratory failure who requires immediate assisted ventilation. Obtaining respiratory rate, listening for air movement, and determining oxygen saturation by pulse oximetry work in concert with the PAT. The primary assessment should allow an evaluation of severity and urgency for treatment and should establish if specific treatment for upper or lower airway obstruction is indicated.

Specific Treatment for Respiratory Distress

After completing the primary assessment, consider specific treatment. The PAT and ABCDE assessment help determine whether the child has upper or lower airway obstruction, lung disease, or disordered control of breathing (from such conditions as brain or nerve injury, poisoning, or sepsis). Snoring or stridor indicates upper airway obstruction; wheezing indicates lower airway obstruction. It can be difficult to separate true stridor from upper airway noise because of nasal congestion. Breath sounds may also make it difficult to tell the difference between upper airway noise and true wheezing. Listen for breath sounds in the second or third intercostal space at the midaxillary line bilaterally (**Figure 3-7**). Consider the auscultation of breath sounds posteriorly between the scapula and spine bilaterally and lower lobes directly above the kidneys. At this location, it is easier to distinguish upper airway congestion from lower airway obstruction. When abnormal airway sounds are loudest with the stethoscope held near the child's nose rather than over the lungs, nasal congestion is the likely cause.

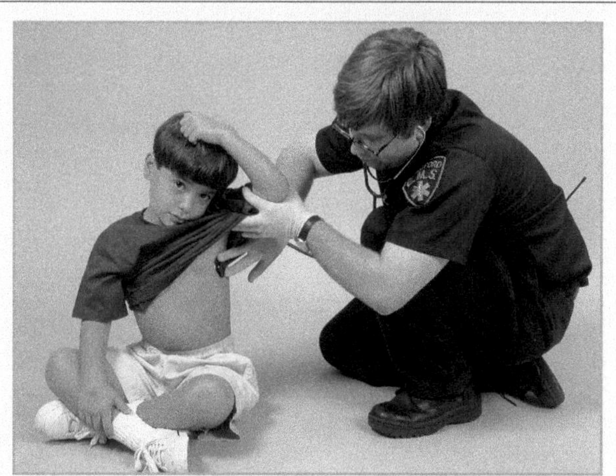

Figure 3-7 Listen for breath sounds in the second or third intercostal space at the midaxillary line bilaterally.

The absence of abnormal airway sounds in a child with hypoxia and increased work of breathing suggests lung disease, such as pneumonia. Lastly, a child with hypoxia and *decreased* work of breathing may have either respiratory failure from airway obstruction or lung disease or disordered control of breathing from another insult to the brain or metabolic system.

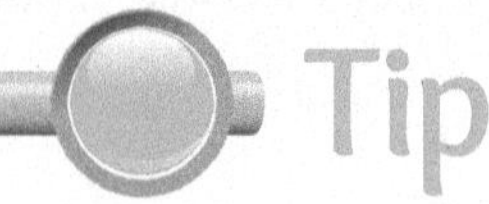

When abnormal airway sounds are loudest with the stethoscope held near the child's nose rather than over the lungs, nasal congestion is the likely cause.

Upper Airway Obstruction

Proximal Airway Obstruction

In a patient with neurologic impairment, loss of oropharyngeal muscle tone may cause upper airway obstruction and stridor because of the tongue and mandible falling back and partially blocking the pharynx. This is a common problem in children during and after seizures. The head-tilt/chin-lift maneuver (**Figure 3-8**) or jaw-thrust maneuver (**Figure 3-9**) may relieve this proximal airway obstruction. At times it may be helpful or even necessary to have two rescuers assist with the jaw-thrust maneuver. The use of airway adjuncts based on level of consciousness may help with keeping the airway open, especially in larger children, children who are actively seizing, or children receiving positive-pressure ventilation (**Figure 3-10**).

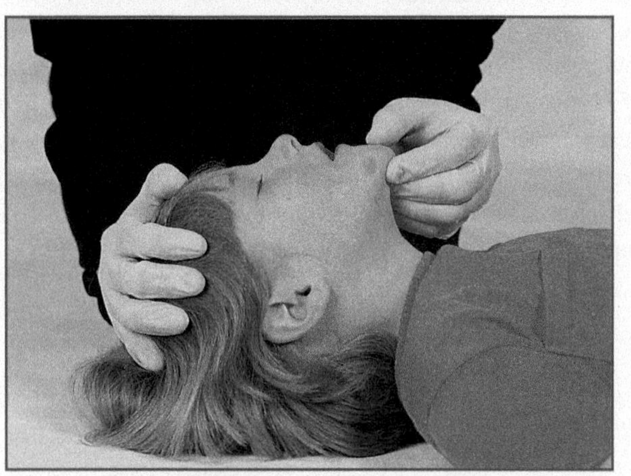

Figure 3-8 Use the head-tilt/chin-lift maneuver to place the airway in a neutral position.

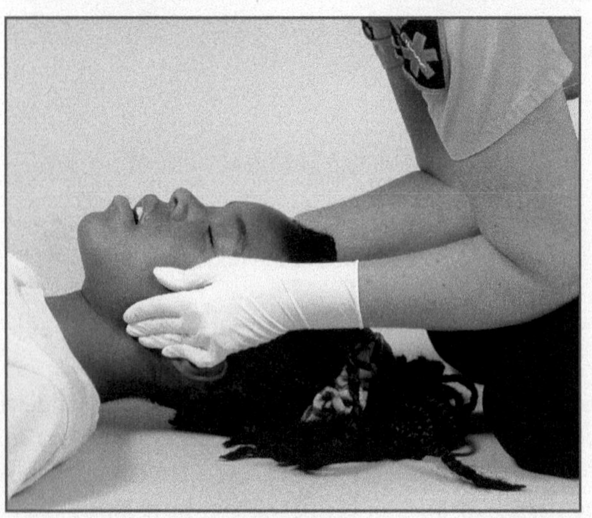

Figure 3-9 Use the jaw-thrust maneuver in a child with possible spinal injury.

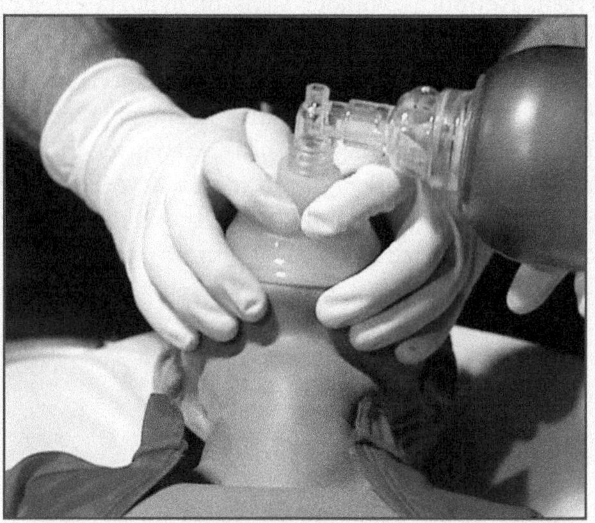

Figure 3-10 Two-rescuer technique for the jaw-thrust maneuver and positive-pressure ventilation.

Sometimes secretions, blood, or foreign bodies block the proximal upper airway. This is an important concern in the child with closed-head injury or seizures. Suctioning alone often relieves the upper airway obstruction caused by fluids or occluding objects in the mouth, pharynx, or nose.

Maintenance of an adequate airway may require placement of an oropharyngeal airway, an NPA, an endotracheal tube, or other approved advanced airways. The role of endotracheal intubation of children in the prehospital setting has been brought into question by data demonstrating significant failure rates, induced hypoxia, airway injury, and endotracheal tube dislodgement. *Bag-mask ventilation is the key lifesaving technique that should be mastered by all prehospital providers and provides adequate airway management for most pediatric patients.*

Alternative advanced airways including supraglottic airways and dual lumen airways can be considered in the early treatment of the child in respiratory failure or arrest. The particular type and brand is based on local emergency medical services (EMS) protocols.

Airway Obstruction Above the Thoracic Inlet

Upper airway obstruction beyond the proximal upper airway may result from a variety of causes. It is not necessary to make an exact diagnosis to provide appropriate management to children with upper airway obstruction.

In most of these cases, simply allow the child to maintain his or her position of comfort and provide supplemental oxygen by the least invasive and least threatening means possible. Causing the child to become more agitated or struggle may worsen the airway obstruction and precipitate the onset of a severe airway obstruction, leading to respiratory failure or respiratory arrest.

In an awake, alert child, upper airway obstruction and stridor are usually caused by croup, a viral disease with inflammation, edema, and narrowing of the larynx or trachea. Croup usually affects infants and toddlers. Most children with croup have had several days of cold symptoms. The cold symptoms are followed by the development of a barking or "seal-like" cough, stridor, and various levels of respiratory distress. There is usually a low-grade fever, and symptoms are often worse at night. The severity of symptoms varies widely among patients, but they usually progress over days, rather than hours.

Treatment. In the prehospital setting, the use of cool mist, either in the form of humidified oxygen or nebulized saline, may provide some comfort for the child. Having the caregiver assist may be of benefit. If the child does not tolerate the treatment, transport in a position of comfort (**Figure 3-11**).

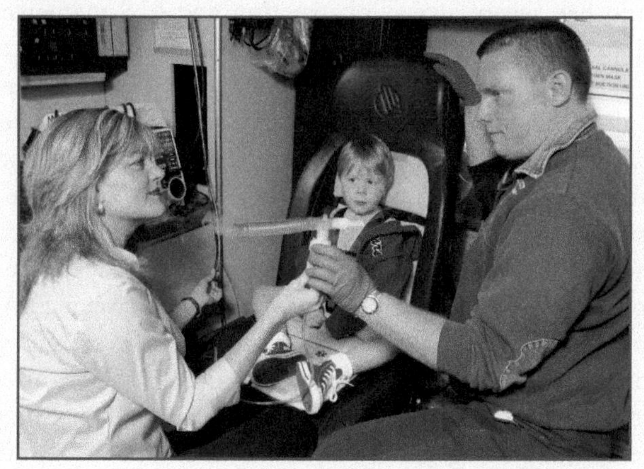

Figure 3-11 Use the caregiver to assist in the administration of oxygen or nebulized saline.

ALS

Pharmacologic Treatment of Croup. Nebulized epinephrine is a specific treatment for the upper airway inflammation associated with croup. Epinephrine is a potent α and β agonist, and works through vasoconstriction to decrease the upper airway edema causing partial obstruction. If local EMS protocols permit, consider nebulized epinephrine therapy for children with stridor, increased work of breathing, poor air movement, blood oxygen saturation less than 94%, or altered appearance. Nebulized epinephrine has two formulations, and either is acceptable: racemic epinephrine and L-epinephrine.

ALS

Side effects of nebulized epinephrine include tachycardia, tremor, and vomiting. Children who receive nebulized epinephrine need a period of observation in the ED because of possible return of stridor after the medicine wears off. Very few children with croup require assisted ventilation in the prehospital setting. In the rare case of a child with croup and respiratory failure, begin assisted ventilation and reassess. Two-person bag-mask ventilation technique may be necessary.

Invasive Airway Management for Croup. Perform endotracheal intubation only in the unusual case of the child with respiratory failure who does not respond to bag-mask ventilation. Preparation for intubation includes choosing an endotracheal tube that is one or two sizes smaller than normal for age or length. Inflammation of the trachea at the subglottic level makes it difficult or impossible to use an endotracheal tube of normal size. Do not use paralytics when attempting endotracheal intubation for upper airway obstruction. Refer to local protocols when making the decision for rapid sequence intubation (RSI). Other advanced airways should also be considered based on local protocols and availability.

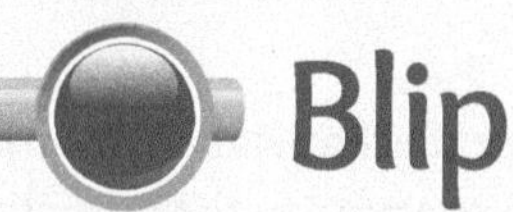

Blip

Stridor is often mistaken for wheezing. Stridor is an inspiratory sign of upper airway obstruction and may improve with an agent with vasoconstrictive properties, such as nebulized epinephrine.

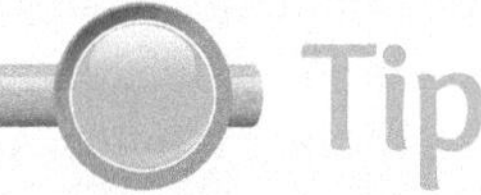

Tip

Position of comfort, humidified oxygen, and avoiding agitation are the best treatments for suspected croup.

Bacterial Upper Airway Infections

Bacterial infections may also cause upper airway obstruction in children. Unlike viral croup, these infections tend to progress rapidly with severe respiratory compromise developing over hours. The child with a bacterial upper airway infection usually is older than 12 months, appears ill or toxic, has pain on swallowing, and may drool. Stridor may be present, but the child does not have the barking cough that is common with croup.

There are several possible causes of bacterial upper airway infections. Epiglottitis, inflammation of the epiglottis, is now extremely rare because of widespread vaccination of infants against the bacteria *Haemophilus influenzae* type B. A retropharyngeal abscess involves swelling of the retropharyngeal nodes that are located between the cervical vertebrae and esophagus. It usually occurs in children younger than 4 years and can mimic the presentation of epiglottitis. The child may have torticollis, and there may be swollen cervical lymph nodes. A peritonsillar abscess is a collection of pus adjacent to the tonsil. It tends to occur more often in adolescents and is often caused by group A streptococcus (so the child may be on antibiotics for a strep throat). The child complains of trouble speaking, is unable to open his or her mouth fully, and often drools. Tracheitis can occur in two forms. In the child without a tracheostomy, it can mimic the presentation of epiglottitis. In a child with a tracheostomy, it results in increased thick airway secretions.

Treatment. When a bacterial upper airway infection is suspected, give only general noninvasive treatment with high-flow oxygen in a position of comfort. Avoid agitating the child by trying to place an intravenous (IV) line or attempting another maneuver, and quickly transport. If the child is in respiratory failure, initiate bag-mask ventilation and consider endotracheal intubation.

Foreign Body Aspiration

Foreign body aspiration may cause mechanical obstruction anywhere in the airway, from the pharynx to the bronchus. A retained esophageal foreign body can also cause respiratory distress in an infant or young child. This happens because the trachea is pliable and can be compressed by the adjacent distended esophagus. A typical history of foreign body aspiration includes the sudden onset of coughing, choking, gagging, and shortness of breath in a previously well child without a fever or other symptoms of upper respiratory tract infection. Older infants and toddlers, who explore their world by placing things in their mouths, are at highest risk.

Treatment. If the child can still cough, cry, or speak, the airway is only partially obstructed. Stridor may be present. Immediately transport such children, who have mild upper airway obstruction. Use only general noninvasive treatment, avoid agitating the child, and keep the child in a position of comfort.

If the child has severe respiratory distress and is at risk for getting worse during transport, be prepared to perform foreign body airway obstruction (FBAO) maneuvers for severe airway obstruction, as illustrated in **Figures 3-12** and **3-13**. **Table 3-3** summarizes these maneuvers. Consider these FBAO maneuvers if the child cannot cough, cry, or speak. *Never perform FBAO procedures if the child has mild airway obstruction (i.e., can cough, cry, or speak).*

Airway Obstruction and Foreign Body Removal

In the setting of severe airway obstruction, prehospital professionals can make the difference between life and death. Immediate removal of an airway foreign body can often be achieved using BLS procedures while the child is still conscious. Sometimes basic maneuvers are unsuccessful. In such cases, pediatric Magill forceps along with direct laryngoscopy may be the only option for removal. For a step-by-step explanation of this procedure, see **Foreign Body Obstruction, Procedure 6.**

Foreign Body Airway Obstruction Maneuvers. If the child has severe airway obstruction and BLS maneuvers fail to dislodge the foreign body to the mouth where it can be easily removed, and the patient loses consciousness, begin cardiopulmonary resuscitation (CPR) with chest compressions, then open the airway. If the foreign body can be seen at or above the level of the larynx, remove it using pediatric Magill forceps if at the level of a paramedic, and if an EMT, continue CPR and look for airway obstruction before delivering ventilations. Finger sweep FBAO only if the object is seen. If the child has severe airway obstruction and neither FBAO maneuvers nor direct laryngoscopy relieve the obstruction, attempt bag-mask ventilation, using the two-person technique whenever possible (**Figure 3-14**). If bag-mask ventilation fails to achieve chest rise, consider endotracheal intubation.

Case Study 2

Your unit is dispatched to a child care center for a child in respiratory distress. On arrival you and your partner find a 23-month-old girl very cyanotic in color grasping her throat. The child care worker states that she believes that the child has a history of asthma and tried giving her an inhaler treatment but the child would not tolerate it. The child is making no audible noises and seems desperate for help.

1. What is the most important thing for you to do at this time?
2. What would you do if your initial steps failed? What would you do next?

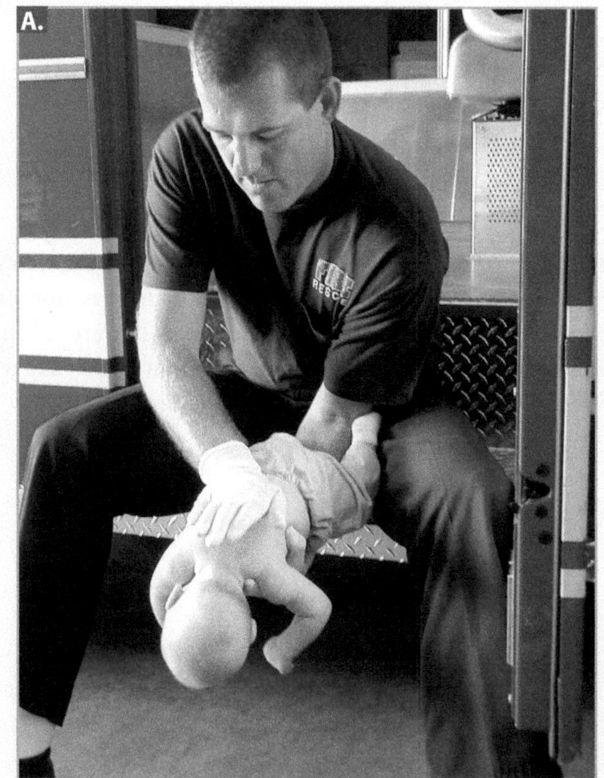

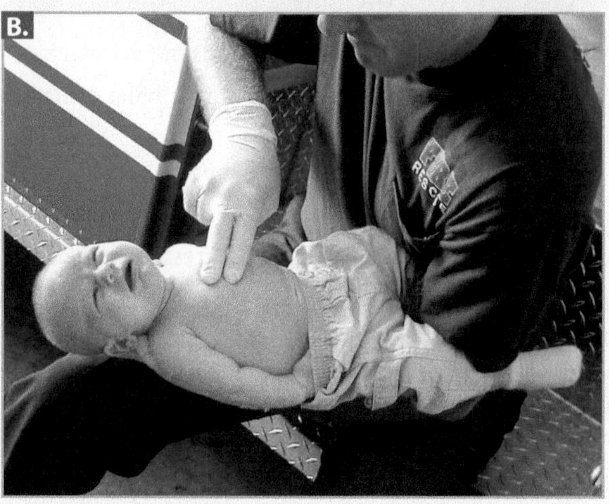

Figure 3-12 Foreign body airway maneuvers for a conscious infant. **A.** Use five back blows (slaps), followed by **B.** five chest compressions in infants with severe airway obstruction.

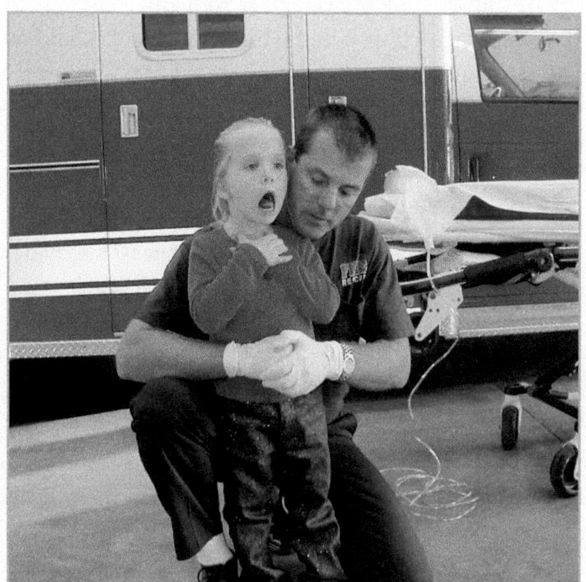

Figure 3-13 Foreign body airway maneuvers for a conscious child. Use abdominal thrusts to treat severe airway obstruction in the conscious child in the standing position.

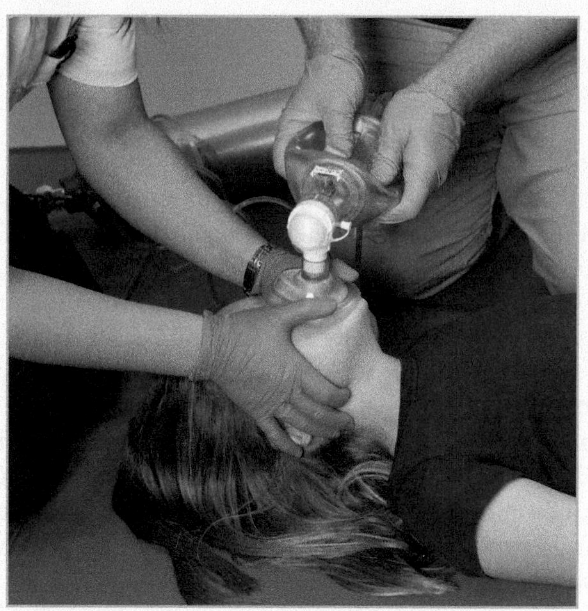

Figure 3-14 Two-person bag-mask ventilation technique.

Table 3-3 Foreign Body Airway Obstruction Maneuvers

Age	Technique
Infant (<12 months)	Five back blows (slaps) followed by five chest compressions until unresponsive, then start CPR
Child (>1 year)	Abdominal thrusts until unresponsive, then start CPR

Suction should be readily available when performing unconscious airway maneuvers.

Based on local protocols, cricothyrotomy might be considered for obstructions that cannot be removed.

Specific Treatment of Upper Airway Obstruction

When transporting any child with suspected mild upper airway obstruction, have airway equipment immediately available.

Consider transporting the caregiver with any conscious child with airway obstruction, because this may keep the child calm. Also, the caregiver can help administer oxygen.

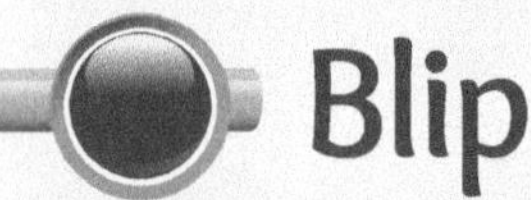

Never perform airway obstruction procedures if the child has only mild airway obstruction and can still cough, cry, or speak.

Lower Airway Obstruction

Bronchiolitis and asthma are the most common conditions causing lower airway obstruction in children. Foreign body aspiration is much less common and usually occurs in toddlers who have been otherwise well, and then suddenly start choking, coughing, or wheezing. *Wheezing is the clinical hallmark of lower airway obstruction of any cause.* Pneumonia can also cause lower airway disease but usually without obstruction. A specific diagnosis of lower airway obstruction in the field is not necessary, and many times it is impossible to tell which of the three main conditions the child is experiencing: (1) bronchiolitis, (2) asthma, or (3) foreign body aspiration. Treatment for all forms of **broncho-constriction** is similar, but asthma is much more likely to respond to bronchodilators than bronchiolitis.

Asthma

Asthma is the most common chronic disease of childhood, affecting almost 5 million children in the United States. The ED admission rate for children with asthma younger than 5 years of age is more than twice the national average for all ages, and the mortality rate for children is rising. Half of all pediatric asthma deaths occur in the out-of-hospital setting. The length of the final attack is less than 1 hour in many children, and less than 2 hours in half of children with asthma who die. Common reasons for an asthma attack include upper respiratory infection and exercise. Exposure to cold air, emotional stress, and passive exposure to smoke also may trigger attacks.

Asthma is a disease of small airway inflammation. The inflammatory reaction leads to bronchoconstriction, mucosal edema, and profuse secretions. These three factors in combination cause airflow obstruction and **ventilation-perfusion mismatch**. Clinically, children having an asthma attack show different degrees of tachypnea, tachycardia, increased work of breathing, and wheezing, which tends to be worse on exhalation. Pulse oximetry may be normal or low.

Carefully assess air movement by auscultation both anteriorly and posteriorly; this helps to distinguish not only sounds but also tidal volume. The person with asthma complaining of shortness of breath, but without wheezing

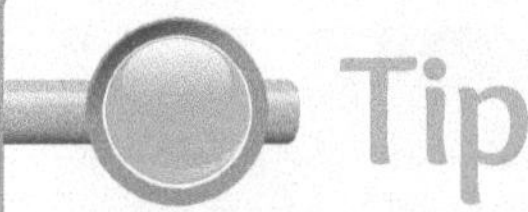

Attempt BLS maneuvers first in a child with suspected foreign body aspiration and critical airway obstruction.

on auscultation, may have too much airway obstruction to wheeze. Aggressive bronchodilator treatment may improve airflow and increase audible wheezing. Beware of the following features of the primary assessment, which suggest severe bronchospasm and respiratory failure:

- Altered appearance
- Exhaustion
- Inability to recline
- Interrupted speech
- Severe retractions
- Decreased air movement

In the focused history, several things suggest that a severe or potentially fatal attack may occur. These include:

- Prior intensive care unit admissions or intubation
- More than three ED visits in a year
- More than two hospital admissions in past year
- Use of more than one metered dose inhaler canister in the last month
- Use of steroids for asthma in the past
- Use of bronchodilators more frequently than every 4 hours
- Progressive symptoms despite aggressive home therapy

Home therapy of asthma has several goals: preventing and controlling asthma symptoms, reducing the number and severity of attacks, and reversing existing airflow obstruction. Some children with a history of severe or frequent asthma attacks are on daily medications, but most children receive treatment only during serious attacks. **Table 3-4** lists the medications frequently used in home asthma therapy for quick relief. Some patients may think they will obtain quick relief from medications that do not have a quick onset of action and delay calling for help.

Treatment of Lower Airway Obstruction

For all children with lower airway obstruction, give general noninvasive treatment as the first field action.

ALS **Asthma Treatment.** Specific field treatment of wheezing includes either inhaled bronchodilators or intramuscular (IM) epinephrine. In patients with asthma, treatment with corticosteroids in the ED has been shown to result in decreased need for admission and more rapid time to resolution of symptoms. Based on this evidence, some prehospital protocols now include corticosteroid treatment as an option in patients with asthma. However, the effect of prehospital corticosteroid treatment on patient outcome is not known.

Table 3-4 Asthma: Common Home Therapy Quick-Relief Medications for Acute Asthma Attacks

Class of Medication	Medication	Mechanism of Action
β_2 agonists	Inhaled bronchodilators (albuterol [salbutamol]), levalbuterol	Relax bronchiole smooth muscle; prevent bronchospasm; rapid onset of action
Anticholinergics	Inhaled anticholinergics (ipratropium)	Relax bronchiole smooth muscle; decrease secretions; rapid onset of action
Anti-inflammatory medications	Oral corticosteroids (prednisone)	Block allergic response; reduce airway hyperresponsiveness; improve response to bronchodilators; delayed onset of action (2–12 hours)

ALS

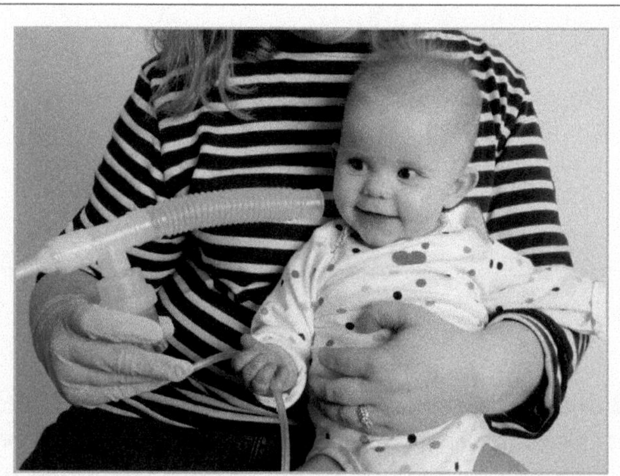

Figure 3-15 A nebulized bronchodilator can also be given without a mask using a blow-by technique.

Figures 3-15, **3-16**, and **3-17** illustrate administration of inhaled bronchodilators.

Bronchodilators

Early bronchodilator therapy, on the scene and on the way to the ED, helps immediately open airways, relieve respiratory distress, and improve oxygen delivery in asthma. In unstable or critical patients, continuous inhaled treatment with a β agonist is the preferred approach, although subcutaneous (SQ) or IM bronchodilators are acceptable in some patients who cannot cooperate with inhalation therapy. For a step-by-step explanation of this procedure, see **Bronchodilator Therapy, Procedure 7**. In-line bronchodilator used with continuous positive airway pressure (CPAP) can be used on older children based on local protocols.

Pharmacologic Treatment of Wheezing. Albuterol (salbutamol) is the most popular inhaled bronchodilator. Because of its selective action on the bronchiole smooth muscles and its minimal effect on cardiac rate, the drug has a high margin of safety. In a critical child with wheezing, treat with the highest dose and give continuous treatment. Unit dose vials of albuterol (salbutamol) premixed with saline are used by most prehospital systems. These vials provide 2.5 mg of albuterol (salbutamol) in a total volume of 3 mL. One vial is an acceptable initial dose for almost all children and adolescents. For critical patients, the nebulizer may be refilled continuously or two vials may be placed in the nebulizer initially and given immediately. Levalbuterol is an isomer of albuterol that has not been studied in the out-of-hospital setting, and has not been shown to offer any benefit over albuterol in the hospital setting.

ALS

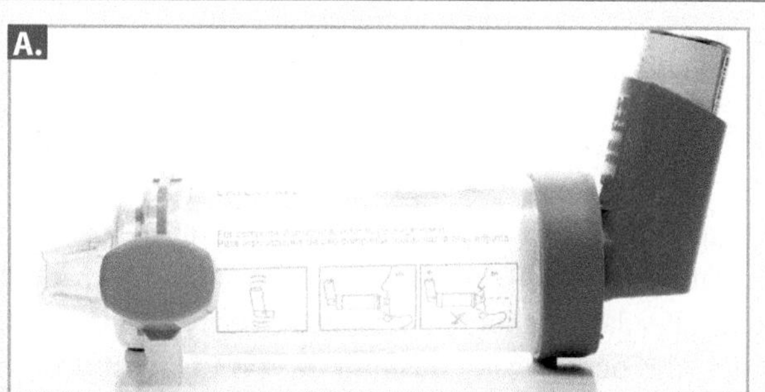

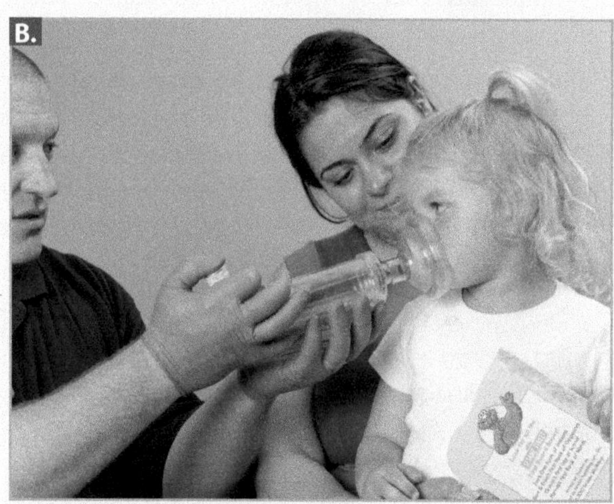

Figure 3-16 **A.** A metered dose inhaler and spacer can be used with or without a mask. **B.** A metered dose inhaler with spacer and mask can be used in children as young as 6 months old.

Depending on local protocols, give ipratropium with albuterol (salbutamol). Ipratropium is an anticholinergic that may provide additional bronchodilatation in addition

ALS

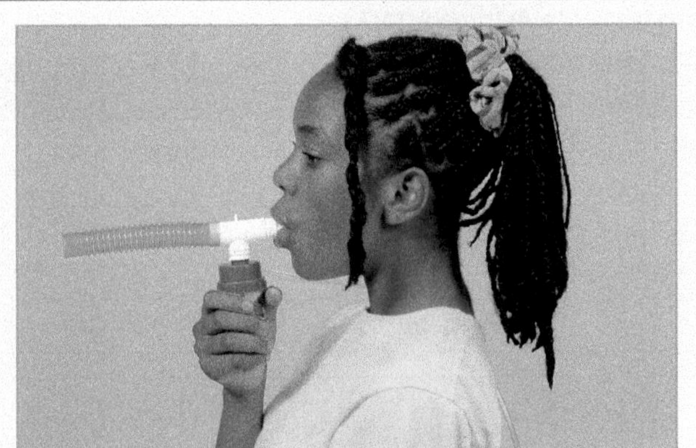

Figure 3-17 One method for delivering a bronchodilator is with an oxygen-powered nebulizer.

to β agonists. Precautions include sensitivity to the effects of ipratropium or atropine. Adverse reactions include dry mouth, headache, cough, hoarseness, blurred vision, tachycardia, and occasionally flushing. Add it to a unit dose vial of albuterol (salbutamol) and administer together by nebulizer. Multiple doses of ipratropium provide added benefit in asthma exacerbations.

If a child cannot tolerate nebulized drug therapy, or is moving air so poorly that the drug is not being inhaled, give IM epinephrine. Transport with cardiac monitoring if frequent nebulized treatments or IM epinephrine is necessary. **Table 3-5** summarizes the drugs and doses for field bronchodilator therapy.

Table 3-5 Management of Wheezing: Bronchodilator Treatment

Bronchodilator	Dose
Albuterol (salbutamol)	Nebulized solution (1.25 mg/3 mL, 2.5 mg/3 mL, 5 mg/mL). 2.5-5 mg every 20 minutes for three doses. Repeat dose every 1–4 hours as needed. If not already prediluted, dilute in minimum of 2–3 mL saline for adequate nebulization. May use continuously for critical patients.
Ipratropium bromide inhalation solution	Nebulized solution (0.5 mg/2.5 mL). *Children* <12 years: 0.25 mg nebulized every 20 minutes for three doses. *Children* >12 years: 0.5 mg nebulized every 20 minutes for three doses.
Albuterol (salbutamol) metered dose inhaler	90 mcg per puff. 4–8 puffs every 15–20 minutes for three doses.

ALS

In most cases of known asthma, begin a bronchodilator on scene before transport, and then give additional doses en route, as indicated.

Unit dose vials of 2.5 mg of albuterol (salbutamol) premixed with saline to a total volume of 3 mL may be used as an initial dose for children and adolescents of all ages. In critical patients, doses may be repeated continuously en route to the ED.

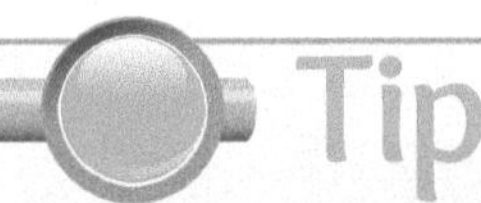

Tip

When a child has a history of increased work of breathing, but now has altered appearance and a slow or normal respiratory rate without retractions, THINK RESPIRATORY FAILURE.

IM Injections. IM is the preferred route of administration for epinephrine in patients with severe respiratory distress due to asthma. SQ absorption is slow and unreliable. The IM route may result in nerve damage, particularly if the injection is in the buttocks of infants and small children. For a step-by-step explanation of this procedure, see **Intramuscular and Subcutaneous Injections, Procedure 14.**

Assisted Ventilation. Because of the severe air trapping associated with bronchospasm, assisted ventilation may be associated with many complications and death. Positive-pressure ventilation requires very high inspiratory pressures and may result in pneumothorax or pneumomediastinum. Consider bag-mask ventilation and endotracheal intubation of a wheezing child only if the child is in respiratory failure and has failed to respond to high-flow oxygen and maximal bronchodilator therapy. While assisting ventilation in any patient with lower airway obstruction, slow rates (12–15 breaths/min in older children and adolescents, and a maximum rate of 20–30 breaths/min in infants) with long expiratory times are useful in minimizing barotrauma and complications.

Bronchiolitis

Bronchiolitis is a viral lower respiratory infection, which usually affects infants and children younger than 2 years of age. Often caused by respiratory syncytial virus (RSV), this disease is widespread in the winter months. The infection leads to destruction of the lining of the bronchioles, profuse secretions, and bronchoconstriction. Infants are particularly likely to develop the disease because of their small airway size, high resistance to airflow, and poor airway clearance. Airway edema and debris from sloughed cells and mucus are much more important in the pathophysiology of this disease than bronchospasm and smooth muscle contraction.

Presenting complaints of bronchiolitis include upper respiratory infection symptoms, fever, cough, vomiting, poor feeding, poor sleep, and trouble breathing. Assessment shows variable degrees of increased work of breathing, tachypnea, diffuse wheezing, inspiratory crackles, and tachycardia.

Historical risk factors for respiratory failure in infants with suspected bronchiolitis include age younger than 2 months, history of prematurity, underlying lung disease, congenital heart disease, and immune deficiency. **Table 3-6** lists important clinical predictors of respiratory failure in children with suspected bronchiolitis. BLS treatment can include nasopharyngeal suctioning with a bulb syringe (see **Procedure 4-1**).

Table 3-6 Predictors of Respiratory Failure in Suspected Bronchiolitis

Respiratory rate >60 breaths/min with increased work of breathing
Heart rate >200 beats/min or <100 beats/min
Poor appearance
Blood oxygen saturation <90% on supplemental oxygen

ALS

It is often difficult to distinguish new-onset reactive airway disease from viral bronchiolitis; therefore, treat with nebulized epinephrine or albuterol (salbutamol) initially.

Foreign Body Aspiration

Children with lower airway obstruction caused by foreign body aspiration usually are only mildly ill. Unlike foreign bodies in the upper airway, it is rare to develop respiratory failure or severe airway obstruction from a small foreign body in the lower airway. Foreign body aspiration is most common in older infants and toddlers (**Figure 3-18**). Often, there is an abrupt onset of coughing or choking that may be followed by a period of relatively few symptoms. Tachypnea, increased work of breathing, and wheezing or decreased breath sounds, which are usually unilateral unless the foreign body is in the trachea, may develop rapidly or over a period of hours to days. The absence of a history of asthma or the symptoms of an upper respiratory infection in a child of the right age should suggest the possibility of foreign body aspiration. General noninvasive treatment, including allowing the child to assume a position of comfort and providing oxygen if tolerated, should be given to all patients. A trial of inhaled bronchodilators is reasonable if the diagnosis is unclear, but do not delay transport. Additional diagnostic tests may be done after arrival at the ED.

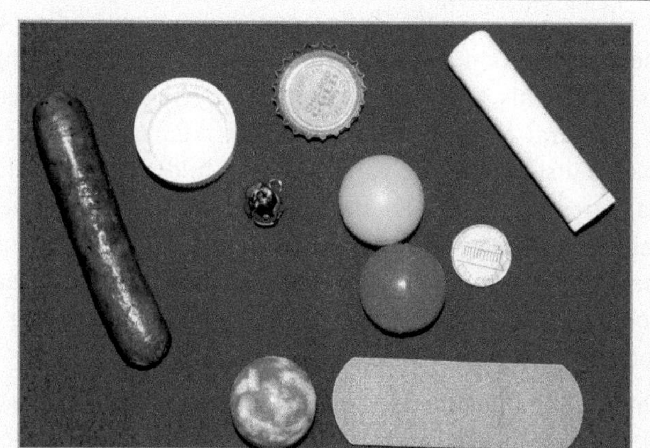

Figure 3-18 Examples of foreign bodies that can obstruct the upper or lower airway.

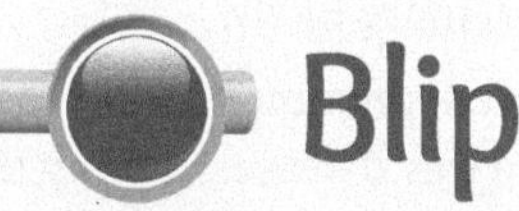

The efficacy of treatment of bronchiolitis with bronchodilators is questionable. If unable to distinguish from new-onset reactive airway disease or asthma, give a dose.

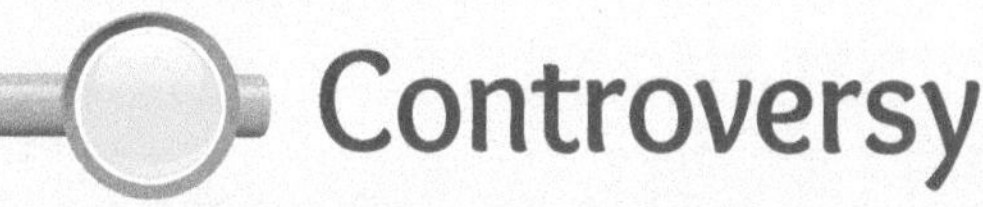

Specific field treatment of infants with wheezing may include bronchodilation with nebulized β agonists or nebulized epinephrine. The relative effectiveness of these treatments for bronchiolitis is controversial.

Lung Disease

In children, most lung disease is caused by pneumonia. Other causes, such as pulmonary edema or pulmonary contusion, are rare. Pneumonia may cause symptoms of lower airway disease and respiratory distress or failure in children. Almost all children with pneumonia have fever or a history of fever at some point in their illness. Most pneumonias in children are caused by viruses. These children generally have less severe symptoms and symptoms of a more gradual onset than children with bacterial pneumonia.

Bacterial pneumonia in children occurs after aspiration or hematogenous seeding of bacteria into the lung. This is followed by an acute inflammatory reaction leading to the accumulation of fluid within the airspaces of the lung. At times, this may be accompanied by the development of a pleural effusion or collection of fluid in the pleural space outside the lung parenchyma. Children with bacterial pneumonia usually have symptoms including fever, chills, tachypnea, and frequently nonspecific complaints including lethargy or irritability, poor appetite, and occasionally chest pain. Cough may not develop until after a period of other more nonspecific symptoms.

Physical findings may include fever, tachypnea, increased work of breathing, decreased breath sounds, and rales. Grunting respirations are relatively common in young children with any form of lung disease. Wheezes may be heard, especially with viral infections, but are not as common as rales or decreased breath sounds. In the absence of underlying illness, disability, or very young age, it is unusual for a child to abruptly develop respiratory failure caused by pneumonia. Respiratory distress is more likely.

Approach children with suspected pneumonia like any patient with symptoms of lower airway disease. Making the diagnosis is not as important as providing good supportive care. Give general, noninvasive treatment to all patients. If the patient has wheezing, try bronchodilators. Patients with signs of respiratory failure may need assisted ventilation. Respiratory failure from lung disease is more commonly seen in young infants, children with underlying neurologic or pulmonary disease, and children who have been ill for several days. There is no specific prehospital therapy for children with pneumonia.

Disordered Control of Breathing

Sometimes hypoxia or respiratory insufficiency is caused by problems in control of breathing. This category of respiratory disease includes brain injury, spinal injury, poisoning, metabolic problems (e.g., botulism, Guillain-Barré syndrome), or sepsis. The hallmark of patients with disordered control of breathing is inadequate minute volume, from poor tidal volume or slow breathing rate. Treatment includes ventilatory support with oxygen, bag-mask ventilation, and occasionally endotracheal intubation or other advanced airways.

Summary of Specific Treatment for Respiratory Distress

After identifying respiratory distress or failure and beginning general supportive measures, assess whether the anatomic level of the respiratory problem is in the upper or lower airway, using the PAT and the hands-on ABCDEs. Stridor is the hallmark of upper airway obstruction; wheezing is the hallmark of lower airway obstruction; grunting is the hallmark of lung disease; and inadequate minute volume and decreased work of breathing are the clinical markers for disordered control of breathing.

The most common cause of upper airway obstruction is croup. Rarely, foreign bodies lodged at or above the vocal cords may be the cause of stridor in infants and toddlers. Specific treatment of croup includes nebulized epinephrine. Frequent causes of lower airway obstruction are asthma and bronchiolitis—a disease of infants. Asthma is the most likely cause of wheezing in all children from infancy to adulthood. A nebulized bronchodilator, delivered

Case Study 3

A caregiver calls 9-1-1 because a 3-month-old girl has had 3 days of cough, runny nose, and low-grade fever. The caregiver is concerned because the child seems to be working harder to breathe and is having a hard time taking feedings. On arrival, the child is found lying on the caregiver's lap. She appears sleepy and does not make eye contact or respond to examination. She has audible wheezing and a deep subcostal and intercostal retractions. There is nasal flaring. Her skin is mottled. Respiratory rate is 70 breaths/min and heart rate is 180 beats/min. Her breath sounds are tight with only fair air movement, but you hear high-pitched, inspiratory and expiratory wheezes throughout. Pulse oximetry in room air is 74% with a pulse that corresponds to the patient's pulse on examination.

1. Is this child in respiratory distress or respiratory failure, and what is the level of airway obstruction?
2. What are the first steps in the management of this child?

continuously if necessary, is the specific treatment for all causes of wheezing. Albuterol (salbutamol) and epinephrine have similar effectiveness as bronchodilators, and the anticholinergic ipratropium provides added benefit in patients with asthma. Start treatment on scene in those with asthma.

Foreign body aspiration and pneumonia may present as lower airway problems, but there is no specific treatment for these conditions in the prehospital setting other than the general noninvasive measures for respiratory distress. Disordered control of breathing has many causes and often requires general ventilatory support.

Management of Respiratory Failure

Regardless of the cause, initially treat every cooperative child in respiratory failure with general noninvasive measures. If upper or lower airway obstruction is present, attempt specific treatment. However, if the child has altered appearance or altered mental status and has signs of increased or decreased work of breathing (e.g., flaring, grunting, gasping, apnea, or cyanosis), or if the child has a documented blood oxygen saturation of less than 90% on 100% nonrebreathing oxygen mask, the child is in respiratory failure or respiratory arrest. For this child, bypass general noninvasive treatment and consider immediately beginning assisted ventilation.

First, position the patient to maintain an open airway. Then use suction. Suctioning is a basic technique to maintain an open airway. Children have tiny airways that are easily obstructed by secretions, vomitus, pus, blood, or foreign bodies. Children of different ages, with different clinical problems, need different types of suction devices and suctioning procedures. For a step-by-step explanation, see **Suctioning, Procedure 4**.

If the patient is unresponsive, use an airway adjunct. Adjuncts may immediately improve the child's spontaneous ventilation. In addition, they may allow more effective bag-mask ventilation, reduce gastric inflation, and avert the need for endotracheal intubation. For a step-by-step explanation of this procedure, see **Airway Adjuncts, Procedure 5**.

Then deliver assisted ventilation or positive-pressure ventilation using bag-mask. Bag-mask is usually the best method for providing oxygenation and ventilation during stabilization and transport. Use an age-appropriate rate of 30 breaths/min in infants and 20 breaths/min in older children. Saying the words, "squeeze, release, release" helps time the ventilations to avoid a rate that is too rapid. Ensure that there is good chest rise. Good bag-mask technique decreases the risk of gastric distention, a common complication leading to elevation of the diaphragm, decreased lung compliance, and increased risk of vomiting and aspiration of gastric contents. With severe, lower airway obstruction, slower rates and longer expiratory times are indicated. Consider placing a nasogastric (NG) tube.

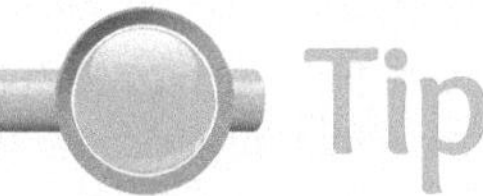

For an older child in respiratory failure who has increased work of breathing, ventilating at a rate of 20 breaths/min may assist the patient's respiratory effort.

Bag-Mask Ventilation

Bag-mask ventilation is one of the prehospital professional's most useful skills in pediatric prehospital care. Although the technique does not provide the definitive airway control that endotracheal intubation does, in most cases bag-mask ventilation is the best technique for providing oxygenation and ventilation during resuscitation and transport. For a step-by-step explanation of this procedure, see **Bag-Mask Ventilation, Procedure 8**.

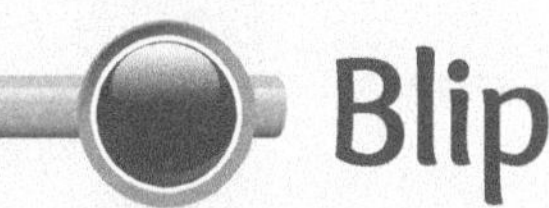

Minimize gastric distention during bag-mask ventilation with good bagging technique.

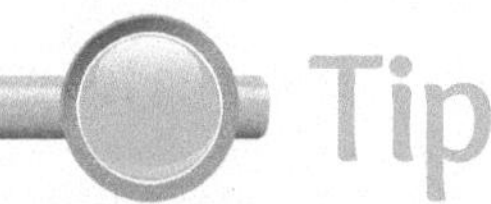

If the child does not respond to bag-mask ventilation, or if there is a long transport time with a critically ill or injured child who has an unstable airway, consider endotracheal intubation.

ALS

Management With Endotracheal Intubation. The indications for endotracheal intubation of a child in the prehospital setting are controversial. Potential advantages of intubation include definitive airway control, decreased risk of aspiration, and ease of assisted ventilation. Potential complications include transient hypoxia and hypercapnia caused by prolonged intubation attempts; unrecognized misplacement of the tube; elevation of intracranial pressure; aspiration of stomach contents; and injury to the

ALS

teeth, mouth, tongue, palate, larynx, and soft tissues of the pharynx and neck.

Dislodgment of the tube from the trachea during patient movement or transport is common and may be catastrophic. If an intubated patient fails to respond with improved color, oxygen saturation, heart rate, and appearance, the DOPE mnemonic may help to identify potential technical problems (**Table 3-7**). Most EMS systems require constant monitoring of proper placement of endotracheal tubes. Alternative advanced airways are also considerations for the treatment of ventilatory support; refer to local protocols and procedures.

Nasogastric and Orogastric Insertion

During positive-pressure ventilation, it is common to inflate the stomach and the lungs with air. Gastric inflation with air slows downward movement of the diaphragm and decreases tidal volume, making ventilation more difficult and necessitating higher inspiratory pressures. In addition, inflation of the stomach with air increases the risk that the patient will vomit and aspirate. Gastric intubation with an NG or orogastric (OG) tube takes air from the stomach and helps

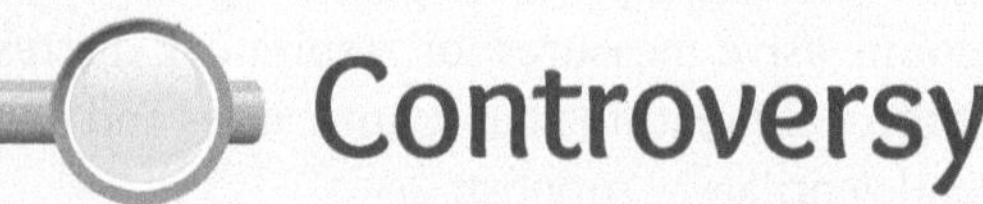

The value of nasogastric and orogastric tubes is unknown. Avoid inserting a nasogastric or orogastric tube unless ventilation is impaired by a distended stomach.

Table 3-7 Troubleshooting the Endotracheal Tube: DOPE

	Problem	Assessment	Intervention
Dislodgment	Esophageal intubation	End-tidal carbon dioxide monitor or detector reads no or low carbon dioxide or has poor waveform, or no color change Oxygen saturation <90% Bradycardia Lack of chest rise with ventilation Auscultation of bubbling over the stomach	Extubate Bag-mask ventilation Reintubate
	Mainstem bronchus intubation	Asymmetric chest rise Asymmetric breath sounds	Pull tube back until breath sounds and chest rise are symmetric
	Accidental extubation	End-tidal carbon dioxide monitor/detector reads no or low carbon dioxide level, or has poor waveform, or no color change Oxygen saturation <90% Bradycardia Lack of chest rise with ventilation Poor or absent air movement on auscultation	Bag-mask ventilation Reintubate
Obstruction	Tube blocked with blood, secretions, or kink	Decreased chest rise Decreased breath sounds bilaterally Oxygen saturation <90% Carbon dioxide monitor has abnormal waveform Increased resistance to bagging	Suction, if no improvement extubate Bag-mask ventilation Reintubate
Pneumothorax	Tension pneumothorax, spontaneous or induced, compromises air exchange and may lead to decreased cardiac output	Asymmetric chest rise Asymmetric breath sounds Shock Oxygen saturation <90% *Jugular venous distention *Tracheal deviation	Needle thoracostomy
Equipment	Big air leak around tube Activated pop-off valve on resuscitator Oxygen tubing disconnected Oxygen tank empty	Oxygen saturation <90%	Check equipment, "patient-to-tank"

* Not always detectable in young children.

ALS

positive-pressure ventilation. However, only use this technique if there is difficulty ventilating the patient. Insertion may be painful and frightening to the child and family. For a step-by-step explanation of this procedure, see **Orogastric and Nasogastric Tube Insertion, Procedure 10**.

Endotracheal Intubation

Successful endotracheal intubation allows optimal oxygenation and ventilation, provides a tube for medication delivery, and decreases the risk of aspiration and loss of airway control. A properly placed and secured endotracheal tube is a good tool for managing critical patients, but the procedure can take a long time, and there can be frequent and serious complications. Every placement of an advanced airway must be confirmed for proper placement of the device. Exhaled carbon dioxide colorimetric devices or in-line capnometry or capnography should be used during the confirmation process. For a step-by-step explanation of this procedure, see **Endotracheal Intubation, Procedure 11**.

ALS

Alternative Breathing and Intubation Techniques

Rarely, standard bag-mask ventilation fails and endotracheal intubation is difficult or impossible. Examples of such patients are children with massive head trauma and airway edema or hematoma of the mouth or upper airway, or infants with significant congenital or acquired airway abnormalities who cannot be ventilated. In such dire circumstances, some EMS systems allow prehospital professionals to perform advanced breathing techniques. These include use of a supraglottic airway or dual lumen airway. Additional adjuncts to assist in endotracheal intubation include the gum elastic bougie, a lighted stylet, and RSI. Needle cricothyrotomy is another option, if necessary. None of these techniques have been well evaluated in children in the out-of-hospital setting.

Table 3-8 summarizes the advantages and disadvantages of these alternative techniques. For a step-by-step explanation of the LMA, Combitube and its recommended removal, gum elastic bougie, lighted stylet, and RSI (should

Table 3-8 Advantages and Disadvantages of Rescue Breathing Techniques

Technique	Advantages	Disadvantages
Supraglottic airway devices (LMA, SALT, King LAD, i-gel)	Simple insertion Good airway seal Adapts to bag-mask equipment	Does not prevent aspiration Fewer size choices
Gum elastic bougie	May facilitate endotracheal tube insertion	No equipment or data in infants and young children Prolonged attempts may worsen hypoxia
Lighted stylet	Does not require airway visualization	Poor information in children Unknown accuracy
Dual lumen airway (e.g., Combitube), pharyngeotracheal lumen airway	Effective isolation of the airway Reduced risk of aspiration More reliable ventilation relative to bag-mask ventilation Does not require visualization of the glottis	Fatal complications may occur if the position of esophageal-tracheal tube is identified incorrectly Potential for esophageal trauma
Laryngeal tube/ supralaryngeal airway (e.g., "King Air")	Effective isolation of the airway Reduced risk of aspiration More reliable ventilation relative to bag-mask ventilation Does not require visualization of the glottis Less complicated to insert than esophageal-tracheal tube	Limited data published on the use of the laryngeal tube in children Potential for esophageal trauma
Rapid sequence intubation	Paralyzes child and eliminates muscle resistance Improves visualization Allows mild hyperventilation	Drugs remove spontaneous breathing Drugs may decrease blood pressure or respiratory rate Succinylcholine may cause high potassium
Cricothyrotomy	Provides tiny airway for lifesaving oxygenation or ventilation Bypasses obstruction	Technically difficult Bleeding Injury to other neck structures

be referred to local protocols), see **Advanced Airway Techniques, Procedure 13.**

Confirmation of Endotracheal Tube Placement

Several products are currently available for confirming proper placement of the endotracheal tube. These include quantitative end-tidal carbon dioxide monitors or capnometers, which read out the blood carbon dioxide tension ($PaCO_2$) (**Figure 3-19**); colorimetric end-tidal carbon dioxide detectors that give a qualitative reading; and syringe and self-inflating bulb devices that distinguish endotracheal from esophageal intubation based on positive aspiration of air from the tube (not approved for children <5 years or 20 kg).

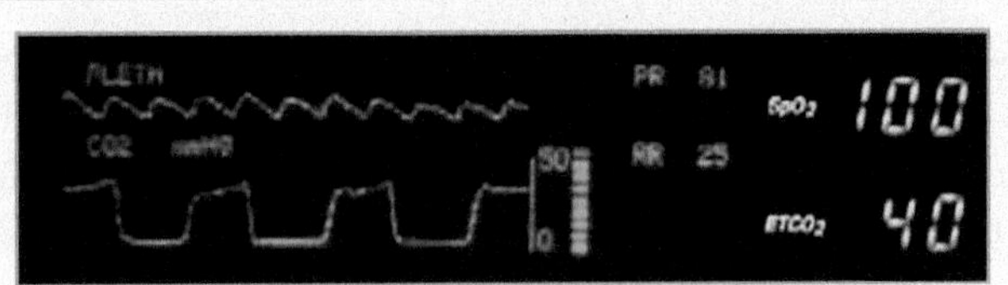

Figure 3-19 Carbon dioxide detector showing normal end-tidal carbon dioxide waveform.

The optimal method for tube confirmation in children in the out-of-hospital setting is not known. Because the child's airway is so short, even slight movement of the endotracheal tube can lead to extubation or mainstem intubation. If capnometry shows no carbon dioxide, if the colorimetric detector fails to change color with ventilation, or if no air is aspirated into the esophageal bulb or syringe, these are indications that the endotracheal tube may not be in the trachea. In such cases, remove the endotracheal tube, perform bag-mask ventilation, and reintubate after 1–2 minutes of oxygenation and ventilation.

The only exception to this approach is the patient in full cardiopulmonary arrest, where pulmonary circulation may be too low to generate detectable expired carbon dioxide. In this case, if the capnometer shows a low or absent end-tidal carbon dioxide reading, or if the colorimetric device shows a tan color (low carbon dioxide), observe for chest rise, auscultate bilaterally for air movement, and attempt to visualize the tube passing through the vocal cords by direct laryngoscopy. If the endotracheal tube seems to be in proper position, leave the tube in place.

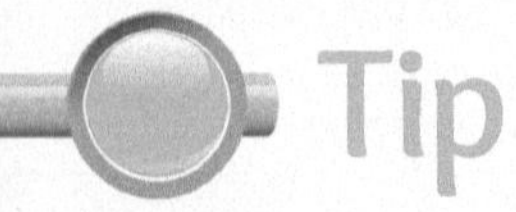

If an esophageal bulb or syringe is used, cardiac arrest and low pulmonary blood flow should not affect the result.

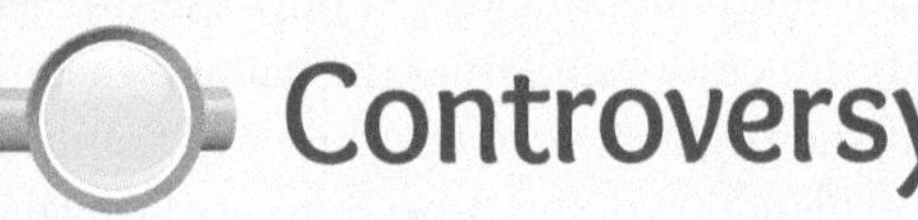

The optimal method for tube confirmation in children in the out-of-hospital setting is not known.

If an esophageal bulb or syringe is used, cardiac arrest and low pulmonary blood flow should not affect the result. If air is aspirated, the tube is in the trachea. Hence, the esophageal bulb or syringe technique for confirmation of endotracheal tube placement may offer an advantage over the other two techniques in the setting of cardiac arrest and low pulmonary blood flow.

For a step-by-step explanation of these confirmation procedures, see **Confirmation of Endotracheal Tube Placement, Procedure 12.**

Summary of Management of Respiratory Failure

Respiratory failure or arrest can result from many different insults to the airway, mechanics of breathing, or gas exchange. Infection, trauma, and bronchospasm are important causes in children. Think respiratory failure when primary assessment reveals a child with altered appearance in the setting of significantly increased or decreased work of breathing. Bradycardia, poor air movement, and low oxygen saturation are key findings. In a child with respiratory failure or respiratory arrest, immediately begin assisted ventilation with a bag-mask device at an age-appropriate rate. Avoid gastric insufflation. Add specific treatment for airway obstruction, such as an inhaled bronchodilator, if indicated. Perform endotracheal intubation cautiously and be alert for the frequent "DOPE" complications in the intubated child who suddenly worsens or fails to respond. Always confirm proper placement of the endotracheal tube with capnometry, colorimetric carbon dioxide detection, or an esophageal bulb or syringe. In some EMS systems, advanced or alternative breathing techniques are options in the child who cannot be ventilated by bag-mask ventilation or endotracheal intubation.

Primary Assessment: The Transport Decision—Stay or Go?

When a child has respiratory distress, begin general noninvasive treatment (position of comfort and oxygen) and consider specific treatment on scene. Never transport a child who is in respiratory failure without assisted ventilations. Also, never transport a child with a severely obstructed airway until after performing FBAO maneuvers. Immediate on-scene care to support breathing improves the outcomes of children with many respiratory emergencies. After opening the airway and providing assisted ventilation when necessary, or after simply giving general treatment, the prehospital professional must decide whether to stay on scene to assess further and treat specifically, or to go.

If the PAT and ABCDEs are normal and the child has no history of serious breathing problems, the child does not usually require urgent treatment or immediate transport. Take the time to get a focused history and physical examination and perform a detailed physical examination (trauma patient) on the scene if possible.

If the child has respiratory distress and signs of upper airway obstruction, transport is usually indicated after general noninvasive treatment. Consider specific treatment of suspected croup with a dose of nebulized epinephrine on the way to the ED, if available. *If the child has asthma and has lower airway obstruction with wheezing, begin specific treatment with bronchodilators on scene, and continue treatment during transport to the closest medical facility.* Call in advance and let the ED know of what kind of patient is being transported to their facility.

For critical children, consider endotracheal intubation or other advanced or alternative airways if the child is in respiratory failure and ventilation by bag-mask device is ineffective, or if an airway is difficult to maintain. However, endotracheal intubation increases scene time and delays the time to definitive care at the ED. There has been a high rate of complications documented in prehospital studies of endotracheal intubation in children. Intubation skills tend to extinguish rapidly because they are used infrequently. In most cases, bag-mask ventilation is probably a better option.

Additional Assessment

If the child has minimal respiratory distress and there are no immediate safety concerns for the child or prehospital professional, consider obtaining the focused history and physical examination and performing a detailed physical examination (trauma patient) on scene. Use the SAMPLE mnemonic to find important features of the complete respiratory history. **Table 3-9** gives examples of a focused history in a child with a breathing problem.

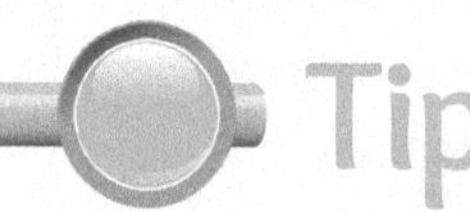

When a child fails to respond to assisted ventilation with improvement in clinical status, quickly assess your equipment—from the oxygen tank to the patient—for mechanical failure.

Perform vigilant ongoing assessment of all children with respiratory distress or failure while on the way to the ED. Use the PAT to recall observational indicators of effective gas exchange, and watch respiratory rate, heart rate, and pulse oximetry. Be prepared to increase the level of respiratory support or to correct complications of therapy if the child worsens or fails to respond.

Table 3-9 SAMPLE Components in a Child With Respiratory Distress

Component	Explanation
Signs and symptoms	Onset and nature of shortness of breath Presence of hoarseness, stridor, or wheezing Presence and quality of cough; chest pain
Allergies	Known allergies: food, medications, environmental Cigarette smoke exposure
Medications	Exact names and doses of ongoing drugs, including metered dose inhalers, and over-the-counter medications Recent use of steroids Timing and amount of last dose Timing and dose of analgesics and antipyretics
Past medical problems	History of asthma, chronic lung disease, or heart problems or prematurity Prior hospitalizations for breathing problems Prior intubations for breathing problems Immunizations
Last food or liquid	Timing of the child's last food or drink, including bottle or breastfeeding
Events leading to the injury or illness	Evidence of increased work of breathing Fever history

CASE STUDY ANSWERS

Case Study 1 — page 50

This child is in respiratory distress but does not seem to have progressed to respiratory failure. He is exhibiting many of the signs and symptoms of upper airway obstruction. His loud, harsh inspiratory breath sounds are consistent with stridor. This sound along with the supraclavicular and suprasternal retractions help localize the obstruction to the upper airway. He has increased work of breathing, but does not show any signs of hypoxia or hypercapnia (carbon dioxide retention). Upper airway obstruction and stridor in a young child after a few days of an upper respiratory infection are most consistent with croup, a swelling in the trachea below the area of the vocal cords caused by a viral infection. Other problems that may cause upper airway obstruction include foreign bodies; bacterial infections (e.g., epiglottitis or retropharyngeal abscess); and airway edema caused by allergic reactions.

Regardless of the cause, the management of children with upper airway obstruction is similar and is based on the severity of the symptoms. Keep this patient in a position of comfort, give oxygen, and transport to an ED for further care.

ALS

Nebulized medications (e.g., epinephrine or racemic epinephrine) act as vasoconstrictors and decrease airway edema. These may be helpful en route to the ED. The child should be closely monitored because his upper airway obstruction may progress and respiratory failure may develop.

Case Study 2 — page 58

This is a choking child who needs first BLS maneuvers and, if unsuccessful, progression to ALS maneuvers by removing the FBAO using pediatric Magill forceps. This cannot be accomplished until the patient becomes unconscious. If the level of training prohibits the use of ALS skills, rapid transport to the ED while continuing chest compressions and ventilation or calling for an ALS intercept should be considered.

Case Study 3 — page 64

Using the PAT, this child has an increased work of breathing, abnormal appearance, and poor circulation to the skin. She is in respiratory failure. Her wheezes and subcostal and intercostal retractions localize her airway obstruction to her lower airways. In the setting of preceding upper respiratory symptoms, fever, and progressive lower airway obstruction, the child probably has bronchiolitis. Open the child's airway, give high-flow oxygen, and begin bag-mask ventilation. Do not delay transport because the child is not likely to have an easily reversible condition. This is unlike the child with asthma, who will likely benefit from a dose of a bronchodilator begun on scene, before transport.

ALS

En route, nebulized albuterol (salbutamol) or nebulized epinephrine may be given based on local protocol. Positive-pressure ventilation has a risk of complications in patients with lower airway obstruction, and it may be wise to wait to see if bronchodilators lead to improvement in this patient.

During transport monitor the child's respiratory status closely. Any evidence of decreased respiratory effort or slowing of the respiratory rate should prompt initiation of positive-pressure ventilation with a relatively slow rate and a long expiratory time.

SUGGESTED READINGS

Textbooks

American Heart Association. *Textbook of Pediatric Advanced Life Support.* Dallas, TX: American Heart Association; 2011.

Gausche M. *Pediatric Airway Management for the Prehospital Professional.* Burlington, MA: Jones and Bartlett Learning; 2004.

Articles

Anders J, Brown K, Simpson J, Gausche-Hill M. Evidence and controversies in pediatric prehospital airway management. *Clin Pediatr Emerg Med.* 2014;15(1):28–37.

Bhende MS, Thompson AE, Orr RA. Evaluation of an end-tidal CO_2 detector during pediatric cardiopulmonary resuscitation. *Pediatrics.* 1995;96(5 Pt 1):983.

Brownstein D, Shugerman R, Cummings P. Prehospital endotracheal intubation of children by paramedics. *Ann Emerg Med.* 1996;28:34–39.

Gausche M, Lewis R, Stratton S, et al. Effect of out-of-emergency department pediatric tracheal intubation on survival and neurologic outcome: controlled clinical trial. *JAMA.* 2000;283:783–790.

Kellner JD, Ohlsson A, Gadomski AM, et al. Efficacy of bronchodilator therapy in bronchiolitis—a meta-analysis. *Arch Pediatr Adolesc Med.* 1999;153(4):430.

Menon K, Sutcliffe T, Klassen T. A randomized trial comparing the efficacy of epinephrine with salbutamol in the treatment of acute bronchiolitis. *J Pediatr.* 1995;126:1004–1007.

Qureshi F, Pestian J, Davis P, et al. Effect of nebulized ipratropium on hospitalization rates of children with asthma. *N Engl J Med.* 1998;339:1030–1035..

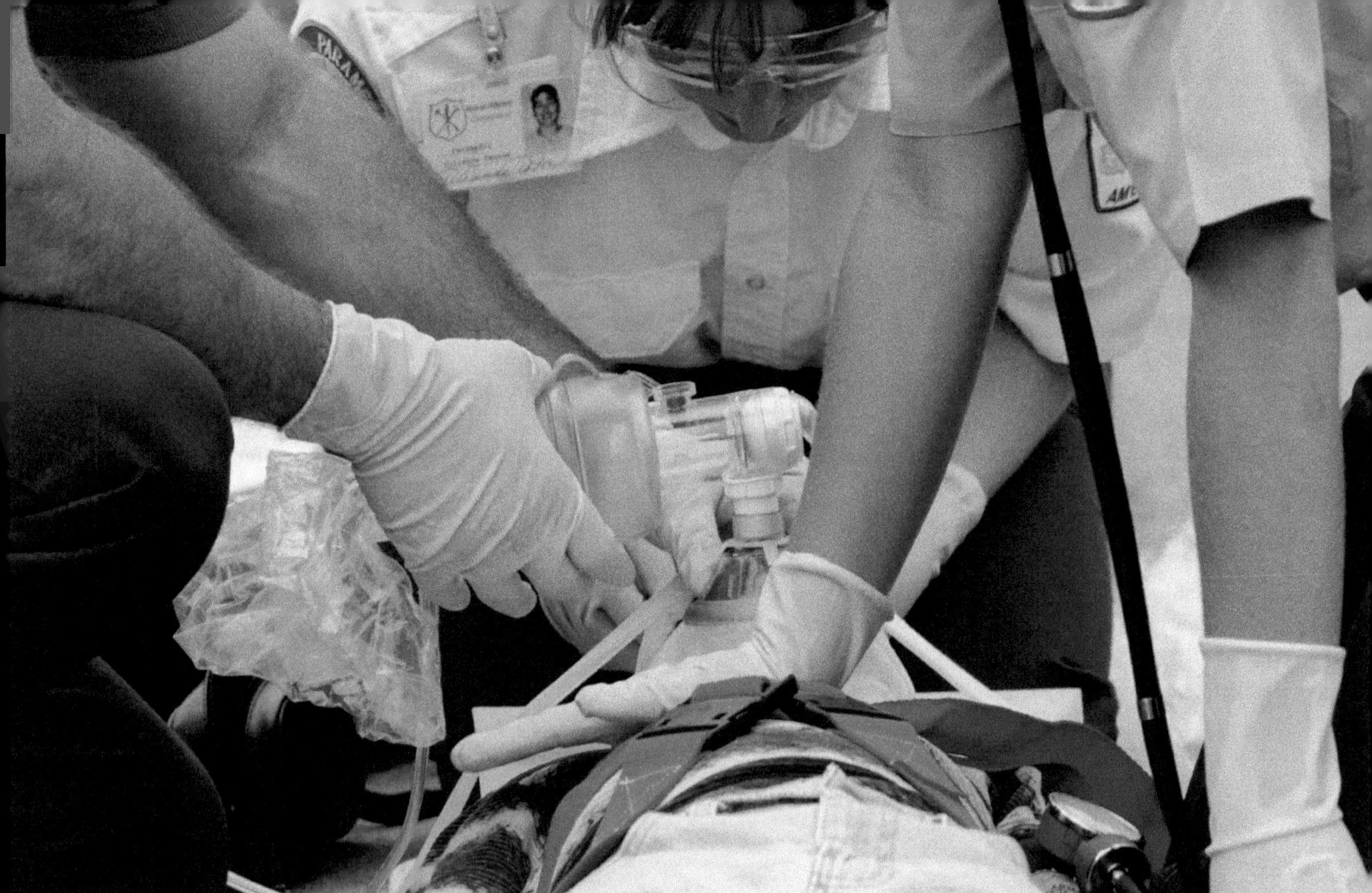

Learning Objectives

1. Describe how to assess circulation using the PAT, ABCDEs, and additional assessment.
2. Explain the relationship between shock and blood pressure.
3. Differentiate between compensated and hypotensive (decompensated) hypovolemic shock, and discuss appropriate management.
4. Distinguish the types of shock (hypovolemic, distributive, cardiogenic, and obstructive) and outline treatment.

Shock

Chapter 4

Introduction

Shock as a pediatric problem is uncommon in the out-of-hospital setting. Emergencies involving shock, or inadequate perfusion, may be the result of hypovolemia, increased vascular permeability, cardiac failure, output obstruction, or a combination of any or all of these causes. Hypovolemia is the usual cause of inadequate perfusion in children, most commonly precipitated by acute gastrointestinal losses from viral illnesses. Traumatic hemorrhage is a less frequent etiology for severe hypovolemia in children. Regardless of the type of emergency involving hypoperfusion, early recognition and timely management can reduce the likelihood for serious morbidity or mortality.

Most perfusion problems in children arise from loss of intravascular fluid. The child's young, healthy cardiovascular system compensates for fluid loss by increasing heart rate and reducing blood flow to nonessential anatomic areas through the mechanism of peripheral vasoconstriction, or "clamping down." Vasoconstriction limits blood flow to less essential peripheral sites, such as the skin, and preserves blood flow to the "core" organs, such as the brain, heart, and kidneys. The physiologic process of restricting circulation to such areas as the skin and mucous membranes results in important physical signs of hypoperfusion.

Distributive shock is less common in children and is usually caused by sepsis. This type of shock primarily involves loss of vascular tone. Additionally, distributive shock can result from anaphylaxis, spinal cord injury, and toxin exposures.

Cardiogenic shock is unusual in pediatrics, except in children with congenital heart disease, dysrhythmias, or acquired viral myocarditis. Cardiogenic shock results from heart rates that are either too fast or too slow to support perfusion, or from primary congestive heart failure. Regardless of the underlying cause, cardiac output is insufficient to meet perfusion requirements.

Obstructive shock is the rarest of all shock types in children. It is caused by pericardial tamponade or tension pneumothorax, secondary to injury to the chest. A third cause, pulmonary emboli, is extremely rare in children.

Identifying the type of shock can be difficult, especially when the pathophysiology is mixed. For example, bacterial toxins or ingested poisons may have adverse effects on vascular tone and myocardial function; sepsis may involve a volume deficit from third spacing (loss of plasma from the vascular space because of leaky blood vessels) and loss of vascular tone and myocardial depression. However, a careful history and physical assessment usually identify the cause of shock and drive appropriate management. Shock from any cause, if unrecognized or inadequately treated, may advance to cardiac arrest. After arrest has occurred, successful resuscitation is unlikely.

Case Study 1

A father calls 9-1-1 about an 18-month-old boy with a fever of 6 hours duration. On your arrival, the child is listless. He will not interact and cries inconsolably when held. There is a purplish rash of the face, trunk, and legs. There are no abnormal airway sounds. Breathing is rapid without retractions or flaring. The brachial pulse is faint, the skin is warm to touch, and capillary refill time (CRT) is about 4 seconds. Respiratory rate is 60 breaths/min, and blood pressure is 60 mm Hg by palpation. The cardiac monitor shows a heart rate (HR) of 190 beats/min.

1. What type of shock is present?
2. What differs in the management of this case versus treatment of pure hypovolemic or cardiogenic shock?

Prearrival Preparation

Based on the dispatch information, prepare mentally for the assessment and management of a child with circulatory problems en route to the scene. Recall appropriate techniques for assessment, the role of vital signs, and the possible equipment, drug, and fluid requirements of the child. Consider when to stay and treat on scene and when to transport immediately.

Scene Size-Up

Be sure that the scene is safe. Evaluate the environment and document potentially important features, especially concerns for child maltreatment.

General Assessment: The Pediatric Assessment Triangle

Evaluating the Presenting Complaint

On arrival, determine the child's presenting complaint. Key questions include the onset of illness, presence of fever, frequency and amount of fluid losses (vomiting and diarrhea), when the child last ate or drank, and prior history of possible congenital or cardiovascular problems. Ask if the child has been injured. In children with mild circulatory compromise who are not in shock, obtain a more complete SAMPLE history (**Table 4-1**) during the additional assessment.

Assessment of Circulation

Using the Pediatric Assessment Triangle

The Pediatric Assessment Triangle (PAT) is the first step in assessment of perfusion, as outlined in Chapter 1. The PAT evaluates three characteristics: (1) appearance, (2) work of breathing, and (3) circulation to skin. Knowing these characteristics helps to determine whether the child is sick or not sick, the type of physiologic abnormality, and the urgency for treatment. Circulatory problems affect each of these characteristics in identifiable patterns.

Appearance

First, assess the child's appearance. A child with decreased core circulation from any shock type may have signs of poor brain perfusion. The abnormality in the child's appearance will be variable, depending on the type of perfusion problem, the degree of circulatory insufficiency, and the presence of associated problems, such as fever, head trauma, or intoxication. Abnormalities in the appearance of a child with decreased core circulation include the following:

- Lethargy or listlessness
- Decreased motor activity
- Diminished interactiveness with caregivers, the prehospital professional, and the environment (**Figure 4-1**)
- Inconsolability
- Poor eye contact
- Weak cry

Sometimes the child in shock is restless and inconsolable. Appearance alone, however, is not a very accurate sign of inadequate perfusion. An abnormal appearance may be caused by many different things, such as poor oxygenation and ventilation, head trauma, hypothermia, drugs, or fever. Assessing appearance is a good way to tell if the child is ill, but not a good way to identify the physiologic cause. Assessment tools other than the PAT, such as the hands-on ABCDE assessment, help distinguish the type of physiologic problem and the presence or absence of abnormal perfusion.

Work of Breathing

Next, assess the work of breathing. If circulation to vital organs is decreased, the child's respiratory rate increases.

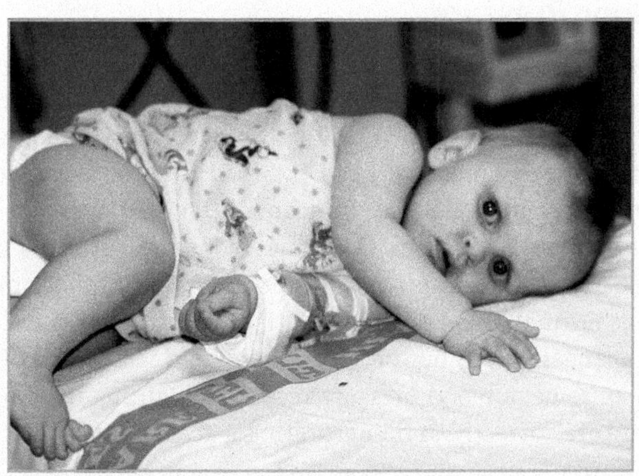

Figure 4-1 A child with decreased core circulation and too little blood and oxygen to the brain has an abnormal appearance. This dehydrated child has listlessness, poor motor activity, and decreased interactiveness.

"Effortless tachypnea," sometimes known as "silent tachypnea," is a fast respiratory rate without increased work of breathing. Effortless tachypnea is a common but nonspecific sign of shock. It reflects the child's attempt to blow off carbon dioxide and reduce the metabolic acidosis created by decreased perfusion to cells. Signs of increased work of breathing, such as abnormal positioning, retractions, flaring, or abnormal airway sounds, such as grunting, stridor, or wheezing, are not usually present in a child without a corresponding respiratory problem. These signs reflect poor gas exchange and hypoxia, typically from a primary lung problem. Although increased work of breathing is most commonly a function of respiratory disease, these signs may also occur with hypoxia and pulmonary edema, when cardiogenic shock results from congestive heart failure, or in anaphylaxis when the respiratory system is a target organ.

Circulation to Skin

After assessing appearance and work of breathing, assess circulation by looking at skin color. This is difficult to interpret if the environmental temperature is low, because vasoconstriction, as a reflexive effort to preserve heat, falsely alters skin findings, especially in infants. Disrobe the child and look for mottling, pallor, and cyanosis, which reflect peripheral vasoconstriction or clamping down of nonessential skin perfusion to maintain essential core circulation. If a child has abnormal appearance and abnormal skin signs in a warm ambient environment, the child may be in shock.

Primary Assessment: The ABCDEs

After the PAT, perform the hands-on ABCDE assessment. After evaluating airway and breathing, as described in the previous chapters, assess circulation. There are four parts to the assessment of circulation: (1) HR, (2) pulse quality, (3) skin temperature and CRT, and (4) blood pressure.

Heart Rate

First, measure HR by feeling a pulse for 30 seconds, and then double the number. A normal HR is between 60 and 160 beats/min, depending on the child's age, as noted in Table 2-3. The radial or brachial areas are preferred sites to measure pulse rate in infants and children. The carotid pulse is acceptable in older children and adolescents, but it is hard to locate in infants. If a pulse is difficult to feel, determine HR by listening to the heart sounds directly with a stethoscope placed on the medial side of the child's left nipple. However, be aware that the presence of a "normal" HR by auscultation does not necessarily reflect adequate cardiac output and perfusion.

Interpreting HR may be difficult, as explained in Chapter 1. Ranges of normal HR change inversely with advancing age. Also, many conditions can increase HR, ranging from serious physiologic problems to noxious stimuli that are rarely life-threatening. Stimuli that can cause tachycardia include pain, fever, fear, cold, and anger. Interpret HR in the context of overall signs of perfusion, age, presence or absence of noxious stimuli, and observed trends. Although a single measurement of HR is usually of limited value in determining the degree of physiologic derangement, a trend of mounting tachycardia, or a HR that is falling below the lower limits of normal, suggests a serious physiologic problem. In addition, sustained tachycardia is a worrisome sign. Finally, be extremely vigilant when the child has bradycardia, because this may mean hypoxia or an advanced state of hypoperfusion.

Pulse Quality

Presence of a strong central pulse (carotid, femoral, or brachial in infants) with a strong peripheral pulse (brachial, radial, or pedal in children) suggests an adequate blood pressure. A strong central pulse with a weak peripheral pulse indicates a shocklike state. If a brachial pulse is not palpable, the child is probably hypotensive and in hypotensive (decompensated) shock.

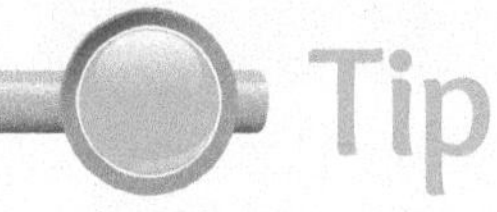

Tip

Tachycardia is often the first sign of shock in a pediatric patient.

Skin Temperature and Capillary Refill Time

The next part of the hands-on cardiovascular assessment involves evaluating skin signs. Check skin temperature for warmth at the hands, feet, thighs, or forearms. Cool hands and feet may be normal, but cool proximal extremities reflect poor perfusion and shunting of blood to the core. Determine CRT by pressing firmly on the skin. CRT should be less than 2–3 seconds in a child who is not cold (**Figure 4-2**). Again, inadequate core perfusion results in peripheral vasoconstriction, which manifests as cool skin and delayed CRT. Although CRT is a good test of circulation in children, it must be interpreted in the context of overall signs of perfusion. The prehospital professional can become comfortable with the technique and interpretation of the key skin findings by practicing on every child.

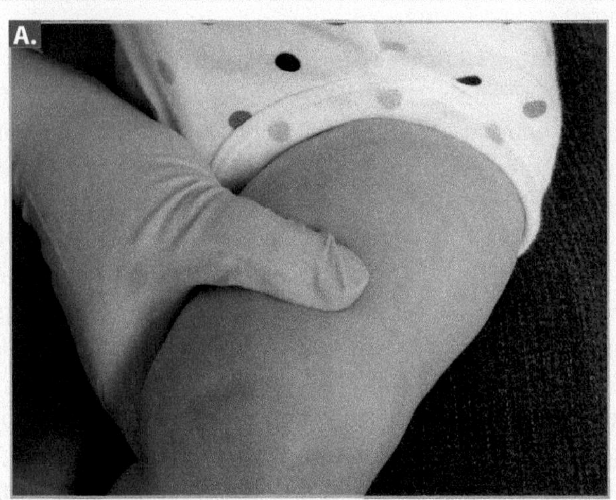

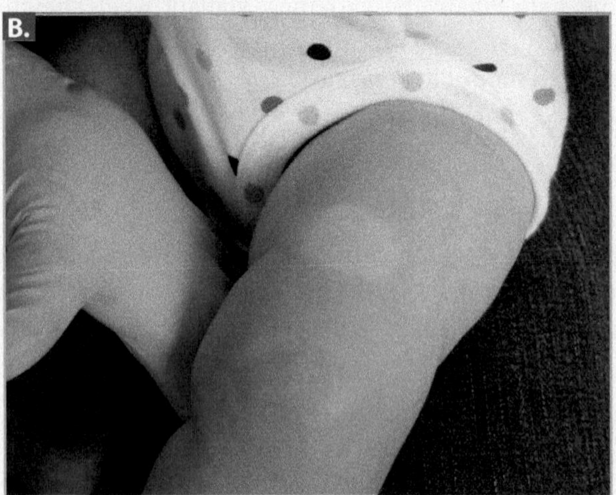

Figure 4-2 To determine CRT, first depress the skin (**A**), and then count the seconds before color returns (**B**). Capillary refill time should be less than 2–3 seconds in a child who is not cold.

Blood Pressure

Last, consider taking a blood pressure. A high blood pressure value is not clinically significant in the field, unless the child has a history of hypertension, known renal disease, or acute head injury. However, a true low blood pressure value is significant and means hypotensive (decompensated) shock. A normal blood pressure does not rule out a shocklike state. Children in significant shock may have normal blood pressures until they decompensate. The challenges in the out-of-hospital setting include knowing when to get a blood pressure reading, obtaining the blood pressure correctly, and interpreting it accurately.

Systolic blood pressure does not accurately reflect intravascular volume status until the acute volume loss is greater than 25%–35% of normal circulating pediatric blood volume. This is because of the efficiency of compensation in a child, including vasoconstriction and an increase in HR. Therefore, a normal blood pressure does not mean the child has a normal blood volume or normal perfusion. A normal minimal systolic blood pressure in a child older than 1 year of age is 70 + (2 × years of age). Proper equipment, technique, and patience are required to obtain an accurate blood pressure in an infant or toddler. Because this can be a time-consuming process and may not contribute greatly to the clinical assessment of perfusion, in a child 3 years old or younger, attempt a blood pressure measurement only once or skip altogether. Inadequate perfusion is better reflected in the other signs of perfusion described previously (skin color, HR, pulse quality, CRT, and skin temperature).

In a child older than 3 years of age, make at least one blood pressure attempt in every patient. Use a cuff with a width two-thirds the length of the upper arm. Applying too large a cuff falsely decreases the blood pressure measurement, and too small a cuff falsely increases the measurement.

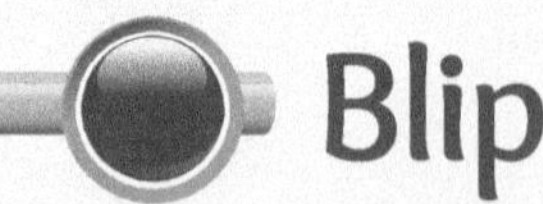

A normal blood pressure does not rule out shock.

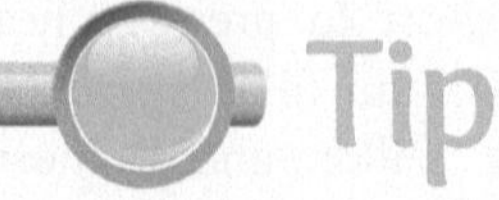

In children, one can use the combination of tachycardia, poor pulse quality, delayed CRT, and decreased mental status to diagnose shock, even with a normal blood pressure.

Additional Assessment

If the child is stable after the primary assessment and does not require immediate treatment, and if there are no immediate safety concerns for the child or prehospital professional, conduct history taking and physical examination and the detailed physical examination (trauma patient) on scene. Use the SAMPLE mnemonic (**Table 4-1**) to recall important features of the history in a child with inadequate perfusion. Use age-appropriate approaches to gain the child's trust and speak directly to him or her. Ask the caregiver to add to the child's history. Obtain the history from the caregiver if the child is too young to speak or is unable to cooperate.

After the history, perform a focused examination of the heart, peripheral circulation, and the abdomen. Then, do an anatomic examination of the entire body, as outlined in Chapter 1. If the child has a traumatic injury, also do a detailed physical examination, searching for other injuries.

Perform an ongoing assessment of all children with perfusion problems while on the way to the emergency department (ED). The child's status may change during transport, so observe and document any physiologic trends. Use the PAT to monitor effective perfusion and watch respiratory rate, HR, blood pressure, and pulse oximetry. Keep a child who is in shock on a cardiac monitor. Be prepared to increase the level of respiratory and cardiovascular support if the child worsens or fails to respond to treatment.

Table 4-1 SAMPLE Components in a Child With Hypoperfusion Problems

Component	Features
Signs/ Symptoms	Presence of vomiting or diarrhea Number of episodes of vomiting or diarrhea Vomiting blood or bile External hemorrhage Presence or absence of fever Rash Respiratory distress or shortness of breath (e.g., in cardiogenic shock with congestive heart failure)
Allergies	Known allergies History of anaphylaxis
Medications	Exact names and dosages of ongoing medications Use of laxatives or antidiarrheal medications Chronic diuretic therapy Potential exposure to other medications or drugs Timing and doses of analgesic/antipyretics
Past medical problems	History of heart problems History of prematurity Prior hospitalizations for cardiovascular problems
Last food or liquid	Timing of the child's last food or drink, including bottle or breastfeedings
Events leading to the injury or illness	Travel Trauma Fever history Symptoms in family members Potential toxic exposure

Summary of Cardiovascular Assessment

The PAT provides a good first-line evaluation of perfusion: abnormal appearance, normal work of breathing, and poor circulation to skin suggest a perfusion problem. Pallor, mottling, and cyanosis all indicate poor peripheral perfusion. The circulatory portion of the hands-on ABCDEs consists of evaluating HR, pulse quality, skin temperature, CRT, and blood pressure. These physical features complement the PAT and help identify the type and severity of circulatory compromise. Vital signs can sometimes be misleading and must be correctly obtained and interpreted for age. Trends in vital signs or persistence in abnormal vital signs, such as tachycardia, are more accurate indicators of real physiologic problems than mild vital sign abnormalities on primary assessment.

Using the Assessment to Identify Shock

Shock is inadequate perfusion at the tissue level, with insufficient oxygen delivery to maintain normal cellular function. Oxygenation and ventilation, HR, intravascular volume, myocardial function, and vascular stability are all determinants of effective systemic cardiovascular function. If any one of these factors is impaired by illness or injury, the body attempts to compensate and normalize perfusion through modification of other physiologic components.

In a child, the same physiologic components are at work as in an adult. However, there are some differences. The physiologic compensatory mechanisms, such as vasoconstriction and tachycardia, are very efficient in a child. Vasoconstriction is so efficient that a line of demarcation can sometimes be seen on extremities and mottling may be evident when circulation to the capillary beds has become stagnant. Sweating as a response to compensation, although common in an adult, does not always occur in a young child. Therefore, most children in shock have cool, dry skin versus pale, cool, diaphoretic skin. By adolescence, sweating as a response to compensation for shock is consistent. The last difference involves the child's energy reserves. A child does not have the amount of energy reserves that are had by an adult. The younger the child, the less is the capacity for energy reserves. Infants in particular have high glucose needs with low energy stores. As a result, compensatory mechanisms, although efficient, cannot last as long as those of an adult. This is one of the reasons why a child tends to decompensate quickly. This is also why checking a blood glucose level is important in any child who is under stress or has an altered mental status.

Because of these differences, clinical signs of decreased perfusion include altered mental status, persistent tachycardia as a compensatory mechanism, and changes in skin color and temperature as a result of vasoconstriction. Do not expect sweating unless the child has increased work of breathing and is building up body heat, as in a congenital cardiac condition. As long as vasoconstriction, increased HR, and increased myocardial contraction are supported by the child's reserves, systolic pressure is maintained and the child compensates. When the body's reserves begin to fail or are exhausted, perfusion to the vital organs, such as the brain, is compromised. Blood pressure falls, mental status is impaired, and organ systems fail.

There are four general classes of shock (hypovolemic, distributive, cardiogenic, and obstructive) (**Table 4-2**) reflecting impairment of the three major functional components of circulation: (1) the blood volume (hypovolemic), (2) the vascular system (distributive), and (3) the heart (cardiogenic and obstructive). Studies of hypovolemia (the most common type of pediatric shock) have allowed researchers to describe the clinical signs that characterize the progression of shock from a compensated state (adequate systolic

Table 4-2 Summary of Different Types of Shock

Shock Type	Physiologic Insult	Common Causes	Treatment
Hypovolemic	Volume loss	Hemorrhage Gastroenteritis (vomiting, diarrhea) Burns Prolonged poor fluid intake	Rapid transport Intravenous fluid boluses
Distributive	Decreased vascular tone	Sepsis Anaphylaxis Drug overdose Spinal cord injury (neurogenic shock)	Rapid transport Fluid administration Epinephrine for anaphylaxis Dopamine or epinephrine for septic shock
Cardiogenic	Heart failure	Congenital heart disease Cardiomyopathy Dysrhythmia Drug overdose	Rapid transport Cautious crystalloid fluid administration, 10 mL/kg Consider a vasopressor, such as dopamine, dobutamine, or epinephrine
Obstructive	Obstructed blood flow	Pericardial tamponade Pneumothorax	Rapid transport Needle thoracostomy Fluid administration

Case Study 2

9-1-1 receives a call about a lethargic 12-year-old boy. On your arrival, he is lying in bed and barely notices your entrance. There is no increased work of breathing, but you do notice that he is breathing fast. His color is pale. Vital signs are as follows: HR, 160 beats/min; RR, 40 breaths/min; BP, 80/40 mm Hg; SpO_2, 99% in room air. His capillary refill is 4 seconds. His mother states that he has been vomiting for 2 days and has had diarrhea for 1 day.

1. **Is this patient in shock?**
2. **If so, what type of shock is this?**
3. **What is the prehospital treatment?**

blood pressure) to an uncompensated state (hypotension). However, the clinical signs characterizing the progression of distributive, cardiogenic, or obstructive shock are not as well defined. This reflects the complex physiology of these other forms of shock.

Hypovolemic Shock

Hypovolemia (loss of fluid) is the most common cause of shock in children in the out-of-hospital setting. Vomiting and diarrhea from gastroenteritis is the most common cause of hypovolemic shock. Bleeding from blunt injuries, such as falls or vehicle collisions with the child as a pedestrian, bicyclist, or passenger, is the most common cause of hemorrhagic hypovolemic shock.

The signs and symptoms of hypovolemic shock vary with the amount, duration, and timing of fluid loss. As intravascular volume is further compromised by ongoing fluid losses (such as profuse diarrhea or continued bleeding), the child may progress from compensated to decompensated shock.

Compensated Hypovolemic Shock

Children who lose bodily fluids through minor blood loss or dehydration from gastroenteritis usually show no clinically significant effects on circulation. However, if fluid losses are more than about 5% of body weight, the body compensates for decreased blood flow by predictable adjustments in cardiovascular physiology. Sympathetic stimulation results in vasoconstriction and an increase in HR or tachycardia. As long as these processes maintain cardiac output to core organ systems, perfusion is maintained. This is compensated shock.

Vasoconstriction causes the following signs of abnormal circulation to the skin: delayed CRT, decreased pulse strength, poor skin color (pallor or mottling), and dry and cool or cold skin temperature. A cold environment or hypothermia may also cause vasoconstriction as a reflex to maintain body heat, which mimics poor perfusion. Systolic blood pressure is normal in compensated shock.

In the compensated stage of hypovolemic shock, appearance may be normal, or the child may appear slightly restless or less interactive. In a child with gastroenteritis, the appearance may be abnormal because of fever, which can alter appearance regardless of the circulatory status.

Hypotensive Hypovolemic Shock

In hypotensive (decompensated) shock, perfusion is profoundly affected because compensatory mechanisms (increased HR and peripheral vasoconstriction) have failed to maintain sufficient circulation to core organs. The clinical signs are those of organ failure. Although a child in hypotensive shock may still be alert on AVPU, assessment of appearance is abnormal because of inadequate brain perfusion. The child may be restless and agitated, or poorly responsive. Hypotension, or low blood pressure for age, develops when there is about a 25% loss of intravascular volume (blood volume). Other late signs are effortless or silent tachypnea, extreme tachycardia, extreme pallor or presence of mottling, and cold skin temperature. If not reversed, hypotensive shock leads to cardiac failure, with bradycardia and respiratory failure, and then to cardiac arrest.

Although the course is less predictable, decreasing perfusion in children with distributive, cardiogenic, or obstructive shock results in progressive changes in appearance, skin signs, and work of breathing. For example, a child with cardiogenic shock may present only with tachycardia and diminished peripheral perfusion, and then progress to respiratory distress and lethargy as cardiac output worsens and congestive heart failure develops. In all shock types, hypotension is an ominous sign. More than one type of shock can occur concurrently in the same patient, as previously described.

Distributive Shock

In distributive shock, the child has decreased vascular muscle tone (peripheral vasodilation), impaired vascular integrity, or both in the presence of a normal circulating blood volume. This creates a relative hypovolemia, and can be thought of as operating with a "less than full" tank. This change in the capacity of the vascular system and relative hypovolemia leads to hypoperfusion to vital organs because of loss of vascular integrity. Patients with distributive shock may also have a component of hypovolemia. This is the case in a patient with sepsis, who in addition to loss of vascular tone has "capillary leak" caused by the effect of bacterial toxins, or in the case of anaphylaxis where capillary leak may occur in the lungs or in the target tissues. In these situations, hypovolemia is the result of "third spacing" of fluid from the vascular space into the surrounding tissues.

The most common cause of distributive shock is sepsis, especially in children younger than 2–3 years of age. In addition to anaphylaxis, chemical intoxication with drugs that decrease vascular tone (e.g., β-blockers, barbiturates) and spinal cord injury (above T6) with interruption of spinal sympathetic nerves to the muscle walls of peripheral arteries can cause distributive shock.

Special Features in Assessment of Distributive Shock

Signs of distributive shock reflect low peripheral vascular resistance (warm skin, bounding pulses, wide pulse pressure, changes in HR, hypotension) and decreased organ perfusion (abnormal appearance and behavior). These signs may vary with the specific cause, as noted in the descriptions of the three major types of shock. Although the progression of physical signs in distributive shock is not as predictable as that in hypovolemic shock, the late findings are indistinguishable from those of hypotensive shock from any cause: abnormal appearance from poor brain perfusion and hypotension.

Major Types of Distributive Shock

Sepsis

Sepsis occurs when any type of infection, usually bacterial or viral, overwhelms the body's defense system and causes a generalized breakdown in core organ function. Distinctive signs of early septic shock are warm skin, tachycardia, and bounding pulses. A septic child's appearance is abnormal and may include listlessness, lethargy, decreased interactiveness, restlessness, and poor consolability. Rash, fever, poor feeding, vomiting, diarrhea, and fussiness may also be present.

Ill children usually like to be held and cuddled. If a child with a fever does not want to be held but is more comfortable when left alone, the child may have paradoxical irritability. This may be a sign of meningitis, where movement irritates the inflamed meninges (membranes covering the spinal cord and brain).

Sometimes, a septic child has a petechial rash or purpura (nonblanching dark red or purple dots or splotches) (**Figure 4-3**). These skin lesions are the result of toxins that cause inflammation of the blood vessels and leakage of blood into the skin. Consider a child with shock in association with a rash and fever to be septic. He or she may require aggressive volume resuscitation in the field, and prehospital professionals should use strict infection-control practices, including masks, to decrease their risk of infection.

Anaphylaxis

Anaphylaxis is a major allergic reaction that involves a generalized, multisystem response to an antigen (foreign protein). The airways and cardiovascular system are important sites of this often life-threatening reaction. Common causes include insect stings by bees, wasps, or fire ants; peanuts; latex; or medication. A child in anaphylactic shock has hypoperfusion and possibly additional signs, such as stridor or wheezing, with increased work of breathing. The child also has altered appearance with restlessness and agitation and sometimes a sense of impending doom. Hives (an intensely itchy skin rash) (**Figure 4-4**) and angioedema (flushed, swollen skin) are also common. Signs and symptoms of anaphylactic shock are dependent on the target organ. This is why some victims of anaphylaxis present with vomiting, diarrhea, and hives, whereas others have angioedema, wheezing, and stridor.

Shock From Drug Intoxication

There are numerous cardiovascular drugs that can cause loss of vascular tone and hypoperfusion when ingested. **Table 4-3** lists common agents. The mechanism usually involves direct depressant effect on the cardiovascular system (slowing of the HR and decreased strength of contraction, and vasodilation).

Neurogenic Shock

Neurogenic shock is rare in children. It results from a mechanism of injury that involves the back, neck, or both, and interrupts nervous system pathways. There is a loss of the autonomic nervous system's sympathetic control of circulation. This is observed when the injury occurs at T6 or above. The result is vasodilation and impaired sympathetic

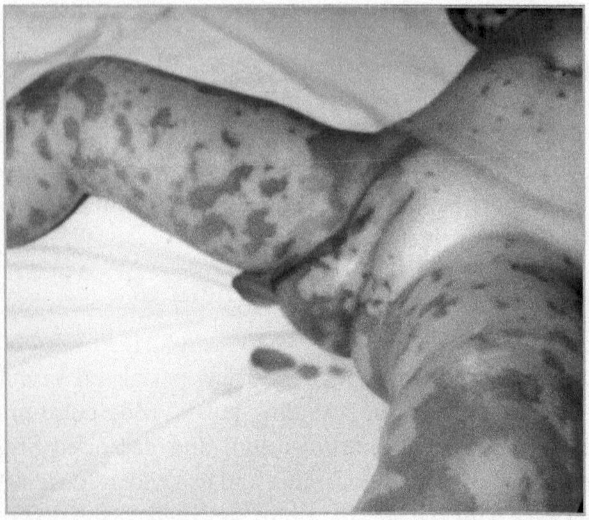

Figure 4-3 Purpura.

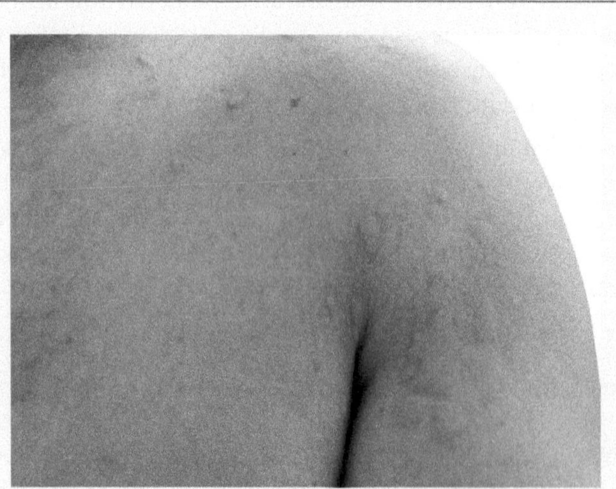

Figure 4-4 Hives suggest an allergic reaction and are usually present with anaphylaxis, the most extreme form of an allergic reaction.

Table 4-3 Drug Intoxications That May Cause Shock

Antihypertensives β-blockers Calcium antagonists Clonidine
Cyclic antidepressants
Iron
Opioids
Phenothiazines

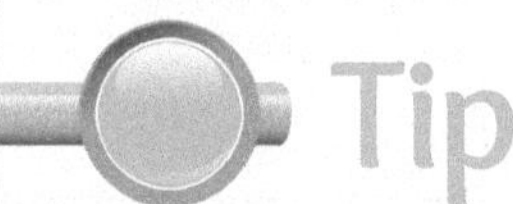

If a trauma patient has a normal or slow HR and low blood pressure, think spinal cord injury and neurogenic shock.

stimulation of the heart. The child has motor paralysis and is hypotensive and bradycardic, with loss of the normal tachycardic response to actual or relative hypovolemia. With loss of the normal vascular reflex to maintain body heat, the body also loses heat to the environment.

Cardiogenic Shock

Cardiogenic shock is uncommon in children and is rarely diagnosed in the prehospital arena unless the child has a known cardiac history (**Figure 4-5**). In fact, the child's condition may be misdiagnosed as septic or hypovolemic shock, resulting in the administration of fluid boluses and adrenergic agents. The most likely cause is either congenital heart disease, dysrhythmia, or cardiomyopathy from myocarditis. Myocarditis is a disease of the heart muscle, usually caused by a virus. A dysrhythmia, such as supraventricular tachycardia (SVT) or bradycardia (<60/min), may also cause cardiogenic shock. Overdose with a cardiac medication, such as a calcium channel blocker or β-blocker, is another possible etiology.

Special Features in Assessment of Cardiogenic Shock

A history from the caregiver usually reveals that the child has had nonspecific symptoms, such as loss of appetite, poor feeding, lethargy, irritability, and inappropriate sweating over a period of days. The sweating is caused by the increased work load (work of breathing or work of the heart) and is an attempt to cool off the body. This is true of children with myocarditis and congenital heart disease. There is often a history of congenital heart disease or the presence of a midline chest scar from heart surgery. **Table 4-4** summarizes the common symptoms and signs of cardiogenic shock.

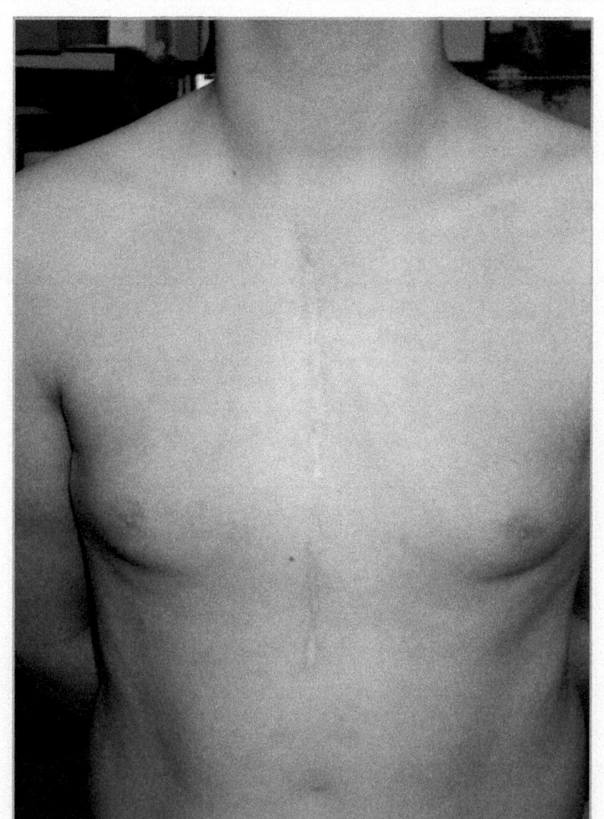

Figure 4-5 A midline sternal scar is an indicator of a cardiac history.

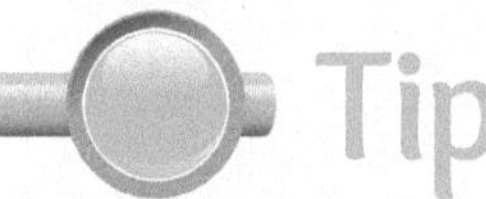

Cardiogenic shock can occur from HRs that are too fast or too slow.

Cardiogenic shock may develop from left heart failure. Impaired left heart function causes decreased core organ perfusion. On physical assessment, the child may appear abnormal: sluggish, irritable, or agitated, and the skin color mottled or cyanotic. Heart rate is rapid; blood pressure may be high (early), normal, or low (late). The skin is cool and the child may be diaphoretic (not dry as with hypovolemic shock) related to the increased work load. Pulmonary edema causes increased work of breathing and inspiratory crackles or wheezing. The increased work load may deplete energy stores resulting in hypoglycemia. Checking blood glucose levels is recommended.

Increased right-sided cardiac pressures are also present in cardiogenic shock and result in liver enlargement (hepatomegaly). Hepatomegaly is an especially useful finding in infants and toddlers. Peripheral edema and jugular venous distention are rare in children. Cardiogenic shock can also

Table 4-4 Symptoms and Signs of Cardiogenic Shock

Possible historical findings in cardiogenic shock
1. Preceding history of chest pain
2. Previous history of flulike symptoms associated with weakness and fatigue
3. Difficulty feeding because of fatigue and sweating during feeding in the breast or bottle fed infant
4. No history of fever
5. No history of volume loss (e.g., diarrhea, vomiting, or blood loss)
6. Positive history of congenital heart disease
7. No history of asthma despite wheezing on examination
8. Persistent wheezing despite the administration of β-agonist (e.g., albuterol [salbutamol])
9. History of cyanosis
10. Recent history of exercise intolerance
Possible physical findings
1. Tachypnea or grunting with clear lungs on examination
2. Unexplained dysrhythmias in the presence of a flulike illness
3. Tachycardia disproportionate to the degree of fever
4. Persistent or worsening tachycardia despite fluid administration
5. Heart murmur, friction rub, or gallop on examination
6. Presence of cyanosis that does not improve with the administration of oxygen
7. Crackles on lung examination
8. Peripheral edema or pitting edema
9. Hepatomegaly

occur from HRs that are too fast or too slow. Because the origin of a rate-related problem is often congenital, assessment and treatment are discussed under congenital cardiac problems.

Obstructive Shock

Several pathologic conditions may obstruct blood flow from the heart and cause shock. Pericardial tamponade and tension pneumothorax are two acute conditions that cause dramatic development of shock after blunt or penetrating injuries to the chest wall. Hemopericardium develops quickly after a gunshot or sharp object penetrates into a blood-filled heart chamber, usually the right ventricle. Blunt trauma to the chest at just the right time during the cardiac cycle can produce pressures great enough to rupture the tendons stabilizing the cardiac valves or rupture the tissue between the chambers of the heart. The hole in the wall of the heart provides a route for blood to escape into the space between the two pericardial membranes. Because the membranes do not stretch quickly, blood collects and collapses the right ventricle (tamponade). This interrupts venous return to the right heart and produces a profound drop in cardiac output.

Rarely, pericardial tamponade may develop after an infectious or inflammatory process in the chest. Cancer or chronic renal failure causes pericardial fluid accumulation. This type of fluid accumulation is slow and the membranes around the heart stretch. Therefore, obstructive shock caused by infectious or inflammatory processes rarely occurs.

Tension pneumothorax develops after a penetration into the pleural space. Sometimes blunt injury to the chest wall can also rupture alveoli, causing a pneumothorax, which may rapidly progress to a tension pneumothorax when vigorous ventilation with a bag-mask device occurs. Air and sometimes blood (hemothorax) collects in between the two membranes of the pleura. When the pressure increases enough to cause a shift of the mediastinum, venous return to the right heart is impaired. This causes a drop in cardiac output and hypoperfusion.

In children or adolescents with cystic fibrosis, the lung may have blebs that rupture spontaneously, resulting in a pneumothorax, which can progress to a tension pneumothorax.

Special Features in Assessment of Obstructive Shock

Penetrating injuries to the chest wall are often deceptive. The appearance of the wound may be benign and seem superficial. Consider all gunshot wounds or stab wounds to the chest as major penetrations into the heart or pleura. Other types of penetrations from sticks or sharp objects may also cause severe internal injury. Be especially vigilant when the penetration has an entry site in the area between the two nipples and the clavicles, because this is a high-risk location for cardiac injury. Blunt chest injury may also cause a pneumothorax that may progress to a tension pneumothorax. Suspect this condition in a child with a significant blunt mechanism of injury and signs of obstructive shock.

The cardinal features of obstructive shock are signs of decreased circulation in an injured child with increased jugular venous distention. The increased jugular pressures reflect the obstruction to venous return to the right ventricle. Sometimes, however, blood loss into the chest (hemothorax) or other related injuries may be associated with hemorrhage, so that jugular venous distention is not apparent. In the case of a tension pneumothorax, lung sounds are unequal or absent on the affected side, and ventilation is increasingly difficult.

General Noninvasive Treatment of Suspected Shock of All Types

Begin general noninvasive treatment of every child with suspected hypoperfusion after completing the PAT and initiating the hands-on ABCDEs. The general treatment is always the same: allow the child to assume a position of comfort if the cause is medical. In the case of trauma, the child needs spinal stabilization. Supply oxygen, as tolerated. This is the only management for most patients.

Positioning

Infants and toddlers may be most "comfortable" in their caregiver's arms or lap during assessment. If the primary assessment indicates that the child is physiologically unstable, place the child in a position of comfort that decreases his or her anxiety and activity. This is usually the supine position (**Figure 4-6**). Elevating the legs when the child is in the supine position is not effective. Putting the child in a head-down position is not known to improve outcome. In a head-down position, the internal organs of the abdomen put pressure on the diaphragm, interfering with breathing. The resulting agitation increases oxygen demand and complicates treatment. In the supine position, alignment of the airway is aided by placing a towel under the shoulders and trunk of the child. This helps with ease of breathing. Keep the child warm because children have a high surface-to-volume ratio and can lose body heat rapidly.

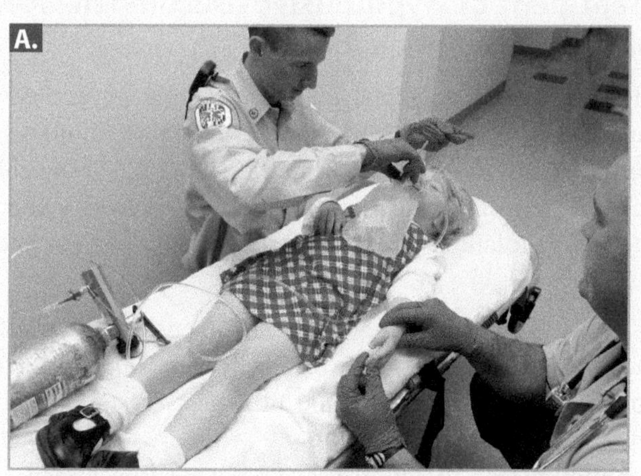

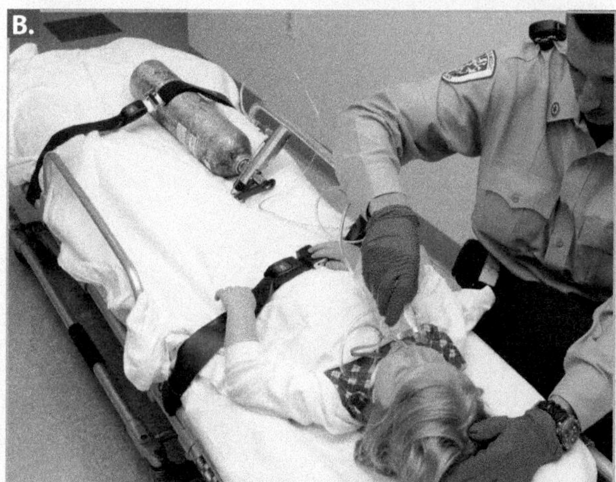

Figure 4-6 A. Treat suspected hypovolemic shock with high-flow oxygen and supine positioning. **B.** Keep the patient warm.

Oxygen

Treat all children in shock with high-flow oxygen. The prehospital professional must weigh the potential benefits of oxygen administration against the risk of agitating the child. "Blow-by" may be the only mechanism for delivering supplemental oxygen without upsetting the child and increasing his or her oxygen consumption.

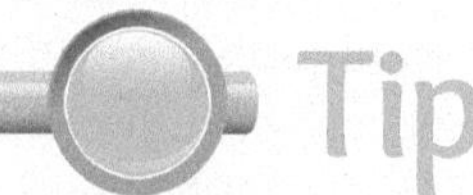

Provide high-flow oxygen to all children in shock.

Specific Treatment of Hypovolemia

After the primary assessment and beginning general supportive measures, provide additional specific treatment of shock. If the child has hypovolemic shock, consider how to stop the child's fluid losses and whether to attempt to replace them. In trauma patients, always look carefully for bleeding sites and assume there may be internal bleeding. Apply direct pressure to stop external bleeding. Consider appropriate immobilization and splinting of injured extremities, as described in Chapter 6.

ALS

If the child has severe fluid losses from vomiting or diarrhea, consider obtaining vascular access to give fluids. If the child has hypotensive shock from illness, attempt an intravenous (IV) placement once in the field. Any further attempts should be made during transport to avoid a prolonged scene time. If the child is in extremis or unconscious, consider an intraosseous (IO) needle insertion.

Intravenous Access

Intravenous (IV) access makes it easier to give medications and provides a way to give fluid therapy in severe blood or fluid loss. IV delivery is the gold standard for giving medication, because it permits rapid drug and fluid treatment and allows titration of important drugs. See **Intravenous Access, Procedure 15.**

ALS

IV Fluid Treatment of Compensated Hypovolemic Shock

If the child has mild-to-moderate volume losses as determined by HR, pulse quality, CRT, and skin temperature, and has a normal blood pressure, he or she is in compensated shock. Do not remain on scene to perform IV insertion and fluid administration. On the way to the hospital, consider obtaining vascular access and giving IV crystalloid fluid at 20 mL/kg boluses to stabilize the patient. The patient may require additional fluid boluses up to a total of 60 mL/kg or the patient has a clinical response.

IV Fluid Treatment of Hypotensive (Decompensated) Shock

If the child has decompensated shock from illness, make one attempt on scene to establish vascular access. If the child is injured, delay all vascular access attempts until en route to the ED. This is in contrast to ongoing traumatic hemorrhage where the value of establishing access and initiating volume resuscitation at the scene may be outweighed by continued blood loss. Once access is established during transport, give 20 mL/kg boluses of IV crystalloid fluid. Consider intraosseous (IO) needle insertion, if vascular access cannot be obtained quickly and the child is unconscious. Repeat boluses (20 mL/kg up to 60 mL/kg) as needed to stabilize perfusion, based on ongoing reassessment of the PAT and vital signs.

IO Needle Insertion

Using an IO needle to give drugs or fluids is an excellent alternative to cannulating peripheral veins. The IO space is highly vascularized and functions as a noncollapsible vein. Needle insertion into this space is quick, simple, effective, and usually safe. Complications are infrequent and usually minor. See **Intraosseous Needle Insertion, Procedure 16.**

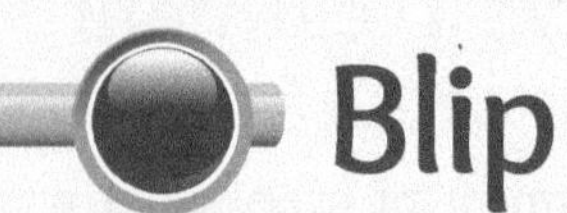

Blip

In a child with hypovolemic shock, crystalloid fluid boluses need to be given as fast as possible. Do not let the fluid just drip in.

Specific Treatment of Distributive Shock

The primary difference between treatment of distributive and hypovolemic shock is the potential need for a vasopressor agent to improve vascular tone and heart muscle function when the child has distributive shock. Treat all shock conditions first with general noninvasive measures. Administer 100% high-flow oxygen and put the poorly responsive child with shock in a supine position.

ALS

Treatment of Hypotensive (Decompensated) Distributive Shock

Attempt a vascular access on scene at least once. Deliver fluid boluses, up to 60 mL/kg of a crystalloid fluid solution in 20 mL/kg boluses on the way to the ED. If the child has lost protective airway reflexes or has refractory shock, support ventilation with bag-mask device or endotracheal intubation.

If cardiovascular instability (hypotension, markedly increased HR, and poor responsiveness) persists after volume therapy with up to 60 mL/kg of crystalloid fluid, try a vasopressor agent (dopamine or epinephrine). Do not administer a vasopressor agent if you suspect untreated hypovolemia.

Case Study 3

A 6-year-old boy in kindergarten is having trouble breathing, so the teacher calls 9-1-1. On your arrival, the boy has swollen eyes, but answers your questions about his name and age. He has increased work of breathing with audible wheezing. There are hives on his face and arms. The teacher says he has a peanut allergy and may have eaten a birthday cake with nuts. Vital signs are as follows: HR, 150 beats/min; RR, 50 breaths/min; BP, 90/50 mm Hg; SpO_2, 90% in room air.

1. Is this child in shock?
2. What is the appropriate prehospital therapy?

ALS

Treatment of Anaphylaxis

A child with anaphylaxis requires fluid and special treatment with epinephrine, a β-agonist if bronchospasm is present, and methylprednisolone. If hives and angioedema are present, diphenhydramine may also be necessary. Unlike a simple allergic reaction, anaphylaxis has dangerous cardiovascular effects (**Figure 4-7**).

Epinephrine is an excellent drug for treatment of anaphylaxis. It stimulates α- and β-adrenergic receptors, leading to two important effects: (1) constriction of the blood vessels to help counter the vasodilation and increased permeability of anaphylaxis (alpha effect), and (2) opening up the airways to help reverse the bronchospasm of anaphylaxis (beta effect). For all children with allergic reactions associated with wheezing, administer epinephrine, 0.01 mg/kg (0.01 mL/kg) of 1:1,000 solution (maximum, 0.3 mg or 0.3 mL) intramuscularly (IM).

Epinephrine is a short-acting drug. Therefore, it is necessary to follow up with a long-acting steroid, such as methylprednisolone. Methylprednisolone (1–2 mg/kg IV/IO; maximum, 60 mg) acts to stabilize mast cell membranes to prevent perpetuation of the reaction by chemicals triggered by the allergic reaction. Research suggests that the earlier the administration of methylprednisolone after treatment of the acute problem, the better the outcome.

If hives or angioedema are present, diphenhydramine (1 mg/kg orally, IV, or IO; maximum, 50 mg) may also be necessary. Diphenhydramine works as a histamine blocker, specific for the histamine receptors that reside in the walls of the blood vessels and in the skin. Administration of this medication eases itching.

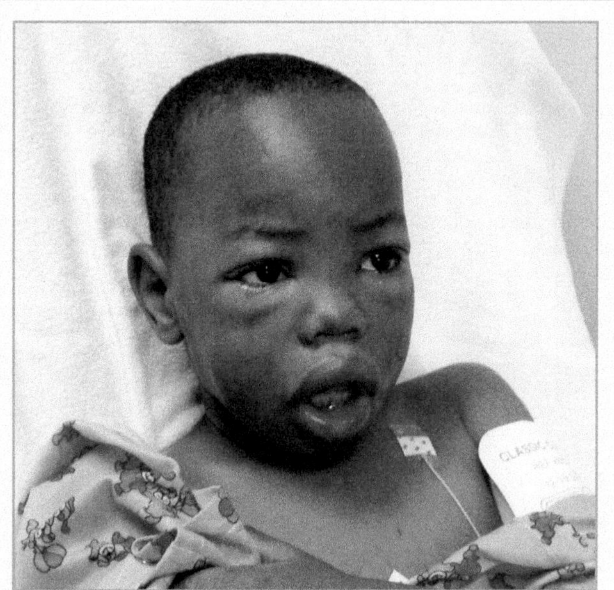

Figure 4-7 An allergic reaction, with edema of face, lips, and tongue.

Treatment of Cardiogenic Shock

If cardiogenic shock is suspected by history or physical assessment, transport after general noninvasive treatment. On the way to the ED, consider vascular access. If the diagnosis of cardiogenic shock is uncertain, give a cautious fluid bolus of only 10 mL/kg of crystalloid fluid, and then reassess appearance, work of breathing, CRT, HR, and blood pressure. If there is no rhythm disturbance on the cardiac monitor (rate-related problems are discussed in Chapter 5) and the child remains poorly perfused after the initial fluid bolus, consider a vasopressor agent (dobutamine, dopamine, or epinephrine) if the transport time is long. Start vasopressors at low doses, based on micrograms per kilogram, and then titrate to achieve acceptable perfusion (improved appearance and skin circulation and decreased HR and respiratory rate). If the child is known to be in congestive heart failure with cardiogenic shock, avoid fluid boluses and consider vasopressor therapy as front-line treatment if perfusion is severely compromised.

The major difference between treatment of hypovolemic, distributive, and cardiogenic shock is the amount of fluid administration and consideration of a vasopressor.

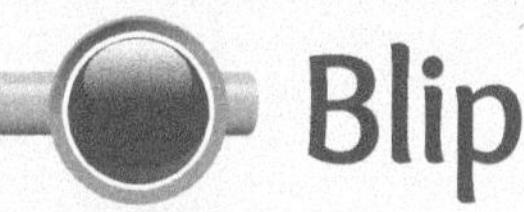

Blip

Do not withhold fluid from a child in cardiogenic shock; just give it in boluses of 10 mL/kg and reassess.

ALS

Treatment of Obstructive Shock

The additional option for treatment of obstructive shock from a tension pneumothorax is needle thoracostomy to decrease air pressure, as explained in **Needle Thoracostomy, Procedure 22.**

This technique does not remove blood, but relieves pressure in the pleural space. Rapid transport is an essential feature of field management of chest injury.

Primary Assessment: Transport Decision

After completing the primary assessment and beginning general treatment when appropriate, the prehospital professional must decide whether to go or stay on scene. If the PAT and ABCDEs are normal and the child has no history of serious illness or injury mechanism, no anatomic abnormalities, and no pain, the child does not usually require urgent treatment or immediate transport. Take the time to get a history and physical examination and perform a detailed physical examination (trauma) on the scene if possible.

If the child has a serious mechanism of injury, a physiologic or anatomic abnormality, severe pain, or if the scene is not safe, transport immediately. With such patients, do the additional assessment and attempt specific treatment on the way to the hospital, if possible.

The transport decision is sometimes difficult in a child with a suspected cardiovascular problem who needs vascular access. If the child is in compensated shock and has a palpable brachial pulse or normal blood pressure, stabilize the spine (if the child is injured), manage the airway and breathing, control hemorrhage, and transport immediately. Attempt vascular access for specific treatment on the way to the ED.

If the child is in hypotensive (decompensated) shock, the prehospital professional has several options, depending on the clinical condition of the child, local EMS system regulations, comfort level, and the time to the nearest ED. If the child is injured, always transport immediately. If the child is ill with abnormal appearance and hypotension, consider attempting a vascular access once on scene, and then transporting without delay.

Summary of Shock States

There are four major classes of shock seen both in children and adults: (1) hypovolemic, (2) cardiogenic, (3) distributive, and (4) obstructive. Hypovolemic shock is commonly the result of trauma and hemorrhage after injury. Vomiting and diarrhea leading to dehydration is the most common medical cause of hypovolemia. Distributive shock may result from sepsis, anaphylaxis, drug intoxication, or spinal injury. Always suspect sepsis in the infant or toddler who has fever and abnormal appearance. A petechial or purpuric skin rash is a red flag for sepsis. Cardiogenic shock caused by inadequate left ventricular contraction is rare in children and difficult to identify in the field, unless the child has a known congenital cardiac problem. Obstructive shock sometimes occurs in conjunction with significant chest wall injury. Clinical findings may reflect more than one type of shock pathophysiology. Treatment of all shock types includes general noninvasive interventions, and then specific treatment based on clinical findings. Consider rapid fluid boluses in children who are hypotensive with an abnormal appearance.

CASE STUDY ANSWERS

Case Study 1 — page 74

This child has septic or distributive shock. He has decompensated shock with hypotension. The rash is an ominous sign and aggressive treatment is necessary to save the child's life. The appropriate first interventions are oxygen and bag-mask ventilation.

Attempt IV or IO access on scene once and give a 20 mL/kg crystalloid fluid bolus as fast as possible. Then transport and deliver 20 mL/kg fluid boluses to a maximum of 60 mL/kg while en route to the ED. Consider giving a vasopressor agent (dopamine, dobutamine, or epinephrine) if perfusion remains poor after fluid administration and the transport time is long. Endotracheal intubation may be necessary.

This case also requires universal precautions to protect the prehospital professional because the child has a serious communicable disease. Direct specific questions about exposures and prophylactic treatment to your infection control personnel.

Case Study 2 — page 78

This child is in hypotensive (decompensated) shock, because his blood pressure is low. The etiology is likely hypovolemia, because of the history of vomiting and diarrhea. His lethargy can be caused by shock, but could also be caused by hypoglycemia. Prehospital treatment is attempt IV or IO access on scene and give a 20 mL/kg normal crystalloid fluid bolus as fast as possible. Then transport and give additional 20 mL/kg fluid boluses to a maximum of 60 mL/kg while en route to the ED. A bedside glucose can also be obtained, and if it is low, 50% dextrose given, in addition to the IV fluids. In this case, his glucose is 50 mg/dL, and his weight is 40 kg, so 40 mL of 50% dextrose (or 80 mL of 25% dextrose) can be administered.

Case Study 3 — page 84

This is a case of anaphylaxis, and although this child is not in shock at this time, it could still develop. Anaphylaxis requires urgent treatment of 0.01 mg/kg of epinephrine 1:1,000 IM. This child weighs 20 kg, so the dose is 0.2 mg (0.2 mL). Administration of albuterol via a nebulizer may help his wheezing. Insertion of an IV now can be useful to give IV diphenhydramine and methylprednisolone (if carried). If his blood pressure begins to drop (anaphylactic shock), a rapid infusion of 20 mL/kg normal crystalloid fluid bolus is indicated.

SUGGESTED READINGS

Textbooks

American Academy of Pediatrics and the American College of Emergency Physicians. *APLS: The Pediatric Emergency Medicine Resource.* 5th ed. Burlington, MA: Jones and Bartlett Learning; 2012.

American Heart Association. *2010 Handbook of Emergency Cardiovascular Care for Healthcare Providers.* Hazinski MF, Samson R, Schexnayder S, eds. Dallas, TX: American Heart Association; 2010.

Hazinski MF, Mondozzi MA, Baker RA. Shock, multiple organ dysfunction syndrome, and burns in children. In: McCance KL, Heuther SE, Brashers VL, Rote NS, eds. *Pathophysiology: The Biologic Basis for Disease in Adults and Children.* 6th ed. St. Louis, IL: Mosby Elsevier; 2010:1727–1752.

Articles

Brierly J, Carcillo JA, Choong K, et al. Clinical practice parameters for hemodynamic support of pediatric and neonatal septic shock: 2007 update from the American College of Critical Care Medicine. *Crit Care Med.* 2009;37(2):666–688.

deCaen AR, Maconochie IK, Aickin R, et al. Part 6: Pediatric basic life support and pediatric advanced life support; 2015 International Consensus and Cardiopulmonary Resuscitation and Emergency Cardiovascular Care Science with Treatment Recommendations. *Circulation.* 2015;132 (suppl 1):S177–S203.

Han Y, Carcillo J, Dragotta, et al. Early reversal of pediatric-neonatal septic shock by community physicians is associated with improved outcome. *Pediatrics.* 2003;112(4):793–799.

Kleinman, ME, Chameides L, Schexnayder SM, et al. Part 14: Pediatric advanced life support: 2010 American Heart Association Guidelines for Cardiopulmonary Resuscitation and Emergency Cardiovascular Care. *Circulation.* 2010;122 (suppl 3):S876–S908.

Morris MC. Pediatric cardiopulmonary-cerebral resuscitation: an overview and future directions. *Crit Care Clin.* 2003;19(3):337–364.

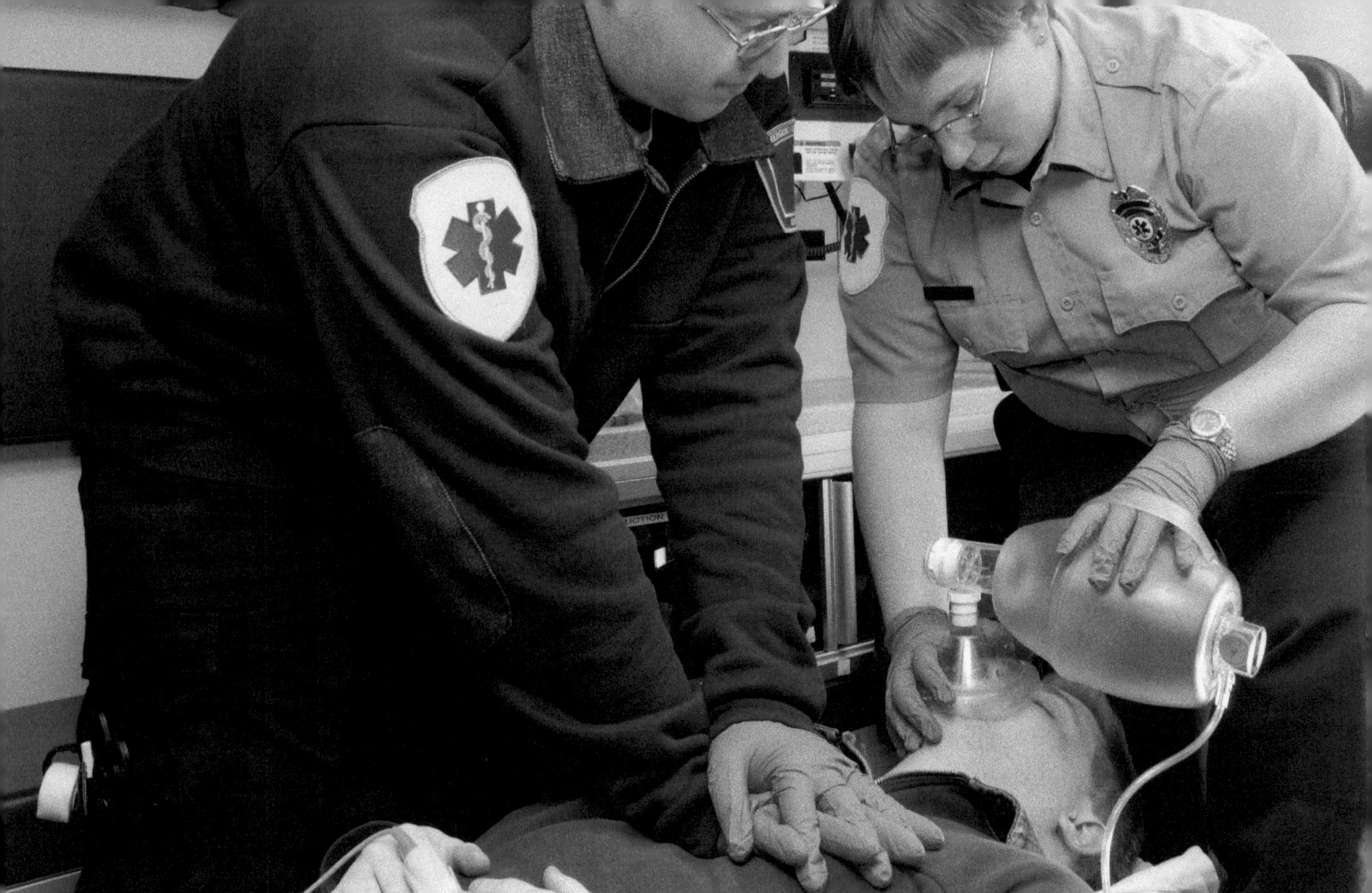

Learning Objectives

1. Describe how to assess circulation using the Pediatric Assessment Triangle (PAT), ABCDEs, and additional assessment.
2. Explain when to treat tachycardia and bradycardia, and discuss management.
3. List the links in the pediatric "Chain of Survival."
4. Order the steps in managing pediatric cardiac arrest caused by asystole, pulseless electrical activity (PEA), ventricular fibrillation (VF), and pulseless ventricular tachycardia (VT).
5. Define indications for the use of the automated external defibrillator (AED) in pediatric patients.
6. Describe the causes of primary cardiac arrest in the pediatric patient.
7. Discuss medical issues in children with congenital heart disease who may present to the prehospital professional.

Resuscitation and Dysrhythmias

Chapter 5

Introduction

Cardiac arrest is uncommon in the out-of-hospital setting. Survival to discharge from out-of-hospital cardiac arrest is 6% (3% for infants and 9% for children and adolescents). The primary cause of arrest in children is usually an asphyxial arrest situation that deteriorates into cardiac arrest.

A large number of patients who present in cardiac arrest demonstrate **ventricular fibrillation (VF)** or **ventricular tachycardia (VT)**. The incidence of acquired cardiac conditions, such as atherosclerotic heart disease, dysrhythmias, or congestive heart failure (CHF), is rare in children. Regardless of the type of cardiovascular emergency, early recognition and timely management can reduce the likelihood for serious morbidity or mortality.

Prearrival Preparation

Based on dispatch information, the provider needs to be prepared to assess, manage, and make transport decisions for a child exhibiting a symptomatic cardiac dysrhythmia, cardiac event, or cardiac arrest. Recall appropriate techniques for assessment, the role of vital signs, and the possible equipment, medications, fluid requirements, AED, and electrical therapy a child may require. Consider when to stay and treat on scene and when to transport immediately.

Scene Size-Up

All providers need to ensure that the scene is safe, and note any significant findings that may be contributing factors to the situation. The provider must also assess the scene, as appropriate, for signs of child maltreatment.

General Assessment: The PAT

Evaluating the Presenting Complaint

On arrival, determine the child's presenting complaint. Gathering a complete patient history is a vital component in determining the cardiac event the patient may be experiencing. Attempt to gather a complete SAMPLE history (see **Table 5-1**) during the primary assessment.

Case Study 1

You have been dispatched for a 7-year-old child who is unconscious and not breathing. You arrive at a soccer complex and find the child lying supine. The child seems to be unconscious, and you note the patient to be cyanotic. The child is unresponsive, not breathing, and has no pulse. You begin CPR while attaching the AED.

1. How does management of VF or VT differ from treatment for pulseless electrical activity (PEA) or asystole?
2. Why should cardiopulmonary resuscitation (CPR) be started as rapidly as possible and continued without interruptions as much as is possible?

Assessment of Circulation

Using the PAT

The PAT is the first step in assessment of circulation, as outlined in Chapter 1. The PAT evaluates three characteristics: (1) appearance, (2) work of breathing, and (3) circulation to skin. Knowing these characteristics helps to determine whether the child is sick or not sick, the type of physiologic abnormality, and the urgency for treatment. Circulatory problems affect each of these characteristics in identifiable patterns.

Appearance

First, assess the child's appearance. A child with decreased core circulation from any cardiac compromise may have signs of poor brain perfusion. The abnormality in the child's appearance will be variable, depending on the type of perfusion problem and the degree of circulatory insufficiency. Abnormal features in the appearance of a child with decreased core circulation include the following:

- Lethargy or listlessness
- Decreased motor activity for infants, poor muscle tone
- Diminished interactiveness with caregivers, the prehospital professional, and the environment
- Inconsolability
- Poor eye contact
- Weak cry

Sometimes the child with hemodynamic instability will be restless and inconsolable. *Appearance alone, however, is not a very accurate sign of circulatory problems.* Assessing appearance is a good way to tell if the child is ill, but not a good way to identify the physiologic problem. Assessment tools other than the PAT, such as the hands-on ABCDE assessment, will help distinguish the type of physiologic problem and the presence or absence of abnormal perfusion.

Work of Breathing

Next, assess the work of breathing. If circulation to vital organs is decreased, the child's respiratory rate will increase. "Effortless tachypnea," or a fast respiratory rate without increased work of breathing, is a common but nonspecific sign of hemodynamic instability. It reflects the child's attempt to blow off carbon dioxide and reduce the metabolic acidosis created by decreased perfusion to cells. Signs of increased work of breathing, such as abnormal positioning, retractions, flaring, or abnormal airway sounds, such as grunting, stridor, or wheezing, are not usually present in a child with a pure circulatory problem. These signs reflect poor gas exchange and hypoxia, typically from a primary lung problem.

Circulation to Skin

After assessing appearance and work of breathing, assess circulation by looking at skin color. This will be difficult to interpret if the environmental temperature is low, because vasoconstriction, as a reflexive effort to preserve heat, will falsely alter skin findings, especially in infants. Disrobe the child and look for mottling, pallor, and cyanosis, which reflect peripheral vasoconstriction or clamping down of nonessential skin perfusion to maintain essential core circulation. If a child has abnormal appearance and abnormal skin signs in a warm ambient environment, the child may be hemodynamically unstable.

Primary Assessment: The ABCDEs

After the PAT, perform the hands-on ABCDE assessment. After evaluating airway and breathing, as described in the previous chapters, assess the circulation. There are four parts to the assessment of circulation:

1. Heart rate
2. Pulse quality
3. Skin temperature and capillary refill time
4. Blood pressure

Table 5-1 SAMPLE Components in a Child With Cardiovascular Problems

Component	Features
Signs/symptoms	Presence of vomiting More cyanotic than usual Lower pulse oximeter reading Number of episodes of vomiting Presence or absence of fever Rash Respiratory distress or shortness of breath (e.g., in cardiogenic shock with CHF)
Allergies	Known allergies and what reaction occurs History of anaphylaxis
Medications	Exact names and dosages of ongoing medications Chronic diuretic therapy Potential exposure to other medications or drugs Timing and doses of analgesics or antipyretics
Past medical problems	History of heart problems or heart surgery History of prematurity Prior hospitalizations for cardiovascular problems
Last food or liquid	Timing of the child's last food or drink, including bottle or breastfeedings
Events leading to the injury or illness	Travel Trauma Fever history Symptoms in family members Potential toxic exposure

Heart Rate

First, measure heart rate by feeling the pulse for 30 seconds, and then double the number. A normal heart rate is between 60 and 160 beats/min, depending on the child's age, as noted in **Table 5-2**. The radial or brachial areas are preferred sites to measure pulse rate in infants and children. The carotid pulse is acceptable in older children and adolescents, but it is hard to locate in infants. If a pulse is difficult to feel, determine heart rate by listening to the heart sounds directly with a stethoscope placed on the medial side of the child's left nipple. However, be aware that the presence of a "normal" heart rate by auscultation does not necessarily reflect adequate cardiac output and perfusion.

Interpreting heart rate may be difficult, as explained in Chapter 1. Ranges of normal heart rates change inversely with advancing age. Also, many conditions can increase heart rate, ranging from serious physiologic problems to noxious stimuli that are rarely life-threatening. Stimuli that can cause tachycardia include pain, fever, fear, cold, and

Table 5-2 Normal Heart Rate for Age

Age	Heart Rate (beats/min)
Infant	100–160
Toddler	95–150
Preschooler	80–140
School-aged child	70–120
Adolescent	60–100

anger. Interpret heart rate in the context of overall signs of perfusion, age, presence or absence of noxious stimuli, and observed trends. Although a single measurement of heart rate is usually of limited value in determining the degree of physiologic derangement, *a trend of mounting tachycardia, or a heart rate that is falling below the lower limits of normal, suggests a serious physiologic problem*. In addition, sustained tachycardia is a worrisome sign. Finally, be extremely vigilant when the child has bradycardia, because this often indicates hypoxia or may be a sign of profound ischemia.

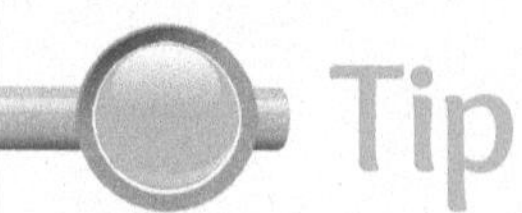

Bradycardia is always a critical sign in a young child and reflects hypoxia or advanced shock.

Pulse Quality

Presence of a strong central pulse (carotid, femoral, or brachial in infants) with a strong peripheral pulse (brachial, radial, or pedal in children) suggests a good blood pressure. A strong central pulse with a weak peripheral pulse indicates compensated shock. If a brachial pulse is not palpable, the child is probably hypotensive and is hemodynamically unstable.

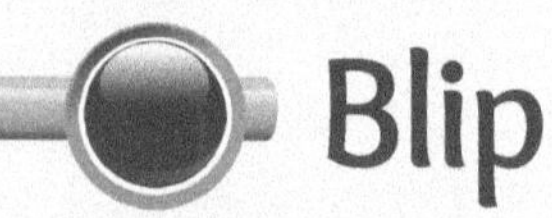

The carotid pulse is an acceptable site for measurement of pulse rate in older children and adolescents, but it is hard to locate in infants.

Skin Temperature and Capillary Refill Time

The next part of the hands-on cardiovascular assessment involves evaluating skin signs. Check skin temperature for warmth at the hands, feet, kneecaps, or forearms. Cool hands and feet may be normal, but cool proximal extremities reflect poor perfusion and shunting of blood to the core. Capillary refill time (CRT) *should be less than 2–3 seconds in a child who is not cold.* Inadequate core perfusion results in peripheral vasoconstriction, which will manifest as cool skin and delayed CRT. Although CRT is a good test of circulation in children, it must be interpreted in the context of overall signs of perfusion. The prehospital professional can become comfortable with the technique and interpretation of the key skin findings by practicing on every child.

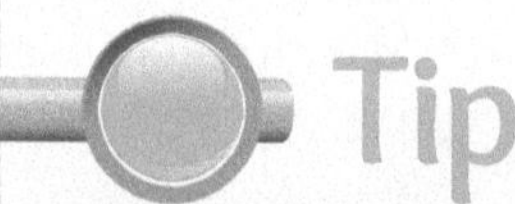

Practice CRT and pulse quality on every child. This will help you to become comfortable with the technique and interpret key findings accurately.

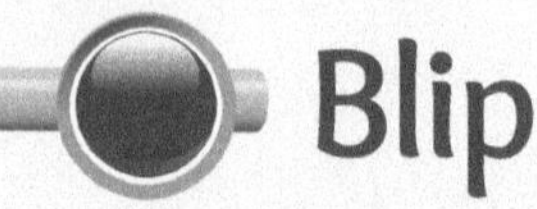

CRT is a good test for circulation in children, but do not place heavy emphasis on this sign alone.

Blood Pressure

Last, consider taking a blood pressure. A high blood pressure value in a child is not clinically significant in the field, unless he or she has a history of hypertension, known renal disease, or acute head injury. However, a true low blood pressure value is significant of hemodynamic instability. The challenges in blood pressure measurement in children in the out-of-hospital setting are: knowing when to get a blood pressure reading; obtaining the blood pressure correctly; and interpreting it accurately.

A normal minimal systolic blood pressure in a child older than 1 year of age is 70 + (2 × years of age). Proper equipment, technique, and patience are required to obtain an accurate blood pressure in an infant or toddler. Because this can be a time-consuming process and may not contribute greatly to the clinical assessment of perfusion, in a child 3 years old or younger attempt a blood pressure measurement only once or skip altogether. Inadequate perfusion will be better reflected in the other signs of perfusion described previously (heart rate, pulse quality, CRT, and skin temperature).

In a child older than 3 years of age, make at least one blood pressure attempt in every patient to provide a baseline for future assessments. Repeated vital signs provide trends that can yield useful information to determine patient severity. Use a cuff with a width that is two-thirds the length of the upper arm. Applying too large a cuff will falsely decrease the blood pressure measurement, and too small a cuff will falsely increase the measurement.

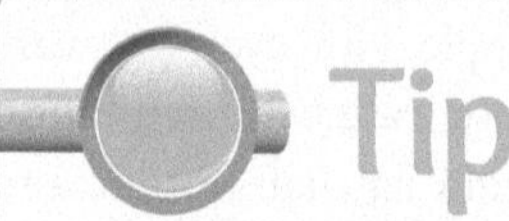

A normal minimal systolic blood pressure in a child older than 1 year of age is 70 + (2 × years of age).

Additional Assessment

If the child is stable after the primary assessment and does not require immediate treatment, and there are no immediate safety concerns for the child or prehospital professional, conduct the focused history and physical examination and the detailed physical examination on scene. Use the SAMPLE and OPQRST mnemonics (**Table 5-3**) to recall important features of the focused cardiovascular history. Use age-appropriate approaches to gain the child's trust and speak directly to him or her. Ask the caregiver to add to the child's history. Obtain the history from the caregiver if the child is too young to speak or is unable to cooperate.

After the focused history, perform a focused examination of the heart, peripheral circulation, and abdomen. Then, do an anatomic examination of the entire body, as outlined in Chapter 1. If the child has a traumatic injury, also do a detailed physical examination, searching for other injuries.

Perform an ongoing assessment of all children with cardiovascular problems while on the way to the emergency department, observing for changes on the cardiorespiratory monitor. The child's status may change during transport, so observe and document any physiologic trends. Use the PAT to monitor effective perfusion and watch respiratory rate, heart rate, blood pressure, and pulse oximetry. Be prepared to increase the level of respiratory and cardiovascular support if the child worsens or fails to respond to treatment.

Table 5-3 The OPQRST of Pain

O—Onset **Key Question:** What were you doing when the pain/discomfort started?
P—Provocation/Palliation **Key Question:** What makes the pain/discomfort better or worse? What have you tried to reduce the symptoms? Did it work? **Support Questions:** Has this ever happened before? If so, when?
Q—Quality **Key Question:** What does the pain feel like?
R—Region/Radiation **Key Question:** Can you point with one finger to the main area of pain/discomfort? **Support Questions:** Do you feel pain anywhere else? If so, can you show me or tell me where it is?
S—Severity **Key Question:** How bad is the pain or chief complaint on a scale of 1 to 10, with 1 being no pain and 10 being extreme pain? **Support Questions:** What is the worst pain you've ever experienced? How does this compare?
T—Time frames **Key Question:** When did you first notice the symptoms? **Support Questions:** Have the symptoms been continuous? If not, has the feeling come and gone?

Summary of Cardiovascular Assessment

The PAT provides a good first-line cardiovascular evaluation: abnormal appearance, normal work of breathing, and poor circulation to skin suggest a perfusion problem. Pallor, mottling, and cyanosis all indicate poor peripheral perfusion. The circulatory portion of the hands-on ABCDEs consists of evaluating heart rate, pulse quality, skin temperature, CRT, and blood pressure. These physical features complement the PAT and will help identify the type and severity of circulatory compromise. Vital signs can sometimes be misleading and must be correctly obtained and interpreted for age. Trends in vital signs, or persistence in abnormal vital signs, such as tachycardia, are more accurate indicators of real physiologic problems than mild vital sign abnormalities on primary assessment.

Dysrhythmias

Bradycardia

In children, bradycardia almost always reflects hypoxia, rather than a primary cardiac problem. It is a prearrest rhythm, and the prognosis is ominous if left untreated. Immediate delivery of high-flow oxygen and assisted ventilation are essential. Untreated bradycardia will quickly cause hemodynamic instability and ultimately death. In children with asthma or respiratory distress, bradycardia means profound hypoxia. Pulse oximetry, when available, will help determine the degree of hypoxia in the field.

Congenital heart block is an extremely rare cause of bradycardia in infancy and early childhood. Drug overdose (e.g., β-blockers, calcium channel blockers, digoxin, clonidine) is another possible cause of bradycardia. Bradycardia may also result from vagal stimulation during medical procedures or gastric tube placement. However, although bradycardia that develops during laryngoscopy or suctioning may be the result of vagal stimulation, hypoxia may be the true cause. If bradycardia does occur in this setting, stop the procedure, administer supplemental oxygen, and reassess the patient.

Bradycardia may also be a normal finding, especially in asymptomatic athletic adolescents. If bradycardia is an isolated finding, without signs of hemodynamic instability in a well-perfused school-aged child or teenager, no treatment is necessary in the field.

Assessment of the Child With Bradycardia

If the child has a heart rate below the normal range for age (see Table 5-2), evaluate carefully for signs of respiratory failure or shock. The PAT and ABCDEs, along with a brief history, will establish the likely cause, the severity of the problem, and the need for urgent treatment.

Treatment of Bradycardia

If the child is asymptomatic, consider no treatment, especially if the child is an adolescent, because slow heart rates are common in athletic teenagers. If the child has bradycardia and a primary assessment demonstrates oxygenation, ventilation, or perfusion abnormalities, provide 100% oxygen with bag-mask ventilation and transport. Check effectiveness of ventilation by observing for chest rise and an improvement in the PAT, heart rate, perfusion, and blood pressure.

In rare situations, chest compressions for bradycardia are necessary. If the heart rate is below 60 beats/min and the child shows signs of poor systemic perfusion after oxygenation and assisted ventilation, begin chest compressions.

ALS

Drug Therapy for Symptomatic Bradycardia. Oxygenation and ventilation are the primary treatments for bradycardia. If the heart rate does not rise in response to assisted ventilation, in most cases administer epinephrine as the first-line drug, give 0.01 mg/kg of the 0.1 mg/mL concentration intravenously (IV) or intraosseous (IO), or 0.1 mL/kg, every 3–5 minutes. If there is increased vagal tone (or poisoning by cholinergic drugs or agents, such as organophosphates) or an atrioventricular heart block, administer atropine, 0.02 mg/kg IV or IO (minimum dose of 0.1 mg, maximum dose of 0.5 mg). When the child has a known reason for cholinergic-mediated bradycardia, such as congenital heart block, give atropine and monitor the response; you may repeat once if indicated.

Before administering vasopressor drugs, always assess for mechanical problems with oxygen delivery and ventilation. Check for disconnected oxygen tubing, poor mask seal, airway obstruction, inadequate chest rise, endotracheal tube blockage, or malposition. Other causes of bradycardia from hypoxia or ischemia are pneumothorax, hypovolemia, cardiomyopathy, poisoning, or increased intracranial pressure.

When oxygenation, ventilation, and drug therapy for bradycardia fail, consider external electrical cardiac pacing of the heart.

Endotracheal Administration of Drugs. If neither IV nor IO access is available for giving drugs during resuscitation, the endotracheal route is an alternative for at least four pediatric drugs: (LEAN) lidocaine, epinephrine, atropine, and naloxone. Although endotracheal drugs are probably not as effective as medications delivered by the IV or IO routes, endotracheal delivery is appropriate in the critical patient until IV or IO access is established. Use the technique for endotracheal drug delivery described in **Endotracheal Tube Drug Instillation, Procedure 19**.

When administering epinephrine through an endotracheal tube to a child who has no vascular or IO access, give epinephrine at the higher concentration of 1:1000, and use the higher dose of 0.1 mg/kg (0.1 mL/kg). Note that this is the same total volume of epinephrine as the IV/IO dose, because the 10-fold dose has 10 times the concentration of 1:10,000. When administering atropine through an endotracheal tube, the dose is two to three times the IV/IO dose (0.04–0.06 mg/kg by endotracheal tube).

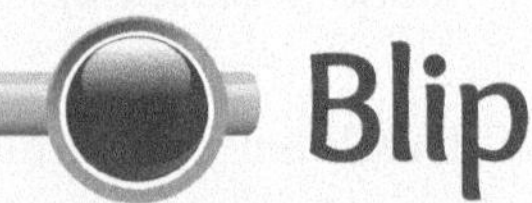

Be extremely careful with IV/IO/ET epinephrine and check doses and concentration.

Tachycardia

Tachycardia may be a nonspecific sign of fear, anxiety, pain, or fever and may not represent serious injury or illness. Tachycardia may also be a sign of a life-threatening problem, such as hypoxia, cardiac abnormality, or hypovolemia. Sinus tachycardia is the most common dysrhythmia in children, and treatment is generally limited to fluid administration, supplemental oxygen, and transport.

Assessment of the Child With Tachycardia

Tachycardia must be assessed in conjunction with the PAT and ABCDEs. Always ask about a history of congenital heart disease and check for midline chest scars from cardiac surgery.

There are two characteristics in the child's rhythm strip to measure and use as a basis for treatment, along with the perfusion assessment: (1) the heart rate per minute and (2) the width of the QRS complex. First, establish an accurate heart rate electronically from the rhythm strip. As in the assessment of bradycardia, interpret the heart rate based on knowledge of the normal range for age (see Table 5-2). Second, establish the width of the QRS from the rhythm strip. If the QRS complex is ≤0.09 seconds (<2¼ standard boxes on the rhythm strip), consider the child to have a narrow complex tachycardia. If the width is >0.09 seconds (>2¼ standard boxes on the rhythm strip), consider the child to have a wide complex tachycardia.

Table 5-4 distinguishes a narrow complex sinus tachycardia from narrow complex supraventricular tachycardia (SVT) and wide complex VT.

Specific Treatment of Tachycardia

If the child presents with tachycardia, determine the appropriate treatment by establishing perfusion status and by assessing the rhythm strip for heart rate and QRS duration.

Narrow Complex Tachycardia. If the child has a narrow QRS tachycardia (≤0.09 seconds), P waves are present, and the heart rate is variable and less than 220 beats/min in an infant or less than 180 beats/min in a child, the cause is usually sinus tachycardia (**Figure 5-1**) from noncardiac conditions (e.g., hypoxia, hypovolemia, hypothermia, hypoglycemia, metabolic abnormalities, toxins, fear, pain, or serious trauma to the chest). No specific cardiac medical management of the sinus tachycardia is needed. Instead, treat with fluids, oxygen, splinting, analgesia, or sedation as indicated by the associated condition. If there is no change in heart rate after treatment, consider other etiologies, such as SVT.

ALS

Specific Treatment of SVT. If the QRS is less than or equal to 0.09 seconds, P waves are absent or abnormal, and the rate is not variable and is ≥220 beats/min in an infant or ≥180 beats/min in a child, consider SVT as the likely etiology. If the child has no previous history of SVT, and the patient is stable, provide oxygen and transport to the emergency department. Delaying specific treatment for SVT until hospital arrival will permit the hospital staff to confirm SVT, and to run a continuous electrocardiogram while actively managing the dysrhythmia. A patient with a confirmed diagnosis of SVT may need long-term treatment with cardiac medications.

If the patient has a prior history of SVT, and is stable, consider a vagal maneuver first. Ice to the face (if available) evokes the "diving reflex" and is an effective management tool for SVT in infants and toddlers. Place crushed ice in a plastic bag, glove, or washcloth and apply firmly over the mid-face (cheeks and bridge of nose) for approximately 15 seconds, until the rhythm changes or the patient's condition dictates immediate cessation of the procedure (**Figure 5-2**). Do not occlude the nose (to allow breathing), and provide constant reassurance to the parent and child. Avoid ocular pressure (pressure on the eyeballs) as a method of vagal stimulation in a child. Only attempt a vagal maneuver once.

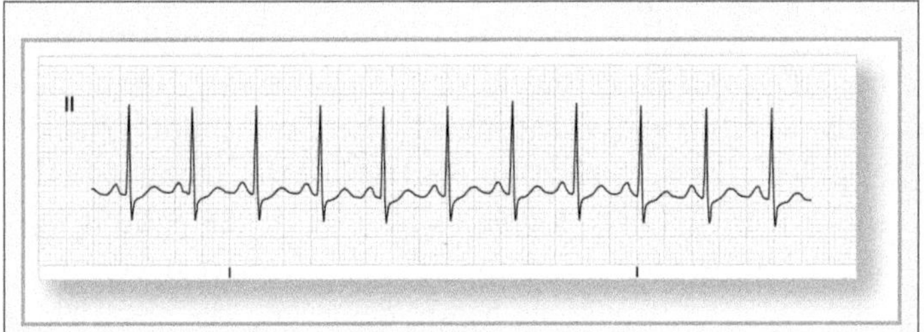

Figure 5-1 ECG of sinus tachycardia.

Table 5-4 Features of Sinus Tachycardia, SVT, and VT

	History	Heart Rate	Variability	QRS Interval	Assessment	Possible Treatments
Sinus tachycardia	Fever Volume loss Hypoxia Pain Increased activity or exercise	<220 beats/min (infant) <180 beats/min (child)	Yes	Narrow ≤0.09 seconds	Hypovolemia Hypoxia Painful injury	Fluids Oxygen Splinting Analgesia/sedation
Supraventricular tachycardia	Congenital heart disease Known SVT Nonspecific symptoms (e.g., poor feeding, fussiness)	≥220 beats/min (often 240–300 beats/min) ≥180 beats/min (child)	No	Narrow ≤0.09 seconds	CHF may be present	Vagal maneuvers (ice to face) Adenosine Synchronized electrical countershock
Ventricular tachycardia	Serious systemic illness	>150 beats/min	Yes	Wide >0.09 seconds	CHF may be present	Synchronized electrical countershock Lidocaine Amiodarone

ALS

If the patient with narrow complex tachycardia is stable, and the heart rate does not convert to sinus rhythm after one attempt at vagal stimulation, give adenosine at 0.1 mg/kg up to a maximum first dose of 6 mg rapid IV or IO push, and follow immediately with a 2- to 5-mL bolus of normal saline. Double the dose to 0.2 mg/kg if the rhythm does not convert after the first dose of adenosine (maximum second dose = 12 mg). Be prepared to treat the untoward effects of adenosine; it is a very potent cardiac drug. If given properly, it is usually effective in the treatment of SVT. Brief runs of bradycardia or even several seconds of asystole commonly occur with adenosine administration, but sustained or fatal dysrhythmias (e.g., asystole, VT, and VF) are rare. Caution should be used when administering adenosine in children on carbamazepine (Tegretol) because it can result in prolonged heart block. Monitor the child closely and have resuscitative drugs and a defibrillator within reach.

If a child with suspected SVT has signs of poor perfusion and hemodynamic compromise (abnormal PAT, poor pulse quality, abnormal CRT and skin temperature, hypotension), is in shock, or is unconscious, immediately administer synchronized electrical countershock at 0.5–1 J/kg as a starting electrical dose. If the initial shock is ineffective, double to 1-2 J/kg. If the child is in shock but still conscious and has vascular access, administer sedation if possible before delivering the electrical countershock. Do not delay electrical therapy for sedation. If electrical therapy fails to convert the child to sinus rhythm, consider using other antidysrhythmic drugs, such as amiodarone (5 mg/kg over 20–60 minutes) or procainamide (15 mg/kg over 20–60 minutes) as per local EMS system guidelines. Do not give amiodarone and procainamide together.

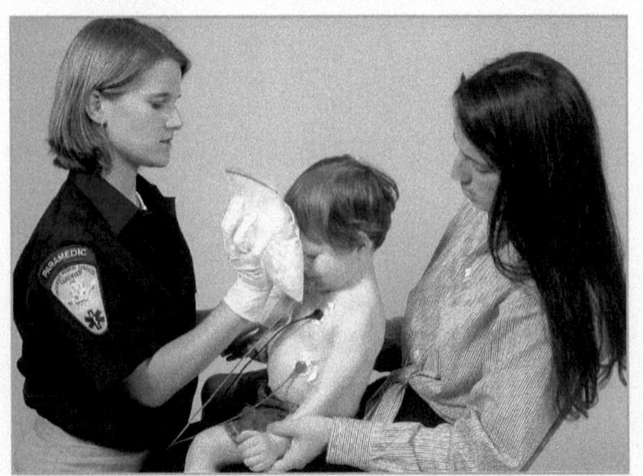

Figure 5-2 Placing a bag of ice on a child's face elicits the "diving reflex" and may convert SVT to sinus rhythm.

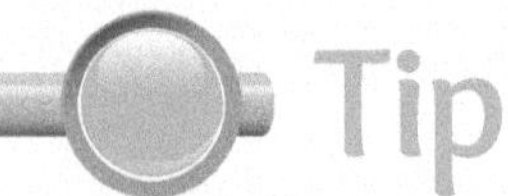

Tip

Prehospital personnel must be prepared to treat the adverse drug effects of all cardiac medications, even if the indication, dose, and route of delivery are correct.

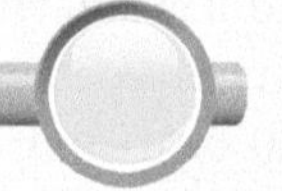

Controversy

Ice to the face for SVT is a controversial field procedure. It has not been evaluated for efficacy or safety in the out-of-hospital setting, especially in children.

Wide complex tachycardia. If the patient is conscious and has adequate perfusion, a heart rate of greater than 150 beats/min, and a QRS interval of greater than 0.09 seconds, he or she is probably in stable VT. Sinus tachycardia with a conduction abnormality (bundle branch block) may look like VT, but usually occurs in a child with a history of heart disease or cardiac surgery. Likewise, SVT with aberrant conduction can result in a wide complex rhythm. In all such stable cases with wide complex tachycardias, provide oxygen and transport the patient to an appropriate emergency department, with close cardiac monitoring and equipment for electrical countershock immediately available.

ALS

If the child has VT, is stable, and the rhythm is monomorphic and regular, try a dose of adenosine first to determine if the rhythm is SVT with aberrant conduction. If the rhythm is VT, an antiarrhythmic can be used per EMS guidelines. If the child has VT and shows signs of poor perfusion, treat with synchronized electrical countershock (0.5 to 1 J/kg). If a second shock (1–2 J/kg) is unsuccessful, or if the tachycardia recurs quickly, consider antidysrhythmic drugs, such as amiodarone (5 mg/kg over 20–60 minutes) or procainamide (15 mg/kg over 30–60 minutes) per local EMS system guidelines. Do not give amiodarone and procainamide together.

If the child has VT and shock, without pulses, treat as pulseless VT/VF.

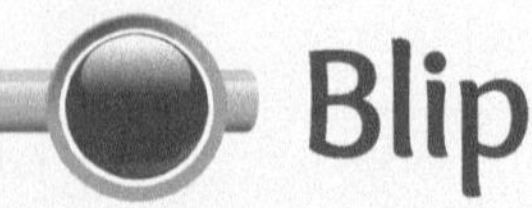

Blip

Most tachycardia in children is a response to noncardiac stimuli (fever, fear, pain) and does not require dysrhythmia treatment.

Automated External Defibrillator

Cardiac arrest in children is usually the result of profound hypoxia or shock, which leads to asystole, the most frequent rhythm of pediatric cardiac arrest. VF, however, does occur in pediatrics. The typical VF case is a child out of the infant age group who has had a witnessed collapse. Etiologies for VF arrest in children include myocarditis, an infection of the heart muscle; the "long QT syndrome," a congenital cardiac conduction problem; and hypertrophic cardiomyopathy (HCM), a hypertrophy of the ventricular septum and ventricles. One other special circumstance for VF arrest is commotio cordis, which develops usually in a young athlete who is struck in the chest by a ball, stick, or other blunt object.

Perform rapid assessment for VF on all unresponsive children, begin CPR, and administer defibrillation if VF is present on the cardiac monitor. Be especially vigilant for VF when the child is older and has suffered a witnessed collapse. There is no demonstrated benefit to defibrillation of asystole, and this procedure will only delay the key interventions of oxygenation, ventilation, and chest compressions.

The AED (**Figure 5-3**) allows early recognition of VF and rapid defibrillation. The 2015 American Heart Association guidelines recommend the use of an AED for treatment of VF in children of all ages, including infants. AEDs have been shown to accurately identify VF and VT in young children and are also accurate in identifying pediatric rhythms that do not require defibrillation. When used with a designated pediatric pad-cable system, these AEDs deliver an energy dose that is smaller than that delivered with adult pads. Use a pediatric AED or pediatric AED pads if available; however, an adult AED can be used on a child or an infant (one may consider putting pads anterior–posterior for an infant). For a pediatric arrest, use the AED as soon as possible. Studies show that even school-aged children with no prior experience or education in defibrillation can successfully operate an AED. **Figure 5-4** illustrates the use of an AED in a child.

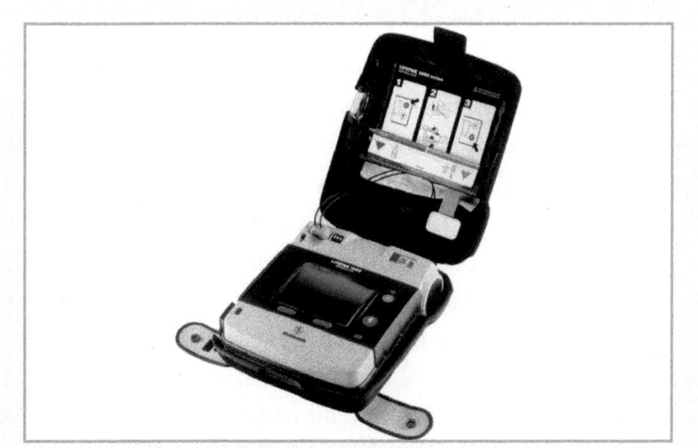

Figure 5-3 An AED.

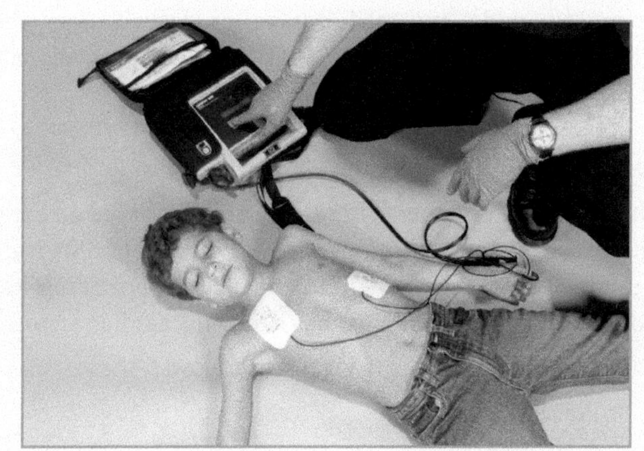

Figure 5-4 Using the AED with CPR in unresponsive children.

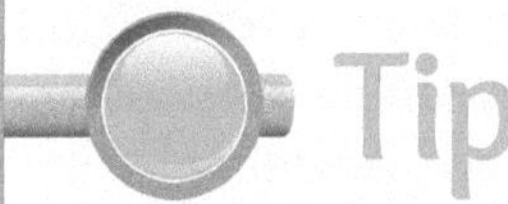

AEDs can be used on anyone. Preferably use a pediatric AED, but an adult AED can be used. For an unwitnessed arrest, begin CPR, and use an AED as soon as it is available.

Case Study 2

You are volunteering as a health care professional at a local high school track meet when a 9-year-old boy collapses while running the 100-meter dash. You rush to his aid and find him apneic and pulseless. You immediately start CPR.

1. What should be the next step in your assessment/management of this child?
2. At what age is it appropriate to apply an AED to assess for VF in a child?

Summary of Dysrhythmias

Unlike adults, primary cardiac rhythm disturbances are rare in children. Bradycardia, a prearrest rhythm, almost always reflects profound hypoxia and bag-mask ventilation should be initiated rapidly. Tachycardia is most commonly a sinus rhythm, but may represent SVT or VT. Although children can develop sinus tachycardia greater than 200 beats/min, do a careful evaluation for hypovolemia and hypoxia and other treatable causes, and then treat the identified causes. Assume all rates over 220 beats/min in infants or over 180 beats/min in children and all wide complex (QRS >0.09 seconds) tachycardias are primary cardiac dysrhythmias. The stable patient may need only general supportive care, regardless of cardiac rhythm. Symptomatic ventricular dysrhythmias may require drug therapy, with amiodarone or procainamide, and cardioversion or defibrillation. The AED is an important adjunct for prehospital professionals in unresponsive children with VF.

Cardiac Arrest

The emphasis for patients in cardiac arrest is based on early and excellent compressions. The new "Chain of Survival" has added a fifth component to enhance the postresuscitation care for the patient who has suffered a cardiac arrest.

The Pediatric Chain of Survival is as follows:

- Prevention
- Early CPR
- Early access
- Early ALS
- Postresuscitation care

Survival from cardiac arrest depends on several factors: time to CPR, with airway and breathing support, and presenting rhythm. The shorter the "downtime" before BLS, the better the outcome. As in adults, pediatric patients who present to EMS personnel in VF are more likely to survive than children who present in asystole, as long as there is early CPR and access to early defibrillation.

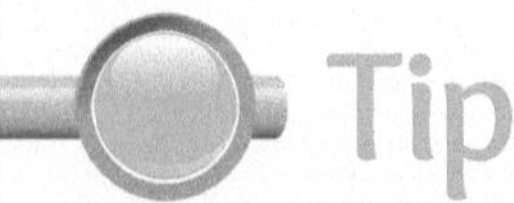
Tip

The only intervention associated with survival in pediatric asystolic cardiac arrest is time to onset of CPR, with airway and breathing support.

Causes

In contrast to adults, pediatric cardiac arrest is almost always a secondary event, the result of profound hypoxia or shock. Cardiac arrest in children usually follows a primary respiratory arrest, often from respiratory failure originating from common conditions, such as pneumonia, bronchiolitis, or asthma. Myocardial infarction and a cardiac dysrhythmia, such as hypertrophic cardiomyopathy (HCM), frequent causes of cardiac arrest in adults, are extremely unusual in young children.

Children can present in arrest from conditions from genetic disorders, such as HCM, which has a high incidence of sudden death, and is the leading cause of cardiac death in both preadolescent and adolescent children. Hypertrophic cardiomyopathy is a condition in which a child has profound hypertrophy of the ventricles and intraventricular septum that causes an outflow obstruction. It also has effects on the coronary arteries, leading to a thickening of the lining of the artery causing a narrowing in the vessel and leading to a decrease of flow to the myocardium.

Long QT syndrome is a congenital problem with the electrophysiology of the heart resulting in an increased risk of dysrhythmias including bradycardia and VF. Another cause of cardiac arrest occurs when a child is struck by a nonpenetrating object in the anterior chest leading to VF and sudden death. Commotio cordis occurs when a child is hit with a baseball, hockey puck, softball, karate blow, or other similar projectile force from sports. The blow is most likely to be critical if it is over the center of the left ventricle. Because this results in VF and collapse, the presence of an AED is critical.

The primary age group for pediatric cardiac arrest is infancy, when sudden unexpected infant death (SUID), infection, or child maltreatment precipitates respiratory failure. In toddlers and school-aged children, however, the causes of cardiac arrest change. In this older age group, the most likely causes are hemorrhagic shock and blunt trauma from either vehicle-related injuries or falls.

Assessment in Cardiac Arrest

A child in cardiac arrest is unresponsive, apneic, and pulseless. The cardiac monitor will show a cardiac arrest rhythm: asystole, PEA, VT, or VF. Asystole is the most frequent rhythm. SVT and VT are rare causes of cardiac arrest.

Asystole reflects profound hypoxia and ischemia. PEA may represent a variety of ischemic, hypoxic, hypothermic, and traumatic insults. Some PEA may arise from low-flow states with blood pressures too low to record in the out-of-hospital setting. VF occurs in children usually older than 2 years from a variety of conditions, including myocarditis, congenital anomalies, poisoning, electrocution, or hypoxia.

Chest Compressions

Chest compressions have become the focus of care in a patient in cardiac arrest. The 2010 American Heart Association (AHA) guidelines has implemented the new C-A-B (circulation–airway–breathing) sequence, which places emphasis on starting compressions more quickly and ensuring that compressions are the primary focus of a patient in cardiac

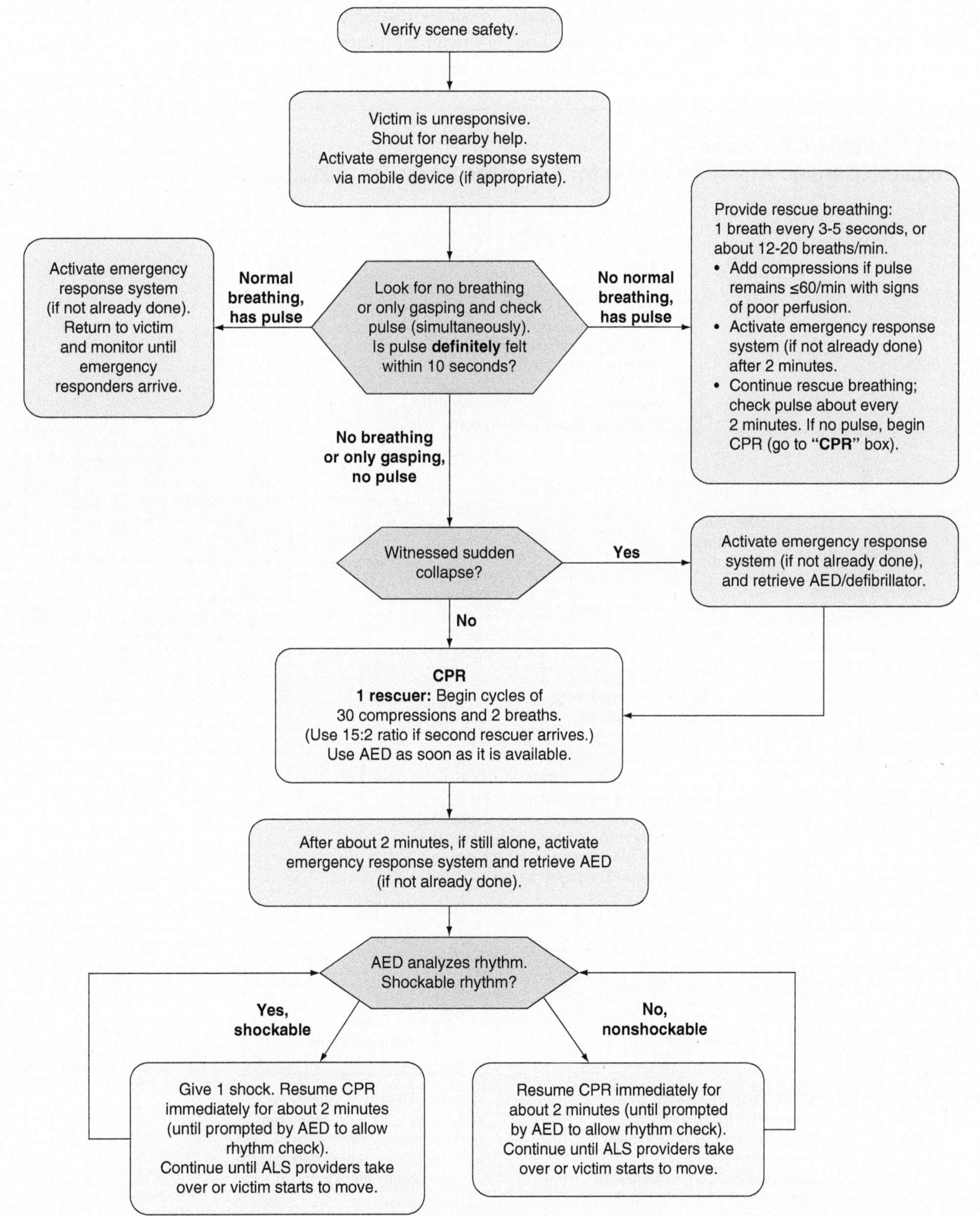

BLS Healthcare Provider
Pediatric Cardiac Arrest Algorithm for the Single Rescuer–2015 Update
Verify scene safety.
Victim is unresponsive. Shout for nearby help. Activate emergency response system via mobile device (if appropriate).
Look for no breathing or only gasping and check pulse (simultaneously). Is pulse definitely felt within 10 seconds?
Normal breathing, has pulse
Activate emergency response system (if not already done). Return to victim and monitor until emergency responders arrive.
No normal breathing, has pulse
Provide rescue breathing: 1 breath every 3-5 seconds, or about 12-20 breaths/min.
• Add compressions if pulse remains ≤60/min with signs of poor perfusion.
• Activate emergency response system (if not already done) after 2 minutes.
• Continue rescue breathing; check pulse about every 2 minutes. If no pulse, begin CPR (go to "CPR" box).
No breathing or only gasping, no pulse
Witnessed sudden collapse?
Yes
Activate emergency response system (if not already done), and retrieve AED/defibrillator.
No
CPR
1 rescuer: Begin cycles of 30 compressions and 2 breaths. (Use 15:2 ratio if second rescuer arrives.) Use AED as soon as it is available.
After about 2 minutes, if still alone, activate emergency response system and retrieve AED (if not already done).
AED analyzes rhythm. Shockable rhythm?
Yes, shockable
Give 1 shock. Resume CPR immediately for about 2 minutes (until prompted by AED to allow rhythm check). Continue until ALS providers take over or victim starts to move.
No, nonshockable
Resume CPR immediately for about 2 minutes (until prompted by AED to allow rhythm check). Continue until ALS providers take over or victim starts to move.

Figure 5-5 A 2015 AHA Guidelines criteria showing the pediatric BLS algorithms.

Reproduced from Atkins DL, et al. Part 11: pediatric basic life support and cardiopulmonary resuscitation quality: 2015 American Heart Association Guidelines Update for Cardiopulmonary Resuscitation and Emergency Cardiovascular Care. *Circulation*. 2015;132(suppl 2): S519–S525

arrest. Compression techniques differ for a child and infant. For a child, the hand(s) should be placed on the lower half of the sternum, rate should be at least 100–120 per minute, and compression depth should be at least 2 inches (5 cm) with complete recoil (to ensure adequate preload). For an infant, as a single rescuer one places two fingers at the nipple line and compresses at a rate of at least 100 per minute with a depth of at least 1.5 inches (4 cm) with complete recoil. When performing two-rescuer CPR for an infant, the recommended technique is the two fingers encircling the chest technique. For the child and infant, when performing single-rescuer CPR, the ratio is 30:2 and changes to 15:2 for two health care provider rescuers. For a step-by-step explanation of this procedure, see **Figure 5-5 A** and **B**.

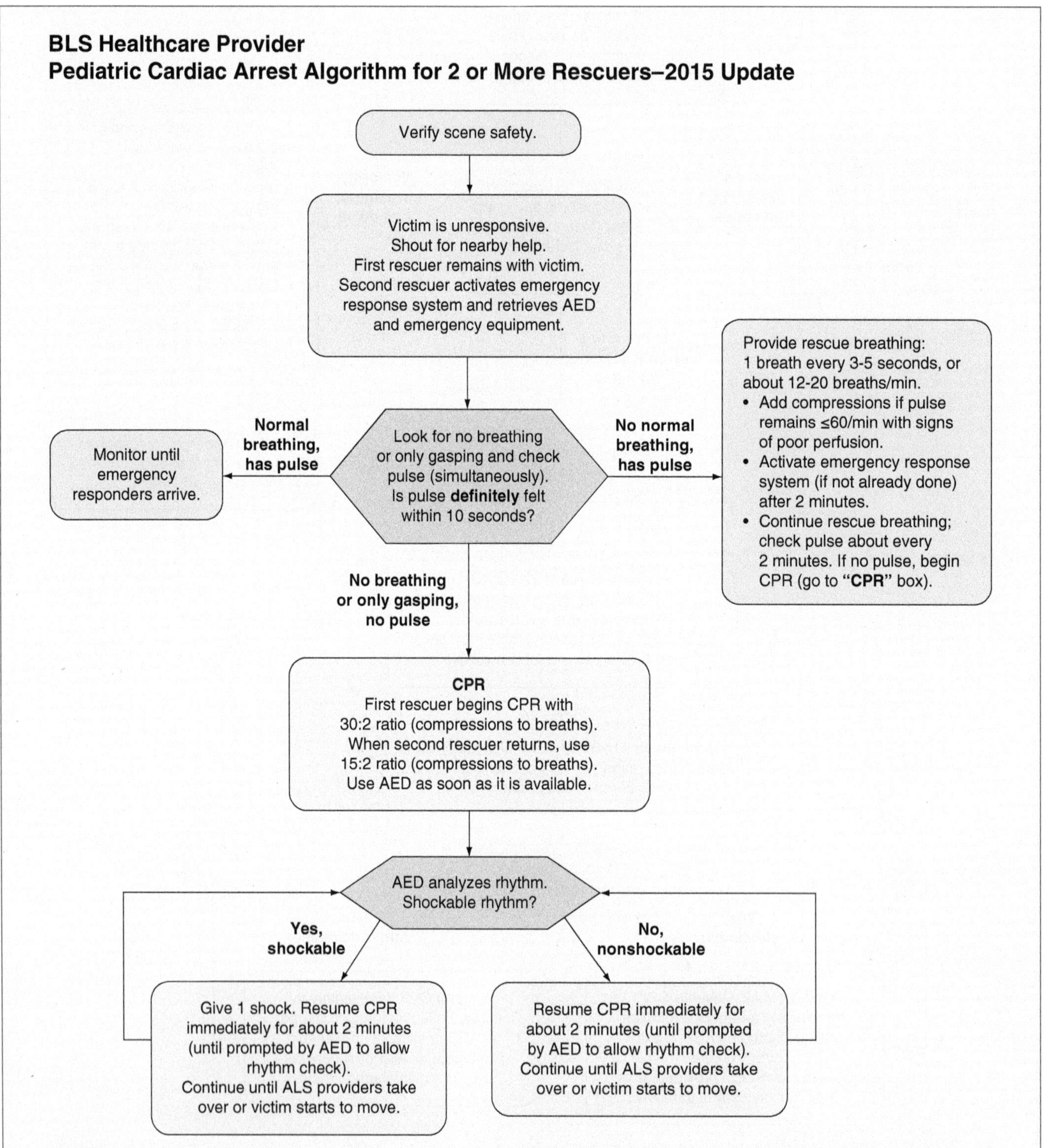
BLS Healthcare Provider
Pediatric Cardiac Arrest Algorithm for 2 or More Rescuers–2015 Update
Verify scene safety.
Victim is unresponsive.
Shout for nearby help.
First rescuer remains with victim.
Second rescuer activates emergency response system and retrieves AED and emergency equipment.
Normal breathing, has pulse
Monitor until emergency responders arrive.
Look for no breathing or only gasping and check pulse (simultaneously).
Is pulse definitely felt within 10 seconds?
No normal breathing, has pulse
Provide rescue breathing:
1 breath every 3-5 seconds, or about 12-20 breaths/min.
• Add compressions if pulse remains ≤60/min with signs of poor perfusion.
• Activate emergency response system (if not already done) after 2 minutes.
• Continue rescue breathing; check pulse about every 2 minutes. If no pulse, begin CPR (go to "CPR" box).
No breathing or only gasping, no pulse
CPR
First rescuer begins CPR with 30:2 ratio (compressions to breaths).
When second rescuer returns, use 15:2 ratio (compressions to breaths).
Use AED as soon as it is available.
AED analyzes rhythm.
Shockable rhythm?
Yes, shockable
No, nonshockable
Give 1 shock. Resume CPR immediately for about 2 minutes (until prompted by AED to allow rhythm check).
Continue until ALS providers take over or victim starts to move.
Resume CPR immediately for about 2 minutes (until prompted by AED to allow rhythm check).
Continue until ALS providers take over or victim starts to move.

Figure 5-5 B 2015 AHA Guidelines criteria showing the pediatric BLS algorithms.

Reproduced from Atkins DL, et al. Part 11: pediatric basic life support and cardiopulmonary resuscitation quality: 2015 American Heart Association Guidelines Update for Cardiopulmonary Resuscitation and Emergency Cardiovascular Care. *Circulation.* 2015;132(suppl 2): S519–S525

Length-Based Drug Dosage

Treatment of infants and children in the out-of-hospital setting is difficult because children of different ages require different sizes of equipment, different doses of medications, and different amounts of fluids (**Figure 5-6**). Length is a good index for drug dosing and equipment sizing during resuscitations. From a measured patient length, either a computerized resuscitation software program or a color-coded tape can provide correct doses and equipment sizes. Computerized programs offer a wider range of drugs and additional safety features. For a step-by-step explanation of this procedure, see **Length-Based Equipment Sizing and Drug Dosing, Procedure 2.**

Presenting Cardiac Arrest Rhythm and Treatment

The top priority in the management of a patient in cardiac arrest is circulation (emphasis on high-quality compressions); airway and breathing (bag-mask ventilation with an airway adjunct is adequate; consider endotracheal intubation as a priority if the cause of arrest is asphyxial in nature); and defibrillation (if indicated). The presenting cardiac rhythm is a major determinant of the treatment of cardiac arrest. When the child is pulseless and apneic, the treatment of asystole and PEA is the same.

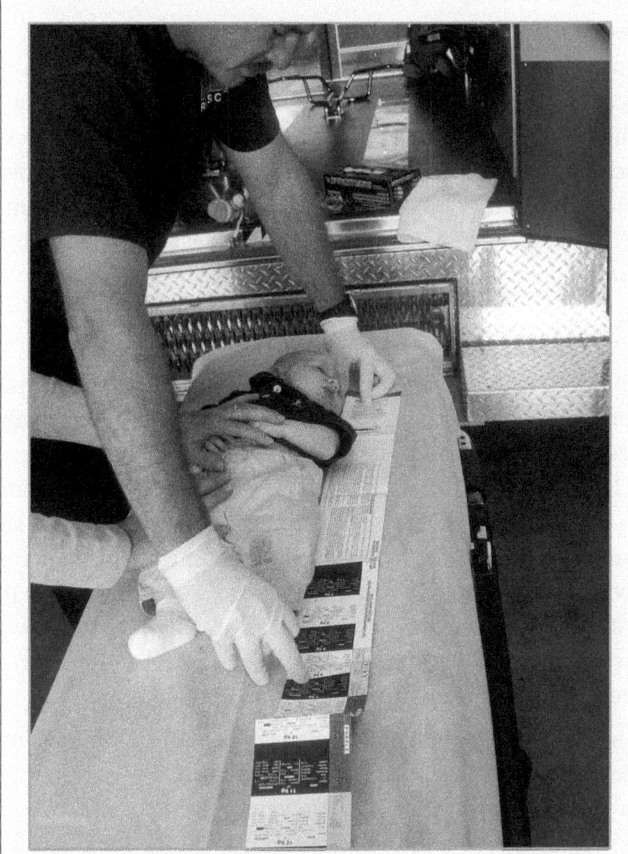

Figure 5-6 Resuscitation tape.

ALS

Asystole/PEA. Resuscitation efforts for nonshockable rhythms begin with high-quality CPR with an emphasis on chest compressions without interruption. Management of airway and breathing may be taken care of with bag-mask ventilation and airway adjunct as primary intervention as long as chest rise and compliance are noted. If the arrest is caused by asphyxia, then an endotracheal tube becomes a priority. The uncuffed endotracheal tube should be sized with the equation of (age in years divided by 4) + 4. Cuffed endotracheal tubes are sized a half size smaller.

Venous access can be accessed by IV or IO. All medications, fluids, and blood products can be administered through the IO.

Epinephrine is the drug of choice administered at 0.01 mg/kg (0.1 mL/kg of 1:10,000 IV/IO). High-quality BLS with adequate airway management is continued throughout the resuscitation with the reassessment every 2 minutes and epinephrine administered every 3–5 minutes.

An important component to the treatment of asystole/PEA is rapidly working to identify the cause; therefore, it is imperative the provider considers the Hs and Ts (**Table 5-5**) while providing care.

ALS

VF/Pulseless VT. VF/VT management should start with quality CPR while attaching the monitor and identifying a shockable rhythm. The initial energy setting for the child should be at 2 J/kg, followed by 2 minutes of excellent CPR. During this time, IV access should be gained. Initial airway management should be maintained with a bag-mask device and oropharyngeal airway (OPA) as long as there is adequate chest rise and good compliance (an advanced airway may be considered further down the algorithm). When an airway is not maintainable with a bag-mask ventilation or the arrest is caused by a hypoxic event, an endotracheal tube should be considered as soon as possible.

After 2 minutes of high-quality CPR, the patient is reassessed and a shock is administered at 4 J/kg. CPR is continued, and the patient is given 0.01 mg/kg of epinephrine (0.1 mL/kg), 1:10,000 IV/IO, repeated every 3–5 minutes. Resume CPR

Table 5-5 Six Hs and Five Ts

Hypovolemia	Tension pneumothorax
Hypoxia	Tamponade, cardiac
Hypoglycemia	Toxins
Hydrogen ion (acidosis)	Thrombosis, cardiac
Hypo/hyperkalemia	Thrombosis, pulmonary
Hypothermia	

ALS

for 2 minutes, then reassess. All subsequent shocks are delivered at 4 J/kg. The patient is given amiodarone at 5 mg/kg, repeated up to 2 times to a total of 15 mg/kg or lidocaine 1 mg/kg as a loading dose with maintenance of 20– 50 mcg/kg per minute by infusion. Repeat bolus if infusion is begun >15 minutes after initial loading dose.

Survival from pediatric cardiac arrest requires good BLS care. IV or IO needle insertion and medication delivery are helpful but not primary determinants of survival. Endotracheal tube insertion offers no known benefit to survival. In addition, "high-dose" epinephrine has shown no increased survival when used in cardiac arrest. It may be considered in exceptional circumstances, such as β-blocker overdose.

The Transport Decision: Stay or Go

Deciding which pediatric cardiac arrest patients require hospital transport is another important controversy. Of all children in out-of-hospital cardiac arrest, only 3% to 5% will survive. Predictors of survival include type of presenting rhythm and early return of spontaneous circulation (<5 minutes) after BLS on scene. Survival from pulseless VT/VF is approximately 15%, versus about 3% for asystole. If children in cardiac arrest fail out-of-hospital resuscitation with BLS and ALS, they will not survive unless there is a special circumstance. Patients who have ingested massive amounts of sedative-hypnotic drugs (e.g., barbiturates) may have a greater chance of survival after prolonged resuscitation and deserve extended treatment before death is declared.

In some cases, field resuscitation attempts can be stopped before transport if permitted by local EMS death-in-the-field policies. Although survival in unwitnessed out-of-hospital cardiac arrest is rare, prehospital professionals may be uncomfortable in discontinuing resuscitative efforts in children. When resuscitation is terminated, skillful communication with the child's caregivers is critical (**Figure 5-7**), as explained in Chapter 12. *Never leave a family member on scene with the deceased child without appropriate supportive personnel.* A system to provide supportive care to the caregivers must be in place if EMS policy permits discontinuation of resuscitative efforts in the field. These services might be provided by social services personnel, pastoral care, or grief counselors.

Cardiac arrest in children is associated with high provider stress. Critical-incident stress debriefing may be helpful for prehospital professionals after such a tragedy.

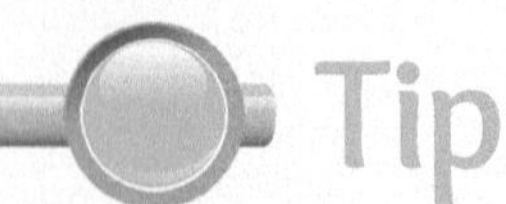

Prehospital cardiac arrest treatment requires good BLS skills.

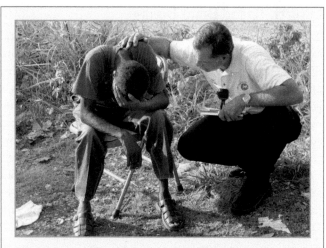

Figure 5-7 Skilled communication with the caregivers and family is imperative after the death of a child.

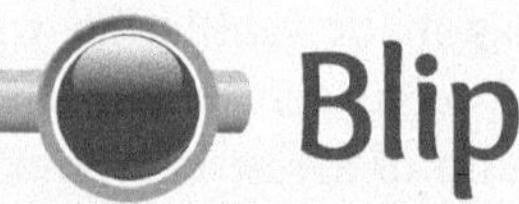

Never leave a family member on scene with the deceased child without appropriate supportive care.

Summary of Cardiac Arrest

Pediatric cardiac arrest is an uncommon event. Survival is unlikely, and asystole has the worst prognosis. VT/VF usually occurs in older children and has higher survival. Meticulous attention to airway, oxygenation, ventilation, chest compressions, and early defibrillation, when appropriate, will improve success. In all cases of pediatric cardiac arrest, grief counseling for the caregivers and critical-incident stress debriefing for the prehospital professionals are extremely helpful.

Congenital Heart Disease

Children with congenital heart disease are at increased risk for the types of cardiovascular emergencies more commonly seen in the adult population, including dysrhythmias and CHF. These complications may present in infancy or as late as the teenage years (**Table 5-6**). Advances in cardiovascular surgery have allowed the medical community to prolong the lives of children who just decades ago would have died in infancy. Many of these children are now living productive lives at home. Prehospital professionals must be prepared to treat "adult problems" in this younger population.

The primary assessment and management of any child experiencing a cardiovascular emergency are the same: airway, breathing, and circulation. However, in any child with a possible cardiac pathology, include a "quick look" at the cardiac rhythm. These children may have treatable cardiac dysrhythmias.

Case Study 3

You are dispatched to the location of an unresponsive 2-year-old boy recently removed from a swimming pool. Estimated downtime is unknown, but the parents are on scene and state that the child had been missing for more than 30 minutes. The parents initiated CPR immediately. Upon arrival you find the child to be cool, blue, apneic, and pulseless.

1. What is the most important intervention for this patient to improve his chances of survival?
2. Should the child be actively rewarmed?

Table 5-6 Congenital Heart Disease Causing Congestive Heart Failure at Different Times During Infancy

Age	Type of Congenital Heart Disease
Newborn	Hypoplastic left heart
	Severe pulmonic insufficiency
	Tetralogy of Fallot
	Severe tricuspid insufficiency
	Third-degree atrioventricular block
	SVT
	Total anomalous pulmonary venous return
	Transposition of the great vessels
First month	Aortic coarctation with patent ductus arteriosus
	Ventricular septal defect
	Tricuspid atresia
	Truncus arteriosus
First 6 months	Ventricular septal defect
	Patent ductus arteriosus
6–12 months	Ventricular septal defect
	Endocardial fibroelastosis

Drowning

Drowning is suffocation after submersion in water. Drowning is the second leading cause of unintentional death in children between the ages of 1 and 4 years, and the third leading cause of death due to unintentional injury in children younger than 14 years (**Figure 5-8**). Unfortunately, drowning is not limited to the summer months. In warmer climates it occurs year-round, and in cooler climates it may occur due to submersion in lakes, buckets, hot tubs, and bathtubs.

Prevention

The best management for near-drowning is prevention. The installation of four-sided fencing prevents up to 90% of childhood residential swimming pool drownings and near-drownings. Eighty-five percent of boating-related drownings are preventable by wearing personal flotation devices.

Treatment

Early recognition of cardiac arrest and immediate bystander CPR has an important association with survival from severe submersion injuries. ALS care has an unproven benefit.

First remove the patient from the water and begin CPR. If the child is pulseless, begin chest compressions, then open the airway and provide two ventilations. Protect the cervical spine if there is potential head or neck trauma. Perform chest compressions, airway management, oxygenation, and ventilation, and follow protocols for drug therapy and electrical countershock depending upon presenting cardiac rhythm.

If the child has a pulse, open the airway and ensure appropriate oxygenation and ventilation, usually with a bag-mask device. Obtain IV or IO access and transport. Provide drug therapy, and rarely electrical countershock, as indicated for shock or dysrhythmias.

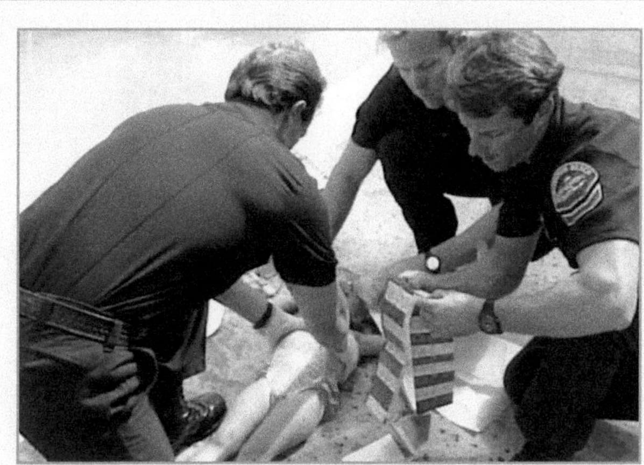

Figure 5-8 Drowning is the third leading cause of death due to unintentional injury in children younger than 14 years.

CASE STUDY ANSWERS

Case Study 1 — page 92

This child could be experiencing VF/pulseless VT, PEA, or asystole. He is in cardiac arrest, and the appropriate first interventions is to provide excellent CPR and BLS care. Treatment for the patient will be based on the type of arrhythmia.

Case Study 2 — page 99

This cardiac arrest appears to reflect a primary cardiac event. Begin 30 chest compressions to 2 ventilations and ask someone to get an AED and call 9-1-1 or the emergency response number. When the AED arrives, attach the AED and let it analyze the rhythm. If it indicates shock advised, deliver a shock and resume CPR for 2 minutes, then reanalyze the rhythm. If shockable, deliver a shock, and resume CPR.

This child was in VF due to a previously undiagnosed disorder known as "prolonged QT syndrome." Survivors from this disease often give a history of "blackouts" associated with exercise and stress. Other family members may also be affected by the same disorder. A look back at the family history can uncover unexplained deaths of relatives at young ages.

The initial treatment for children in VF, as in adults, is rapid defibrillation. With the increasing availability of AEDs, many of these children will receive rapid recognition and defibrillation by bystanders.

Case Study 3 — page 105

After removal from the water, begin CPR, starting with chest compressions, then provide bag-mask ventilation with 100% oxygen. Rushing to intubate this child, before providing effective bag-mask ventilation with 100% oxygen, may result in worsened hypoxia and hypercarbia. Most drownings cause airway spasm with little or no water entering the lungs, so bag-mask may be effective. The best anatomic location for palpating a pulse in a 2-year-old child is over the brachial artery, which is located just proximal to the elbow and medially to the biceps muscle.

Although there have been promising results in adult studies of hypothermia after cardiac arrest, pediatric studies have found no benefit. The hypothermic state may be protective of brain function, and rapid rewarming can introduce dysrhythmias. Therefore, remove wet clothing and provide rapid transport.

SUGGESTED READINGS

References

Atkins DL, Berger S, Duff JP, et al. Part 11: Pediatric Basic Life Support and Cardiopulmonary Resuscitation Quality: 2015 American Heart Association Guidelines Update for Cardiopulmonary Resuscitation and Emergency Cardiovascular Care. *Circulation.* 2015;132(suppl 2):S519–25.

deCaen AR, Maconochie IK, Aickin R, et al. Part 6: Pediatric basic life support and pediatric advanced life support: 2015 International consensus on Cardiopulmonary Resuscitation and Emergency Cardiovascular Care Science with Treatment Recommendations. *Circulation.* 2015;132 (suppl 1): S177–S203.

Dieckmann RA, et al. *Pediatric Education for Prehospital Professionals.* 2nd ed. Burlington, MA: Jones and Bartlett Learning; 2006:76–103.

Hauda WE II. Resuscitation of Children. In: Tintinalli J, Stapczynski J, John Ma O, Cline D, Cydulka R, Meckler G, eds. *Tintinalli's Emergency Medicine*, 7th ed. New York, NY: McGraw-Hill; 2010:80–90.

Kleinman ME, Chameides L, Schexnayder SM, et al. *Pediatric Advanced Life Support.* Part 14. 2010 American Heart Association Guidelines for Cardiopulmonary Resuscitation and Emergency Cardiovascular Care. *Circulation.* 2010;122 (suppl 3):S876-S908.

Moler FW, Silverstein FS, Holubkov R, et al. Therapeutic Hypothermia after Out-of-Hospital Cardiac Arrest in Children. *N Engl J Med.* 2015;372:1898–1908.

Perondi M, Reis A, Paiva E. A comparison of high-dose and standard-dose epinephrine in children with cardiac arrest. *N Engl J Med.* 2004;350(17):1722–1730.

Raghavan SS. *Pediatric long QT syndrome.* Available at http://emedicine.medscape.com/article/891571-overview. Accessed September 12, 2012.

Shah SN. *Hypertrophic cardiomyopathy.* emedicine. http://emedicine.medscape.com/article/152913-overview. Accessed September 13, 2010.

Sirbaugh P, Pepe P, Shook J, et al. A prospective, population-based study of the demographics, epidemiology, management and outcome of out-of-hospital pediatric cardiopulmonary arrest. *Ann Emerg Med.* 1999;33(2):174–184.

Yabek SM. *Commotio cordis.* Available at http://emedicine.medscape.com/article/902504-overview. Accessed September 12, 2012.

Yee LL, Meckler GD. Pediatric Heart Disease: Acquired Heart Disease. In: Tintinalli J, Stapczynski J, John Ma O, Cline D, Cydulka R, Meckler G, eds. *Tintinalli's Emergency Medicine*, 7th ed. New York, NY: McGraw-Hill; 2010:827–830.

Young K, Gausche-Hill M, McClung C, et al. A prospective population-based study of the epidemiology and outcome of out-of-hospital pediatric cardiopulmonary arrest. *Pediatrics.* 2004;114(1):157–164.

Young K, Seidel J. Pediatric cardiopulmonary resuscitation: a collective review. *Ann Emerg Med.* 1999;33(2):195–205.

Zevitz ME. Hypertrophic cardiomyopathy. emedicine. 2012. http://emedicine.medscape.com/article/152913-overview. Accessed September 13, 2010.

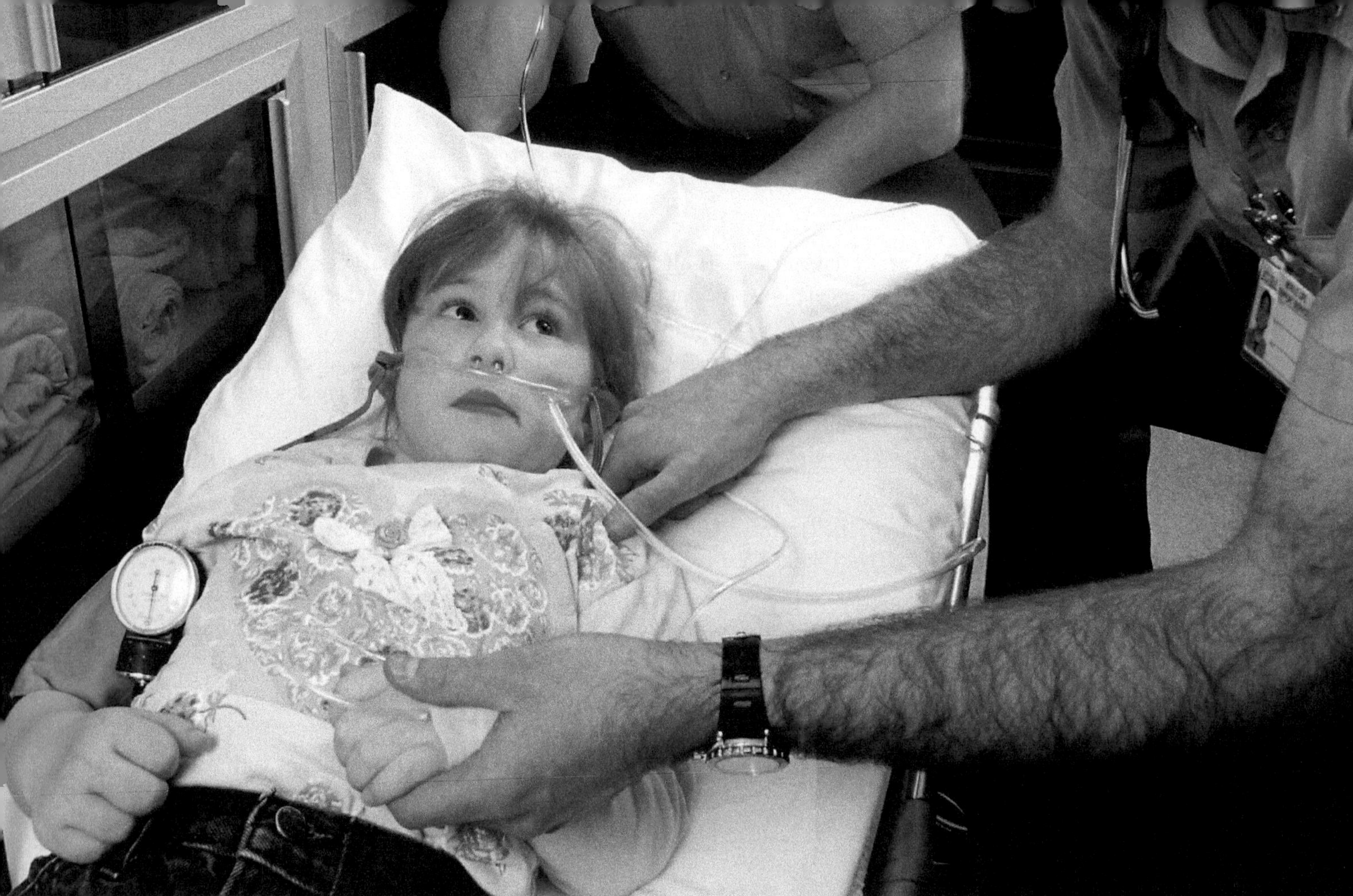

Learning Objectives

1. Describe the major types of seizures and the management priorities for each.
2. Compare the advantages and disadvantages of various benzodiazepines and their routes of administration in status epilepticus.
3. Distinguish the common causes of altered mental status in infants and children, and outline management priorities.
4. Describe signs and symptoms of hypoglycemia and outline management priorities.
5. Discuss the association of fever and serious illness.
6. Outline the assessment and management of common environmental emergencies, including temperature emergencies, bites, and stings.

Medical Emergencies

Chapter 6

Introduction

Approximately 50% of all pediatric 9-1-1 calls are illness (or "medical") complaints, and half are injury (or "trauma") complaints. Calls involving children with pediatric medical complaints tend to be more serious as a whole, and the varied nature of these complaints makes this group especially challenging to assess and treat. This chapter reviews common out-of-hospital pediatric medical emergencies: seizures, altered mental status (AMS), fever, endocrine disorders, gastrointestinal (GI) illness, and environmental emergencies.

Respiratory illness (covered in Chapter 3) and seizures are the two most common out-of-hospital pediatric medical emergencies. Fever is a common medical complaint, but is rarely an emergency in isolation. Fever is usually a symptom of an underlying illness. Although most children with fever have relatively benign, self-limited conditions (e.g., ear infection, croup, viral syndrome), it is important to identify those febrile children with potentially more serious conditions (e.g., meningitis, sepsis) who require immediate prehospital management. Fevers may be associated with seizures in infants and preschool-aged children. AMS is a less common characteristic of pediatric 9-1-1 patients, but the presence of an AMS usually means the child has a serious or life-threatening medical emergency. Endocrine emergencies in childhood frequently involve AMS and altered blood glucose levels.

Environmental emergencies occurring during childhood include heat- and cold-related emergencies and envenomation by bites and stings. The young child is at increased risk for these environmental emergencies because of physiologic, behavioral, and developmental characteristics.

Accurately assessing a child with a medical illness requires an age-based approach to history taking and physical examination, as discussed in Chapters 1 and 2. Communicating with the child and family is essential. Effective communication is fundamental to good clinical care, establishment of trust, and development of comfortable interactions with the child.

Seizures

Seizures are caused by abnormal, sustained electrical discharges from a cluster of cerebral neurons. Seizures have varied physical manifestations, depending on the location of the abnormal electrical seizure activity in the brain and the age of the child. Seizures in the infant, whose central nervous system (CNS) is immature, can be very subtle, consisting only of abnormal gaze, horizontal nystagmus, sustained muscle contractions, sucking motions, or "bicycling" (pedaling

Case Study 1

A 2-year-old boy playing on a floor mat at preschool develops jerking of his arms and legs for 1–2 minutes. The teacher calls 9-1-1. On arrival at the scene, you find a child who appears drowsy, opens his eyes but does not answer questions, and cries when touched. There are no abnormal airway sounds, work of breathing is not increased, and skin color is normal. Respiratory rate is 30 breaths/min, heart rate is 100 beats/min, blood pressure is 110/58 mm Hg, and the oxygen saturation is 95%. There are no focal neurologic findings. The child's temperature is 38.6°C (101.5°F). He becomes more responsive during your assessment and begins to ask for his father.

1. How should you manage this patient?
2. Should the child be transported?

movements of the legs). In the older child, who has a more mature CNS, seizures are usually more obvious, and typically manifest as repetitive muscular contractions (tonic-clonic activity) and unresponsiveness. Sustained or repetitive muscular contractions may be associated with upper airway obstruction, resulting in poor air exchange, hypercarbia, and hypoxia. As a result, cyanosis is common.

"Generalized" seizures are the most common type in children. These seizures are divided into convulsive (with motor activity, such as tonic-clonic movements) and nonconvulsive (no motor activity, such as an absence seizure). "Partial" seizures are classified based on whether consciousness is maintained. Partial seizures with no loss of consciousness are known as "simple partial seizures"; those associated with a loss of consciousness, are known as "complex partial seizures." Partial seizures are further subdivided based on signs and symptoms, such as motor activity (can be focal and then spread), sensory (paresthesias, vertigo, visual, or auditory symptoms), or autonomic changes (sweating, pupillary changes). During a complex partial seizure, the child may have motor automatisms, such as chewing or bicycling movements of the legs. There are also epilepsy syndromes, and these infants and children may demonstrate a variety of seizure types. The term epilepsy refers to a chronic disorder that causes recurrent seizures over time, with or without a known underlying cause. Although caregivers of children with epilepsy may be very calm at the scene of a 9-1-1 call, those who are witnessing a first-time seizure are usually very frightened, may fear that the child is dying, and may have initiated cardiopulmonary resuscitation efforts.

Febrile Seizures

The most frequent type of seizure in childhood is the febrile seizure. About 5% of all children have at least one seizure by 6 years of age. More than half of these children never have another seizure. By definition, a simple febrile seizure is a generalized, tonic-clonic seizure of less than 15 minutes duration that occurs in a febrile child between 6 months and 5 years of age with no underlying neurologic abnormalities. "Simple" febrile seizures do not cause brain injury, even if the child has repeated febrile seizures. Most simple febrile seizures stop spontaneously before the arrival of prehospital professionals. Risk factors for recurrence include age less than 1 year at the time of the first febrile seizure, a family history of febrile seizure, and complex nature of seizure.

Complex febrile seizures last longer than 15 minutes, are focal rather than generalized, and occur more than once in 24 hours. This type of seizure has a higher association with serious illness and requires evaluation in the hospital. Most children with febrile seizures have relatively benign etiology of the fever (otitis media, viral syndrome). Although there may be a brief postictal period, these children generally have improving level of conscious and appear to be well. Children with more serious etiologies (meningitis) usually

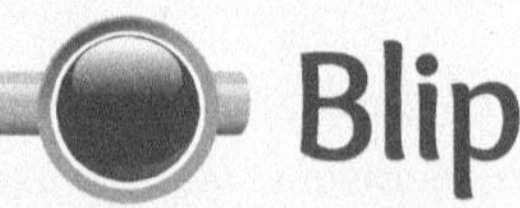

A prehospital professional cannot make a diagnosis of a febrile seizure.

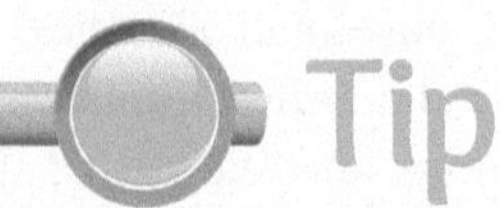

If the child begins to have another seizure, ensure ABCs. If the seizure does not stop in 5 minutes, begin medication administration.

appear ill after the seizure resolves or may have associated symptoms (petechiae, neck stiffness). A child who has a seizure and a fever may not necessarily have had a febrile seizure, and requires physician evaluation to exclude a serious disease. *A prehospital professional cannot make a diagnosis of a febrile seizure.*

Afebrile Seizures

Although childhood seizures are frequently associated with fever, there are many other possible causes of seizures. These include trauma, especially head injury (including child abuse), hypoxia, hypoglycemia, infection, toxic ingestion, CNS bleeding, metabolic disorders, and congenital neurologic problems. A common group of children with afebrile seizures are those with known epilepsy who have not received therapeutic doses of their anticonvulsant medication and experience "breakthrough" seizures. There is a significant group of children who have breakthrough seizures despite medication compliance. In this group, parents call when normal methods of controlling seizure activity are unsuccessful.

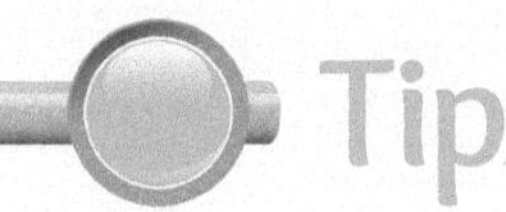

Tip

A seizure with a fever is not the same as a febrile seizure.

Status Epilepticus

The classic definition of status epilepticus is either a series of two or more seizures without recovery of consciousness, with the child unable to carry on verbal communication between the seizures; or a continuous seizure more than 20 minutes long. A newer "operational" definition of status was developed in the late 1990s by a group of neurologists specializing in seizure management. Based on data indicating that most seizures stop spontaneously in less than 5 minutes, they redefined the term "status epilepticus" and set a threshold for initiating pharmacologic treatment as a seizure lasting longer than 5 minutes. Accordingly, consider any child who is actively seizing on arrival of the prehospital professional to be in status epilepticus, and treat with drug therapy to stop the seizure. Such patients inevitably have been seizing for at least 15 minutes, given the average response times in most emergency medical services (EMS) systems.

Status epilepticus may occur as the child's first seizure. The age of the child in status epilepticus helps forecast the likely cause of the seizure. Children younger than 3 years of age tend to have acute, sometimes progressive causes of status epilepticus, such as hypoxia, infection, or toxic ingestion. Children older than 3 years of age who present with status epilepticus tend to have chronic, static causes (e.g., epilepsy, neurologic disorder, an inborn metabolic disorder, or inadequate anticonvulsant treatment). Therefore, be especially vigilant in care of infants and young children with status epilepticus, especially if they do not have a history of fever or epilepsy.

Status epilepticus is a medical emergency. Early treatment in the field is critical because prolonged seizure activity is difficult to control pharmacologically. Stopping the seizure also facilitates airway management and support of oxygenation and ventilation, and transport. However, the risk of long-term neurologic injury is most closely associated with the underlying *cause* and associated complications (hypercarbia, hypoxia) rather than with the *duration* of the seizure. For example, a child who has a 20-minute febrile seizure is unlikely to sustain brain injury, whereas a child with meningitis who has a seizure of the same duration is at high risk for long-term neurologic problems.

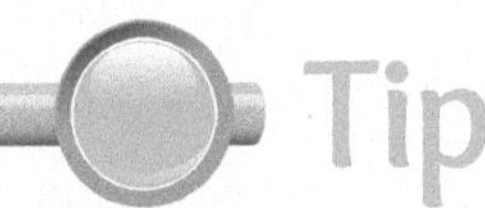

Tip

During status epilepticus, the risk of brain injury is most closely related to the cause of the seizure, not the length of the seizure.

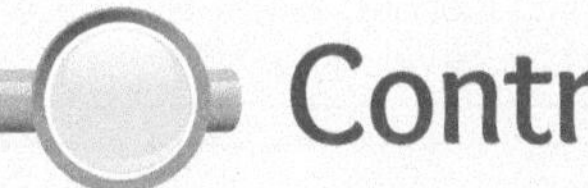

Controversy

When to treat a seizure is a matter of debate. Although most seizures stop spontaneously and do not need any treatment, some untreated children go on to the dangerous condition of status epilepticus. The best practical approach is to treat if the child is seizing on arrival.

Classification of Seizures

The type of abnormal motor activity and the age of the child are factors important to classify seizures, as shown in **Table 6-1**. The main distinction is whether the seizure involves the entire body (generalized seizures affect both hemispheres of the brain) or only one part of the body (focal seizures affect only one hemisphere of the brain). A generalized seizure usually involves abnormal muscle jerking (tonic-clonic or grand mal seizure), but may be nonconvulsive with only a loss of attention or eye blinking (absence or petit mal seizure). When the child has had

Table 6-1 Classification of Seizures

Type	Description
Generalized	
Tonic-clonic (*grand mal*)	• Trunk rigidity and loss of consciousness, with sudden jerking of both arms and/or both legs; may be only tonic (muscle contraction, rigidity), or clonic (muscle relaxation, jerking)
Absence (*petit mal*)	• Brief loss of awareness without any abnormal body movements; the child may appear to be staring or may be blinking his or her eyes repetitively
Partial	
Simple	• Focal motor jerking, without loss of consciousness; may be sensory, autonomic, or psychic; may progress to complex seizure activity
Complex	• Focal motor jerking, with loss of consciousness; sometimes there is secondary generalization to a tonic-clonic seizure
Tonic	• Rigid posturing of trunk and extremities, may have fixed eye deviation
Clonic	• Rhythmic twitching of muscle groups, particularly the extremities and face
Multifocal	• Similar to clonic with multiple muscle groups involved
Myoclonic	• Brief focal or generalized jerks of extremities or parts of the body with distal muscle groups, may occur as a single jerk or series of repetitive jerks
Neonatal	
Subtle	• Chewing motions, excessive salivation, blinking, eye deviation, swallowing, swimming arms, pedaling legs, apnea, or color change

a partial seizure, establish whether consciousness and verbal interaction are preserved (simple partial seizure) or impaired (complex partial seizure). Simple partial seizures can progress to complex partial seizures or to generalized seizures. When a partial seizure evolves to a generalized seizure, it is called "secondary generalization." Neonatal seizures tend to be more subtle, because tonic-clonic activity may not occur during the first month of life. Deviated gaze or horizontal nystagmus and myoclonic seizures (a sudden, single muscle jerk) may be the only evidence of seizures in infants.

Complications

Seizures may cause hypoxia from airway obstruction, aspiration, or inadequate respiratory drive. Good prehospital management minimizes these complications. A second concern is brain injury from prolonged seizure activity in a child with a serious underlying condition, such as infection, intoxication (including toxic exposures), hemorrhage, or congenital neurologic problems. Children have fewer energy reserves than adults. Active seizure activity uses those reserves. Hypoglycemia can cause and prolong seizure activity.

Support of airway and breathing, control of seizure activity, checking and treating for hypoglycemia, and rapid transport to a facility with pediatric intensive care capability are the best strategies for minimizing morbidity in this population of critically ill children.

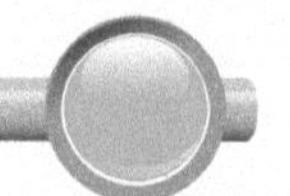

Tip

Be especially vigilant in care of infants and young children with status epilepticus if they do not have a history of fever or epilepsy.

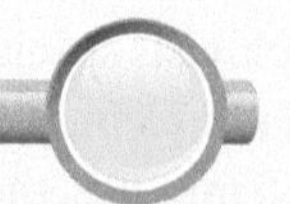

Controversy

The best position in which to place the child during a seizure is controversial. A supine position may increase aspiration risk but allows easy airway and breathing management. The lateral decubitus position provides some protection against aspiration but makes it more difficult to give oxygen and aid breathing.

Assessment and Treatment of the Actively Seizing Child

If a child is actively seizing when the prehospital professional arrives, there are several essential steps:

1. *Open the airway.*

   Managing the airway is the most important initial action (**Table 6-2**).

Table 6-2 Initial Airway Management in Seizing Children

Position the head to open the airway.
Clear the mouth with suction.
Consider the lateral decubitus position if the child is actively vomiting and suction is inadequate to control the airway (**Figure 6-1**).
Provide 100% oxygen by nonrebreathing mask or blow-by.
Consider a nasopharyngeal airway.

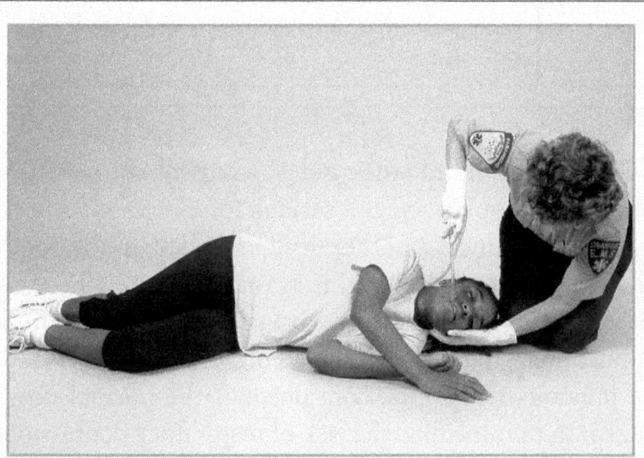

Figure 6-1 Position the head to open the airway, place the child in the lateral decubitus position, and clear the mouth of vomitus with suction.

ALS

Positioning is the easiest method to maintain a clear airway in a young child. For an infant, toddler, or preschool-aged child, perform the chin lift or jaw thrust. If there are a lot of secretions, open the airway while placing the child in the lateral decubitus position (recovery position). The insertion of a nasopharyngeal airway is the most useful tool after doing chin lift or jaw thrust. It provides an open airway around clenched teeth. Although an oropharyngeal airway can also be used, it is more difficult to insert if the teeth are clenched, and may cause vomiting if the patient has a gag reflex. Suction the mouth of secretions, if possible.

Without the use of neuromuscular blockade agents, successful endotracheal intubation during a seizure is extremely difficult, and complication rates are high. *Do not attempt to intubate a seizing child.* If the airway is not maintainable, attempt to stop the seizure through the administration of anticonvulsant medications. After the seizure is stopped, perform airway management as needed.

Consider spinal stabilization as part of airway management in a posttraumatic seizure, although it is not very effective until the seizure activity has stopped.

2. *Ensure adequate breathing.*

   All seizures are associated with some degree of hypoventilation. Attempt to assist ventilation if the child is cyanotic, or has an oxygen saturation less than 90% on supplemental oxygen. Be aware, however, that it is difficult to obtain an accurate pulse oximetry reading in a child who is having a seizure. Again, stopping the seizure is the key to successful ventilation. Opening the airway, coordinating positive-pressure ventilations with the patient's spontaneous respiratory effort, and expanding a rigid chest wall are technically difficult procedures during a generalized seizure. Often the result of assisted ventilation is stomach inflation with air. Advanced life support (ALS) providers should consider a nasogastric tube to decompress the stomach if bag-mask ventilation visibly distends the abdomen.

3. *Safeguard circulation.*

   Unless a child has seizures associated with sepsis or trauma, fluid resuscitation in the field or in transport is not necessary. Signs of poor perfusion are most likely associated with prolonged seizure activity, hypoxia, and metabolic acidosis. Once again, treating the seizure addresses these problems.

4. *Manage any disability.*

   Check the bedside glucose level and treat documented hypoglycemia, as described in **Table 6-3**.

Table 6-3 Dextrose Administration Guidelines During Seizures

Indications • Infant and child with glucose level <60 mg/dL • Newborn with glucose level <40 mg/dL
Treatment • Newly born: give $D_{10}W$, 2 mL/kg IV or IO • Neonate: give $D_{10}W$, 5 mL/kg IV or IO bolus (1 part $D_{50}W$, 4 parts sterile water or normal saline) • Child <2 years old: give $D_{25}W$, 2 mL/kg IV or IO bolus (1 part $D_{50}W$, 1 part sterile water or normal saline) • Child ≥2 years old: give $D_{50}W$, 1 mL/kg IV or IO bolus

ALS

Although most seizures stop before the arrival of prehospital professionals, the child who is still actively seizing usually benefits from pharmacologic treatment. Consider options for anticonvulsant administration, in terms of medications approved in the EMS system and available routes of administration. The goal is to stop the seizure, while minimizing medication side effects.

Benzodiazepine drugs are excellent first-line anticonvulsants. Common drugs in this class are lorazepam, diazepam, and midazolam. **Table 6-4** provides doses and routes of administration.

Although each of the benzodiazepines has the same mechanism of action, differences in specific agent and route of administration lead to significant clinical differences in the time to peak effect and the duration of action.

Lorazepam. Of the benzodiazepines, lorazepam, 0.05–0.1 mg/kg, probably has the best pharmacologic profile for

ALS

Table 6-4 Benzodiazepine Administration During Seizures

Generic Name	Initial Dose	Route	Pros	Cons
Diazepam	0.1 mg/kg	IV, IO	Rapid onset Inexpensive No refrigeration	Sedating Respiratory depression Short duration of action for seizure control (15 min)
Diazepam	0.5 mg/kg	PR	Rapid onset No IV required	Sedating Respiratory depression
Lorazepam	0.05–0.1 mg/kg	IV, IO	Rapid onset Long duration of action for seizure control (12–24 hr)	Must be stored away from heat and extreme temperature
Midazolam	0.1 mg/kg	IV, IM, IO	Rapid onset	Medium duration of action for seizure control (30–120 min)

prehospital seizure management. It has a rapid onset of action, can be given intravenously (IV) or intraosseously (IO), and has a long half-life. Lorazepam is used to stop a seizure and can help to prevent further seizure activity for up to 8 hours, depending on dose. There is little experience with out-of-hospital PR lorazepam administration in children, and drug doses are not well established. In general, this drug has not been widely used by prehospital professionals because of the manufacturer's recommendation regarding refrigeration. Lorazepam may be stocked unrefrigerated on prehospital ALS units if it is replaced every 30 days.

Diazepam. Diazepam is a time-honored drug for status epilepticus. IV diazepam, at 0.1 mg/kg, is an effective treatment for status epilepticus or prolonged seizures, but rapid IV administration may cause respiratory depression. Do not give diazepam intramuscularly (IM), because it is not well absorbed and is irritating to muscle tissue. Sublingual and intranasal administrations have been described, although there is little out-of-hospital experience.

The requirement for cannulating a peripheral vein in a seizing child often slows down delivery of essential ALS drugs, especially in infants and toddlers. *The rectum is an effective alternative route for emergency diazepam administration.* PR diazepam is effective, causes less respiratory depression and is easy to administer. Use a higher dose of 0.5 mg/kg. Rates of respiratory depression associated with PR diazepam are lower than for IV diazepam. However, onset of action is longer, with time to clinical effect in the range of 5 minutes. For a step-by-step explanation of the rectal diazepam administration procedure, see **Rectal Administration of Benzodiazepines, Procedure 20.**

A common home medication is Diastat, a form of rectal diazepam. Caregivers may have already administered Diastat to the child and called for assistance when the seizure did not stop. Administering an additional IV, IO, or IM dose of a benzodiazepine to stop the seizure may be necessary.

ALS

Diazepam begins to work quickly but its anticonvulsant action does not last long, a serious limitation in long field or transport times. Another dose of diazepam (or another anticonvulsant medication, if available) may be necessary within 10–20 minutes if the drug is given. If the child is on phenobarbital or has received other benzodiazepines in the previous few hours, consider half the normal dose of diazepam to minimize the risk of respiratory depression.

Midazolam. IM midazolam is another benzodiazepine that can be given to a patient without IV access. The dose is 0.1 mg/kg IM. Although onset of action is delayed compared to IV diazepam, the time to cessation of seizure activity may be less, when comparing time to start an IV. Midazolam can also be administered IV and IO (dose is 0.1 mg/kg) and also works intranasally. The intranasal dose is 0.2 mg/kg with a maximum dose of 10 mg, best administered by a nasal mucosal atomizer. The buccal route may also be used to stop seizures, but buccal administration procedures and doses have not yet been well studied.

When administering any benzodiazepine by any route, watch closely for respiratory depression, a common side effect of this class of drugs, and be prepared to provide bag-mask ventilatory support. Even in the case of apnea after benzodiazepine administration, a bag-valve-mask device usually suffices, because the respiratory depressant effects of the drugs are transitory. Endotracheal intubation is rarely necessary.

If the seizure does not stop after two doses of a benzodiazepine, further doses are unlikely to terminate the seizure. Consider a second drug if the local EMS system permits. Common choices for second-line anticonvulsants include phenytoin, fosphenytoin, and phenobarbital, the dosing and administration of which are described in **Table 6-5.**

Phenobarbital is preferred as the first-line drug in neonates at a dose of 20 mg/kg, and is a second-line drug for infants and children.

ALS

Table 6-5 Second-Line Anticonvulsant Drug Administration

Generic Name	Initial Dose	Route	Rate of Infusion	Maximum Rate of Infusion
Phenytoin	20 mg/kg	IV, IO	1 mg/kg/min	50 mg/min
Fosphenytoin	20 mg/kg (phenytoin equivalents or PE)	IV, IO, IM	3 mg (PE)/kg/min	150 mg (PE)/min
Phenobarbital	20 mg/kg	IV, IO	1 mg/kg/min	50 mg/min

Fosphenytoin, a recent "prodrug" or metabolic precursor to phenytoin, is a second-line option. Although fosphenytoin can be administered more quickly than phenytoin IV or IO and can also be given IM, it then takes about 15 minutes to metabolize to phenytoin, the active metabolite. *Hence, the total time it takes to get an effective drug level in the blood and brain to stop the seizure is approximately the same with phenytoin and fosphenytoin.* A disadvantage of fosphenytoin is that the drug is much more expensive than phenytoin.

Phenytoin is another second-line drug in neonates, infants, and children. Phenytoin should be administered only in normal saline at a rate no faster than 50 mg/min in adults and 1 mg/kg/min in children. The child should be placed on a cardiac monitor and watched carefully for bradycardia and hypotension, the most common serious complications of IV or IO phenytoin. Complications are caused by the diluent or mixing solution, propylene glycol.

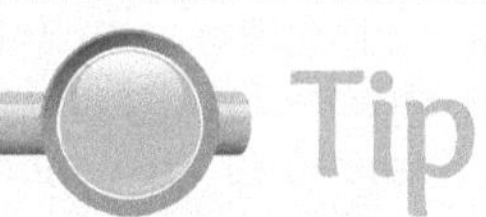

Always give oxygen to a child who is having a seizure or who is postictal.

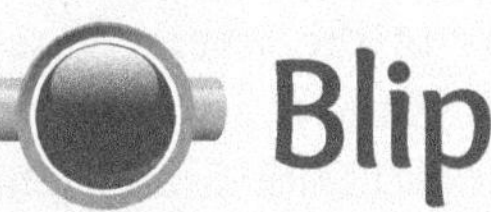

When phenytoin comes in contact with glucose, a gel forms that occludes the IV.

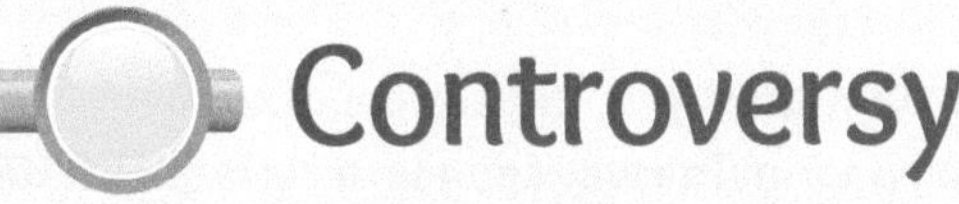

Lorazepam and midazolam may be effective when given buccally or intranasally. However, the exact doses and the relative effectiveness and safety of benzodiazepines given by this route are unknown.

Transport

After providing airway and breathing support and administering a benzodiazepine, transport should be initiated. Some EMS regions allow second-line anticonvulsant medications during transport. Perform history taking and physical examination and the detailed physical examination (trauma patients), if possible, on the way to the hospital. During transport, ongoing assessments should be performed using continuous cardiac monitoring and pulse oximetry, if available. If a patient has not stopped seizing after administration of several doses of a benzodiazepine and a second-line drug (e.g., fosphenytoin, phenytoin, or phenobarbital), the risk for a prolonged seizure is high. Consider options in terms of transport destination because this subset of children is likely to require intensive care.

Assessment of the Postictal Child

Usually the child's seizure is already over when the prehospital professional arrives. This "postictal" state is characterized by abnormal appearance with sleepiness, confusion, irritability, and decreased interactivity that may last from minutes to hours.

If the child is physiologically stable, perform a complete assessment in the field, including history taking and physical examination, observing particularly for any rash or discoloration of the skin, and the detailed physical examination (trauma patients). Check blood glucose levels and correct hypoglycemia if present.

An example of a stable postictal patient is the child with a previous diagnosis of epilepsy who experiences a brief grand mal seizure or the child younger than 6 years of age with fever and a possible febrile seizure. Most children who have had a brief seizure show steady improvement in level of alertness, muscle tone, and interactivity within 15–30 minutes. Failure to reach normal mental status over a 30- to 60-minute period after the seizure may reflect a serious underlying problem and trigger early transport with completion of the assessment en route to the hospital. **Table 6-6** lists some of the conditions that might lead to

Table 6-6 Worrisome Circumstances With the Postictal Child

Posttraumatic seizure
Postingestion seizure
Seizure and sustained hypoxia
Seizure in a neonate (<4 weeks of age)
First seizure in a child >6 years
More than one seizure
Seizure time >5 minutes
Low glucose level

a prolonged postictal state that require urgent treatment in the emergency department (ED). If the child has had a seizure after closed head injury, always stabilize the **cervical** spine, as discussed in Chapter 7.

If the postictal patient has a previous diagnosis of epilepsy, include the name and dosage of anticonvulsant medications and when the last dose was given in the history. Inquire when the last blood levels were obtained and whether the levels were adequate. Determine the duration of the seizure and ask for a description of the motor activity, including where it started, how it progressed, and how long the child was unconscious. From this information, determine the type of seizure (e.g., generalized or partial, or partial with secondary generalization). Ask carefully about head trauma. Consider the possibility of ingestion or overdose especially in toddlers and adolescents. Keep in mind that overdose of many nonprescription medications (e.g., antihistamines) can cause seizures.

Attempt to allay the caregiver's fears. If this was the child's first seizure, the caregiver may be extremely frightened.

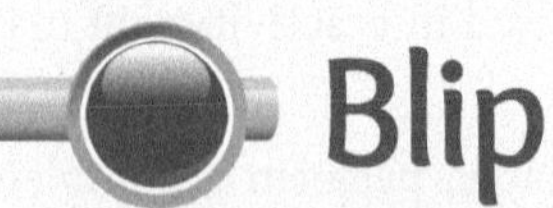

Blip

Calm parents' fears about the seizure, but do not diagnose or provide them uncertain information about the cause of the seizure or chance of recurrence.

Summary of Seizures

Seizures are common in children, and frightened caregivers frequently call 9-1-1 to assist in managing this problem. Usually the seizure has stopped before ambulance arrival, in which case the tasks include only assessment of the postictal child and transport to the hospital with supportive care.

Sometimes the child is seizing on arrival and requires medical management. The treatment includes opening and clearing the airway; giving oxygen; and then administering a benzodiazepine medication, usually diazepam, midazolam, or lorazepam. Rectal diazepam stops most seizures in children. Effective alternatives are IV or IO lorazepam; IV, IO, IM, or intranasal midazolam; or IV or IO diazepam. The benzodiazepine medications often cause temporary respiratory depression, which requires bag-valve-mask ventilation support without endotracheal intubation in most cases. If treatment with a benzodiazepine is unsuccessful, second-line drugs, such as phenobarbital, phenytoin, and fosphenytoin, are good options, based on local EMS protocol.

Altered Mental Status

AMS is an abnormal neurologic state in which the child is less alert and interactive than is age-appropriate. The term AMS refers to a range of abnormal appearances, from irritability to total unresponsiveness. Sometimes the concern of the caretaker is vague, and the complaint is simply that the child is "not acting right." Understanding normal developmental or age-related changes in behavior and listening carefully to the caregiver's opinion about alterations from an individual's normal state are key features in the assessment. A mnemonic recalls many of the severe causes of AMS (**Table 6-7**). The mnemonic is the five vowels in the alphabet (AEIOU), followed by tips (TIPPS), and reflects the major causes of AMS.

Case Study 2

You respond to a call about an unresponsive child. The caregiver states that the 3-year-old boy could not be awakened from his nap. The child is "sleeping" on your arrival, with no abnormal airway sounds or retractions. He is pale. Respiratory rate is 20 breaths/min, cardiac monitor shows a narrow complex with a rate of 160 beats/min, and blood pressure is 80/50 mm Hg. Pupils are small and slow to constrict to light, and the child withdraws to pain. There is no sign of trauma. The caregiver states that the child was playful and appeared healthy before his nap.

1. What are the immediate treatment priorities for this child?
2. What additional history may be helpful?

Table 6-7 AEIOU TIPPS: Possible Causes of AMS

Alcohol
Epilepsy, endocrine, electrolytes
Insulin
Opiates and other drugs
Uremia
Trauma, temperature
Infection, intussusception
Psychogenic
Poison
Shock, stroke, space-occupying lesion, subarachnoid hemorrhage

Assessment

Use the Pediatric Assessment Triangle (PAT) and the disability component of the hands-on ABCDEs to quickly assess neurologic status. These two parts of the primary assessment work in concert to evaluate both cortical and brainstem functions, as described in Chapter 1. There is a difference between "abnormal appearance" and AMS. Abnormal appearance is a more subtle measure of brain function and is evaluated using the TICLS mnemonic (Table 1-1). AMS is a more severe signal of mental status alteration and is evaluated with the alert-verbal-painful-unresponsive (AVPU) scale. Although AMS is always associated with an abnormal appearance, some children with more subtle abnormalities in appearance would not have AMS using the AVPU. For example, a child who is irritable or listless and has abnormal appearance on the PAT may be "alert" on the AVPU scale of disability during the ABCDE hands-on evaluation.

The AVPU system is a quick way to determine level of consciousness and to assess major changes in mental status during transport. A child with sepsis or brain hemorrhage from inflicted injury, for example, has a serious degree of brain dysfunction and may score "verbal" or lower on the AVPU.

Finally, observe motor activity and check the pupils. In the assessment of motor activity, watch for purposeful and symmetric movement of extremities, ataxia, seizures, posturing (decorticate or decerebrate), or flaccidity (hypotonia). In the assessment of pupils, check size (small or large), equality, and response to light. Pupils may have abnormal size or reactivity in the presence of drugs, ongoing seizures, hypoxia, or impending brainstem herniation. The presence of a deviated gaze is abnormal and should be noted and reported.

Look for a Medical Alert Bracelet, and ask about important medical history that may account for the child's AMS, such as diabetes or a seizure disorder (**Figure 6-2**).

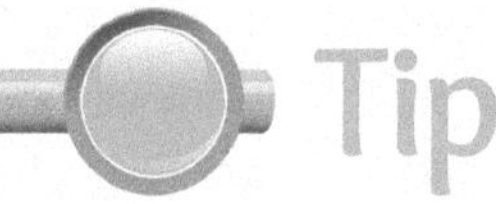

There are many causes of AMS, but management must focus on the ABCs.

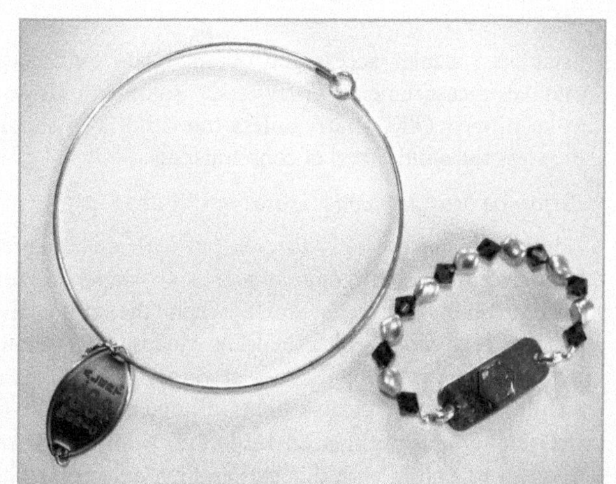

Figure 6-2 In a child with AMS, look for a bracelet with his or her medical history.

Management

Regardless of the cause of AMS, focus on the ABCs.

1. *Open the airway.*

   In the poorly responsive patient with compromised airway reflexes, suction the mouth to relieve potential obstruction from secretions or vomitus. If there is no gag reflex or if the patient is totally unresponsive, position the head and insert an oropharyngeal or nasopharyngeal airway. Keep the spine stabilized if there is a suspicion of head or neck injury.

2. *Ensure adequate breathing.*

   Patients with AMS may have inadequate breathing despite spontaneous respiratory effort, based on inadequate respiratory rate or inadequate tidal volume. Administer 100% oxygen by nonrebreathing mask. Start

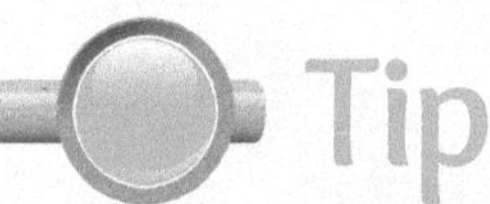

There is a difference between abnormal appearance and AMS. Abnormal appearance is a more subtle measure of brain function and is evaluated using the TICLS mnemonic. AMS is a more severe signal of mental status alteration and is evaluated with the AVPU.

bag-valve-mask ventilation with 100% oxygen if the patient is cyanotic, has oxygen saturation less than 90% on 100% oxygen by nonrebreathing mask, is breathing at a rate too slow for age, or has shallow or irregular respiratory effort.

Consider endotracheal intubation to protect the airway and to avoid aspiration. Ventilate the patient with suspected brain injury, but do not hyperventilate the patient (see Chapter 3). Use end-tidal CO_2 ($EtCO_2$) or capnography to guide ventilations. Place the patient on a cardiac monitor and a pulse oximeter.

3. *Safeguard circulation.*

   Establish vascular access and obtain blood for serum glucose measurement. Always start isotonic fluids at a to-keep-open (TKO) rate, unless the child is in shock. Reassess the child's level of consciousness.

4. *Perform a bedside blood glucose test* (**Figure 6-3**).

   Administer glucose only to children with documented hypoglycemia. Neurologic outcome in patients with diffuse brain injury is worse when the child also has hyperglycemia. If a bedside glucose test shows hypoglycemia (<40 mg/dL in a newborn, <60 mg/dL in a child), give an IV glucose bolus, diluted as directed, or IM glucagon as outlined in **Table 6-3**. Administer oral glucose to a child with diabetes and hypoglycemia who is conscious and has a gag reflex.

5. *In the child with AMS and depressed respirations, consider naloxone administration.*

   The naloxone dose is 0.1 mg/kg, with maximum doses up to 2 mg. Naloxone may be given by a variety of routes: IV, IM, IO, subcutaneous (SQ), intranasal, or endotracheal (ET) tube. Caution must be exercised when giving naloxone to a depressed newly born of a narcotic-addicted mother, because it may induce acute withdrawal symptoms and seizures. Instead of giving naloxone, consider supporting ventilation and transporting the newborn to the hospital. Outside of the newly born, narcotic overdose is an unlikely cause of AMS in

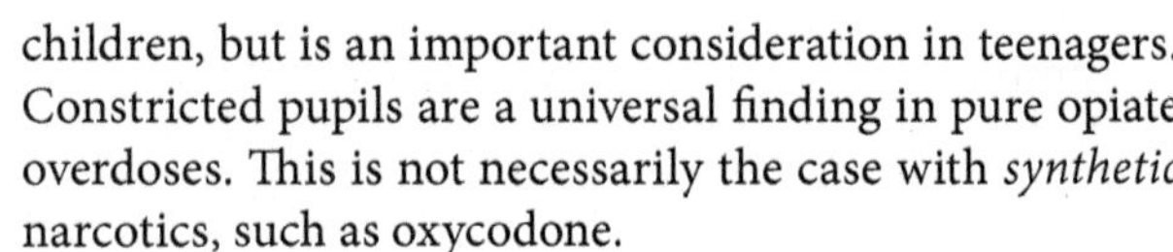
children, but is an important consideration in teenagers. Constricted pupils are a universal finding in pure opiate overdoses. This is not necessarily the case with *synthetic* narcotics, such as oxycodone.

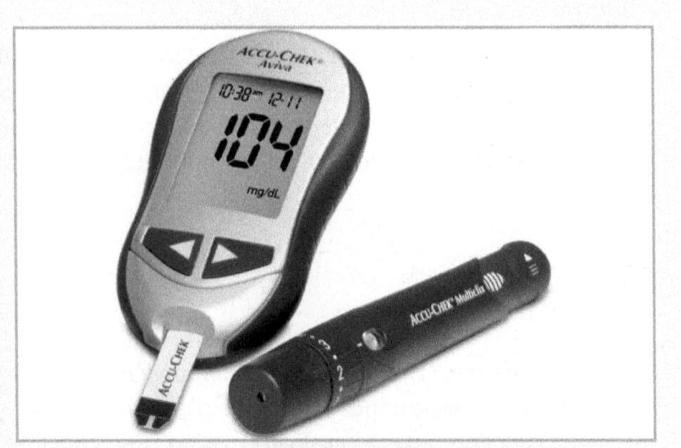

Figure 6-3 Perform a bedside blood glucose test.

Endocrine Disorders

In children, endocrine disorders include diabetes, congenital adrenal hyperplasia (CAH), panhypopituitarism, and cortisol deficiency. Of these disorders, diabetes is the most common.

Diabetes Mellitus

Diabetes is a disorder of the hormone insulin. Insulin, produced by the pancreas, helps regulate blood glucose levels. Glucose is needed in the production of energy by the cells in the body. Without adequate amounts of insulin, muscle cells cannot access circulating glucose and thus cannot create energy. The disease called diabetes mellitus is a result of a lack of functioning insulin.

Diabetes mellitus is a disease of children and adults. Of the two types, Type 1 (insulin-dependent diabetes mellitus, IDDM) and Type 2 (non–insulin-dependent diabetes mellitus, NIDDM), younger children are more likely to have Type 1 diabetes, which is insulin-dependent. These children are more prone to develop antibodies to the cells in the pancreas that produce insulin. The underlying cause is unknown.

There is an increasing prevalence of Type 2 diabetes (NIDDM) in childhood. Such children are usually adolescents, often with associated obesity. The child may be on oral hypoglycemic agents, rather than insulin.

Regardless of the type of diabetes, the onset of symptoms is relatively slow, over days (as in Type 1 diabetes) to weeks (as in Type 2 diabetes). The disease process begins as insulin production is diminished. Diminished amounts of insulin increasingly impair the availability of glucose to the muscle cells. The diminished amounts of glucose available for energy production stimulate the release of fat stores. As fat stores are mobilized, they are converted to ketones and other metabolic acids. Together the accumulation of glucose and metabolic acids cause the symptoms of diabetic ketoacidosis (DKA).

If the blood glucose level exceeds the renal threshold for reabsorption, an osmotic diuresis is created. This results in frequent urination (polyuria) with corresponding loss of body water. The higher the blood glucose level, increasing amounts of body water are lost in the urine. Loss of body water causes intense thirst (polydipsia). Fat breakdown leads to increased hunger (polyphagia) in the presence of abdominal pain along with the hallmark symptom of Kussmaul respirations. These respirations are rapid and deep, and have the odor of ketones or rotten fruit. These children may fall asleep in school, begin wetting the bed and have abnormal thirst, and the odor of ketones is often prevalent.

EMS may be called for a child with AMS with a history of abdominal pain, vomiting, and excessive thirst. The child is often severely dehydrated. In the presence of abdominal pain, nausea, and vomiting, sepsis may be suspected. The presence of a blood glucose level higher than 300 mg/dL or hyperglycemia may lead one to suspect the presence of DKA.

Assessment

Signs and symptoms of hyperglycemia can be hard to detect, especially because the onset is relatively slow. The primary sign of hyperglycemia is dehydration. Depending on the blood sugar level, signs and symptoms may range from mild to severe hypoperfusion. Tachycardia, rapid/deep respirations, and dry skin are all signs of volume depletion. In general, the higher the blood glucose level, the more extreme the dehydration.

Management

After general treatment measures are implemented, initiate an IV and administer fluid at 20 mL/kg. Care must be taken when administering IV fluid because children with high blood glucose levels are prone to develop cerebral edema in the presence of excess fluid. Therefore, repeat fluid boluses only if the child is hypotensive. If not hypotensive, keep IV fluids at maintenance rate.

Hypoglycemia

Hypoglycemia is defined as a serum glucose concentration of less than 40 mg/dL in a newly born infant, or less than 60 mg/dL in a child. The most frequent scenario for out-of-hospital hypoglycemia is a child with known diabetes who uses too much insulin; exerts himself or herself excessively; or delays a meal (transient hypoglycemia) after taking insulin. Hypoglycemia may also occur in children with a history of almost any endocrine problem.

In nondiabetic infants, hypoglycemia may occur when the child has been working so hard that glycogen reserves become depleted (e.g., when compensating for a cardiac defect or for an extreme respiratory rate). This is more common in infants and toddlers.

Hypoglycemia may also occur in children with sepsis. Check a bedside glucose level in any acutely ill appearing child, especially in the presence of abnormal appearance or AMS. Other causes of hypoglycemia in children are poor food intake in the face of an acute illness, such as gastroenteritis, especially in infants and toddlers with limited glycogen reserves.

Assessment

Signs and symptoms of hypoglycemia can be hard to detect, especially in younger infants who have mild hypoglycemia.

Table 6-8 Signs and Symptoms of Hypoglycemia

Mild	Moderate	Severe
Hunger, irritability, weakness, agitation, tachypnea, tachycardia	Anxiety, blurred vision, stomach ache, headache, dizziness, sweating, pallor, tremors, confusion	Seizure, coma

The changing signs and symptoms are noted in **Table 6-8**. Depending on the blood sugar level, signs and symptoms may range from mild to severe. Tachycardia, tachypnea, sweating, agitation, and tremor all reflect increased catecholamine release as the body responds to inadequate sugar supplies to support cellular metabolism. When blood sugar is dangerously low, seizures, coma, and death can occur.

Management of Hypoglycemia in Diabetes Mellitus

Children with Type 1 IDDM are often well aware of the signs and symptoms of hypoglycemia, based on past experiences with insulin. If a patient with diabetes is at least physiologically stable and cooperative but is hypoglycemic by blood sugar testing, allow him or her to attempt oral glucose replacement. Give 0.5–1.0 g/kg of sugar. There are 20 g glucose in 8 oz of regular (not dietetic) soda, as well as orange or apple juice. Milk may be the preferred replacement with a balance of 12 g glucose, 8 g protein, and 8 g fat in 8 oz of whole milk.

Children taking oral hypoglycemic agents (Type 2 diabetes) are also prone to hypoglycemia, although not as frequently. When present in the child with Type 2 diabetes, hypoglycemia can be more difficult to stabilize. Give the child oral glucose replacement if signs and symptoms of hypoglycemia occur and the child is physiologically stable and cooperative, or treat with IV dextrose or IV or IM glucagon if the child has AMS.

Treatment of Hypoglycemia

Treat hypoglycemia if the child has AMS and measured serum glucose of less than 40 mg/dL in a newborn or less than 60 mg/dL in a child, as outlined in **Table 6-3**. Children have different tolerances to hypoglycemia, so a child may be alert and cooperative with a blood sugar level between 40 and 50 mg/dL. A child in this condition can take oral glucose or an infant can breastfeed.

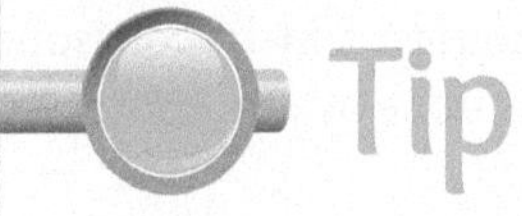

Signs and symptoms of hypoglycemia can be nonspecific.

For the physiologically unstable patient with hypoglycemia and AMS, IV or IO dextrose should be administered immediately. Recheck the serum glucose if scene time or transport is prolonged and repeat glucose doses as needed. It is important to dilute 50% IV glucose to either D25% for a child <2 years or D10% for a neonate and infuse the diluted solution by slow IV push, and avoid infiltration, because the solution, even when diluted, is quite irritating to skin tissues.

If there is no IV access, glucagon should be administered (0.03–0.1 mg/kg IV, IO, IM, or SQ up to 1 mg). Repeat in 20 minutes as needed. Glucagon stimulates a transient increase of the blood glucose level as long as there are liver stores of glycogen (long chains of stored glucose molecules). It is important to note that the incidence of vomiting is increased in children when glucagon is administered. Take care to position the child to ensure airway patency within the first 15–20 minutes after administration.

Congenital Adrenal Hyperplasia

CAH is another endocrine disorder. This disorder involves the hormones of the adrenal glands. The adrenal glands help keep the body in balance by making the right amounts of cortisol, aldosterone, and androgens. Although there are many different types of CAH, the most common type (95%) results in a deficiency of cortisol and sometimes aldosterone. As a result, the body cannot adjust to illness or injury. Hypotension, hypoglycemia, and dehydration may be severe and a threat to life.

Most children with this disorder carry emergency medication with them at all times. Usually, the medication includes dexamethasone or hydrocortisone. Parents should be asked if they have given the needed medication, such as hydrocortisone. If not, have them administer the medication if possible. Because the body is unable to adjust to a stress, checking blood glucose level and administering dextrose as needed, monitoring blood pressure and replacing fluids as necessary are all part of assessment and treatment.

Cortisol Deficiency

This deficiency occurs when the adrenal glands do not produce enough cortisol. This may occur for a variety of reasons, including CAH, pituitary gland malfunction, and failure of the adrenal gland itself or when steroids are already present. When children are prescribed steroids for a period of time, they must be gradually withdrawn to give the adrenal glands a chance to resume function. Normal management includes oral hydrocortisone or IM injections. In certain circumstances, the amount of hydrocortisone should be increased quickly. This is done by administering either oral or IM hydrocortisone.

In any case, when a child with cortisol deficiency becomes sick, many body systems are affected, including the ability to balance blood glucose and regulate body water. These children should always have a blood glucose check. Asking the parent or caregiver if the child's normal medication has been administered is very appropriate. If the medication has not been administered, calling the receiving facility or following the care plan (found with the rescue medication) is also encouraged.

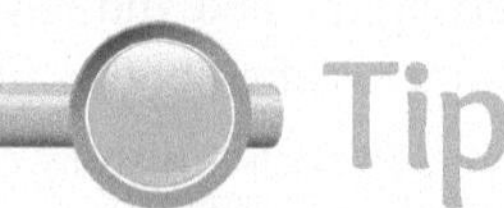

In a child with impaired adrenal gland function, administration of steroids (dexamethasone or hydrocortisone) can be lifesaving.

Panhypopituitarism

This condition affects the pituitary gland, particularly the anterior pituitary where thyroid-stimulating hormone (TSH), adrenocorticotropic hormone (ACTH), growth hormone (GH), and others are produced. As a result, many other glands of the child's endocrine system are also affected. These children are usually diagnosed in infancy, or can develop the condition after removal of certain brain tumors, and parents or other caregivers are well educated in their child's condition. When a child suffering this condition becomes ill, hypoglycemia is common and dehydration may also be present.

Transport

With any child having an endocrine issue, transport is important. If the child is suffering from hyperglycemia, do not delay transport for administration of fluid. The child needs to be transported, so IV/IO starts en route are appropriate.

However, if a low blood glucose level is present, treatment should be initiated immediately. After giving IV or IO dextrose or IM glucagon, reassess. Watch for a return to normal appearance and behavior. If the child with AMS does not return to normal in a few minutes after IV or IO administration or 15–20 minutes after IM glucagon, transport immediately and conduct additional assessment on the way to the ED. If the child returns to normal, consider doing additional assessment on scene. If the child has no history of diabetes or other endocrine problems, and has either hyperglycemia or hypoglycemia, transport is indicated.

Additional Assessment

Perform history taking when possible. Ask key questions, such as:

- How quickly did the symptoms progress?
- Does the patient have diabetes or any other known illness?

- If the patient is a diabetic, or has another endocrine problem, has there been a recent change in medication or meals?
- Is the child on insulin, an oral hypoglycemia drug, or any other replacement medication?
- Is this the first episode? If not, how often does this happen?
- Is it possible that the child was exposed to drugs or alcohol?
- If the patient is a newborn, has the mother received prenatal care?
- Has the mother had any medical problems with the pregnancy?
- Is the mother a diabetic?
- What is the newborn being fed and how often?
- When was the last time the child had medication?
- How many caregivers are giving medications? Are they doubling up doses?

After the history, a physical examination should be performed. It is important to continually reassess the patient's status. If the child has diabetes and received too much insulin, and there are no physiologic or anatomic abnormalities on reassessment, or if the child has another endocrine problem, consider contacting medical control. In some EMS systems, the child with Type 1 diabetes, who is not in DKA, may be left at the scene with management directed by the primary care physician in consultation with the caregiver. However, the circumstances with Type 2 diabetes are somewhat different, because the oral drugs that are taken for this condition have a longer duration of action than most insulin and the child may need ongoing administration of glucose to maintain blood sugar. *Patients with Type 2 diabetes on oral agents, who have experienced hypoglycemia, should not be left on the scene.* If the child has an emergency medication that needs to be administered, or if the child is a Type 2 diabetic with an episode of hypoglycemia, transport the child to the ED.

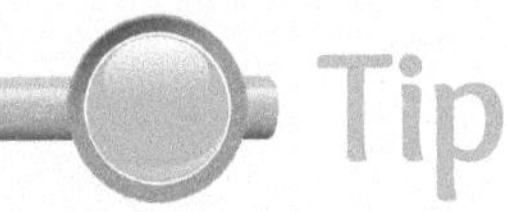

Do not leave patients with Type 2 diabetes on oral agents, who have experienced hypoglycemia, on the scene.

Summary of Altered Mental Status and Endocrine Disorders

There are many causes of AMS in children. The caregiver may be the best judge of AMS, especially in the infant or toddler where developmental assessment is more challenging. Appearance and the AVPU scale work in concert to help assess AMS. Address the ABCs first and especially consider causes of dehydration, such as hyperglycemia, and reversible causes, such as hypoglycemia. Transport the child with hyperglycemia immediately.

Fever

Fever is a sign of infection or inflammation, rather than a problem itself, and is often misunderstood. Most infections in childhood are systemic and result in fevers. Children can run high fevers in response to either bacterial or viral infections. High fever (>40°C or 104°F) can be caused by minor illness, such as a cold, or serious problems, such as pneumonia, meningitis, or sepsis. Fever of any cause leads to an increase in basal metabolic rate, causing a more rapid respiratory rate, increased cardiac output, higher oxygen consumption, and a greater need for fluids and calories. The ill child frequently is not interested in eating or drinking and, with the increased metabolic demands of fever, may be at risk for volume depletion and hypoglycemia. A body temperature less than 41.1°C (106°F) is not itself harmful. However, body temperatures greater than 41.1°C (106°F) may have the potential to be harmful, and the child should be carefully evaluated. In general, fevers are a common cause of concern for most parents, and high temperatures are a cause of concern to caregivers who fear brain damage as a result of a high fever despite the fact that there is no evidence to support that concern.

Determine the presence of fever by history and field evaluation. Knowing the temperature, however, usually does not change field management.

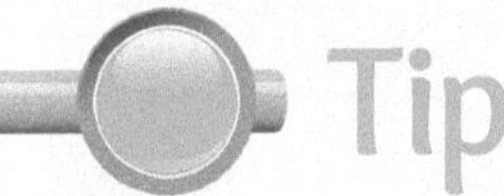

Fever less than 41.1°C (106°F) by itself does not cause brain damage.

Assessment

The primary assessment helps determine the severity of the child's illness and the urgency for treatment. If the primary assessment is normal, take a history and perform a physical examination. Ask about important signs and symptoms of infection, such as chills, malaise, poor feeding, lethargy, pulling of ears, vomiting, diarrhea, abdominal pain, presence of a rash or skin discoloration, stiff neck, headache, and irritability.

Ask about exposure to known childhood communicable diseases. Many childhood illnesses begin with a fever before any other symptoms are present. Determine if the child has any significant medical history, because febrile children who may be immune deficient (e.g., patients with sickle cell disease, cancer, human immunodeficiency virus [HIV], or post-organ transplantation) are at higher risk for serious infection as the cause of fever.

Febrile respiratory infections are very common in children and are characterized by fever, tachycardia, tachypnea, nasal congestion, cough, and respiratory distress. Fever may make a child with a minor illness appear sicker than he or she really is, and parents often report a marked improvement in symptoms after administration of antipyretics, such as acetaminophen or ibuprofen. After the history, if the child has no physiologic abnormalities, a physical examination should be performed to look for possible sources of infection.

Although the height of fever is not reflective of the degree of illness, certain findings suggest a serious underlying illness and must prompt rapid transport. These include a bulging fontanelle (if <12 months of age, palpate with the child sitting up), photophobia (sensitivity to light), nuchal rigidity (stiff neck), paradoxical irritability (an infant who is crankier when picked up and held than when left alone) (**Figure 6-4**), seizures, prolonged capillary refill time, or a petechial or purpuric rash (**Figure 6-5**).

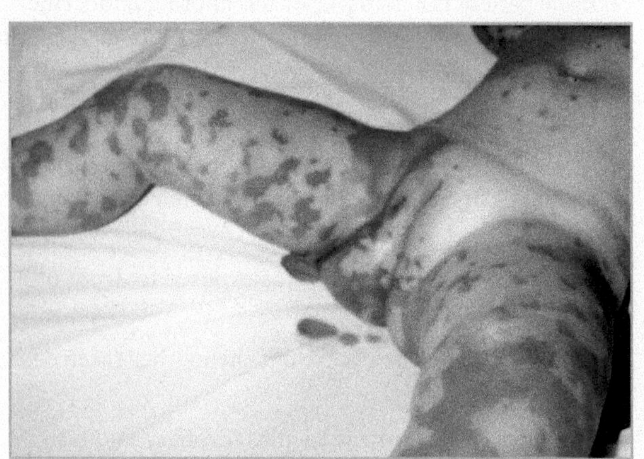

Figure 6-5 Purpuric rash in a child with meningococcemia.

Age and Fever

In addition to signs and symptoms, the age of a child is important in assessing the significance of fever. A fever in an infant less than 6 months old may be the only indication of serious infection, but the degree of temperature may be lower in comparison to the severity of illness or in comparison to older children with the same problem. The symptoms of serious bacterial infection in a young infant may be nonspecific, such as fussiness, poor feeding, and sleepiness. Because these very young infants have an immature immune system and are difficult to assess because of their limited range of behaviors and activities, any infant less than 4 weeks old with fever greater than or equal to 38°C (100.4°F) requires blood, urine, and spinal fluid cultures and empiric antibiotics in the ED. In the first few days of life, jaundice may be a sign of serious bacterial infection. Infants 28 days to 2 months of age usually require a similar evaluation but may be discharged from the ED if the physical examination and laboratory evaluation are normal. A seizure in the presence of a fever in a child less than 6 months of age also warrants transport.

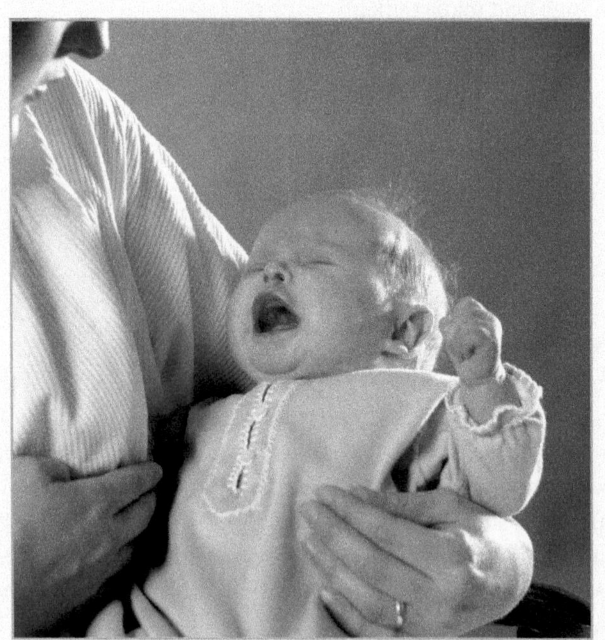

Figure 6-4 An infant suffering from paradoxical irritability.

Management

Management of fever in the child who has a normal primary assessment includes the following:

1. *Prevent transmission of disease to the prehospital professional.*

   Use standard precautions for infection control.

2. *In a febrile child who is older than 6 months, consider administration of antipyretics if none have been administered in the past 4 hours.*

   Give acetaminophen at a dose of 15 mg/kg orally or rectally. Another option for the alert pediatric patient is ibuprofen at 10 mg/kg orally if awake. Ibuprofen is not recommended by the manufacturer for infants less than 6 months of age. A pediatric patient's level of consciousness or history of recent vomiting should be considered before administering anything by mouth. Aspirin should be avoided in a febrile infant or child because prior studies suggest that there is an increased incidence of Reye syndrome in children who receive aspirin for a viral illness. Parents may need explanation that overbundling a febrile child retains heat and may increase fever.

3. *Cool the feverish child by undressing him or her, but avoid hypothermia.*

   Do not use cold water, fans, ice, or alcohol baths to lower temperature.

4. *Transport with ongoing reassessment for deterioration.*
5. *Explain to the caregiver that fever alone is not dangerous to the child.*

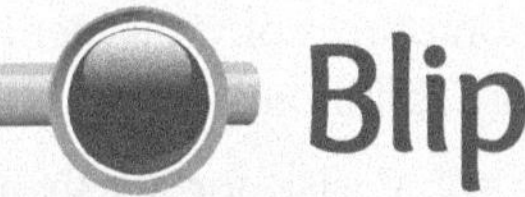

Blip

Never use ice, cold water, fans, or alcohol baths to cool a feverish child.

Summary of Fever

Fever is usually a response to any type of infection. It is rarely a problem in and of itself. However, the longer the child has sustained a fever the more likely the child is dehydrated. The age of the child and other associated signs and symptoms are important in determining probability of serious illness. The presence of a petechial or purpuric rash, stiff neck, light sensitivity, and/or AMS in a child with a fever is highly suspicious for a more serious problem. In most cases, simple cooling measures and transport are the primary actions for the prehospital professional.

Communicable Diseases

Many communicable diseases are common during childhood. Although most are viral in origin, and mild in terms of severity, infectious diseases on occasion cause significant compromise in the pediatric patient, resulting in the need for prehospital transport. Many childhood diseases have a respiratory component, a GI component, or both. Respiratory diseases are addressed in Chapter 3. This chapter concentrates on the GI signs and symptoms of nausea, vomiting, and diarrhea.

Nausea, Vomiting, and Diarrhea (Gastroenteritis)

Collectively, nausea, vomiting, and diarrhea are termed gastroenteritis. Gastroenteritis is an inflammation of the GI tract that presents as vomiting and diarrhea in the pediatric patient. There are numerous causes of gastroenteritis ranging from food and waterborne diseases, viruses, bacteria, side effect of antibiotics, and parasites, many carried by animals, especially pets. Of all the causes, viral agents are most common, with the Norwalk virus being especially contagious. No matter the cause, this infectious illness can result in volume depletion, particularly in younger children. Beware that signs and symptoms most commonly associated with gastroenteritis, such as fever, abdominal pain, or vomiting, can also herald more serious abdominal emergencies, such as appendicitis and bowel obstruction.

It is important to determine the presence and sequence of nausea, vomiting, diarrhea, and/or fever. Conditions of malrotation of the gut (in newborns) and pyloric stenosis (vomiting shortly after nursing but no diarrhea or fever) are conditions more common in young infants. Food poisoning, such as salmonella, usually occurs after eating (sometimes as much as 6–8 hours) and causes vomiting and diarrhea in that order, then followed by a fever. The diagnosis of gastroenteritis requires exclusion of more serious causes, and this determination is not possible in the field.

Assessment

Focus the assessment of a child with presumed gastroenteritis on the child's state of hydration.

The history should include questions regarding:

- The onset, sequence of events, and frequency of vomiting or diarrhea
- Relationship to eating
- Amount of oral intake
- Number of wet diapers or times of urination in the past 8 hours
- Character of stool including the presence of blood
- Last urination or wet diaper

The physical examination should include attention to:

- Presence or absence of fever
- Level of consciousness
- Hydration of mucous membranes (moist or dry)
- Presence or absence of tears
- Extremity warmth and pulse quality
- Abdominal tenderness or distention

Always check a bedside glucose level in a child with a history of vomiting, diarrhea, and poor oral intake.

Management

Management of the pediatric patient with presumed gastroenteritis depends on the degree of dehydration. Prevention of disease transmission to the prehospital professional is an additional component of care.

1. *Use standard precautions to reduce the likelihood of disease transmission.*

   Gastroenteritis, whether bacterial, viral, or parasitic in origin, is transmitted by the fecal-oral route. Ingestion of even a few pathogenic organisms can lead to disease in some cases. Some organisms can survive on examination instruments and surfaces for hours, so special care of clothes and instruments and careful hand washing are essential.

2. *Provide supplemental oxygen and airway management for the unstable pediatric patient.*

ALS

3. *Provide fluid replacement for severe clinical dehydration.*

   Establish vascular access, IV or IO, and initiate fluid replacement using crystalloid fluid at 20 mL/kg initial bolus if the child has severe clinical dehydration as evidenced by elevated heart rate, poor pulses, delayed capillary refill time, cool extremities, and abnormal coloration. Repeat the bolus to a total of 60 mL/kg until perfusion is stabilized.

4. *Treat documented hypoglycemia.*
5. *Reassess vital signs.*
6. *Transport.*

   Transport decisions depend on the degree of dehydration and local resources. A child with mild to moderate dehydration and ongoing vomiting and diarrhea may require transport alone without treatment. Provide oral fluids in the field to children with dehydration, if permitted by the EMS system. The child with signs of severe dehydration or shock benefits from immediate fluid replacement before hospital transport.

Sepsis and Meningitis

Sepsis implies an overwhelming, life-threatening bacterial bloodstream infection. Some children with sepsis also have **meningitis**, resulting from infection and inflammation of the meninges, the membranes that cover the brain and spinal cord. Other children present with sepsis or meningitis alone. The causative agent of meningitis may be aseptic (nonbacterial) or bacterial. Although children with viral or aseptic meningitis may appear quite ill, the infection is not often life-threatening. However, bacterial meningitis is rapidly progressive, with death sometimes following the onset of symptoms within hours to days. Although fever is usually present, except occasionally in the neonatal period, other symptoms may vary from stiff neck and headache to impending brainstem herniation.

Infants in the first year of life are at highest risk for sepsis and bacterial meningitis, and the organisms vary with age. Since the introduction of the *Haemophilus influenzae* type B vaccine in the late 1980s, this previously common cause of childhood illness has almost disappeared. Bacterial sepsis and meningitis in the first month of age is most commonly caused by bacteria acquired from the maternal vaginal area during delivery. These include *Escherichia coli*, group B streptococcus, and *Listeria monocytogenes*.

Outside of the youngest age group, community-acquired infection is the source of sepsis and meningitis, with common bacterial causes in immune-competent children including *Streptococcus pneumoniae* (also the most common cause of bacterial ear infections, sinusitis, and pneumonia in children) and *Neisseria meningitidis* (meningococcus). The pneumococcal vaccine recently available throughout the United States is significantly reducing the incidence of childhood bacteremia and sepsis from the pneumococcal organism. *H. influenzae* type B meningitis has also decreased significantly because of widespread vaccine use. The **enteroviruses** are also common causes of viral meningitis, especially during summer and fall months.

Another group of children who are at risk for sepsis are those who are immunodeficient (e.g., cancer, post-organ transplantation), especially if they have an indwelling central line.

Meningococcal sepsis or meningitis is a life-threatening emergency that presents acutely with high fever, AMS, and a characteristic **petechial rash** or **purpura**. The presence of such a rash should always trigger rapid transport by the highest level of provider to the highest level of care available, because these children can deteriorate very quickly, requiring aggressive life support.

Assessment

In a physiologically unstable child with presumed sepsis or meningitis, limit the scene assessment. Perform the focused history and physical examination during transport, if possible. The focused history should include:

- Known exposure to illness
- Perinatal history for infants <1 month of age
- Onset of symptoms and rapidity of progression
- Presence or absence of fever
- Associated symptoms and signs, such as irritability, vomiting, nuchal rigidity, rash (petechiae or purpura)
- Immunization history

The physical examination should include attention to:

- Fever
- Level of consciousness
- Adequacy of perfusion
- Nuchal rigidity
- Presence of a rash (petechiae or purpura)
- Photophobia

Because children with sepsis and meningitis are in a hypermetabolic state, they can develop hypoglycemia and dehydration. Check a bedside glucose level on any patient with presumed sepsis or meningitis.

Management

Management of the pediatric patient with sepsis or meningitis must include infection control precautions. Interventions vary based on the patient's clinical presentation.

1. *Prevent disease transmission.*

   The prehospital professional should use standard and respiratory precautions, including gowns, gloves, and masks to avoid contact with patient secretions.

2. *Provide supplemental oxygen.*

   Unstable patients may need assisted ventilation or airway management.

3. *Establish vascular access.*

4. *For inadequate perfusion, initiate fluid replacement.*

   For the pediatric patient with inadequate perfusion, initiate fluid replacement using crystalloid fluid at 20 mL/kg initial bolus as fast as possible. Because of the effects of fever, dehydration may be present. Because of the effects of bacterial toxins on the blood vessels, children with sepsis may develop distributive shock requiring aggressive fluid resuscitation. Therefore, repeat fluid boluses of 20 mL/kg up to 60 mL/kg of crystalloid fluid may be required.

5. *Treat hypoglycemia.*

6. *Reassess vital signs frequently.*

   Use continuous cardiorespiratory monitoring and pulse oximetry, if available. Anticipate deterioration in transport.

7. *Transport.*

   Because these children are at risk for rapid deterioration and may need ALS intervention, transport by the highest level of service available. Children with sepsis or meningitis generally require intensive care. Consider this when determining a transport destination.

Environmental Emergencies

Common pediatric environmental emergencies include temperature-related problems, bites, and stings. Each of these emergencies can range from mild to severe. Match the intensity of the intervention to the severity of the illness or injury.

Heat-Related Emergencies

Heat-related emergencies involve two separate and distinct processes leading to three main heat-related emergencies: (1) heat cramps, (2) heat exhaustion, and (3) heat stroke. Heat cramps and heat exhaustion are caused by a combination of fluid deficit and electrolyte imbalance. Heat stroke, however, is a result of a resetting of the heat-regulating mechanism in the hypothalamus of the brain, resulting in **hyperthermia**.

Heat cramps are a combination of electrolyte imbalance and dehydration where the electrolyte imbalance precipitates spasms of the muscle, typically of the long bones. These children complain of pain in their legs, arms, and sometimes the abdomen. Because this has occurred, usually during activity, the skin is warm and sweaty. Tachycardia may be present and may be caused by pain.

Heat exhaustion is a combination of electrolyte imbalance and dehydration where the dehydration precipitates dizziness and/or syncope. Because a volume deficit is present, the skin is often pale, cool, and diaphoretic. Tachycardia and tachypnea are also common. Hypoglycemia is not common but should be assessed for and treated as necessary.

Heat stroke occurs when the temperature-regulating mechanism is reset to a higher set point, usually higher than 40.6°C (105°F). As a result, the basal metabolic rate is greatly increased and every body organ is affected. Because the enzymes within the organs and body systems are designed to work between a relatively narrow temperature range, organ failure occurs. AMS, heart failure with pulmonary edema, kidney and liver failure, and profound hypotension are evident. Because of the increased metabolic rate, hypoglycemia is common. The skin is usually dry and red; tachycardia is extreme (usually >150 bpm); and tachypnea is present.

Heat-related emergencies, however, are rarely as clear-cut as they are described. The child with heat exhaustion may have AMS, or the child with heat stroke may be sweating. Regardless of the type of heat-related emergency, it is very important that a heat-related emergency is recognized and treatment implemented. In the pediatric population, heat-related emergencies occur most commonly when young children are left in a closed car or older children who are not heat-acclimated participate in sports during periods of high environmental temperatures and do not hydrate adequately. Because of the difficulty of obtaining temperature readings in the field, the assessment of such patients often occurs without the benefit of an objective temperature.

Physiologic considerations in infants and toddlers with heat-related emergencies include immature thermoregulatory systems, greater body surface area-to-mass ratio, and a lesser ability to dissipate heat (**Table 6-9**). These characteristics predispose infants and toddlers to heat-related emergencies, particularly heat stroke, much more quickly than in older children.

Assessment

The history should include:

- Environmental temperature
- Duration of environmental exposure
- Activities and events before symptom development
- Preexisting medical conditions

Table 6-9 Typical Clinical Presentation of Heat-Related Emergencies

Clinical Presentation	Signs and Symptoms
Heat cramps	• Normal level of consciousness • Slightly elevated body temperature • Painful muscle spasms
Heat exhaustion	• Mild AMS • Tachycardia, tachypnea, hypotension • Core temperature 38°–40°C (100.4°–104°F) • Fatigue • Headache • Diaphoresis
Heat stroke	• Severe AMS; confusion to coma • Tachycardia, hypotension • Core temperature >40.6°C (105°F) • Flushed, dry skin • Nausea and vomiting

Management

The management of heat-related illness depends on the severity of symptoms, especially the patient's level of consciousness and cardiovascular status. Because the mechanism is different, use of antipyretics is not effective.

Heat Cramps

- Cool environment
- Remove excess clothing
- Oral rehydration with an electrolyte-containing solution
- Establish vascular access with normal saline at TKO rate

Heat Exhaustion

- Cool environment
- Cool mist or light sponging with tepid water and allow moisture to evaporate
- Establish vascular access and initiate fluid replacement with crystalloid fluid at 20 mL/kg for treatment of shock

Heat Stroke

- Airway management, assist ventilations, intubate if indicated
- Establish vascular access and fluid replacement with crystalloid fluid at 20 mL/kg
- Cool mist or light sponging with tepid water and allow moisture to evaporate
- Aggressive cooling measures: wet sheets, ice bags to axilla, groin, and neck
- Frequent remeasurement of core temperature
- Treat hypoglycemia
- Avoid shivering
- Treat for shock

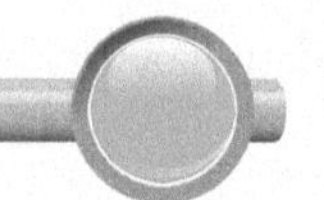

Tip

Early recognition and frequent reassessment of a heat-related emergency is important, because the patient's temperature may continue to rise despite initial management techniques.

Summary of Heat-Related Emergencies

Rapid recognition of heat-related emergencies is essential to effective management. Reassess vital signs frequently to evaluate the patient's response to treatment. Aggressive cooling measures are required for heat stroke.

Cold-Related Emergencies

Hypothermia is a core temperature of less than 35°C (95°F). Infants and toddlers are at especially high risk for hypothermia because of their greater body surface area-to-mass ratio, decreased body fat, increased permeability of thin skin, and limited ability to shiver and produce heat. Extended exposure to a cold environment and immersion in cold water are the two most common causes of hypothermia in young children. Children with severe illness or injury may also develop hypothermia. Finally, infants and young children may become hypothermic while being exposed for medical evaluation, especially in cold environments. The presence of hypothermia may precipitate or extend shock and complicate resuscitation, regardless of the underlying condition.

Assessment

History taking should include recent illness or injury and circumstances of exposure. The physical examination should include special attention to airway and breathing. Because hypothermia leads to a slowing of metabolism, the child may hypoventilate, with slow or shallow respirations.

Circulation

Bradycardia and hypotension may be present because of hypothermia itself or because of a concurrent hypoxic insult. Hypothermia may also lead to cardiac dysrhythmias. The skin is often pale and cool.

Disability

Mental status may range from confusion to coma, depending on the degree of hypothermia. Again, hypoxia may be the underlying cause of AMS, especially in submersion victims, so ensure the adequacy of oxygenation and ventilation. Depending on the circumstances, hypoglycemia may also be present.

Core Body Temperature

Obtain core body temperature, when possible, with a thermometer that registers less than 34°C (94°F).

Determine degree of hypothermia:

- Mild: 35°–36°C (93°–95°F)
- Moderate: 30°–34°C (86°–93°F)
- Severe: less than 30°C (<86°F)

Loss of the compensatory mechanism of shivering to generate heat is characteristic of moderate to severe hypothermia.

Management

Management of the patient with hypothermia depends on the core temperature.

1. *Support airway, breathing, and circulation as indicated.*
2. *Prevent heat loss.*

   It is crucial to prevent further heat loss. Remove wet clothing, dry the skin, and cover the patient after the examination is completed (**Figure 6-6**). Apply a hat or head wrap because a high proportion of heat is lost through the head.
3. *Rewarm.*

   External, passive rewarming is appropriate for mild to moderate hypothermia. In the case of severe hypothermia, external rewarming may shunt cold blood to the core, leading to further complications. Core rewarming in the ED is the appropriate therapy for these patients.

   a. Mild hypothermia: apply warm blankets, increase ambient temperature of the ambulance. Prehospital professionals should be uncomfortably warm!

   b. Moderate hypothermia: warm blankets, heat packs to axilla and groin.

   ALS

   c. Severe hypothermia: cautious movement with gentle handling; warmed, humidified oxygen; warmed IV solution; treat hypoglycemia if present; rapid transport to a definitive care facility for core rewarming.

ALS

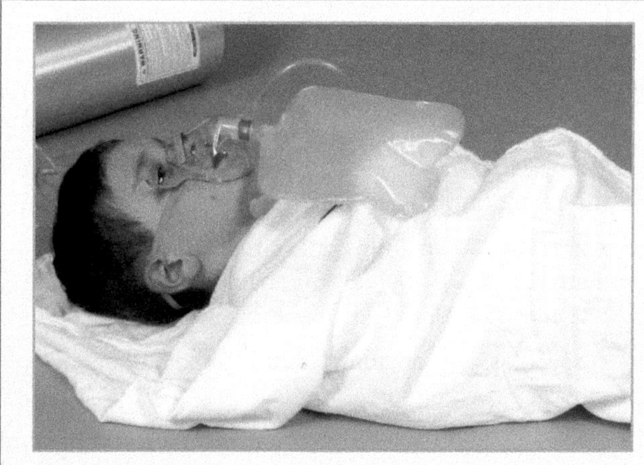

Figure 6-6 Cover patient after examination.

Summary of Cold-Related Emergencies

Pediatric patients' physiologic and developmental characteristics place them at risk for the development of cold-related emergencies. Accurate assessment of the degree of hypothermia is essential to effective management of children in the prehospital environment.

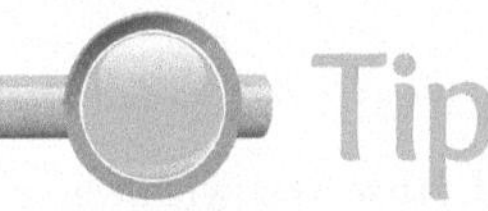

Use caution when rewarming the severely hypothermic pediatric patient in the prehospital environment, because cold acidemic blood from the periphery could lead to further deterioration. Focus instead on preventing further heat loss and supporting the ABCs.

Bites and Stings

Bites and stings typically result in a puncture-type wound or laceration. Most of these injuries are minor. However, some stings, such as from a bumblebee or fire ant, may produce a severe allergic or anaphylactic reaction. Some bites, such as from a rattlesnake, spider, or scorpion, can cause life-threatening envenomation or bleeding problems. Bites and stings may pose a greater risk to the pediatric patient because of his or her smaller body weight and higher metabolic rate.

Assessment

History taking should include:

- Time and type of bite or sting
- Activities since the injury

- Known allergies to bites or stings
- Immunization history

The physical examination should include special attention to:

- Clinical presentation varies depending on the type of bite, the presence or absence of envenomation, and the time since the bite occurred.
- Assess airway, breathing, and circulation; respiratory distress and anaphylaxis may be the initial signs of a bite envenomation.
- Inspect for type, anatomic location, and number of punctures or wounds.
- Assess for swelling, discoloration, and pain at or around the site.

Management: Bites

Management depends on the type of insect, snake, or animal involved in the envenomation.

General Management

- Support airway, breathing, and circulation; establish vascular access.
- Treat anaphylaxis if present (see Chapter 4, page 85).

Local Management

- Stop bleeding and perform wound care.
- If an envenomation is suspected, rinse area with water and consider cool compresses to the affected area to reduce spread of venom.
- Minimize the activity level of the pediatric patient. Most venom is transported through the lymphatic system, and increased physical activity increases the rate spread throughout the body.
- Immobilize an affected extremity at or below the level of the heart.
- Transport rapidly to evaluate for possible antivenin administration and for definitive care.
- Remove any clothing or jewelry on the affected area or limb.

Management: Stings

General Management

- Support airway, breathing, and circulation; establish vascular access.
- Treat anaphylaxis if present (see Chapter 4, page 85).

Local Management

- Apply cold compresses.
- Consider medications based on clinical presentation: epinephrine in the case of anaphylaxis, albuterol in the case of wheezing, or diphenhydramine hydrochloride in the case of hives, itching, or swelling.

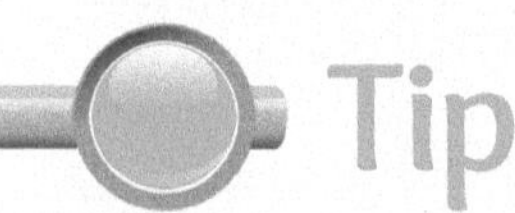

Abnormal behavior may be the first clue that the pediatric patient has been bitten or stung. A thorough inspection of the patient's skin, particularly around the waist, distal extremities, axillae, and neck, may reveal the location of the bite or sting.

Summary of Bites and Stings

Insect bites are common in children and may result in complications ranging from mild local reaction to life-threatening anaphylaxis. Other types of envenomation, such as snake or scorpion stings, are more regionally specific. Early recognition of the nature of the injury is important. Field treatment of anaphylaxis may be lifesaving. Prompt transport to a definitive care facility is crucial if antivenin treatment is needed.

Case Study 3

A 6-year-old boy with a known allergy to bee stings has been playing outside in the garden. The caregiver calls 9-1-1 when the child develops noisy breathing. On arrival at the scene, the PAT reveals a pale, irritable child, with audible wheezing, and supraclavicular and subcostal retractions. Respiratory rate is 32 breaths/min, heart rate is 140 beats/min, and blood pressure is 90 mm Hg by palpation. His skin is covered in pink welts.

1. What are the possible causes of respiratory distress in this child?
2. What are the immediate management priorities?

CASE STUDY ANSWERS

Case Study 1 — page 110

The child is physiologically stable and can be further assessed on the scene. As you manage the child, allay the caregiver's fears. Use the opportunity to provide the caregiver with education regarding seizures and fever. Take a history, which suggests a possible febrile seizure.

All children with a history of seizure activity should be transported to the hospital because it is impossible to diagnose a febrile seizure in the field. There are many causes of seizures, including serious infections, such as meningitis.

Field treatment should be limited to simple cooling methods, such as a cool towel to the forehead if the child is still febrile. There is no need to apply ice packs to the body, unless the child has heat stroke. Reassess the patient frequently and be prepared for repeat seizures.

ALS

If multiple seizures occur or a seizure lasts longer than 5 minutes, treat with a benzodiazepine: rectal or IV diazepam; IV lorazepam; or IV, IN (intranasal), or IM midazolam. Although brief seizures do not require pharmacologic treatment, prompt treatment of seizures lasting longer than 5 minutes have the greatest success in terms of seizure cessation. Continuous, careful monitoring during transport is especially important if drug therapy has been given, because administration of benzodiazepines and phenobarbital can result in apnea or respiratory depression.

Case Study 2 — page 116

The etiology of the child's AMS is wide and includes head trauma, toxin, hypoglycemia, or postictal period after a seizure, yet the initial treatment is the same. Open and manage the airway with positioning. Administer 100% oxygen by nonrebreathing mask. If there is no trauma, place the patient in the sniffing position and use the jaw-thrust maneuver to maintain the airway. If respirations are shallow or irregular, or if oxygen saturation is less than 90% on supplemental oxygen, assist ventilation with the appropriate-sized bag-mask device. Insert an oropharyngeal or nasopharyngeal airway as needed to maintain a patent airway.

ALS

Use a length-based resuscitation tape or computer software program, as described in Length-Based Equipment Sizing and Drug Dosing, Procedure 2, to determine drug doses.

Rapidly assess the serum glucose. If the glucose level is less than 60 mg/dL, establish an IV and give D_{50} 1 mL/kg by IV bolus. If there is no IV access, give glucagon IM 0.7 mg. If bedside glucose determination is normal, consider other causes of AMS and consider administering naloxone, 0.1 mg/kg (maximum 2 mg).

Case Study 3 — page 128

A previously healthy child playing outdoors with an acute onset of respiratory distress should be assessed for bites and stings. This child's prior history of hymenoptera (bumblebee) allergy, the presence of hives in addition to respiratory distress, and the sudden onset of symptoms all suggest anaphylaxis.

Supplemental oxygen and inhaled bronchodilators for wheezing should be provided. In addition, IM epinephrine should be administered.

ALS Establish vascular access and give IV diphenhydramine.

Even if the child shows marked improvement with these treatments, transport urgently, because symptoms may recur as the medication effect wears off. Monitor carefully during transport.

SUGGESTED READINGS

Textbooks

American Academy of Orthopaedic Surgeons. *Emergency Care and Transportation of the Sick and Injured.* 10th ed. Burlington, MA: Jones and Bartlett Learning; 2011.

American Academy of Pediatrics and the American College of Emergency Physicians. *APLS: The Pediatric Emergency Medicine Resource.* 5th ed. Burlington, MA: Jones and Bartlett Learning; 2012.

Baram T, Shinnar S. *Febrile Seizures.* San Diego: Academic Press; 2002.

Baren JM, Rothrock SG, Brennan JA, et al. *Pediatric Emergency Medicine.* Philadelphia: Saunders/Elsevier; 2008.

Bledsoe B, Porter R, Cherry R. *Essentials of Paramedic Care.* Upper Saddle River, NJ: Prentice Hall; 2003.

McCance KL, Heuther SE, Brashers VL, et al, eds. *Pathophysiology: The Biologic Basis for Disease in Adults and Children.* 6th ed. St. Louis: Mosby Elsevier; 2010.

Articles

Freedman S, Powell E. Pediatric seizures and their management in the emergency department. *Clin Pediatr Emerg Med.* 2003;4;195–206.

Holsti M, Sill BL, Firth SD, et al. Prehospital intranasal midazolam for the treatment of pediatric seizures. *Pediatr Emerg Care.* 2007;23;148–153.

Reuter D. Common emergent pediatric neurologic problems. *Emerg Med Clin North Am.* 2002;20(1):155–176.

Warden CR. Evaluation and management of febrile seizures in the out-of-hospital and emergency department settings. *Ann Emerg Med.* 2003;41(2):215–222.

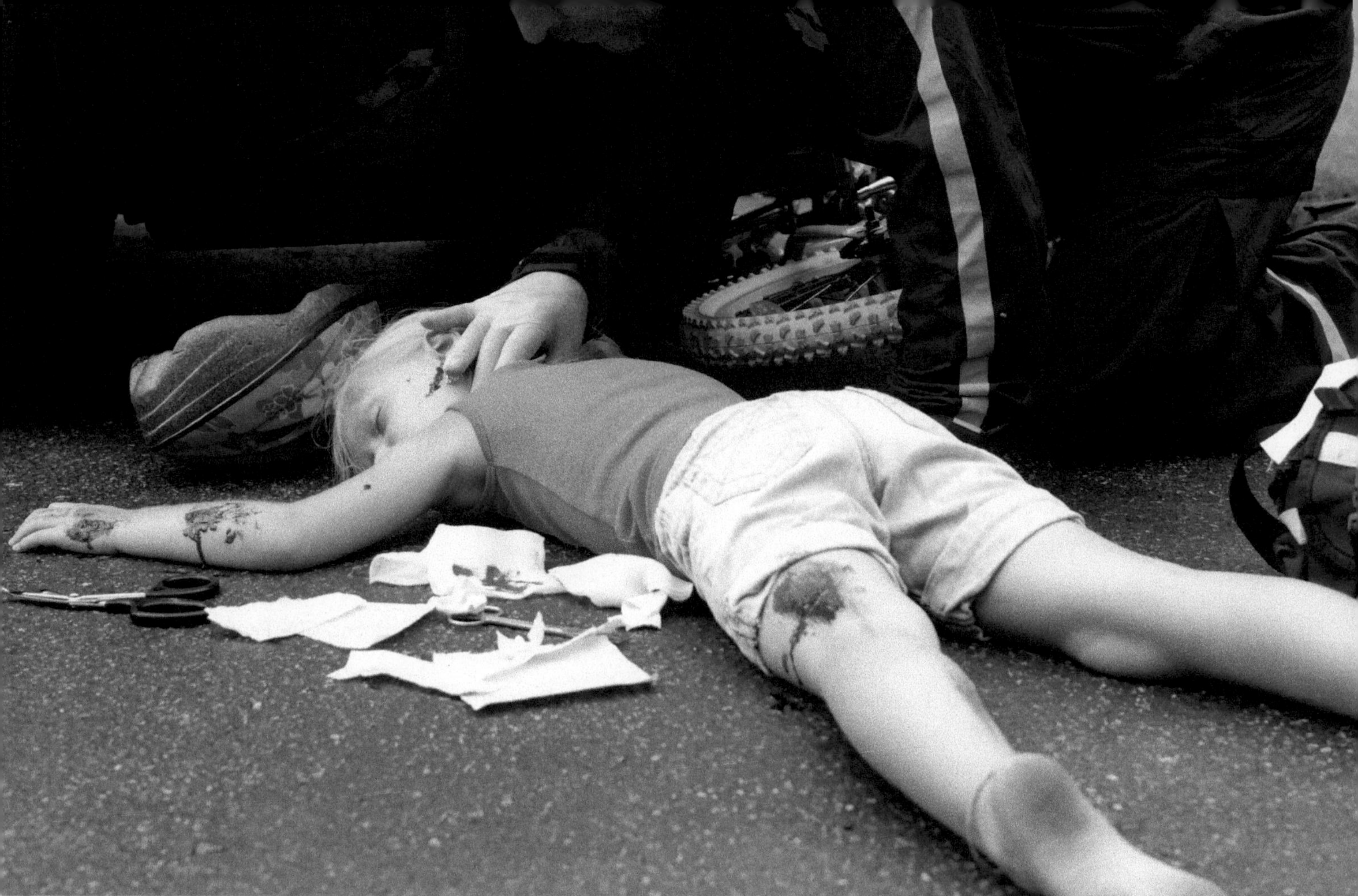

Learning Objectives

1. Explain the unique anatomic features of children that predispose them to injuries.
2. Sequence the primary assessment of the injured child.
3. Integrate the essential trauma interventions into the hands-on ABCDEs.
4. Distinguish different approaches in airway management of injured children.
5. Discuss assessment and treatment of pediatric burn patients.

Trauma

Chapter
7

Introduction

Half of the children transported by emergency medical services (EMS) have an acute injury. Fortunately, the most common injuries are minor problems, such as lacerations, minor or superficial burns, mild closed head injuries, and extremity fractures. In minor trauma, the role of the prehospital professional is straightforward: Perform a scene size-up, assess for physiologic or anatomic problems, and transport to the emergency department (ED). Treatment usually entails only wound care, spinal stabilization, and splinting when necessary.

Multisystem trauma, in contrast, provides the prehospital professional with a great challenge, and demands a disciplined assessment and a child-specific approach to treatment. Most principles of adult trauma management can be effectively and safely applied to children. Important modifications in assessment are related to differences in mechanisms of injury, anatomy, and physiologic responses. Modifications in treatment are related to differences in equipment sizes and emergency procedures.

From infancy through adulthood, injuries are the most common cause of death. From 1–44 years of age, unintentional injuries are the most common cause of death. Intentional injuries, primarily child abuse in younger children and suicide and homicide in adolescents, are also among the leading causes of death.

Most injuries are preventable. Child restraint devices in automobiles, bicycle helmets, swimming pool fences, and window barriers have significantly reduced the incidence of blunt injuries and drowning. Stricter building codes have reduced the incidence of fires, although burns continue to be a leading cause of death in children under 12 years of age. Pediatric trauma challenges the prehospital professional to manage not just the injury and related physiologic abnormalities, but also to treat the child's pain and communicate with and support the injured child and the "injured family."

Death or serious injury of a child from trauma causes tremendous emotional stress on prehospital professionals, who may project feelings and fears about their own children's vulnerability onto the situation. This common provider response may lead to difficulty in maintaining an appropriate emotional distance, and it may compromise objective performance. Experience and education in the care of ill and injured children helps the prehospital professional have a greater sense of confidence, competency, and control in these stressful situations. Critical incident stress management or employee assistance programs (EAP) may be valuable to the prehospital professional after treating a seriously injured child.

Case Study 1

Your unit is dispatched to a residential neighborhood where a child has had a fall. You are greeted in the street by a teenage girl who leads you to a 7-year-old boy who is lying face up on the grass next to a tall tree. The teenager indicates that she observed the child fall about 20 feet out of the tree. No one has moved him. Your primary assessment reveals a child who is only responsive to painful stimuli. His breathing is shallow, with audible snoring sounds. His color is pale with slight cyanosis. Respiratory rate is 12 breaths/min, heart rate is 130 beats/min, and blood pressure is 80 mm Hg/palp. His skin is cool, the radial pulse is weak, and capillary refill time is greater than 3 seconds. Pupils are equal and reactive, lung sounds are absent on the right and decreased on the left. The oxygen saturation is 82%. He has a hematoma on the right side of his head. His abdomen feels rigid. His right upper leg is swollen, with an obvious deformity of the right femur.

1. Based on the primary assessment and mechanism of injury, what are the child's most likely injuries?
2. Discuss the initial stabilization and prehospital management of this child.

Fatal Injury Mechanisms

Table 7-1 summarizes the most frequent fatal mechanisms of injury in children and adolescents. Vehicular trauma (including automobile occupant, pedestrian, all-terrain vehicles [ATVs], and bicyclist injuries) is the most common cause of death in all age groups. Drowning is the second leading cause. House fire is a significant cause of death, especially in the eastern United States. Falls are common, but rarely cause major injury unless the height of the fall is greater than the child's height and the stopping surface is unyielding, such as concrete.

Table 7-1 Leading Mechanisms of Injury-Related Death

Preschoolers	School-Aged Children
Vehicular trauma	Vehicular trauma
Drowning	Drowning
Fires	Nonaccidental trauma
Nonaccidental trauma	Fires
Falls	Gunshot wounds

Unique Anatomic Features of Children: Effect on Injury Patterns

Head

Head injury is the most common cause of serious trauma in children. Even in multisystem trauma, the severity of traumatic brain injury (TBI) usually defines the patient's medical and functional outcome. Many of the essential interventions in managing pediatric trauma are directed at preserving brain function.

Until early school age (5–6 years old), the child's head is disproportionately large in relationship to overall body mass and surface area compared to adults. Because of this anatomic feature, in a fall or in an acceleration-deceleration event, such as a motor vehicle crash, the head functions like the heavy end of a lawn dart, becoming the lead point (**Figure 7-1**). Consequently, the head and brain of a child are more commonly injured in blunt trauma compared to adults.

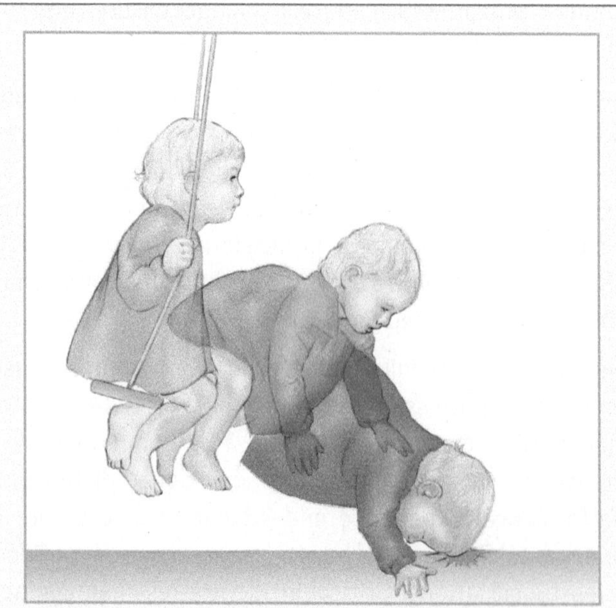

Figure 7-1 A disproportionately large head size in children explains their tendency to fall "head first," leading to a high rate of TBI.

Spinal Column

As a group, children do not suffer many vertebral fractures or dislocations. When vertebral fractures do occur, the event typically involves a high-energy mechanism (e.g., motor vehicle crash or diving incident) with axial loading of the spine or extreme flexion or extension. Traumatic spinal cord injury, or disruption of the central nerve pathways, is also uncommon in children.

The most common cervical spine injuries in children occur at the level of the high cervical spine. Weaker neck muscles and spinal ligaments, in conjunction with a "heavy" head, create greater vulnerability to acceleration-deceleration forces common in motor vehicle crashes and falls. In reality, most children with high cervical injury are in full arrest on the scene and die despite all medical interventions.

The most common lower spine injuries occur in the mid to lower thoracic spine. Mechanisms include direct blows, falls, or spinal compression during a motor vehicle crash from improper seat belt use. The use of booster seats in vehicles may reduce these types of injuries by allowing proper fitting of the lap and shoulder belt.

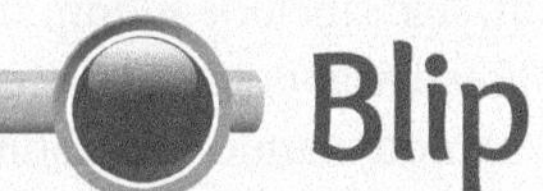

It is difficult to find a cervical collar that really fits an infant or toddler. When a properly sized collar is not available, stabilize the child's spine on a long board with padding to prevent movement.

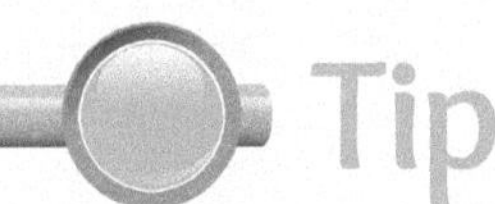

Injuries cause almost half the deaths among children from 1–4 years of age and outrank all other causes of death combined among older children and adolescents.

Chest

The ribs of the child are more pliable and compressible than those of the adult because they are comprised mainly of cartilage. For this reason, rib fractures and flail chest are uncommon in younger children, even with high-energy transfers. However, this bony compressibility in conjunction with a chest wall that is poorly protected by fat or muscle leads to direct transfer of energy to the lungs and heart on impact (**Figure 7-2**). Serious injuries of the thoracic organs can be present with or without external signs of injury, such as abrasions, bruises, or tenderness.

Pulmonary contusion, or bruising of the lung tissue itself, is the most common form of serious lung injury in children. You may suspect this condition in a child who sustains blunt chest trauma and has hypoxia or respiratory distress; however, pulmonary contusions may take time to fully develop and can only be diagnosed by X-ray, which makes the distinction between pulmonary contusion and pneumothorax impossible in the field.

If a child has a blunt injury mechanism, be careful about placing a needle in the pleural space because a contusion is more likely than a tension pneumothorax. In contrast, a child with progressive hypoxia and respiratory distress after a penetrating injury probably does have a tension pneumothorax, and needle decompression is indicated.

Penetrating chest trauma may cause serious problems in oxygenation and ventilation. When the chest wall, back, or high abdomen is penetrated, look for tension pneumothorax and sucking chest wounds. These injuries are unusual in children but, if present, require specific immediate lifesaving treatment in the field. Needle decompression may save the life of a child with a tension pneumothorax. The procedure is similar for a child and adult, the major difference being the size of the catheter. The procedure is illustrated in **Needle Thoracostomy, Procedure 22.**

The diaphragm of a child can rise as high as the nipple line during full expiration. When there is blunt or penetrating

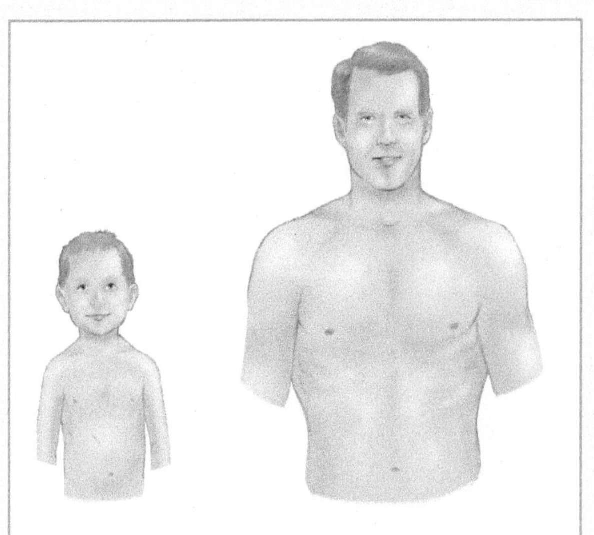

Figure 7-2 The child's chest wall is not well muscularized, so it lacks the soft tissue protection from injury that is present in adolescents and adults.

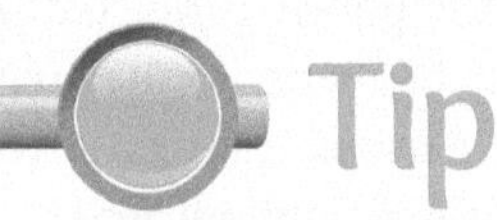

Because the child's chest wall is smaller, thinner, and less muscular than an adult's, lung sounds may be transmitted throughout the chest cavity, making it difficult to appreciate asymmetric breath sounds. Listening along the lateral sides of the chest wall under the axillas (armpits) may improve the ability to distinguish sound variability between the right and left lungs.

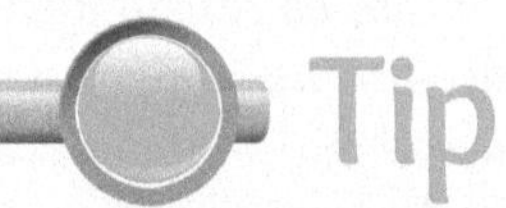

If there is penetration of the chest wall below the nipple, or below the scapula, anticipate abdominal injury as well as tension pneumothorax.

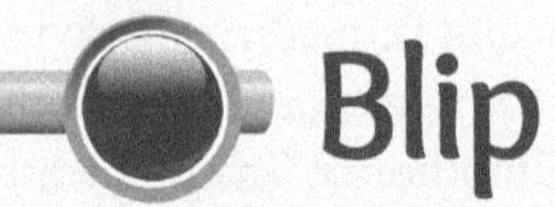

Remember that young children rely heavily on their diaphragm to breathe. Do not restrict the abdomen when stabilizing the patient's spine.

trauma to the chest below the nipple line or below the scapula, internal injury may include chest and abdominal organs (**Figure 7-3**).

Abdomen

The abdomen is often the site of serious blood loss in pediatric patients and is the most common site of injury causing shock. The solid organs of the upper abdominal cavity are the liver, spleen, and kidneys. These organs are disproportionately larger and more exposed than in adults and are poorly protected by the child's softer ribs and relatively undeveloped abdominal muscles (**Figure 7-4**). The liver is the largest abdominal organ, located in the right upper quadrant of the abdomen, and extends below the rib cage in infants, toddlers, and preschool-aged children. It is the most commonly injured abdominal organ in young children. The spleen, located in the left upper quadrant, is also commonly injured. Injuries to the hollow organs of the abdomen—the stomach, small bowel, and bladder—are less common than solid organ injuries. Although pelvic fractures are uncommon in children, they become more frequent in adolescents, who have adult anatomy.

Assume that every child with a serious trauma has a life-threatening abdominal injury. Many children with abdominal injury have no localizing signs and may not complain of pain. Fear, young age, or other distracting injuries may hide signs and symptoms. When present, signs include abdominal wall contusions or abrasions, progressive abdominal distension, tenderness, rigidity, and hemodynamic instability. Serial examinations in timed intervals (5–10 minutes) may improve the accuracy of abdominal assessment.

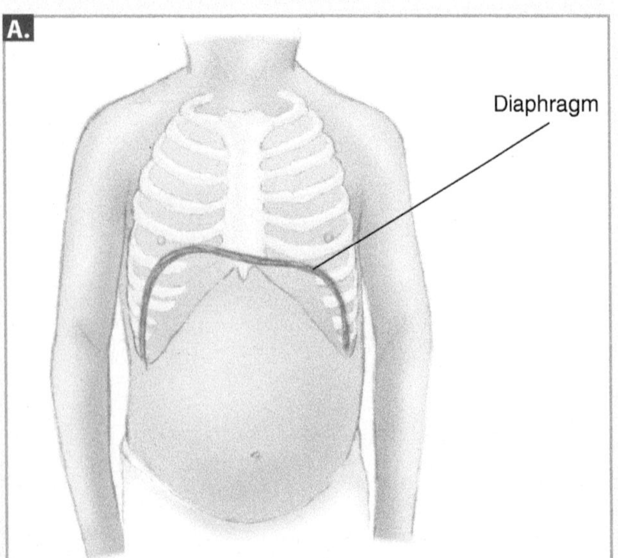

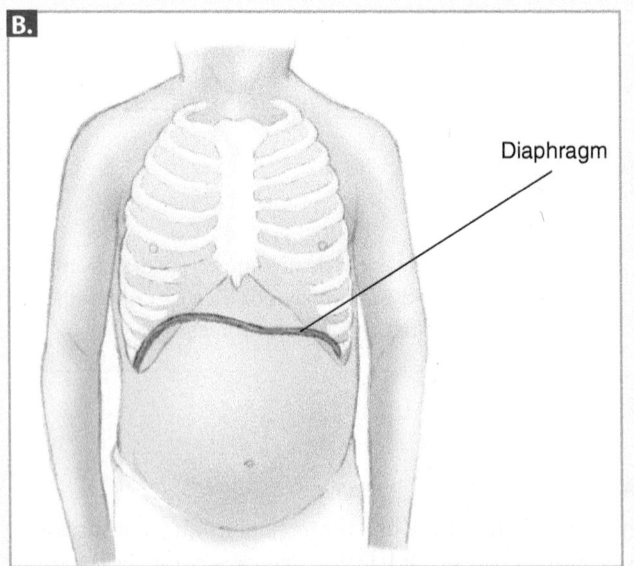

Figure 7-3 The diaphragm can rise as high as the nipple line during full expiration **A.** and can flatten to the level of the lowest ribs during full inspiration **B.** Therefore, injuries to the abdominal organs may occur after chest trauma.

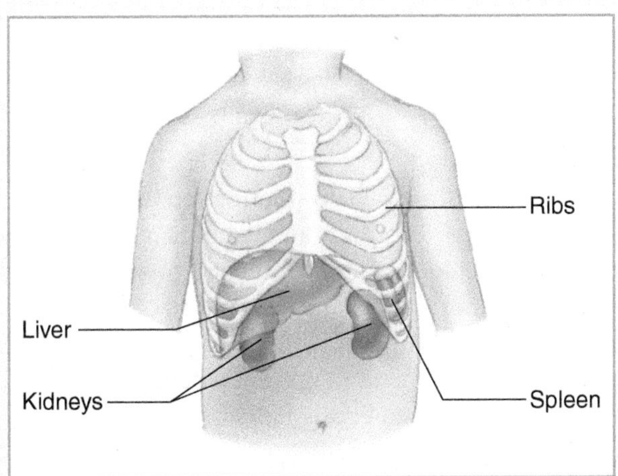

Figure 7-4 The solid organs of the upper abdominal cavity are disproportionately large and more exposed in children than in adults. They are poorly protected by the thin chest wall and undeveloped abdominal muscles.

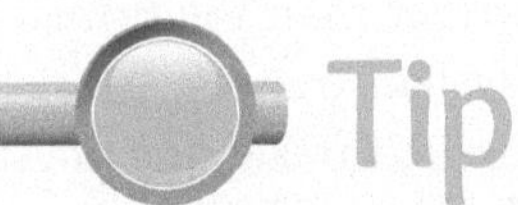

Tip

The abdomen is the most frequent site of injury causing shock. Serial examinations greatly improve the accuracy of assessment of abdominal injury.

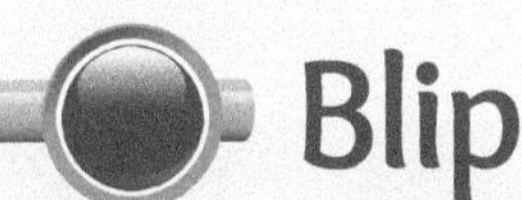

Blip

Never overlook the possibility of solid organ injury when there has been blunt injury, because fear, young age, or other distracting injuries may mask signs and symptoms.

Extremities

Children's bones are more flexible, and their muscles are not as well developed as those of adults. They are especially vulnerable to fractures at the weak, cartilaginous growth plates near the ends of the bones (**Figure 7-5**). Fractures that disrupt the periosteum on only one side of the bone (often called greenstick fractures) are common, as are "buckle fractures" in which the pliant bone is compressed with axial loading. These fractures may be present in the absence of significant swelling, bruising, or deformity. *Suspect a fracture whenever there is point tenderness or limited range of motion, especially around a joint.*

The most serious complications of extremity injuries are neurovascular problems and blood loss into the soft tissues at the fracture site. Blood loss may be severe in long-bone fractures (e.g., fractures of the femur) or in pelvic fractures. The symptom usually associated with serious extremity injuries is pain.

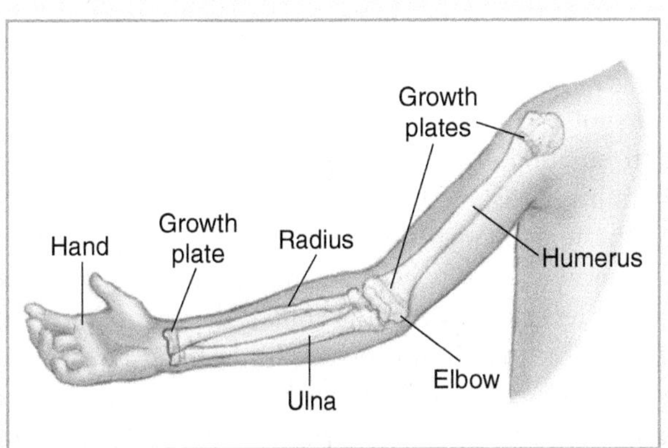

Figure 7-5 The physeal (growth) plates at the ends of children's bones are easily fractured.

ALS

Pain is frequently underestimated and undertreated in children! Consider analgesia for pain management in children with isolated extremity fractures. Morphine sulfate or fentanyl is the medication of choice. Repeat with half doses as needed for pain control. Be extremely careful with morphine administration in children with a serious injury mechanism or signs of compensated or decompensated shock. Morphine can rapidly drop the child's blood pressure and critical perfusion when it is administered to a hypovolemic patient. Fentanyl is faster acting than morphine, and also has a shorter duration of action. In addition, Fentanyl can be administered intranasally, which may be preferable in children. Always be alert for signs of respiratory depression, especially if multiple doses of a narcotic are administered.

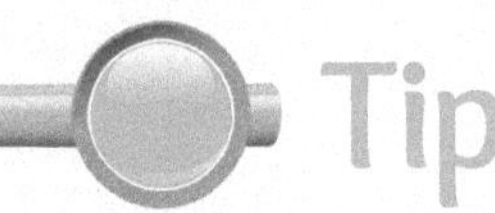

Tip

Suspect an extremity fracture whenever findings include point tenderness or limited range of motion.

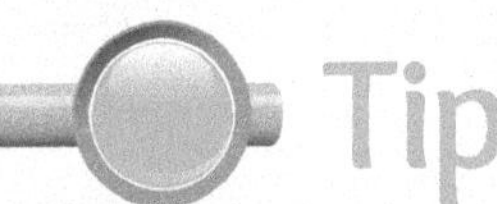

Tip

Injuries to the physeal plate or growth plate of a long bone can be permanently damaging to the limb.

Skin

The skin provides temperature regulation. Children's skin is thinner and has a greater surface area in relation to their overall size and weight than does the skin of adults.

Because of this, heat transfer (loss or gain) from the skin can be rapid. Even without injuries that damage the skin, such as burns, injured children are at increased risk for hypothermia, which can in turn compromise core organ function. The signs and symptoms of hypothermia can mimic those of hypovolemia and shock. In infants, hypothermia may deplete vital glucose stores. To avoid hypothermia, especially in an infant and toddler, prevent heat loss by ensuring that the child is dry and covered, and limiting time that the undressed child is exposed for assessment and procedures. Turn up the heat in the ambulance! For the temperature to be warm enough for an infant who is disrobed, it must be uncomfortably hot for an adult. In extremely hot environments, beware of hyperthermia.

Mechanism of Injury: Effect on Injury Patterns

The different mechanisms of injury in children in combination with their unique anatomic features lead to predictable patterns of injury. Head injury caused by blunt trauma is very common in children. Although there are many cases of minor closed head injuries associated with play that do not have neurologic consequences, high-energy impacts are often associated with TBI. Because of a child's small size, high-energy blunt impacts can lead to **multisystem trauma**, including the head, chest, abdomen, and long bones.

Table 7-2 lists the common mechanisms of pediatric injury and the associated patterns of injury. **Figure 7-6** illustrates several typical injury sequences in children.

Assessment of the Injured Child

The initial steps in assessing the injured child follow the generic approach for all children outlined in Chapters 1 and 2. This includes prearrival mental preparation based on dispatch information and a scene size-up on arrival. Always use **universal precautions** or personal protective measures and equipment to prevent potentially harmful or infectious exposures to bodily fluids.

The on-scene trauma evaluation includes (1) general assessment using the Pediatric Assessment Triangle (PAT); (2) the primary assessment with the hands-on ABCDEs; and then (3) additional assessment consisting of a focused history and physical examination and a detailed physical examination (trauma). A child with multisystem injuries needs a prioritized, efficient on-scene approach to assessment and treatment, and rapid transport to the ED. Typically, the prehospital professional gets no further than the primary assessment of a child with multisystem trauma, because the recognition and management of life-threatening physiologic problems is the focus of field care. The anatomic problems identified in the additional assessment are generally not life-threatening and can be treated in the hospital when the child is physiologically stable.

Table 7-2 Common Mechanisms and Associated Patterns of Pediatric Injury*

Mechanism of Injury	Associated Patterns of Injury	
Motor vehicle crash (child is passenger)	• Unrestrained	Multiple trauma, head and neck injuries, scalp and facial lacerations
	• Air bag	Head and neck, facial and eye injuries
	• Restrained	Chest and abdominal injuries, cervical and lower-spine fractures
Motor vehicle crash (child is pedestrian)	• Low speed	Lower-extremity fractures
	• High speed	Chest and abdominal injuries, head and neck injuries, lower-extremity fractures
Fall from a height	• Low	Upper-extremity fractures
	• Medium	Head and neck injuries, upper- and lower-extremity fractures
	• High	Chest and abdominal injuries, head and neck injuries, upper- and lower-extremity fractures
Fall from a bicycle	• Without helmet	Head and neck injuries, scalp and facial lacerations, upper-extremity fractures
	• With helmet	Upper-extremity fractures
	• Hitting handlebar	Internal abdominal injuries

*Adapted from *Teaching Resource for Instructors in Prehospital Pediatrics (TRIPP)*. Version 2.0. New York, NY: Center for Pediatric Emergency Medicine; 1998.

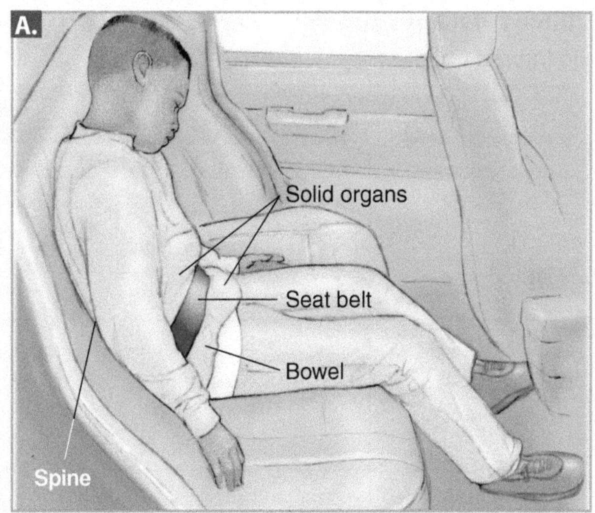

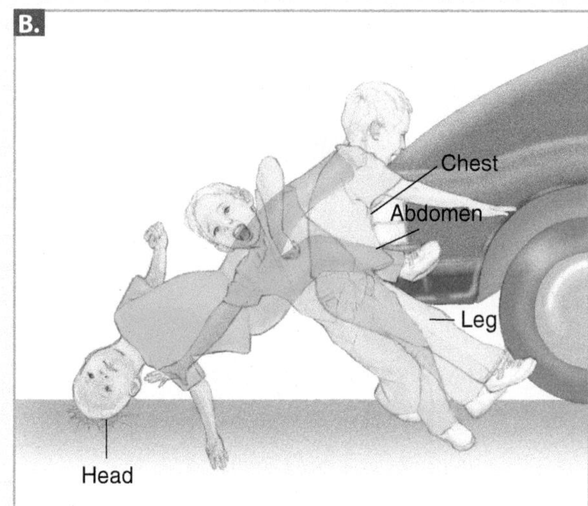

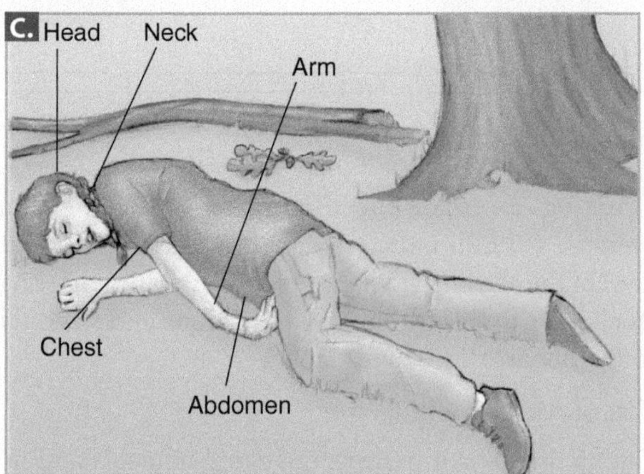

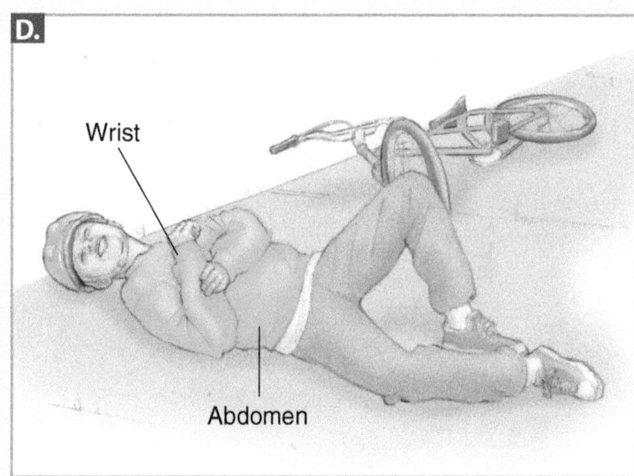

Figure 7-6 **A.** A restrained child in a motor vehicle crash may have a lap belt injury involving solid organs, bowel, and spine. **B.** Children frequently sustain multisystem injuries involving the head, chest, abdomen, and long bones. **C.** A fall from height frequently involves injuries to the head and neck, chest, abdomen, and the extremities. **D.** A fall over the handlebars of a bike may result in injuries to the abdomen and extremities.

The General Assessment

The PAT

The PAT is the first part of the primary assessment of trauma as well as medical patients, and allows rapid determination of the type of physiologic disturbance, severity of injury, and urgency of treatment.

Appearance

Appearance reflects brain function, which may be abnormal in injured children because of primary brain injury (caused by direct trauma to the brain tissue itself) or secondary brain injury (caused by an indirect insult to the brain tissue by hypoxia or ischemia). The most likely causes of abnormal appearance in a pediatric trauma patient are closed head injury, hypoxia, hemorrhage, and pain from fractures, burns, and soft-tissue injuries.

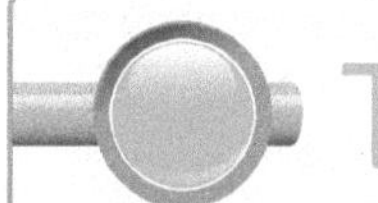

There are many potential causes of abnormal appearance in a pediatric trauma patient, including closed head injury, hypoxia, hemorrhage, and pain from fractures, burns, and soft-tissue injuries.

Toxins may also cause an abnormal appearance, but are uncommon causes of poor responsiveness in the preschool- and school-aged trauma patient. However, toxins (most often alcohol or recreational drugs) are an important contributor to trauma in the adolescent, who may incur injuries caused by high-risk behaviors while "under the influence." **Table 7-3** lists common causes of abnormal appearance in injured children.

Table 7-3 Common Causes of Abnormal Appearance in Injured Children

Category of Injury	Examples
Primary brain injuries	• Closed head injury • Brain edema • Concussion • Contusion • Intracranial hematoma • Intracranial hemorrhage • Penetrating brain injuries
Secondary brain injuries	• Hemorrhage with hypoperfusion/shock due to: - Solid organ abdominal injury - Hemothorax - Pelvic fracture • Hypoxia due to: - Aspiration of gastric contents - Failure of central respiratory drive - Pulmonary contusion - Smoke inhalation - Tension pneumothorax
Pain	• Burns • Fractures • Soft-tissue injuries
Toxins	• Alcohol • Recreational drugs • Carbon monoxide

Work of Breathing

Work of breathing is increased by injuries that affect the airway, lungs, pleura, or chest wall. **Table 7-4** summarizes the causes of increased work of breathing in pediatric trauma patients. Effortless tachypnea, or a rapid respiratory rate in the absence of increased work of breathing, may be seen in a child with traumatic shock. This is a reflexive mechanism to compensate for metabolic acidosis caused by hypoperfusion by "blowing-off" carbon dioxide.

Listen for abnormal airway sounds, such as stridor or change of speech, which may reflect tracheal injury or obstruction. Wheezing reflects lower airway irritation and bronchospasm. This may occur from inhalation of vaporized toxins. When children are confined in a house fire, this type of inhalation should always be suspected.

Table 7-4 Injury Causes of Increased Work of Breathing in Injured Children

Cause	Examples
Airway injuries	• Hematomas or lacerations of the tongue, mouth, or neck • Smoke and hot gas inhalation • Penetrations into the upper airway
Chest injuries	• Pulmonary contusion • Sucking chest wound • Tension pneumothorax/hemothorax
Abdominal injuries	• Diaphragmatic injury • Solid or hollow viscus injury with pain and "splinting"

Grunting, an infant's method of positive end-expiratory pressure (PEEP), indicates decreased gas exchange at the level of the alveoli, and may be seen with pulmonary contusion. After listening, look for retractions and nasal flaring to further assess for hypoxia.

Circulation to Skin

Circulation to skin reflects the blood flow to the skin and mucous membranes. If skin color and skin temperature are abnormal in an injured child who is not in a cold environment, it suggests hypovolemia and poor perfusion. Hemorrhage from abdominal solid organ injury is the most common cause of hypoperfusion and shock in pediatric trauma patients. The use of tourniquets in children with exsanguinating hemorrhage from an extremity to prevent blood loss should be based on local protocols. An isolated closed head injury cannot account for signs of hypoperfusion or shock in children outside of infancy, because the closed space of the skull cannot accommodate a significant volume of blood. However, infants can lose large volumes of blood based on intracranial bleeding, because the plates of their skull (sutures) are not yet fused, and the skull can expand under pressure.

Figure 7-7 and **Figure 7-8** show the PAT findings for the two most common patterns of major pediatric trauma: closed head injury and multisystem injury.

The Primary Assessment

Hands-on ABCDEs

The ABCDEs are the hands-on primary assessment. The trauma ABCDEs have a special focus on spinal precautions and control of blood loss.

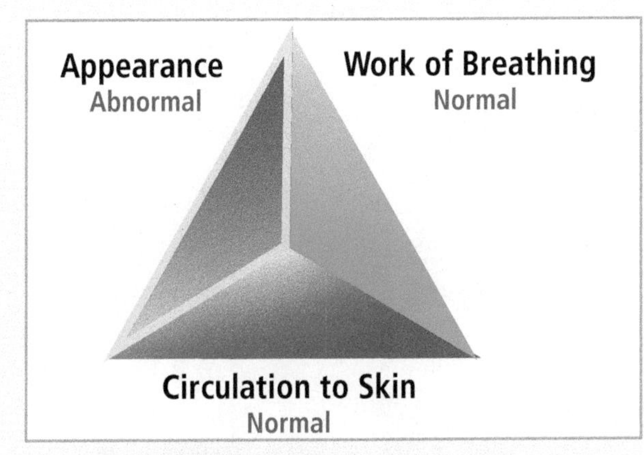

Figure 7-7 A patient with closed head injury has an abnormal appearance, but normal work of breathing and normal circulation to skin.

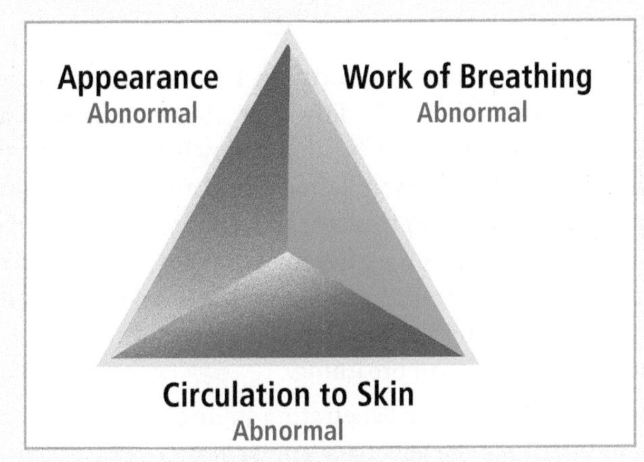

Figure 7-8 A patient with multiple system injury has an abnormal appearance, abnormal work of breathing, and abnormal circulation to skin.

Table 7-5 Pediatric Trauma ABCDEs

Element of Assessment	Special Interventions
Airway	Modified jaw-thrust maneuver while maintaining cervical spine stabilization Consider airway adjunct
Breathing	Needle thoracostomy Dressing to sucking chest wound
Circulation	External hemorrhage control Splinting of fractured extremity
Disability	Elevated intracranial pressure management (head midline, head of backboard or stretcher up, assisted ventilation to maintain normal CO_2 levels)
Exposure	Prevent heat loss

The pediatric assessment, including the PAT and ABCDEs, does not require any specialized equipment. Potentially life-threatening problems should be treated as they are identified in the ABCDE sequence. **Table 7-5** lists the key features of the pediatric trauma ABCDEs and interventions specific to the trauma patient.

Airway

Airway is always the first priority. Trauma victims are at risk for airway obstruction from bleeding, emesis, edema, or foreign objects. TBI may cause loss of protective airway reflexes or impair central respiratory drive.

Consider spinal injury in a child with any of the following:

- A mechanism of injury involving high-velocity forces transmitted to the head or spine (e.g., fall from a height, ejection from a motor vehicle)
- Physical evidence of trauma to the head or spine (e.g., scalp hematoma, tenderness to palpation of the cervical spine); altered mental status (AMS)
- Neck or back pain
- Weakness or numbness

If the child has any of these findings, stabilize the entire spine while managing the airway. Although great care must be taken to prevent further injury in the unlikely event of an unstable spine injury, these concerns must not take precedence over appropriate management of the child's airway. *An injured child is far more likely to die from untreated hypoxia or shock than spinal trauma.*

Actions. If airway obstruction is present, use a modified jaw-thrust maneuver combined with manual spinal in-line stabilization (**Figure 7-9**) to establish and maintain airway patency. Insert an airway adjunct if unable to maintain an open airway and the child has no gag reflex. Use suction to clear any fluid from the mouth, nose, or upper airway, or Magill forceps to remove foreign bodies. Be prepared to turn the child on his or her side and suction if he or she vomits to prevent aspiration of stomach contents. Quickly but carefully logroll the patient if vomiting occurs before he or she is secured to a spine board or stretcher. After the spine is fully stabilized, the entire backboard can be turned if necessary to protect the child from aspiration.

Spinal Motion Restriction. The spinal column is made of 33 articulating bones, the vertebrae, and its structure changes significantly during childhood growth. The incidence and type of spinal injuries depend on the age of the child and the

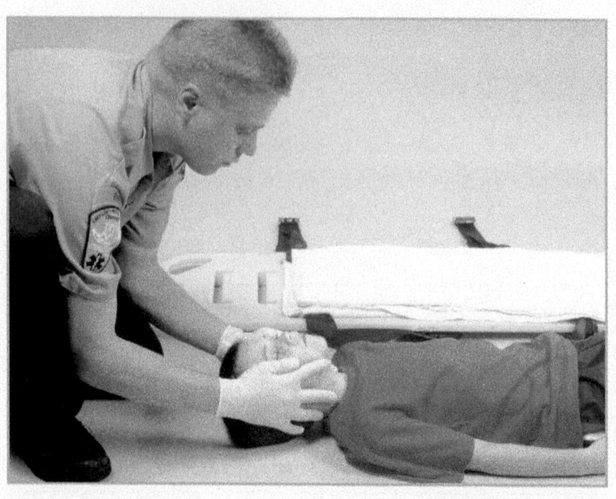

Figure 7-9 If airway obstruction is suspected in a child with possible spine injuries, use the modified jaw-thrust maneuver combined with manual spinal in-line stabilization.

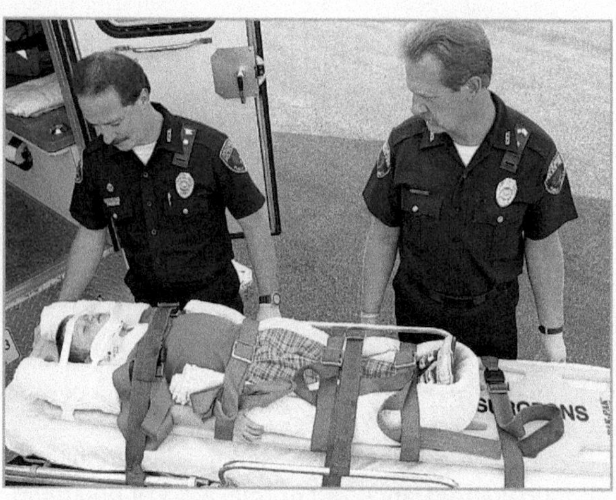

Figure 7-10 Spinal motion restriction with the use of a cervical collar, towels, straps, and a backboard.

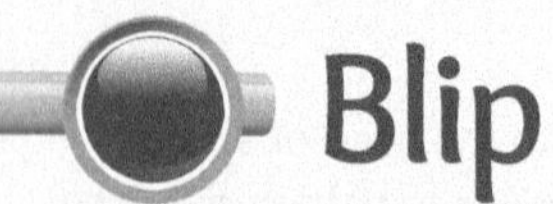

Never let concern for spinal injury compromise appropriate management of the child's airway.

mechanism of injury, and in turn are influenced by the child's developmental level and activity. Cervical spine trauma can lead to quadriplegia, the most devastating type of spinal injury. If cervical spine injury is suspected, an appropriately-sized cervical collar should be applied. The use of a backboard should follow local protocols (**Figure 7-10**). Spinal cord injuries and lifelong paralysis may follow thoracic or lumbar trauma. For a step-by-step explanation of this procedure, see **Spinal Motion Restriction, Procedure 21.**

Breathing

Breathing is the second priority in the ABCDEs. Injuries to the airway, chest wall, lungs, or abdomen as well as gastric distention caused by air swallowing may compromise oxygenation and ventilation. Head and cervical spine injuries sometimes depress central respiratory drive mechanisms or diminish protective airway reflexes. Pulmonary aspiration of gastric contents is a common and potentially serious complication of head injuries that results in hypoxia and increased work of breathing.

Look for soft-tissue or penetrating injuries of the chest or back. Watch for the adequacy and symmetry of chest rise, and then listen with a stethoscope to assess air entry and equality of breath sounds. Feel the chest wall for crepitus, pain, or instability. Apply a pulse oximeter to assess for hypoxia, because pallor and cyanosis can be late findings. A normal pulse oximetry reading does not, however, rule out respiratory distress. A child with profound tachypnea or increased work of breathing may need assisted ventilation regardless of the reading on the oximeter, before he or she exhausts compensatory mechanisms.

Case Study 2

You are dispatched to a local recreation field where a 4-year-old boy was struck in the head by a baseball that was hit into the stands. The child has a large hematoma on his forehead and is crying inconsolably in his father's arms. The child did not lose consciousness but is not making eye contact with you or his dad. Other than his altered appearance, the PAT is normal and the hands-on ABCDEs reveal normal vital signs and no other apparent injuries. The child becomes increasingly somnolent during your assessment, and is difficult to arouse.

1. What is the child's greatest threat to life?
2. What interventions are required?

Actions. If breathing is inadequate, position the child and assist ventilation. Lift the jaw into the mask. Pushing the mask onto the face to make a seal may cause cervical spine movement. The E-C clamp technique (**Figure 7-11**) helps with proper hand placement for good mask-to-face seal. Consider inserting an airway adjunct to help maintain an open airway, although an oral airway is not tolerated by a child with an intact gag reflex.

Give 100% oxygen or bag-mask ventilation. Use a properly fitted oxygen mask. Provide assisted ventilation with a bag-mask device if the child's respiratory effort is inadequate or if he or she has deteriorating cardiopulmonary or mental status. Use the "squeeze-release-release" timing technique, because the tendency is to bag too fast. Allow a brief pause between each breath to minimize the chance of gastric distention. *Only hyperventilate children who are experiencing brainstem herniation.* Be extremely careful, because hyperventilation may decrease perfusion to the brain. The best gauge is by using capnography to keep the $ETCO_2$ 30–35 mmHg. The pupillary reactions can also help guide rate of ventilation in a child with suspected brainstem herniation.

If capnography is not available, **Table 7-6** can help provide guidance. In each breath, provide only enough tidal volume to just achieve chest rise.

Table 7-6 Using Pupils to Guide Ventilation Rates in Closed Head Injury

Patient Category	Rate of Ventilation
Pupils equal	Normal for age[a]
Both pupils fixed and dilated	Above normal rate[b] until pupils constrict
Pupils asymmetric	Above normal rate[b] until pupil constricts
Child posturing	Above normal rate[b] until posturing stops

[a] 30 breaths/min for infants; 20 breaths/min for toddlers and children

[b] 35 breaths/min for infants; 25 breaths/min for toddlers and children (if capnography is not available)

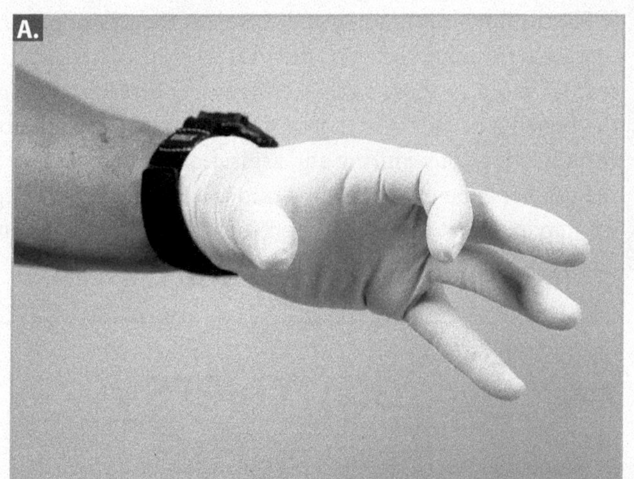

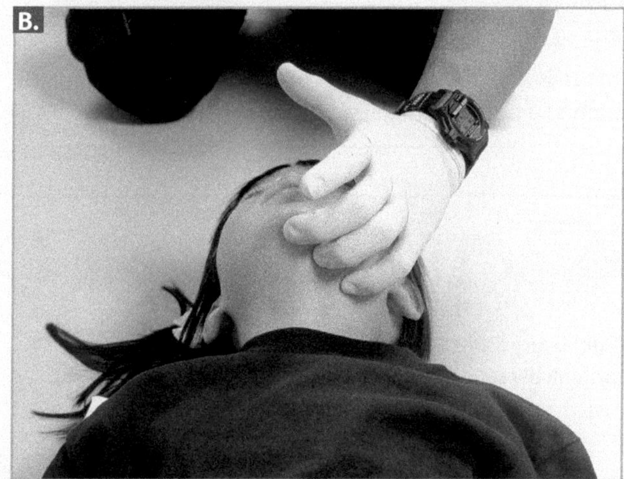

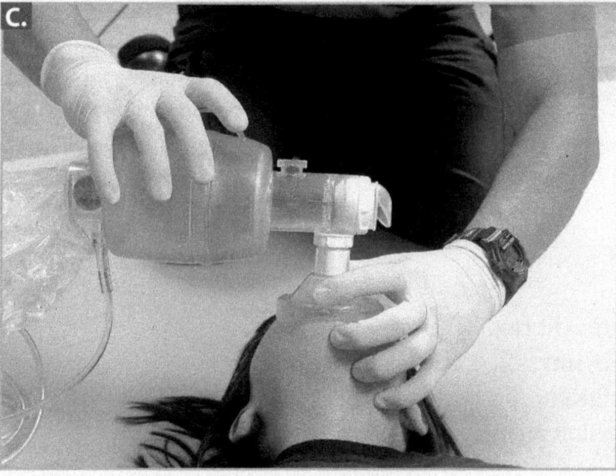

Figure 7-11 The E-C clamp technique facilitates proper hand placement for good mask-to-face seal. **A.** Hand displaying E-C shape. **B.** Fingers resting on bony ridge of jaw. **C.** Bag-mask ventilation in place.

Treating penetrating chest injuries, sucking chest wounds, impaled objects, and tension pneumothorax in pediatrics is the same as in adults. Cover sucking chest wounds with an occlusive dressing, such as petrolatum gauze, taped on three sides (**Figure 7-12**) or a specially designed bandage/seal for sucking chest wounds. This technique allows trapped air to escape while helping to prevent the entrance of air and development of tension pneumothorax. Do not remove impaled objects. Instead, stabilize them in place.

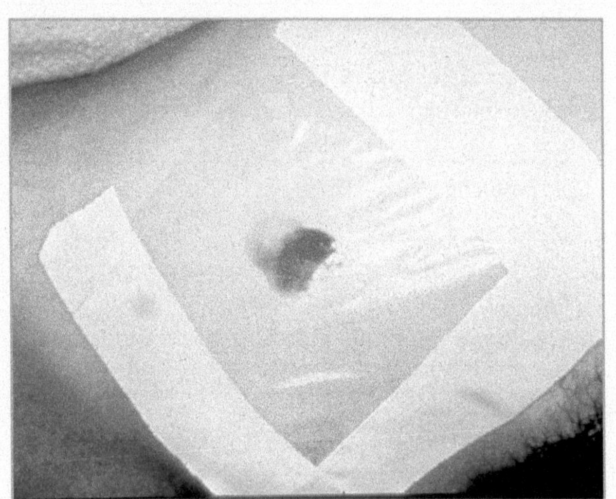

Figure 7-12 Management of a sucking chest wound. Cover sucking chest wounds with an occlusive dressing, such as a petrolatum gauze, taped on three sides.

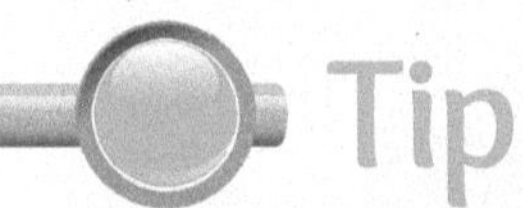

Tip

Pulmonary aspiration of gastric contents is a common and potentially serious complication of head injuries.

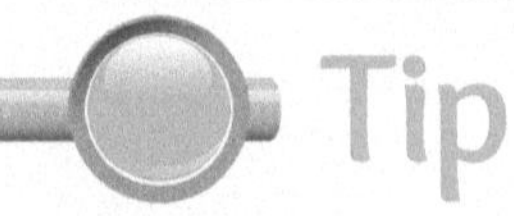

Tip

If a patient with penetrating chest trauma also has respiratory distress, hypoxia, and hypoperfusion, perform needle decompression to treat possible tension pneumothorax.

ALS

Management of Tension Pneumothorax. If a patient with penetrating chest trauma has increasing respiratory distress, hypoxia, and hypoperfusion, perform needle decompression to treat possible tension pneumothorax.

Needle decompression may also be necessary in the child with blunt chest injury if the child has serious blunt chest-wall injury and respiratory distress, especially if he or she worsens with assisted ventilation. In this situation, when there is a closed pneumothorax, positive pressure ventilation quickly increases the air pressure in the pleural space, creating a dangerous level of "tension." Tension pneumothorax not only compromises ventilation of the affected lung, but impairs venous return to the heart. This can lead to shock unresponsive to fluid resuscitation. Needle decompression of the tension pneumothorax improves oxygenation, ventilation, and perfusion. For a step-by-step explanation of this procedure, see **Needle Thoracostomy, Procedure 22.**

Management of Gastric Distention With a Nasogastric/Orogastric Tube. Assisted ventilation or prolonged crying can cause air swallowing and gastric distention. Nasogastric (NG) or orogastric (OG) tube placement may improve ventilation by decreasing the upward pressure on the diaphragm caused by the distended stomach, and reduce the risk of vomiting. If possible, insert an NG or OG tube after endotracheal intubation of a comatose patient, because positive pressure ventilation can cause gastric inflation even in an intubated child. Contraindications for NG insertion include midfacial trauma and suspected basilar skull fracture (raccoon eyes, Battle sign, or suspected cerebrospinal fluid [CSF] rhinorrhea or otorrhea) because of the risk of passing the tube through the disrupted cribriform plate into the cranial vault. In these cases, perform OG insertion. Weigh the benefits of gastric decompression against the possible complications of vomiting and aspiration during passage of the tube or tube misplacement into the trachea. For a step-by-step explanation of this procedure, see **Orogastric and Nasogastric Tube Insertion, Procedure 10.**

Controversy

Studies suggest that rapid administration of crystalloid fluids to adult patients with internal bleeding caused by penetrating trauma may worsen outcome. These studies have not been confirmed in children, who usually sustain blunt trauma. In the absence of data to change practice, provide aggressive volume resuscitation of the pediatric trauma patient with signs of shock.

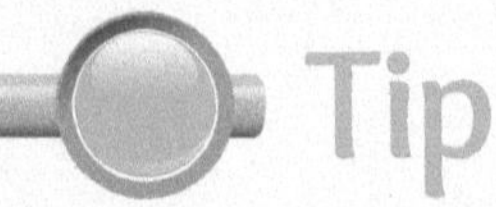

Tip

Frequently reassess heart rate, preferably with an electronic monitor. Tachycardia may be a response to pain, fear, cold, or anxiety, but a trend of rising heart rate suggests ongoing blood loss.

Circulation

Multisystem pediatric trauma more often involves respiratory failure than shock. Sometimes, however, shock develops because of external or internal bleeding, tension pneumothorax, spinal injury, or pump failure caused by cardiac contusion or tamponade. The combination of the PAT and the hands-on ABCDEs allows ongoing perfusion evaluation. Measure heart rate continuously with a cardiac monitor, or with frequent pulse checks. Tachycardia may be caused by pain, fear, cold, or anxiety, but a trend of rising heart rate suggests ongoing blood loss. Blood pressure measurement is not a good indicator of hypovolemia, because a child can be in compensated shock with a normal blood pressure. When there is frank hypotension, assume the child is in decompensated shock. If it is significantly higher than normal in a child with possible TBI, consider possible intracranial hypertension.

Because of the technical challenges of obtaining a reliable blood pressure (mainly because of having the proper cuff size) and because skin signs, capillary refill time, and pulse quality are good signs of perfusion, make only one attempt at obtaining a blood pressure in children older than 3 years of age. Make sure the blood pressure cuff size is correct, or the measurement is inaccurate. In children younger than 3 years of age, taking the time on scene to get a blood pressure is of limited value.

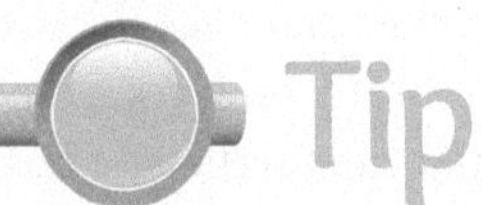
Tip

Remember, the systolic blood pressure for a child older than 1 year should be greater than 70 + 2 × age in years. If not, the child is hypotensive and in decompensated shock.

Actions. Stop any visible external bleeding with direct pressure on the wound. Use sterile gauze compresses, and use gloves and personal protective equipment. Splint any extremities with obvious deformity. Apply oxygen and place the child in a supine position for transport.

Begin transport when the airway is properly secured, ventilation is adequate, and the child's spine is appropriately stabilized.

ALS

Volume Resuscitation. If the child has signs of shock or significant ongoing blood loss, obtain vascular access and start volume resuscitation on the way to the ED. Look first for peripheral intravenous (IV) sites in the upper extremities. Attempt to secure two lines. Insert an intraosseous (IO) needle if IV access is problematic and the child has signs of decompensated shock.

In a poorly perfused patient, administer 20 mL/kg of isotonic crystalloid fluid as quickly as possible. Use a pressurized system or the pull-push method, with an in-line, three-way stopcock and a large syringe to maximize the infusion rate (**Figure 7-13**). Repeat 20-mL/kg boluses as needed to improve appearance and stabilize vital signs.

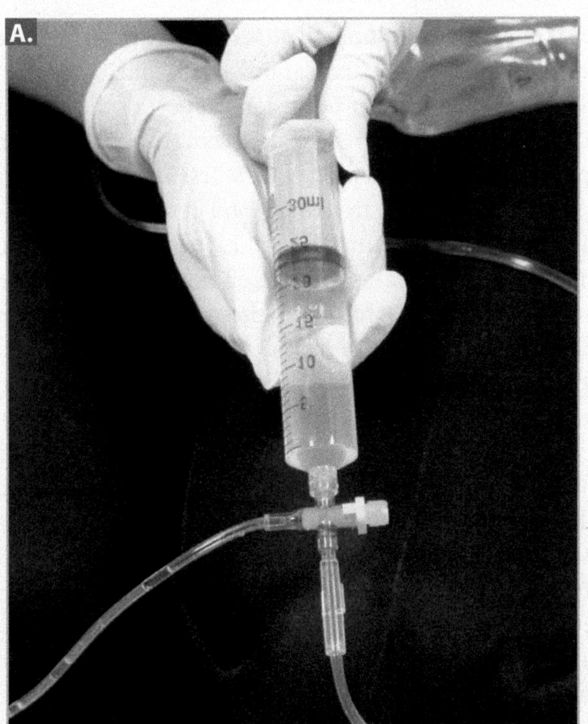

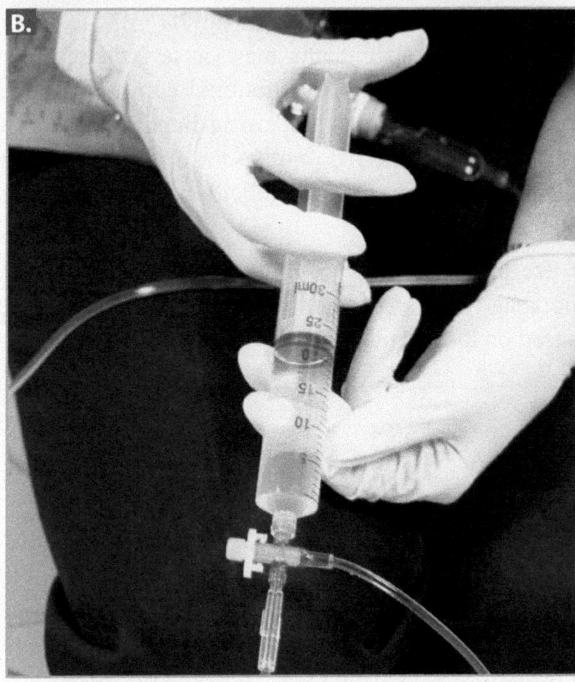

Figure 7-13 Infuse boluses using a pressurized system or the pull-push method with an in-line, three-way stopcock and a large syringe. **A.** Pull fluid bolus into syringe after turning stopcock off to patient. **B.** Push fluid bolus into patient after turning stopcock off to IV bag.

Never delay transport in an effort to establish vascular access. Only about one-third of crystalloid remains in the vessels after administration, and crystalloid has no useful oxygen-carrying capacity. The benefits of crystalloid administration are outweighed by the risks of ongoing hemorrhage with prolonged scene time.

Controversies in Volume Resuscitation of the Pediatric Trauma Patient. The indications, technique, and rate of volume resuscitation for perfusion support of the pediatric trauma patient are controversial. Recent studies suggest that rapid use of crystalloid fluids may worsen outcome in adult patients with bleeding from blunt and penetrating injury. In this circumstance, volume resuscitation increases perfusion, which in turn increases the rate of bleeding. Dislodgment of a clot may be a factor. Also, progressive dilution of red cells with crystalloid may further decrease oxygen-carrying capacity. The applicability of adult research in penetrating injury on volume resuscitation in pediatric blunt trauma victims is unknown. Treat traumatic shock in children with isotonic fluids. However, a child with ongoing hemorrhage is likely to lose more blood during prolonged attempts to establish vascular access at the scene than can be replaced during transport with crystalloid. Therefore, crystalloid treatment is detrimental if transport is delayed. If an IV is started without delaying transport, infuse enough fluids to maintain core perfusion. Reassess fluid status frequently, and stop hemorrhages if possible.

ALS

Do not use military anti-shock trousers (MAST) in children. The leg compartments may cause ischemia to the lower extremities, and the abdominal compartment may compromise ventilation by impairing diaphragmatic movement. In adults, MAST do not seem to improve outcome from multiple trauma. No controlled studies in children are available at this time.

The use of tourniquets in children with exsanguinating hemorrhage from an extremity to prevent blood loss should be based on local protocols.

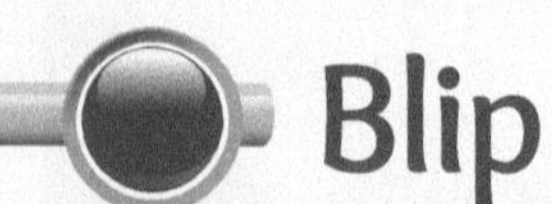

Blip

MAST have not been proved to be useful, and may be dangerous in children. They may cause ischemia to the lower extremities or limit ventilation.

Disability

Disability in the context of trauma care relates to TBI or spinal cord trauma. Injuries may be open or closed. Children may have primary or secondary brain injuries, or both.

Primary brain injury is the direct result of the traumatic insult and may include brain hemorrhage, cerebral edema (brain swelling), or diffuse axonal shearing. Increased intracranial pressure may develop quickly after primary brain injury. Untreated, the downward spiral of increased intracranial pressure can lead to brainstem herniation, cardiopulmonary arrest, and brain death. By the time the prehospital professional reaches the scene, any damage incurred from the primary brain injury is complete.

Secondary brain injury results from central nervous system hypoxia or ischemia and disorders of blood glucose. The prehospital professional has a key role in preventing secondary brain injury. Hypoxia may be the result of airway or chest injury, or of compromised central respiratory drive caused by the primary brain injury. Brain ischemia may result from hemorrhage, usually in the abdomen or chest. Central nervous system (CNS) cells cannot survive without sufficient blood glucose levels.

Ensuring adequate oxygenation, ventilation, perfusion, and normal blood glucose are the keys to preventing secondary brain injury.

A 9-1-1 call sometimes involves an infant with AMS, apnea, or seizures with no report of preceding trauma. Assessment of these infants may not reveal any physical examination findings suggestive of head trauma or TBI, despite the fact that they have sustained severe TBI. This is a typical scenario in shaken baby syndrome/abusive head trauma, where the infant is forcibly shaken by a caregiver, sometimes with impact of the baby's head against a fixed object. This mechanism involves severe acceleration-deceleration forces to the infant's brain and consequent diffuse axonal injury or intracranial hemorrhage. Shaken baby syndrome/abusive head trauma is further discussed in Chapter 13.

Assess the injured child's degree of neurologic disability with the AVPU scale (see Table 1-7). Disability, as categorized in the AVPU scale, is not the same as "abnormal appearance" in the PAT. An injured child may have an abnormal appearance for many reasons other than brain or spinal cord injury, such as pain, fear, shock, hypoxia, or intoxication. Appearance may be quite abnormal in a child who is "alert" on the AVPU scale. Appearance is a more subtle indicator of overall physiologic function in children than AVPU. The AVPU scale is more helpful in categorizing children with severe neurologic insults, including critical primary or secondary brain injuries.

Some EMS systems use a Pediatric Glasgow Coma Scale (PGCS) to assess neurologic injury (**Table 7-7**). Neither the AVPU score nor the PGCS has been validated in young children. Although both systems attempt to objectively assess neurologic function, the AVPU is less complex and easier to remember. When using the PGCS, pay special attention to the motor component of the score, which has the highest value in predicting neurologic outcome from TBI.

Table 7-7 Pediatric Glasgow Coma Scale

Score	Child	Infant
Eyes		
4	Opens eyes spontaneously	Opens eyes spontaneously
3	Opens eyes to speech	Opens eyes to speech
2	Opens eyes to pain	Opens eyes to pain
1	No response	No response
_______ = Score (Eyes)		
Motor		
6	Obeys commands	Spontaneous movements
5	Localizes	Withdraws to touch
4	Withdraws	Withdraws to pain
3	Flexion	Flexion (decorticate)
2	Extension	Extension (decerebrate)
1	No response	No response
_______ = Score (Motor)		
Verbal		
5	Oriented	Coos and babbles
4	Confused	Irritable cry
3	Inappropriate words	Cries to pain
2	Incomprehensible words	Moans to pain
1	No response	No response
_______ = Score (Verbal)		
_______ = **Total Score (Eyes, Motor, Verbal). Scores will range from 3 to 15.**		

Source: James HE, Anas NG, Perkin RM. *Brain Insults in Infants and Children.* Orlando, FL: Grune & Stratton; 1985. Reprinted with permission.

After evaluating the level of consciousness with AVPU or the PGCS, note abnormal positioning (including posturing) and seizures, and check for pupil size, symmetry, and reactivity. Seizures are common with head injury in children. Beware of persistent horizontal nystagmus, which may indicate persistent seizure activity.

The pupils provide important information about brainstem function, and the pupillary examination helps determine the need for hyperventilation in patients who are comatose.

Concussion, a form of mild TBI, can result from rotational and acceleration forces on the brain, or a bump, blow, or jolt to the head. A direct blow to the head is not needed. Frequently sports-related, loss of consciousness is seen in only 10% to 15% of concussed patients. Symptoms of confusion, amnesia, loss of coordination, slow reaction time, and delayed thought processing put the player at increased risk for further injury. Recovery requires physical and cognitive rest and may take weeks to months. A "second impact" during the recovery phase may lead to rapid brain swelling and death.

Actions. In pediatric trauma patients with AVPU scores of P or U, provide assisted ventilation to maintain good oxygenation and adequate ventilation. Hypoxia is an important cause of secondary brain injury in these children with TBI. Hypoxia may be associated with increased intracranial pressure, a situation that may occur rapidly and sometimes deceptively in a child with a primary brain injury.

Children with TBI require careful oxygenation and ventilation, but the rate of ventilation is controversial. Although hyperventilation was widely recommended in the past as a way of rapidly decreasing intracranial pressure, extreme hyperventilation can itself cause decreased brain perfusion and secondary brain injury. In addition, there are no data that demonstrate improved neurologic outcomes for patients who have been hyperventilated. Reserve hyperventilation for victims of TBI who have signs of impending brainstem herniation, and use appropriate breathing rates and tidal volumes, as outlined in Table 1-4.

If the patient with TBI has impending herniation syndrome, use mild hyperventilation. Consider this intervention if the child has a severe neurologic disability, as defined by a rating of P or U on the AVPU scale, a score of less than 9 on the PGCS, and a fixed and dilated pupil, asymmetric pupils, or posturing (decerebrate or decorticate). Provide mild hyperventilation as guided by capnography to keep $ETCO_2$ 30–35 mmHg. When the pupils constrict or the posturing stops, resume the normal ventilation rate for age.

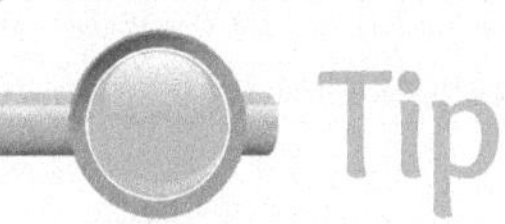

A child with head trauma has impending brainstem herniation if the AVPU score is P or U, or if the PGCS is less than 9, or there is a fixed dilated pupil, asymmetric pupils, or active posturing.

ALS

Management of Elevated Intracranial Pressure If the child has AMS (not alert on AVPU or <15 on the PGCS), anticipate elevated intracranial pressure. Take a graded approach to intracranial pressure management, always balancing risks and benefits of treatment.

- Support the patient's head in a midline position to facilitate jugular venous return to the heart.
- If the patient is not in shock, elevate the head of the backboard or stretcher. Ensure adequate oxygenation and ventilation.
- Consider hyperventilation only in patients with signs of impending herniation syndrome.
- If there is head injury and hypovolemia, administer fluid to maintain brain perfusion. The injured brain hates ischemia!
- Mannitol may be useful to acutely decrease intracranial pressure in the child with asymmetric pupils or posturing, but must be used with caution in a child with associated injuries who is at risk for hemorrhagic shock.

Exposure

Exposure is the last step in the primary assessment. Good exposure allows full assessment of the child's entire anatomy, including the extremities. Quickly examine the back during the spinal stabilization procedure for soft-tissue or penetrating injuries. Assess circulation and neurologic function distal to obvious or suspected extremity injuries. Although not usually life-threatening, complicated extremity injuries (e.g., open fractures of the humerus or femur) may cause significant blood loss and pain. Remember to cover the patient after the examination to prevent heat loss and hypothermia.

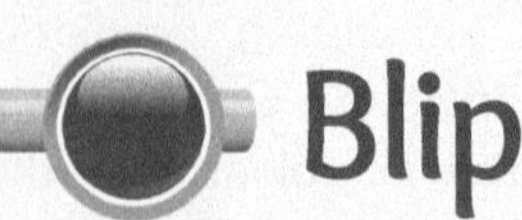

Administration of mannitol can acutely decrease intracranial pressure through changes in CNS fluid distribution and diuresis. Do not administer mannitol to patients with hypovolemic shock.

Summary of Primary Assessment

The assessment of the injured child requires knowledge of anatomic and developmental differences that lead to pediatric-specific patterns of injury. The child's airway is small and easily obstructed, the lungs are vulnerable to contusion, and the solid organs and long bones are poorly protected. The prehospital professional's primary role in multisystem trauma is to ensure an open airway, assist ventilation, and minimize secondary brain injury. Treatment goals are to avoid hypoxia and hypotension. Short time on scene and rapid transport to the ED are overriding priorities for all children who are physiologically unstable or have concerning mechanisms of injury. Vascular access and volume resuscitation are secondary tasks to be considered on the way to the hospital.

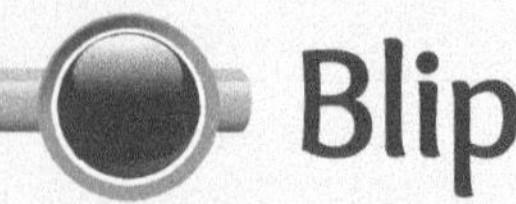

Mannitol is temperature sensitive. Do not store in temperatures less than 45°F.

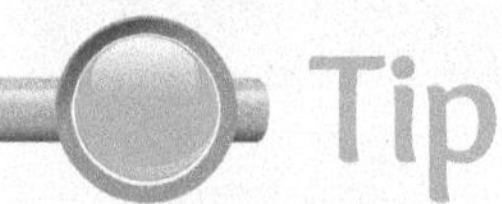

Use assisted ventilation to maintain oxygenation and to avoid carbon dioxide retention in pediatric trauma patients with AVPU scale scores of P or U.

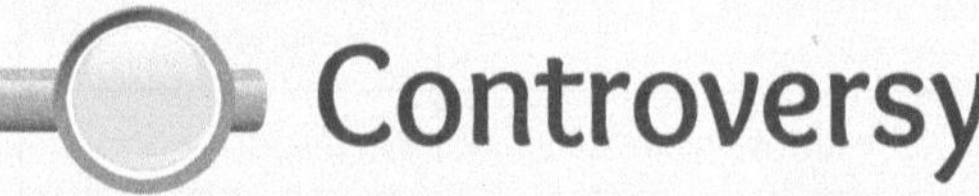

The rate of ventilation in patients who are comatose is controversial. No one has studied enough children with serious closed head injury to know at what point the benefit of hyperventilation and reduction of cerebral blood flow to decrease intracranial pressure outweighs the associated risk of brain ischemia.

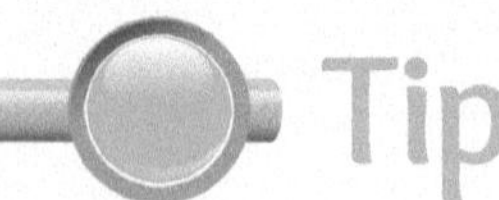

In the out-of-hospital environment, endotracheal intubation is not always the optimal airway management tool.

Special Airway Considerations in Pediatric Trauma

Children with severe head injuries with neurologic disability and impending herniation often require field interventions to:

- Protect the airway and prevent aspiration
- Improve or control ventilation
- Improve or control oxygenation

Optimal airway management balances the potential risks of the procedure against the potential benefits to the patient. Although endotracheal intubation has long been considered the best method for airway management in a critically injured patient, the procedural risks are significant. These risks may include prolonged scene time, worsened hypoxia, vomiting and aspiration, elevation of intracranial pressure during laryngoscopy, or a misplaced tube. The decision to support ventilation using a bag-mask device versus an endotracheal tube (ET) is a complex one, and must take into consideration the following factors:

- Risk of increasing intracranial pressure (by increasing the child's combativeness or inducing gagging during intubation procedure)
- Ability to access the airway
- Length of on-scene and transport times
- Personnel availability and experience
- Ability to perform rapid sequence intubation (RSI)

Table 7-8 lists the factors that the prehospital professional must consider to choose the optimal airway management approach for each patient.

Table 7-8 Factors Influencing Optimal Airway Management Decisions

Factors Favoring BLS (bag-mask ventilation)
Combativeness, strong gag reflex
Presence of **trismus** (spasm of jaw muscles)
Short on-scene and transport times
Factors Favoring ALS (endotracheal intubation)
Inability to ventilate with a bag-mask device
Unresponsive child
Absent gag reflex
Apnea, poor muscle tone
Long extrication or transport times
Limited personnel to assist during transport
Availability of RSI

Advanced Airway Management of the Pediatric Trauma Patient

If a severely injured child needs endotracheal intubation, the preferred path is orotracheal, with manual neutral stabilization of the cervical spine (see **Endotracheal Intubation, Procedure 11**).

Although blind nasotracheal intubation may cause less cervical spine motion in the adult than the orotracheal technique, the procedure is not applicable to children because of the anterior location of the larynx and the increased risk of adenoidal bleeding. *Do not attempt blind nasotracheal intubation in a child.*

RSI for pediatric endotracheal intubation, with sedatives and paralyzing drugs, is standard practice in many EDs and in a limited number of EMS regions. Its effectiveness, safety, and feasibility are controversial. Further study is required to determine its safety and effectiveness as a tool for out-of-hospital pediatric airway management. See **Advanced Airway Techniques, Procedure 13**, for a detailed explanation of this procedure.

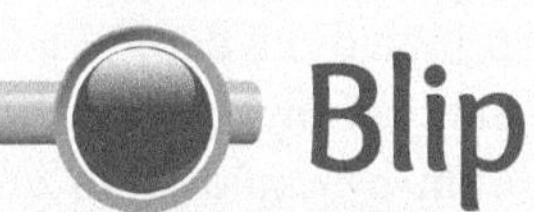

Do not attempt blind nasotracheal intubation in children.

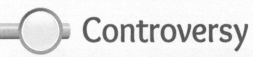

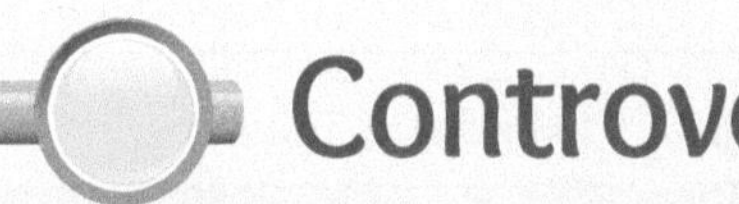

RSI for pediatric endotracheal intubation, with sedatives and paralyzing drugs, is standard practice in many EDs and in a limited number of EMS regions. Its effectiveness and safety in the field are controversial.

The Primary Assessment

The Transport Decision: Stay or Go?

After the primary assessment and initiation of life support, consider the timing for transport. *Immediately transport every pediatric trauma patient who has any abnormal physiologic or anatomic findings, severe pain, or a serious mechanism of injury.* Stable trauma patients with apparently minor injuries may undergo further evaluation and treatment on scene. If the scene size-up suggests circumstances that could be dangerous to the child or prehospital professional, transport immediately. Potentially dangerous conditions that warrant immediate transport and completion of assessment in the ambulance include proximity to fire or hazardous materials, threatened violence, angry bystanders or caregivers, and suspected nonaccidental trauma.

Additional Assessment

The additional assessment consists of the focused history and physical examination and the detailed physical examination (trauma patient). This part of the assessment is directed at anatomic problems. Perform the focused history and physical examination, and the detailed physical examination in the field only if the patient is physiologically normal and the conditions are safe. Otherwise, address these components of the assessment in the ambulance while on the way to the ED. In physiologically unstable patients, defer the additional assessment altogether.

When obtaining the focused history, use the SAMPLE template, as outlined in Chapter 1. Focus only on points likely to affect primary trauma assessment and interventions. **Table 7-9** provides a SAMPLE template oriented to pediatric trauma patients.

The focused physical examination includes a careful look at the anatomy in the suspected areas of injury. This may involve a conscientious examination by exploration and palpation of the head and scalp for a child with closed head injury, observation and palpation of the back and axillae in a child with a penetrating chest injury, or inspection and palpation of the neck in a child with a strangulation injury.

Table 7-9 SAMPLE History in Pediatric Trauma

Component	Explanation
Signs/symptoms	• Time of event • Nature of symptoms or pain • Age-appropriate signs of distress
Allergies	• Known drug reactions or other allergies
Medications	• Chronic medications—timing and dose of last dose • Timing and dose of **analgesic**/antipyretic
Past medical problems	• Prior surgeries • Immunizations
Last food or liquid	• Time of the child's last food or drink, including bottle or breastfeeding
Events leading to the injury	• Key events leading to the current incident • Mechanism of injury • Hazards at the scene

The detailed physical examination (trauma) is a head-to-toe sequence or (in infants, toddlers, and preschool-aged children) toe-to-head, then front-to-back complete physical examination of the patient. This examination uses the traditional assessment tools of observation, palpation, and auscultation, as outlined in Chapter 1.

After the child is on the way to the ED, perform ongoing reassessments, especially with patients with abnormal physiology. This includes serial evaluations of the PAT, ABCDEs, pulse oximetry, vital signs (including heart rate and rhythm on the cardiac monitor), anatomic problems, and response to treatment. Be sure to monitor and treat pain, if possible. When the child arrives in the ED, diagnostic testing with blood tests and imaging studies may assist with continued assessment.

Summary of Additional Assessment

After the primary assessment, determine the timing of transport and the appropriate destination. Do an additional assessment, or on-scene focused history and physical examination, then a detailed physical examination, only on stable patients in safe scene circumstances. All other patients deserve immediate transport with continuation of assessment on the way to the ED. Frequent reassessment is important in all injured patients. Transport severely injured pediatric patients to trauma centers rather than community hospitals when possible. Many state trauma programs have algorithms for directing patients, including children, to the appropriate level of care.

Spinal Motion Restriction and Splinting for Transport

Indications for spinal protection for children are the same as for adults and are indicated for any child with a concerning mechanism of injury, signs of significant head injury, or multisystem trauma. Stabilize the neck using a properly sized pediatric extrication collar and a head immobilizer when available. Otherwise, use properly secured towel rolls and tape. For a step-by-step description of this procedure, see **Spinal Motion Restriction, Procedure 21.**

Preschool-aged children may not be able to localize or communicate the presence of neck or back pain. Anatomic differences, specifically the large size of an infant's or toddler's head, require modification of spinal stabilization procedures. For example, placing a thin (1 inch) layer of padding beneath a child's body from shoulders to hips before securing the child to the stretcher or spine board (**Figure 7-14**) helps to properly align the airway and spinal column.

The spine does not stop at C-7, and spinal stabilization is not complete unless the entire body is secured. Secure the patient against all axes of motion on the stretcher or spine board. Near vertical positioning may be necessary during extrication. Secure the patient against lateral movement by padding along the sides of the body to eliminate all space between the patient and the straps.

Avoid chin straps and other spinal stabilization aids that might impair ventilation. Leave room for chest expansion during breathing when tightening chest straps or flaps. Make sure cervical collars fit properly, or use manual spinal stabilization until the child can be secured to the board or stretcher if a properly sized collar is not available. Ensure that spinal stabilization equipment does not interfere with assessment and access to the patient. A child who does not have severe injuries may be frightened and fight the process vigorously. Reassure the child and offer relaxation or distraction techniques to minimize discomfort.

Splinting deformed or painful extremities is also an important prehospital intervention. Splinting has several important functions: pain control, hemorrhage reduction, and preservation of neurovascular function. Unless the extremity shows signs of neurovascular compromise or there is severe pain, splint bones that may be fractured or dislocated in an "as is" position (**Figure 7-15**). An open femur fracture should be reduced by traction ONLY if the traction can be maintained. This controls the bleeding at the fracture site and helps to control pain. Otherwise, unless circulation is compromised, leave exposed bone out to avoid introducing further contamination by forcing fractured bone fragments back under the broken skin (**Figure 7-16**).

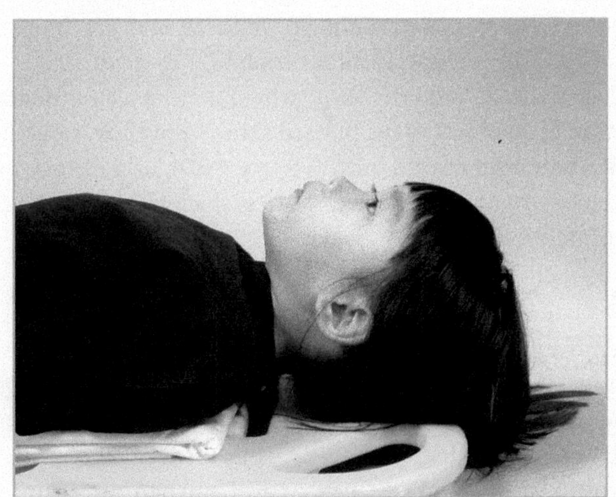

Figure 7-14 Keep the airway and spine in a neutral position by placing a layer of padding beneath the child's body from shoulders to hips before securing the child to the spine board.

Restraint of Children During Transport

Make sure all persons riding in an ambulance are appropriately restrained. Secure children with possible spinal injury in a supine position on a stretcher or backboard (and secure the board to the stretcher) (**Figure 7-17**). If the child has mild to moderate trauma without suggestion of spinal injury, use EMS system guidelines for age-appropriate restraint. All states have well-defined regulations on proper child restraint in a passenger vehicle. However, these regulations may not extend to ambulance transport. The appropriate use of a child restraint seat in an ambulance is controversial. When "car seats" are used for EMS transport, both the device and the method of securing the seat to the gurney must conform to industry standards and meet local requirements. If EMS local policy allows, have the child's caregiver remain within view or speaking distance of the child, if the caregiver's presence does not compromise the child's treatment or crew safety. This is comforting for the conscious and hemodynamically stable child.

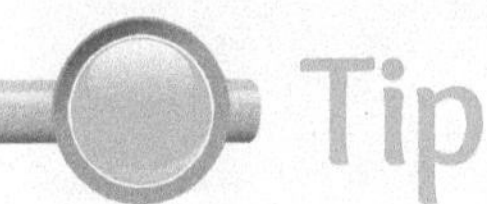

Tip

Although spinal injuries are not common in children, the high frequency of head injury means that spinal stabilization should be part of the care of many pediatric patients with a significant mechanism of blunt trauma.

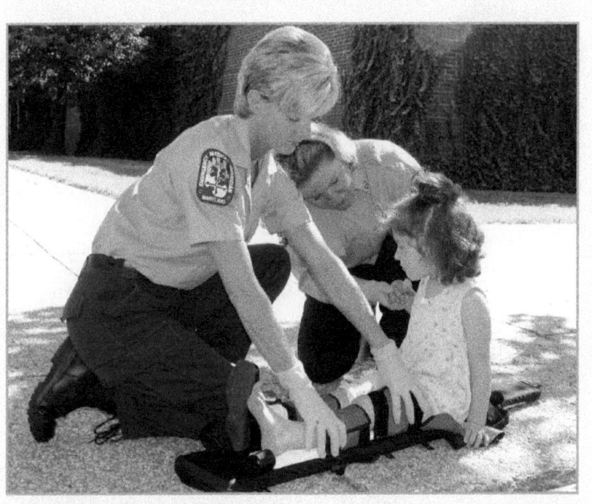

Figure 7-15 Splinting.

Pediatric Burn Patients

The assessment and management priorities for the burn patient are the same as for any other trauma patient. Make sure the scene is safe before approaching the child. Always anticipate exposure to hazardous materials and carbon monoxide, and use protective measures. Get technical help, if needed, from authorities on hazardous materials.

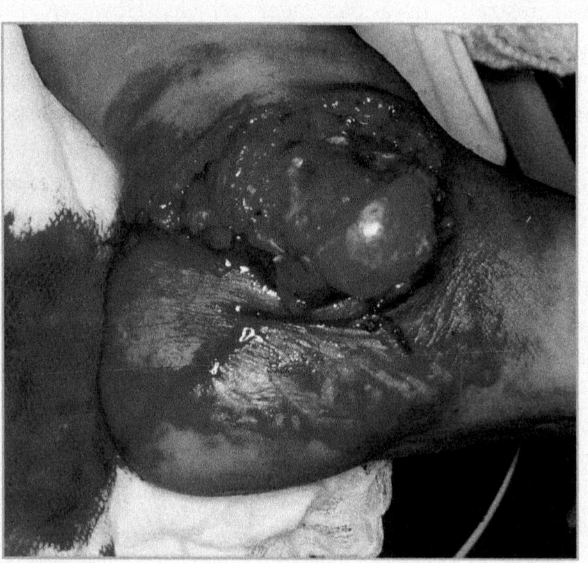

Figure 7-16 Leave exposed bone out. Do not attempt to reduce open fractures, unless circulation is compromised.

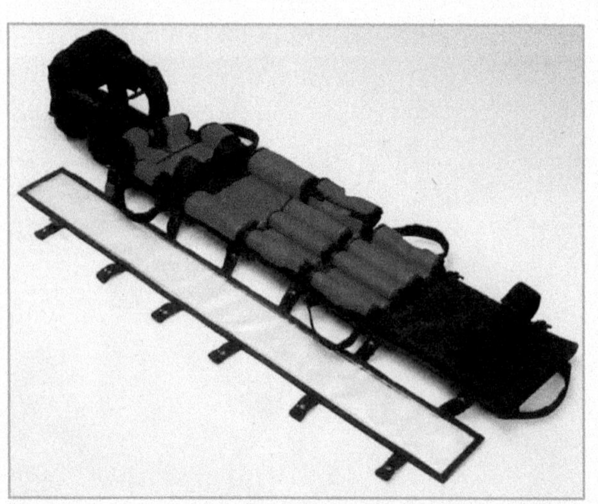

Figure 7-17 A pediatric spine board is an excellent stabilization device.

Assessment

Assess the scene for risk factors for airway and breathing. Important considerations in patients with fire and smoke exposures include the following:

- Enclosed space
- Heavy smoke
- Fumes
- Steam
- Hot vapors
- Chemical hazards
- Explosions with blunt or penetrating injury

Assess the patient for signs of smoke or particle inhalation and thermal burns of the airway. Give 100% oxygen for suspected carbon monoxide poisoning in children with abnormal appearance or AMS, or in children exposed to fire or smoke in an enclosed space. Anticipate hidden injuries (especially abdominal) from a fall or a blast injury.

Make a quick estimation of burned body surface area. A modified anatomic diagram of children of different ages gives an approximation of burned body surface area, as shown in **Figure 7-18**. If such a diagram is not available, use the "rule of palms," which states that the patient's palm plus fingers equals 1% of body surface area (**Figure 7-19**). The percentage of burned body surface area is therefore roughly equal to the number of patient palm plus fingers-sized areas burned.

Although most burns are unintentional, assess all burn patients for risk factors for intentional injury. Scald and contact burns are common in children and are frequent findings in nonaccidental trauma, as explained in Chapter 13. A "pattern" burn (where there is a clear demarcation of an object in the burned skin), "glove" or "stocking" distribution of a scald burn (**Figure 7-20**), or a history that is inconsistent with the injury are suspicious circumstances for intentional injury.

Management

Remove any burning clothes. Give 100% oxygen to all patients with flame or blast burns. High-flow oxygen therapy is the only field treatment for suspected carbon monoxide poisoning. Because of the risk of hypothermia, do not flush or wet burned areas unless necessary to decontaminate or stop the burning process. Cover burned areas with clean dry sheets or nonstick dressings. Covering helps to reduce pain by minimizing exposure to air currents. *Do not apply ointments or creams to burn areas.*

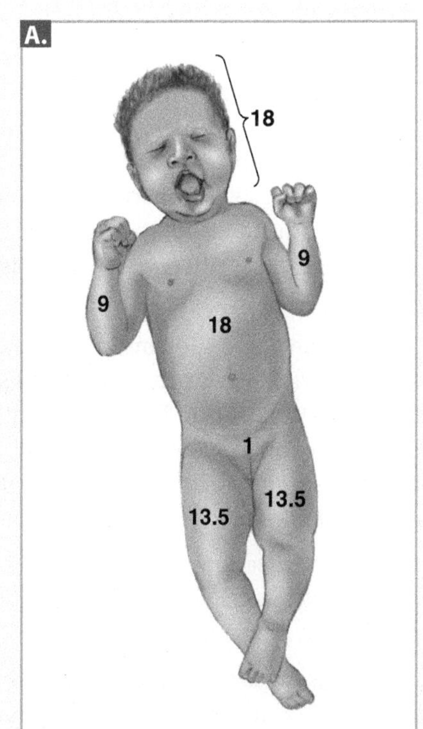

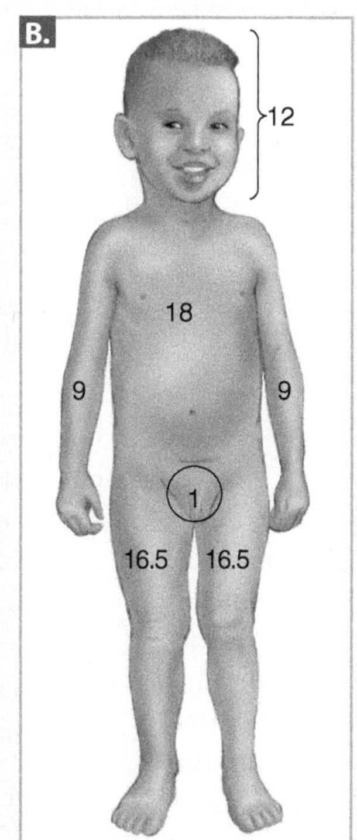

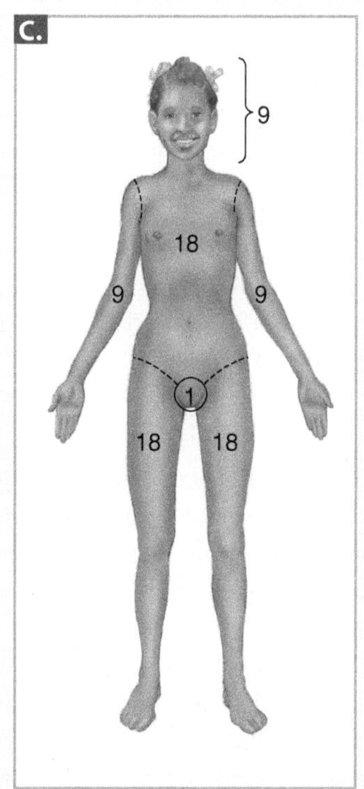

Figure 7-18 Modified anatomic diagrams of children of different ages give an approximation of involved body surface area for calculation of extent of burn in **A.** infant, **B.** child, and **C.** adolescent.

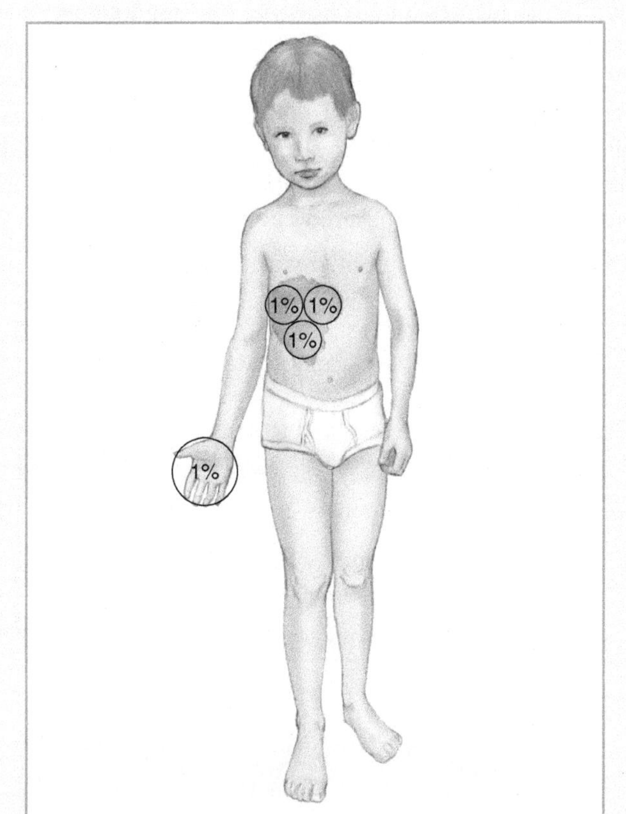

Figure 7-19 The palm plus fingers is approximately 1% of the body surface area.

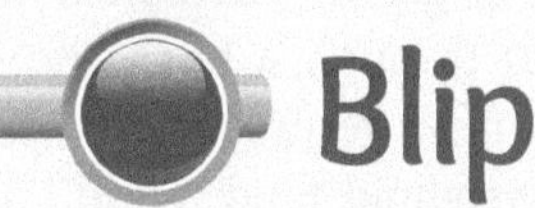

Blip

Do not apply ointments or creams to burn areas.

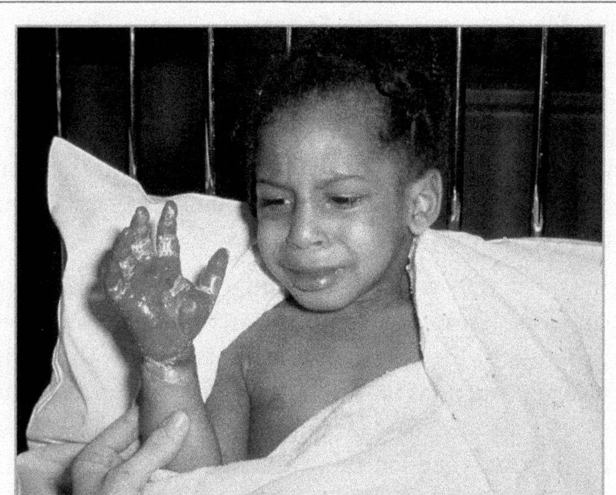

Figure 7-20 Consider intentional injury with a suspicious pattern of the burn, especially a "stocking" or "glove" distribution.

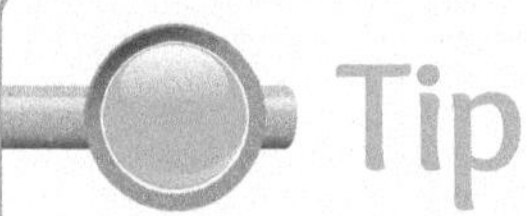

The Parkland formula (or a modification thereof) is the most common method of determining fluid resuscitation after a burn. It is intended only as a guide for fluid resuscitation. Based on this formula, the patient receives 2 to 4 mL/kg of crystalloid multiplied by the percentage body surface area burned of crystalloid for the first 24 hours.

ALS

Advanced Airway Management of the Pediatric Burn Patient. Consider early (before edema starts) endotracheal intubation in any patient exposed to a fire in an enclosed space with a suspected inhalation injury to the airway. Such patients may have abnormal airway sounds, abnormal positioning, and respiratory distress or failure. Singed or burned nasal hairs and carbonaceous sputum may also indicate airway injury. Smoke inhalation may cause bronchospasm. If wheezing is present, give a bronchodilator, either intramuscular (IM) epinephrine or inhaled albuterol.

Pharmacologic Management of the Pediatric Burn Patient. Try to establish at least one IV line in patients with partial or full-thickness burns greater than 5% body surface area. Insert IV catheters through a burn site if necessary. If indicated, initiate fluid resuscitation with 20-mL/kg boluses of isotonic crystalloid fluid. Fluid and heat are rapidly lost through disrupted skin, with the rate of loss proportionate to the percentage body surface area burned. Provide early analgesia and sedation, and titrate to effect. For longer transports, contact the medical control to determine IV infusion rates.

Pain Management and Sedation. Fear and pain in children are frequently ignored or misinterpreted. Pain management is an important out-of-hospital priority, especially in trauma and burn patients with long transport times. Infants and young children experience the same degree of pain as older children and adults; they just cannot express it in words.

Pain and anxiety are different things and require different treatments. Treat pain with a narcotic analgesic drug, such as morphine or fentanyl. Treat anxiety with a sedative drug, such as a benzodiazepine (e.g., diazepam or midazolam). For example, a child with continued pain after stabilization of an isolated extremity fracture needs morphine or fentanyl to control the principal problem, which is pain. Narcotics, such as morphine or fentanyl, are pain killers but also provide some sedation. However, a child who is anxious or a child who has been intubated and is fighting the ET needs a medication, such as diazepam or midazolam, because anxiety is the problem, not pain.

IV narcotic analgesics are appropriate in hemodynamically stable trauma patients with burns or with isolated long-bone fractures or dislocations. If serious blood loss or bleeding is suspected, or if assessment suggests hypoperfusion, avoid the use of narcotics because of the tendency to contribute to hypotension. Compared to morphine, fentanyl may cause less hypotension.

Consider sedative drugs when transporting an awake, intubated child or a child who has received neuromuscular blocking agents (paralytics) during RSI to help with endotracheal intubation. Benzodiazepine drugs can also contribute to hypotension, so give them only to patients who are hemodynamically stable.

Table 7-10 lists common medications to treat pain or anxiety in a hemodynamically stable child after consultation with medical control as per local EMS protocol.

All IV sedatives and narcotics cause respiratory depression. Give by slow IV push over 3–5 minutes. Another option is to give intranasal Fentanyl. Give supplemental oxygen to all children receiving these medications. Place the child on a cardiac monitor and use pulse oximetry and end-tidal CO_2 when available. Be ready to begin positive pressure ventilation with a bag-mask device if the child develops respiratory depression. Naloxone (0.1 mg/kg/dose to a maximum single dose 2 mg IV/IM/IO/subcutaneously [SQ]/ET) may temporarily reverse respiratory depression caused by narcotic administration. Keep in mind that use of naloxone also negates any analgesic effect and prevents further positive effects of narcotics until the naloxone has been metabolized by the child's body.

Treat circulatory compromise with IV fluid boluses.

Table 7-10 ALS: Pharmacologic Management of Pain and Anxiety

Pain	
Morphine sulfate	• *Neonates*: 0.05 mg/kg IM, IV, IO, or SQ • *Infants and children*: 0.05–0.1 mg/kg IM, IV, IO, or SQ • *Adolescents*: 3–4 mg IV, IM, or IO
Fentanyl	• 1–2 mcg/kg/IV, IO, IM, or IN every 30–60 minutes
Anxiety	
Diazepam	• 0.1 mg/kg IV (max 5 mg/dose)
Midazolam	• 0.05–0.1 mg/kg IV, IM, or IO or 0.2 mg/kg IN

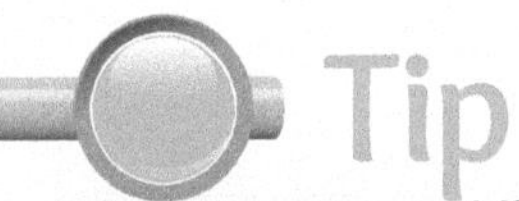

Pain and anxiety are different things and require different treatments.

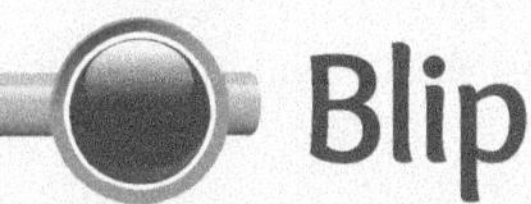

Avoid narcotics in the multiple trauma patient because they may contribute to hypotension.

Summary of Burns

Burns are common pediatric injuries, but usually are small and require only first aid. Burns involving the airway, or more than 5% of body surface area, or of full thickness require important field interventions, including possible airway protection and fluid administration. Closed-space burns raise the possibility of carbon monoxide poisoning. Pain is a universal feature of burns, and analgesia is usually a primary intervention.

Case Study 3

You are dispatched to a child who has been run over by a vehicle. On your arrival you notice a full-sized SUV parked in the middle of the road, and a 6-year-old girl, conscious and alert with a small laceration on her chin, being held in her father's arms. She has no abnormal airway sounds or increased work of breathing, and her skin is pale. You notice the odor of alcohol on the man's breath. According to bystanders, the child was walking behind the car when her dad backed up. The patient is cool and clammy to the touch. Respiratory rate is 40 breaths/min, heart rate is 146 beats/min, and you are unable to obtain a blood pressure. Lung sounds are decreased in lower fields. While exposing the child, you notice a tire track impression across the abdomen and sternum area. Pulse oximetry is 90% on room air.

1. What critical injuries do you suspect?
2. What are your treatment and transport priorities?

CASE STUDY ANSWERS

Case Study 1 — page 134

This patient requires immediate treatment and transport. The patient has sustained multisystem trauma to the head, chest, abdomen, and right lower extremity, and the primary assessment confirms respiratory failure and shock. Snoring respirations are likely caused by airway obstruction by soft tissues or blood. Positioning the airway and suctioning may alleviate the problem. Perform rapid spinal stabilization.

The patient is hypoxic with abnormal breath sounds from either pulmonary contusion or tension pneumothorax.

ALS If the child does not respond to oxygen at 100% by positive pressure ventilation, consider needle decompression on the right side.

Stabilize the femur with a splint. Start IVs en route to the hospital and initiate fluid resuscitation. Transport rapidly to a trauma center with pediatric expertise.

Case Study 2 — page 142

This child appears to have an isolated head injury and TBI. The child's rapid deterioration suggests an expanding intracranial hematoma, which may be life-threatening. As with any serious head injury, consider the risk of associated spinal injury. Stabilize and protect the child's spine and be prepared for vomiting. Apply 100% oxygen. Rapidly transport.

ALS Establish an IV en route for the administration of medications and leave at TKO.

Transport to a facility with pediatric neurosurgical capability, or consider rendezvous with an air ambulance service if such care is not available in your community. This is a surgical emergency and immediate access to operative care may make the difference between the life and death of this child.

Case Study 3 — page 155

The injuries to this child are life-threatening and she appears to be in shock. Transport immediately after spinal stabilization and 100% oxygen.

ALS Do not prolong scene time with IV attempts. Give fluid resuscitation during transport.

This child is at risk for massive internal injury, including abdominal solid organ hemorrhage (liver, spleen, and kidneys); viscus rupture of the stomach, small bowel, and large bowel; hemothorax; pneumothorax; pulmonary contusion; and pelvic fracture. The source of bleeding is not relevant to field care, but the recognition and treatment of compensated shock is critical.

Transport to the highest level of trauma care available in your community, based on local trauma triage protocol. This child requires rapid radiologic assessment of the extent of injury and possibly early operative intervention.

SUGGESTED READINGS

Textbooks

American Academy of Orthopaedic Surgeons. *Emergency Care and Transportation of the Sick and Injured*. 10th ed. Burlington, MA: Jones and Bartlett Learning; 2011.

American Academy of Pediatrics and the American College of Emergency Physicians. *APLS: The Pediatric Emergency Medicine Resource*. 5th ed. Burlington, MA: Jones and Bartlett Learning; 2012.

Barss P, Smith G, Baker S, et al. *Injury Prevention: An International Perspective*. Oxford University Press; 1998.

Bledsoe B, Porter R, Cherry R. *Essentials of Paramedic Care*. Upper Saddle River, NJ: Prentice Hall; 2003.

Campbell J. *BTLS for Paramedics and Other Advanced Providers*. 5th ed. Upper Saddle River, NJ: Pearson-Prentice Hall; 2004.

Articles

Adelson PD. Guidelines for the acute medical management of severe traumatic brain injury in infants, children, and adolescents. Chapter 4. Resuscitation of blood pressure and oxygenation and prehospital brain-specific therapies for the severe pediatric traumatic brain injury patient. *Pediatr Crit Care Med*. 2003;4(suppl 3):S12–S18.

Gausche-Hill M, Brown KM, Oliver ZJ, Sassoon C, Dayan PS, et al. (2014). An evidence-based guideline for prehospital analgesia in trauma. *Prehosp Emerg Care*. 2014;18(suppl 1):25–34.

Morrison W. Pediatric trauma systems. *Crit Care Med*. 2002;30(suppl 11):S448–S456.

Sadow KB. Prehospital intravenous fluid therapy in the pediatric trauma patient. *CPEM*. 2001;2(1):23–27.

Stafford PW. Practical points in evaluation and resuscitation of the injured child. *Surg Clin North Am*. 2002;82(2):273–301.

Stallion A. Initial assessment and management of pediatric trauma patient. *Respir Care Clin N Am*. Mar 2001;7(1):1–11.

White IV CC, Domeier RM, Millin MG, and the Standards and Clinical Practice Committee, National Association of EMS Physicians. EMS spinal precautions and the use of the long backboard-resource document to the position statement of the National Association of EMS Physicians and the American College of Surgeons Committee on Trauma. *Prehosp Emerg Care*. 2014;18:306–14.

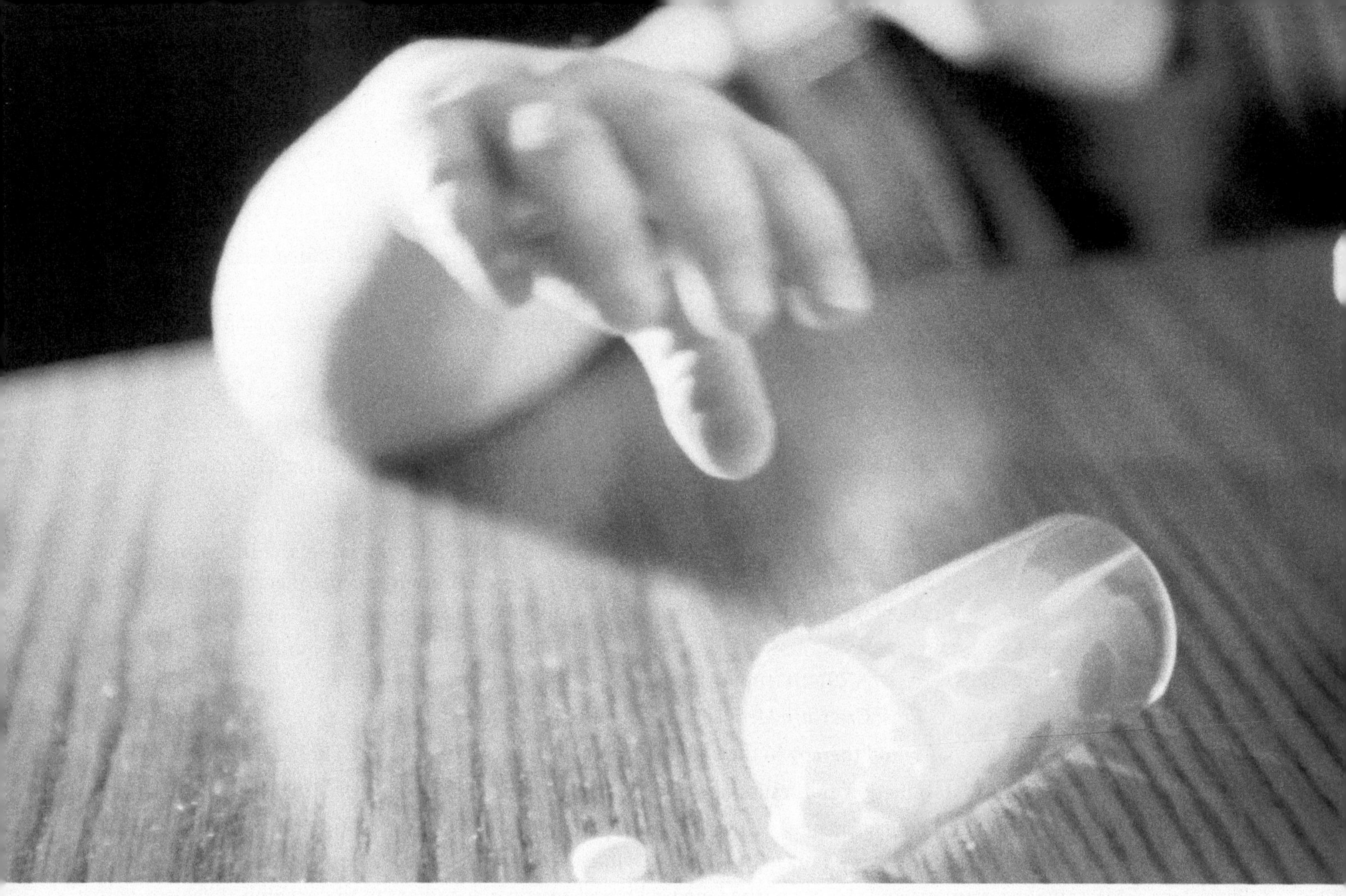

Learning Objectives

1. Identify the age groups at risk for toxic exposures, and the substance and management issues unique to each group.
2. Describe the physical assessment of the child with a suspected toxic exposure.
3. Discuss the risk assessment of the child with a suspected toxic exposure.
4. Explain the risks and the benefits of different forms of gastric decontamination.
5. Identify situations where online contact with the regional poison center might influence the assessment and treatment of toxic exposures.

Toxic Emergencies

Chapter 8

Introduction

A toxic exposure is an ingestion, inhalation, injection, absorption, or application of any substance that causes illness or injury. There are a myriad of reasons that children experience such exposures, including unintentional ingestions of poisons, environmental misadventures, and deliberate intoxications. An example of an unintentional exposure is a toddler who ingests a caregiver's medication. An environmental misadventure might be a child who inhales carbon monoxide during a house fire, or a child with a systemic reaction to a skin contact with an insecticide. Deliberate intoxications include recreational exposures and attempted suicides.

Age-Related Differences

Toxic exposures are a common pediatric out-of-hospital complaint. Although children younger than 6 years of age account for most of the total exposures for all age groups, according to 2013 data from the American Association of Poison Control Centers, the percentage of fatalities in this age group remains low at 2.1% of all fatalities, similar to statistics from previous years (**Table 8-1**). Although the number of reported exposures for the adolescent population (13–19 years) is relatively low, the mortality rate is much higher (2.6% of all fatalities or approximately 10 times that of children <6 years), and is usually caused by intentional exposure.

Most exposures in infants and preschool children younger than 6 years of age are asymptomatic. The toddler is a fearless, curious individual who explores the world by placing objects in his or her mouth (**Figure 8-1**). Because toddler ingestions are unintentional, and most nonfood items ingested are not very palatable, poisonings in this age group often involve small volumes of a single substance. The most common ingestions in young children include cosmetics and personal care products, cleaning substances, and analgesics. The great majority of toddlers are initially asymptomatic; however, toddlers may also present with significant symptoms without a known history or witnessed ingestion. It is important that providers consider this possibility and survey the scene to better understand possible causes. In addition, it is important to keep in mind, that the initially asymptomatic child may have dangerously high levels of a toxin in his or her body that may not become apparent until much later. In the absence of any apparent life threats, obtaining a thorough history before making a transportation decision is absolutely imperative. In this age group, analgesics, button batteries, and hydrocarbons cause the most fatalities.

Button (disk) batteries usually pass through the digestive tract without a problem but can get stuck in the esophagus or anywhere else in the body. If there is suspicion that a child has ingested a battery (or one is stuck in the nose, ear, or elsewhere), attempt to find out exactly what kind of battery it is and bring the child to the emergency department (ED). More than one-third of patients with disk batteries lodged in the esophagus are initially asymptomatic. Symptoms develop when the battery begins to erode and damages surrounding tissues. Although battery ingestion can be fatal, most pass through the gastrointestinal (GI) tract in 1–4 days.

Case Study 1

A mother calls 9-1-1 because her 2-year-old toddler is drooling and having trouble breathing. On arrival at the home, you find a young boy crying but consolable by the mother. He has no abnormal airway sounds, no flaring, and no retractions. His skin is pink. The respiratory rate is 32 breaths/min, the pulse oximetry is 98%, and the heart rate is 120 beats/min. His lungs are clear. On further assessment, you note that the child has very red, swollen lips, and a mouth odor that smells like bleach. His mother states that she was doing the laundry when she received a telephone call and left her son briefly.

1. What are key aspects of the scene size-up?
2. Outline transport and management priorities.

Children 6–12 years of age are less likely to ingest nonfood articles or nonprescribed medications (**Table 8-2**). Although most exposures continue to be unintentional in this age group, intentional exposure begins to play a role, particularly among the middle-school age group. Unintentional fatal exposures are mostly caused by smoke inhalation and carbon monoxide poisoning. Intentional exposure, nonfatal and fatal, is seen with "huffing," the intentional inhalation of volatile chemicals.

Among adolescents (13–19 years), toxic exposures are usually intentional, either as recreational abuse or as a suicide gesture or attempt. Intentional exposures lead to more ED visits and hospital admissions than unintentional exposures. In suicide attempts, adolescents usually ingest two or more substances, often in large quantities (polypharmacy). Recreational abuse often involves alcohol in addition to another recreational drug. The number of fatalities in this age group is increasing. Statistics represent an underestimation of the true incidence, because statistics only include those cases reported to the poison control database. Many adolescents would have difficulty getting the resources to purchase illicit drugs were it not for the ever-evolving creative ways they find to get high. Huffing usually involves common household products, such as markers, glue, aerosol air freshener, spray paint, correction fluid, gasoline, and other products. These substances are inexpensive, easy to find in many homes, and give the teenager an easy-to-hide substance because it would not normally seem out of place to have these items in one's home. Botanical substances including salvia and jimson weed are also easy to grow or obtain. Other drugs, often sold inexpensively and legally on the Internet, in head shops, and in convenience stores, include what are commonly known as "bath salts," a group of synthetic drugs that mimic the symptoms of methamphetamine, hallucinogens, and synthetic marijuana, often known as "spice" or "K2," which can cause tachycardia, elevated blood pressure, and nausea. It is important to remember crew member safety first because some of these substances can cause delusional and violent behavior in the teenage patient.

Another problem continues to be the exposure of young children to the chemicals used in methamphetamine laboratories, and the use of methamphetamines. Crew safety in these situations is critical because of explosion hazards.

An unusual form of abuse involves deliberate intoxication of infants or young children, a condition called Munchausen syndrome by proxy. This condition is a complex form of deliberate poisoning of a child by a caregiver. In these cases, the caregiver frequently possesses more than average medical information and is trying to induce a state of illness in the child in an attempt to bring attention to himself or herself. Children with such exposures may be especially difficult to identify because the intoxication is secretive and often chronic.

Common Substances Responsible for Serious Poisonings in Children

Most poisonings occur in the home. Table 8-2 lists common substances responsible for serious poisonings.

Summary of Age-Related Differences

Most toxic exposures in children are minor and involve household products. The most common patient is the toddler who unintentionally ingests a single agent in small quantity and is asymptomatic. The second most common patient is the adolescent who uses recreational drugs or who is making a suicide attempt or gesture. Adolescent exposures often consist of more than one drug and often involve large quantities. Common serious exposures in young children involve analgesics, whereas those in

Table 8-1 Toxicological Cases 2013, American Association of Poison Control Centers Toxic Exposure Surveillance System

Total reported cases	2,079,090 (excludes 108,923 cases of unknown age)
Patients <6 years	1,019,297 (49%)
Patients 6–12 years	127,569 (6%)
Patients >19 years	581,432 (28%)

Source: Mowry JB, Spyker DA, Cantilena LR, et al. *2013 Annual Report of the American Association of Poison Control Centers' National Poison Data System (NPDS): 31st Annual Report,* Clinical Toxicology (2014), 52,1032–1283.

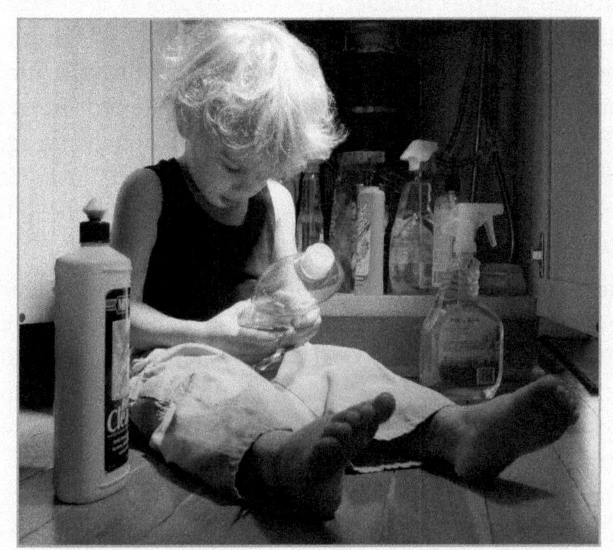

Figure 8-1 Toddlers are "oral explorers;" they will try to taste or swallow almost any substance.

adolescents involve analgesics, alcohol, and recreational drugs. An unusual form of intoxication in young children involves a condition called Munchausen syndrome by proxy, a complex form of deliberate poisoning or abuse of a child by a caregiver.

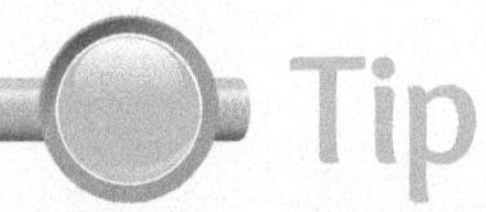

Most patients with toxic exposures are toddlers or preschool-aged children. There is usually only one poison involved, the exposure is usually small and unintentional, and the child is asymptomatic.

Table 8-2 Top 10 Substances Involved in Toxic Exposures by Age Group

All Human Exposures		Pediatric (≤5 years) Exposures	
Analgesics	13%	Cosmetics/Personal Care Products	15%
Cosmetics/Personal Care Products	9%	Household Cleaning Substances	11%
Household Cleaning Substances	9%	Analgesics	10%
Sedative/Hypnotics/ Antipsychotics	7%	Foreign Bodies/Toys/Misc.	7%
Antidepressants	5%	Topical Preparations	6%
Antihistamines	5%	Vitamins	5%
Cardiovascular Drugs	5%	Antihistamines	4%
Foreign Bodies/Toys/Misc.	5%	Pesticides	3%
Pesticides	4%	Gastrointestinal Preparations	3%
Topical Preparations	4%	Plants	3%

Modified from the 2014 Annual Report of the American Association of Poison Control Centers' National Poison Data System. To locate your local poison center call 1 (800) 222-1222 or visit aapcc.org.

Prearrival Preparation and Scene Size-Up

Sometimes at the time of dispatch the toxin has already been identified by the caregiver, the poison center, or another health professional. In such cases, immediately contact medical control or the poison center, depending on local emergency medical services (EMS) protocol. They help clarify the toxicity of the agent and priorities in assessment and treatment. In other cases, where the dispatch involves a toddler or adolescent with a sudden change in behavior, consider a toxic exposure.

On arrival, first perform the scene size-up. Note if there are potentially hazardous toxins in the area or on the patient's clothes or skin. If so, assess the scene and whether immediate patient decontamination is safe to perform. The poison center or other public health agency may assist in defining risk and the need to mobilize other personnel (e.g., hazardous materials team). Pay close attention to scene safety when dealing with adolescents with sudden behavioral changes, because some common substances of abuse can lead to paranoia and sudden violent actions.

If there is a possible toxin or hazardous material, secure the scene and minimize the risk of toxic exposures to the EMS crew through the skin, eyes, or lungs by use of personal protective equipment. Use all your senses to gather information at the scene. Pay particular attention to your initial impression with smell on the scene. Some dangerous toxins quickly overwhelm the sense of smell, rendering it useless after just a few sniffs ("olfactory fatigue"). Other toxins have an odor only at low levels, such as hydrogen sulfide. The "rotten egg" smell given off by this chemical overwhelms the sense of smell and one cannot smell it at the high toxic levels. Other key smells include bitter almonds (cyanide) and garlic (organophosphates, arsenic). Pay attention to confined spaces, and remember that some toxic gases are heavier than air and may affect children first or may only be in low-lying areas, such as cesspools or ditches.

Be aware of the possibility of a mass exposure to a toxic substance, either because of unintentional or deliberate action (e.g., bioterrorism). If a disaster or mass-casualty event is suspected, implement disaster response preparedness (see Chapter 9).

Next, look over the surrounding area. Bring any bottles, containers, or plastic bags containing possible toxins and samples of ingested plants or syringes to the ED along with the patient (**Figure 8-2**). If the caregiver refuses to let a poisoned child be transported to the hospital, ask medical control to talk to the caregiver over the telephone or radio. If this strategy does not work, then request assistance from law enforcement personnel.

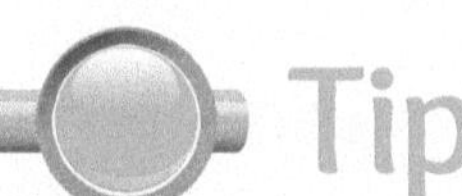

Bring bottles, containers, plastic bags, suspicious substances, plants, or syringes to the ED.

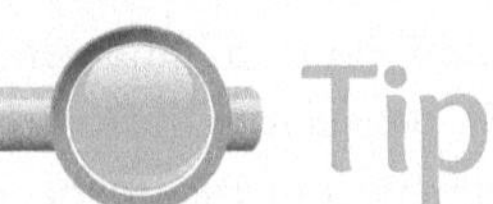

The adolescent who makes a suicide attempt or gesture must be transported to the ED for medical and psychologic assessment, even if the child refuses. This is true even if the injury or immediate medical risk is assessed as trivial.

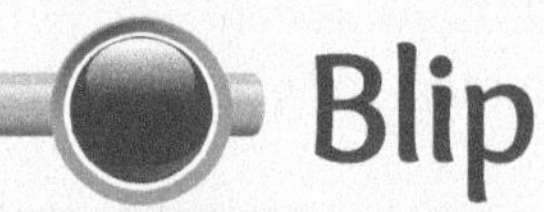

Never forget about toxic hazards on scene. Watch out for absorbable toxins and protect skin and eyes by using gloves and other personal protective equipment.

Role of the Poison Center

Almost every state in the United States has at least one regional poison center. The telephone number within the state is usually toll-free. For ease of access, there is also a national toll-free number (1-800-222-1222) that forwards calls to the state poison center, when available. At the other end of the telephone is a specialist who can provide information about the potential toxicity of an item or adverse effects, and can recommend home or hospital management. Caregivers often call the poison center for advice before or while awaiting the arrival of the prehospital professional.

The regional poison center can also be a valuable resource to the prehospital professional when managing children with a toxic exposure. Local EMS system protocol should define the circumstances when contact with the poison center must be made by online medical control, and when the call can be made directly.

Assessment of the Child With a Possible Toxic Exposure

General Assessment

After the rapid scene size-up and environmental evaluation for toxins, assess the child. Use age-appropriate techniques to approach the patient, as outlined in Chapters 1 and 2, and conduct a general assessment (pediatric assessment

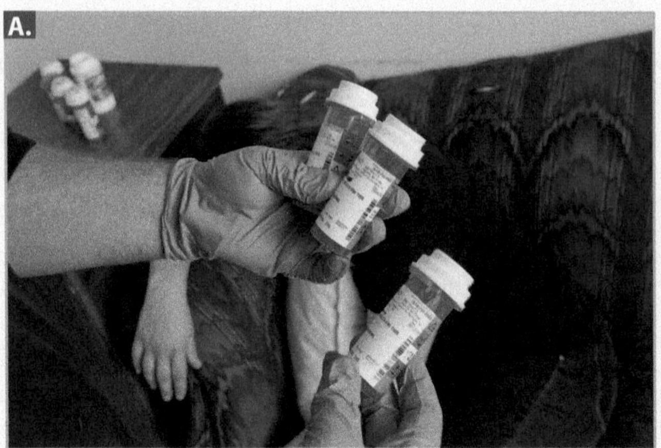

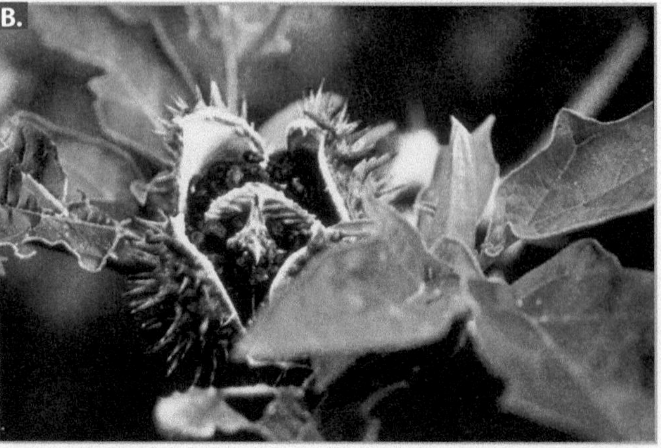

Figure 8-2 Bring any bottles or plant samples to the ED. **A.** Bottles and containers. **B.** The poisonous plant jimson weed.

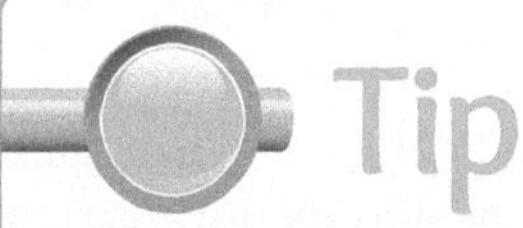

The poison center has a key role in individual and community prevention and treatment of toxic exposures. Have the toll-free number (1-800-222-1222) posted near or on your telephone.

triangle [PAT]), a primary assessment, and then an additional assessment when appropriate. If the child is unstable, treat the physiologic abnormalities detected in the general (PAT) and primary assessment, and then transport. En route, do a reassessment and the additional assessment, if possible.

History is the best tool for overall assessment of risk and for determining urgency for treatment in pediatric poisoning. It is usually more accurate than a physical evaluation in determining the specific type of toxic exposure. In the first few minutes, the important questions are: (1) the identity of the agent; (2) the route of exposure (ingestion, inhalation, injection, absorption); (3) the time since the exposure occurred; and (4) the amount of the agent involved in the exposure, but if unknown, assume the worst case scenario. Using the acronym TART can help one to remember: T = Toxin, A = Amount, R = Route, T = Time. See **Table 8-3**, TART Chart.

Special Considerations in the Primary Assessment

After the PAT, do the hands-on ABCDEs to complete the primary assessment, and then immediately treat any

Table 8-3 TART Chart

Toxin	Amount	Route	Time
Name of substance Type (pill, capsule, liquid, seed, root, flower, suppository, patch, etc.)	Milligrams or other amount if known. Include approximate number of pills, seeds, amount of liquid, and so forth (note if any spilled on floor or clothes). Any vomitus? Take with you if possible.	By mouth, snorted, smoked, injected, rectal, skin absorption, eyes, nose, other.	Approximate time of first exposure or ingestion. Include duration and whether confined space, if applicable.

Table 8-4 Common Toxidromes

Toxidrome	Agents	Signs and Symptoms
Anticholinergics	Antihistamines, cyclic antidepressants*	"Hot as a hare, red as a beet (hot dry skin, hyperthermia), blind as a bat (dilated pupils), mad as a hatter (delirium, hallucinations)"
Cholinergics	Organophosphates	DUMBELS: diarrhea, diaphoresis, urination, miosis, bradycardia, bronchoconstriction, emesis, lacrimation, salivation
Narcotics	Morphine, methadone	Hypoventilation, bradycardia, hypotension, miosis
Sympathomimetics	Cocaine, amphetamines	Tachycardia, hypertension, hyperthermia, mydriasis (dilated pupils), diaphoresis (sweating)
Specific Agents		
γ-Hydroxybutyrate	GHB, "date rape drug"	Initially drowsiness, dizziness, and disorientation; High doses result in bradycardia, hypoventilation, and apnea
Ecstasy/"Bath salts"	3,4 Methylenedioxy-methamphetamine, mephedrone and/or methylenedioxypyrovalerone (MDPV)	Euphoria, increased energy, intense visual perceptions; Complications: hyperthermia, hypertension, seizures, dehydration, myocardial infarction, intracerebral hemorrhage
K2	Spice, "synthetic marijuana"	Elevated mood, relaxation, and altered perception; agitation, hallucinations, severe paranoia, seizures, vomiting, tachycardia, hypertension, and myocardial ischemia

*Cyclic antidepressants have anticholinergic properties, as well as other effects.

physiologic abnormalities. Special elements of the physical assessment that may help identify the type of poison include breath odor, vital signs, pupillary size, skin temperature, and skin condition. An odor of bitter almonds may be caused by cyanide, whereas garlic odor may be caused by organophosphates. Also, look for stains and powders on the skin or clothes. Use assessment information to match the patient's signs and symptoms with possible "toxidromes," identifiable clinical patterns of single-agent intoxications. **Table 8-4** outlines the signs and symptoms of important toxidromes in pediatrics.

Airway

Clear, maintain, and control the airway in the child with a suspected toxic exposure who has altered mental status (AMS). This may happen in a child exposed to a sedative or hypnotic drug, such as a benzodiazepine or a barbiturate. Beware of the child who has ingested a caustic agent, such as lye. This child may have severe burns of the esophagus and present with drooling, dysphagia, and signs of upper airway obstruction. Have a suction unit on hand; if using it becomes necessary, do so gently.

Breathing

Give 100% supplemental oxygen by a nonrebreathing mask if there is AMS, respiratory distress, or a history of exposure to a toxic substance known to cause breathing problems. One example of this type of toxic exposure is hydrocarbon inhalation. Obtain pulse oximetry, but be aware that the reading is not accurate for some toxic exposures, notably carbon monoxide poisoning. Sedative or hypnotic drugs, opiates, and γ-hydroxybutyrate (GHB) may decrease the respiratory rate, whereas sympathomimetic agents (cocaine, amphetamines), phencyclidine (PCP), and aspirin may increase the respiratory rate.

Close monitoring of the airway is essential to evaluate the adequacy of breathing so that intervention with a bag-mask device with supplemental oxygen can be started without delay should breathing become inadequate.

Circulation

If the child has eaten or swallowed a possible cardiopulmonary toxin, place him or her on a cardiac monitor to watch for dysrhythmias. Such drugs as β-blockers, digoxin, or calcium channel blockers may decrease the heart rate, whereas sympathomimetic agents and anticholinergic agents (scopolamine, antihistamines, and jimson weed) may increase heart rate. Skin can be warm and dry because of such drugs as antihistamines and anticholinergics, whereas the skin may be hot and sweaty from sympathomimetics, organophosphates, aspirin, and PCP.

Disability

AMS is a common effect of many different chemical exposures. Recreational drug use with sedatives or hypnotics depresses the central nervous system (CNS). Sympathomimetic drugs may stimulate the CNS and cause excitement, agitation, paranoia, or hallucinations. Cyclic antidepressants may cause seizures or coma. In the comatose or unresponsive patient, always consider the other common causes of AMS, such as a head injury, seizure, or hypoglycemia (which may accompany alcohol or β-blocker ingestion). Check the bedside glucose level in any patient with AMS, even if toxins are suspected.

Exposure

Undress the child and look for evidence of toxic exposure to the eyes and skin. Many substances, such as hydrocarbons, irritate the eyes. Other toxic substances, such as hydrochloric acid, are caustic to skin. Organophosphate insecticides can be inhaled and also enter through the skin and can cause a severe cholinergic crisis with diaphoresis (sweating); urination; miosis (small pupils); bradycardia; bronchoconstriction; emesis; tearing; and salivation. The mnemonic DUMBELS (Table 8-4) helps identify signs of cholinergic drug intoxication. In some systems, the mnemonic SLUDGEM is used: Salivation, Lacrimation, Urination, Defecation, Gastrointestinal pain, Emesis, and Muscle twitching (seizures or coma). These signs coupled with agitation and respiratory distress signal a severe exposure, as you will read in Chapter 9.

Initial Management of Toxic Exposures

After the primary assessment, determine the need for treatment and transport of the poisoned child by combining the physical assessment with a risk assessment. The physical assessment is a way to determine the child's physiologic stability and the overall urgency for treatment and transport. The risk assessment evaluates the probability of serious toxicity (early and delayed) from the exposure. *Perform the risk assessment with knowledge of the identity of the drug involved, time since ingestion* or *exposure, and amount of poison involved. The child's weight should also be considered* (see **Table 8-5**). Contact with the poison center can provide much of this information.

Table 8-5 Risk Assessment

Assess the chances of serious toxicity from the following five pieces of information:
1. The agent involved and its lethality, usually identified through consultation with medical control or the poison center
2. Amount of the toxin, in milligrams when possible
3. Child's weight
4. Route of exposure
5. Time since the exposure

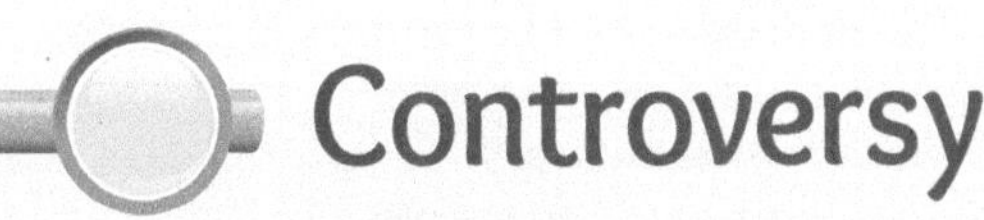

If the child is stable and has a history of a single small ingestion of a low-risk agent, some EMS systems allow the transport to be canceled after agreement from medical control. Although this approach may be medically sound, it eliminates an opportunity for assessment of psychosocial risk factors in the ED.

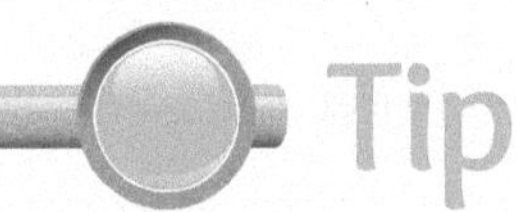

In suspected toxic exposures, perform risk assessment to determine the chances of serious toxicity.

Table 8-6 One Pill Can Kill: Potentially Lethal Toddler Ingestions

Medicine	Lethal Dose
Camphor	One teaspoon of oil
Chloroquine	One 500-mg tablet
Clonidine	One 0.3-mg tablet
Glyburide	Two 5-mg tablets
Imipramine	One 150-mg tablet
Lindane	Two teaspoons of 1% lotion
Diphenoxylate/atropine	Two 2.5-mg tablets
Propranolol	One or two 160-mg tablets
Theophylline	One 500-mg tablet
Verapamil	One or two 240-mg tablets

Common toxic agents, such as aspirin, acetaminophen, or iron, have predictable physiologic effects that are determined by how much of the drug was taken, time since exposure, and amount of drug per kilogram. By collecting information and evidence at the scene, the prehospital professional serves an important role in later ED testing and treatment. Be sure to ask about *all* medications (prescription and over-the-counter), preparations, and other substances to which the child may have been exposed. Caregivers may not realize that some topical preparations (e.g., Bengay or wart treatments) contain salicylate and can contribute to the potential salicylate toxicity when a child ingests aspirin or some common herbal preparations and oils, many of which also contain salicylates.

Sometimes the prehospital professional's risk assessment determines that a child has had a potentially lethal exposure, although the child is physiologically stable. Indeed, in a small child, one ingested pill or teaspoon of some common medications can kill. **Table 8-6** lists potentially dangerous agents where a tiny toxic exposure (e.g., one pill) may be fatal to a toddler.

Iron poisoning is one of the leading causes of fatal poisonings in young children. Tasty chewable children's vitamins have, on average, 17 mg of iron, and the tempting new chewable gummy prenatal vitamins have 27 mg each. A young child can easily mistake either of these for candy and eat excessive amounts. Consider that seriously toxic doses begin at 60 mg/kg of iron and as the ingestion climbs toward 120 mg/kg and higher, the poisoning can easily be lethal without prompt treatment. Gather up all bottles and assume that when pills are missing, the child has eaten them until proved otherwise.

Case Study 2

You respond to a call for a 4-year-old that just ingested all of her mother's prenatal iron tablets (approximately 30). On your arrival, the child is active, running around the room, but complaining that her "tummy hurts." She has no increased work of breathing, and her skin is pink. Her respiratory rate is 24 breaths/min, heart rate is 110 beats/min, and blood pressure is 90/60 mm Hg. Her physical examination reveals no abnormalities. The mother hands you the empty bottle of fruit-flavored chewable prenatal vitamins. Reading the label, you learn that each vitamin contains 27 mg of iron.

1. Do you need to transport this child to the hospital?
2. Should you give activated charcoal?

The Transport Decision: Stay or Go?

After the primary assessment, initial treatment, and risk assessment, consider whether to transport immediately, performing additional assessment and treatment on the way to the ED, or to stay on the scene. If the results of the physical assessment and the risk assessment reveal an asymptomatic child and the ingestion of a small amount of a single low-risk agent, consider canceling transport after appropriate consultation with medical oversight or the poison center. This is controversial, however, because some EMS systems consider hospital transport necessary in all toxic exposure cases. Other systems allow the poison center to manage minor ingestions exclusively over the telephone.

If the physical assessment indicates that the child has any physiologic abnormality, or if the risk assessment indicates that the toxic exposure is potentially harmful, transport and perform additional assessment on the way to the ED, if possible. The onset of symptoms varies with the substance involved. A child without symptoms on arrival of EMS may have ingested a lethal dose of a substance. For example, ingestions of acetaminophen, a common household over-the-counter medicine, may be extremely dangerous but cause no early symptoms. History from the scene is critical to the management in the ED.

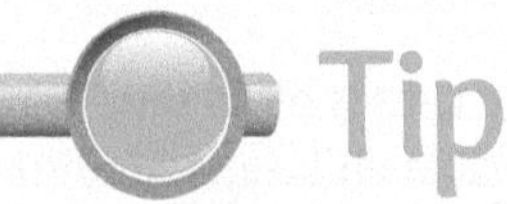

Most preadolescent pediatric poisonings do not require any treatment in the field.

Additional Assessment

If the child has no physical abnormalities and is asymptomatic, and if the risk assessment indicates no serious toxicity, perform a complete assessment on scene. Additional assessment includes the focused history and physical examination and the detailed physical examination (trauma). Sometimes it is more appropriate to perform this additional assessment on the way to the ED. **Table 8-7** lists important history in a suspected toxic exposure, presented in the standard SAMPLE format. During the primary assessment and the risk assessment, the prehospital professional will have already obtained some of the SAMPLE history.

Table 8-7 The Pediatric SAMPLE for Toxic Exposures

Component	Explanation
Signs and symptoms	Time of suspected exposure Behavior changes in child Emesis and content of vomitus
Allergies	Known drug reactions or other allergies
Medications	Identity of suspected toxin Amount of toxin exposure (count pills or measure volume) Pill or chemical containers on scene Exact names and doses of prescribed medications
Past medical problems	Previous illnesses or injuries
Last food or liquid	Timing of the child's last food or drink Type and time of home treatment
Events leading to the exposure	Key events leading to the exposure Type of exposure (inhaled, injected, ingested, or absorbed through the skin) Poison center contact

Summary of Assessment of the Child With a Possible Toxic Exposure

Every child with a toxic exposure needs a careful physical assessment and risk assessment. The physical assessment includes all of the features of the standard assessment, with an emphasis on the history, which is usually the most important part of the toxicologic evaluation. Preparation begins on the way to the scene with dispatch information about the age of the patient, the type and potential toxicity of exposure, and the need for personal protective equipment. Preparation then continues with the scene size-up and environmental assessment. If multiple patients are involved, consider disaster plan activation.

After the physical assessment, the risk assessment helps determine if there might be serious toxicity based on the type of toxin involved, the amount of the toxin, the weight of the child, route of exposure, and the time since the exposure. The risk assessment gives important information about expected physiologic effects, need for treatment, and timing of transport. The poison center often plays a key role in helping decide about treatment and transport.

Toxicologic Management

The prehospital professional has three possible options for toxicologic management of serious or potentially lethal exposures: (1) decontamination to reduce local or systemic exposure to the toxin; (2) enhancement of elimination, or increasing the speed of removal of the toxin; or (3) antidote administration to reverse the actions of the poison directly. In most cases, documenting a thorough history, evaluating the risk assessment, and appropriate transport supporting the ABCs are usually the best treatment.

Decontamination

After the treatment and transport decision, consider decontamination. There are several ways to decontaminate, depending on the toxin and the type of exposure.

Skin

If there is a chance that the poison was absorbed through the skin, remove the child's clothing. The prehospital professional must protect his or her own skin and eyes by using gloves and protective gear. Flood the skin with large amounts of warm water for 15–20 minutes (if time allows and no apparent life threats take priority), and then wash it well with mild soap and water, avoiding harsh scrubbing.

Eyes

Immediately wash out the eyes if there has been direct eye contact (**Figure 8-3**). Alkali burns with caustic agents, such as lye, are the most dangerous. Flush the eyes for 20 minutes using normal saline or water. Attach intravenous (IV) tubing to the bag of normal saline and flush the eye with the end of the IV tubing. If this is not possible, hold the patient's head under the sink and pour water into the eye from a pitcher or cup. When the eyes are the main point of exposure, continue flushing during transport if possible.

Gastrointestinal Decontamination

Before any gastrointestinal (GI) decontamination, contact medical control or the poison center, depending on EMS protocol. In some cases, it may be beneficial to dilute mild acid or alkali ingestions by asking the alert patient to drink an 8-ounce glass of milk or water. Dilution is contraindicated when there is absent gag reflex, airway compromise, diminished level of consciousness, or ingestion of a hydrocarbon corrosive or caustics (strong alkalis and acids).

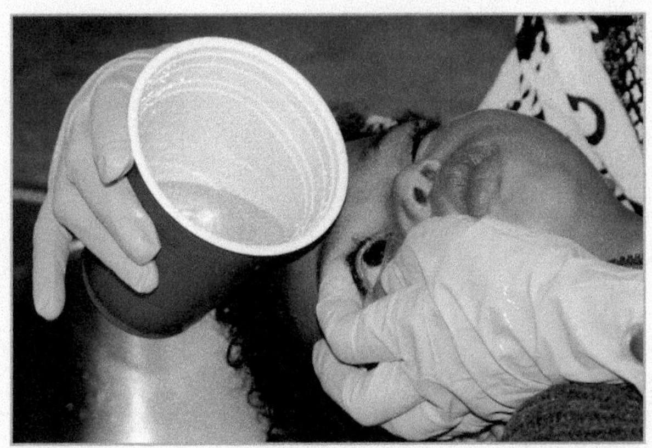

Figure 8-3 Immediately wash out the eyes if there has been direct eye contact.

Ipecac, an old-time remedy for ingestions, although *no longer recommended for home, EMS, or hospital use*, may have been given in the home by the caregiver. Make note of this and the time it was given. The vomiting induced by ipecac does not remove significant amounts of ingested toxins from the stomach and may cause prolonged emesis, delaying the administration of activated charcoal (**Figure 8-4**).

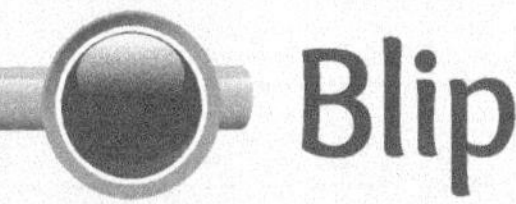

Blip

Do not give ipecac to a child with a suspected ingestion.

Activated Charcoal. Most high-risk ingestions in toddlers and preschool children do not require any out-of-hospital treatment. In cases where GI decontamination is necessary, consider using activated charcoal. Activated charcoal is made from burned wood products. Its surfaces are "activated" by steam or chemical treatment, so the material can irreversibly adsorb ingested toxins in the stomach and small bowel, and reduce bloodstream absorption of the toxins. Charcoal itself is not absorbed from the GI tract, nor is it metabolized. Activated charcoal has no odor or taste, but has a granular consistency that makes many children unwilling to drink it. Charcoal administration is messy, even with a cooperative child. In a child with altered or deteriorating mental status, aspiration of charcoal can lead to serious pulmonary consequences. There are limited data on the use of activated charcoal in the prehospital setting, and the risks of prolonged scene time must be weighed against the potential benefits of rapid transport and early ED management. Some agents are not adsorbed by activated charcoal, as noted in **Table 8-8**.

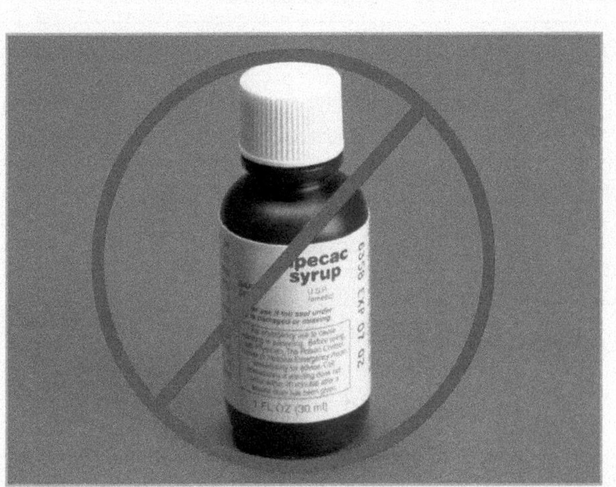

Figure 8-4 Ipecac has no role in prehospital professional treatment of pediatric poisoning.

Table 8-8 Toxins Poorly Adsorbed by Activated Charcoal

"PHAILS"
Pesticides, potassium
Hydrocarbons
Acid, alkali, alcohol
Iron
Lithium
Solvents

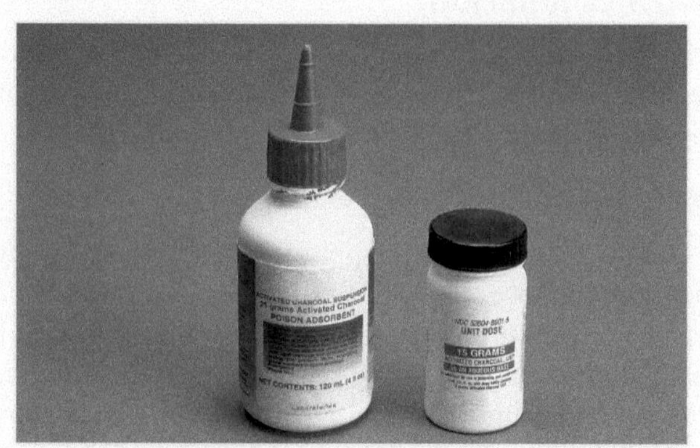

Figure 8-5 Activated charcoal is a treatment option for potentially serious ingestions of bindable toxins.

Administration of Activated Charcoal. The activated charcoal dose is 10 times the mass of the ingested substance. However, because the actual amount of ingested material is usually not known, use 1–2 g/kg of the child's body weight. Activated charcoal begins working immediately, and it is most effective when given within an hour of ingestion (**Figure 8-5**).

Never force a child to take activated charcoal because this may lead to aspiration and pulmonary complications. If local EMS policy allows, consider adding a flavoring agent (e.g., cola, juice, milk) to make the mixture more acceptable to drink, then transport the child. Some formulations of activated charcoal also contain sorbitol. However, there are dangers in giving charcoal with sorbitol to infants less than 1 year of age because of the induction of electrolyte abnormalities and dehydration from diarrhea. **Table 8-9** summarizes activated charcoal and guidelines for use.

ALS

The child must be stable and cooperative to receive activated charcoal. Because young children or adolescents may not want to drink the activated charcoal, some EMS systems use a nasogastric tube as an alternative method of delivery if the ingestion is potentially serious or lethal. Delivery of activated charcoal by nasogastric tube can be dangerous and must be reserved for highly unusual circumstances where transport time is long and risk assessment indicates severe toxicity.

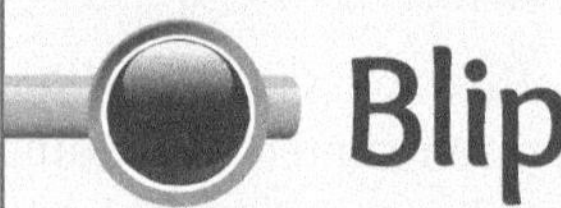

Delivery of activated charcoal by nasogastric tube can be dangerous and must be reserved for highly unusual circumstances where transport time is long and risk assessment indicates severe toxicity.

Table 8-9 Activated Charcoal: Guidelines for Use

Product Information	• A highly adsorbent, harmless, tasteless material made from wood pulp.
Indication	• To limit amount of drug absorbed by the body in most toxic ingestions (i.e., intestinal decontamination). • Repeated doses may enhance the elimination process.
Technique	• Mix 1–2 g/kg patient weight with water to form a **slurry**. If the quantity of ingested substance is known, give 10 times the ingested dose of toxin by weight (maximum dose, 100 g). Administer orally (or by nasogastric tube in rare situations). Consider adding a flavoring agent to make the slurry more acceptable.
Contraindications	• Loss of gag reflex. • Altered mental status. • Unwillingness voluntarily to take the drug. • **Corrosive** substance ingestion. • Drugs not adsorbed by charcoal.
Adverse effects	• **Constipation** or intestinal **bezoar** (large foreign-body mass in gut). • Pulmonary aspiration. • Diarrhea and dehydration may occur in young children given a combined **cathartic** (e.g., sorbitol) and activated charcoal.

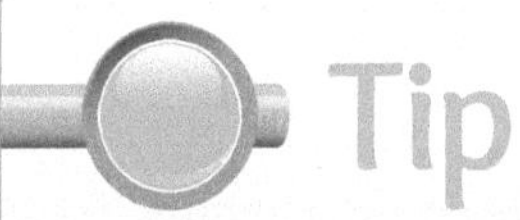

The biggest problem with field use of activated charcoal is the difficulty getting children to take it.

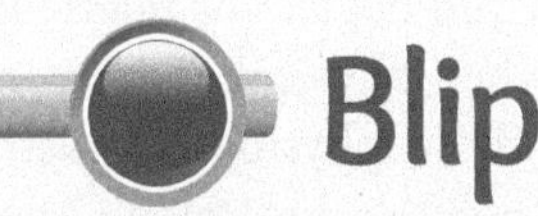

Sorbitol may cause nausea, vomiting, abdominal discomfort, and diarrhea in children, and therefore should not be used in pediatric patients.

Enhancement of Elimination

Sorbitol is a cathartic that is mixed with many commercial activated charcoal preparations. Cathartics have been promoted to clear the bound toxin from the gut and help speed up elimination. The effectiveness of cathartics has not been proved. Sorbitol is not an approved drug in most EMS systems. Prehospital professionals may think they are giving pure activated charcoal when the preparation actually is a mixture of activated charcoal and sorbitol. Sorbitol may cause nausea, vomiting, abdominal discomfort, diarrhea, and electrolyte disturbances in young children. *Therefore, never use a cathartic in children in the prehospital setting.*

Antidotes

Antidotes are medications that reverse or treat the side effects of toxic ingestions. Prehospital providers carry several antidotes that may be lifesaving for poisoned patients. Use these medications with knowledge of the type of ingestion or exposure, patient's clinical status, and possible adverse effects associated with the antidote.

Naloxone is an antidote used frequently in adult patients with suspected opioid overdose. It can have a therapeutic and diagnostic effect in selected pediatric patients. If the child has signs of an opioid ingestion or overdose (bradycardia, coma, small pupils, respiratory depression), administer 0.1 mg/kg. Maximum single dose is 2 mg. Although IV is the preferred route, it can be given intramuscularly (IM), intraosseously (IO), intranasally (IN), endotracheally (ET), or subcutaneously (SQ). However, ET or SQ administration is less effective. The child may then awaken slightly or fully, with improvement in vital signs. The duration of action of naloxone is 20–60 minutes, so repeat doses may be necessary if a longer-acting narcotic (e.g., methadone, Lomotil®) is involved. When administering naloxone, as with adults, give the lowest effective dose and administer slowly. In adolescents chronically addicted to opioids, too rapid administration may induce undesired acute withdrawal symptoms. Have suction on hand in case vomiting should occur.

Although flumazenil is an effective benzodiazepine antagonist, do not use this antidote routinely for patients with AMS of unknown cause. One of the most common causes of AMS in children is the postictal state after a seizure. If flumazenil is given and the child has further seizures, benzodiazepines are not effective. Also, flumazenil may precipitate seizures if administered to the patient who is on chronic therapeutic doses of a benzodiazepine.

Sodium bicarbonate helps reverse the adverse cardiac effects seen with cyclic antidepressant overdoses, including conduction abnormalities. It alkalinizes the blood to reverse the sodium channel blockade caused by the drugs. The dose is 1–2 mEq/kg IV slowly.

β-Blockers are drugs commonly used for treatment of hypertension and adult cardiac disease. Overdose in children can cause bradycardia and hypotension. Glucagon, a familiar drug to prehospital professionals because of its role in treatment of hypoglycemia, helps reverse toxicity from β-blocker overdose. Although there are no good pediatric studies, the suggested dosage of glucagon is 0.03–0.15 mg/kg followed by 0.07 mg/kg/hr (maximum 5 mg/hr). β-Blocker overdose can also cause hypoglycemia in young children, so check the bedside glucose level and treat hypoglycemia if present.

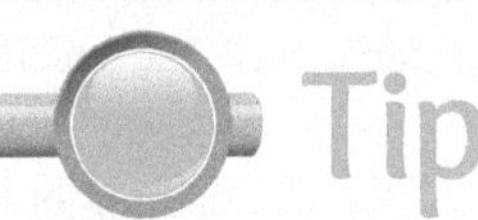

Poison centers have the capability to follow up with continuing reassessment by telephone.

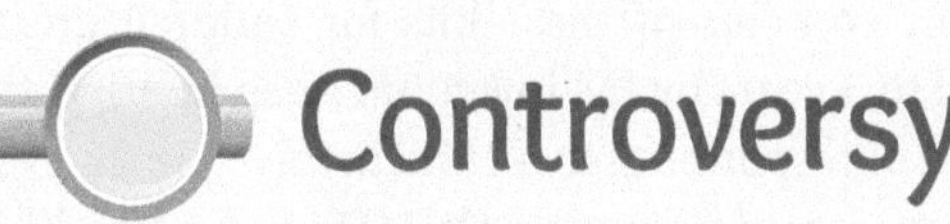

The value of activated charcoal for out-of-hospital treatment of ingestions is unproven. Although the drug has a possible advantage of early binding of toxins in the gut, there are potential complications, such as aspiration and bowel obstruction.

Calcium channel blockers are another frequently prescribed medication for hypertension in adults. Pediatric ingestions may result in severe toxicity that is similar to β-blocker overdose, including bradycardia and hypotension. There can be secondary respiratory and neurologic effects (respiratory depression, decreased level of consciousness). IV fluids are the first line of therapy, and calcium can be beneficial. Give either IV calcium chloride 10% (20 mg/kg = 0.2 mL/kg) or IV calcium gluconate 10% (60 mg/kg = 0.6 mL/kg) slowly. The patient needs to be on a cardiac monitor during administration of these drugs and during transport. Glucagon is another potential therapy for refractory hypotension in such patients.

Organophosphates

DUMBELS (Table 8-4) is the mnemonic that summarizes the clinical hallmarks of organophosphate poisoning toxidrome. Treatment involves several steps:

1. Ensure your personal protection (use gloves and other protective clothing to prevent exposure).
2. Remove contaminated clothing and place them in a bag.
3. Perform the primary assessment and ensure adequate oxygenation and ventilation.
4. Decontaminate the patient (flush the skin with large amounts of water; wash the skin, hair, and under the nails well with soap and water).
5. Flush exposed eyes with large amounts of warm water or saline.
6. If the child has refractory bradycardia, consider treatment with the antidote atropine. The drug helps reverse the "muscarinic" organophosphate effects (salivation, bronchorrhea, bronchospasm, bradycardia, respiratory depression, seizures, coma). The initial pediatric atropine dose is 0.01–0.02 mg/kg IV. Repeat doses until the airway is dry and the child has adequate perfusion. The specific antidote is pralidoxime (2-PAM).

With the advent of possible chemical terrorism incidents, there has been much attention to the side effects of organophosphates, which are the same as those for such nerve agents as sarin gas. Because some EMS agencies have distributed MARK 1 or MARK 2 kits to their providers for management of chemical terrorism, it is important to realize that the medication doses in these autoinjector kits are for adults. However, in severe, life-threatening pediatric cases, administer the contents of these kits for children greater than or equal to 3 years by IM injection. Keep in mind that the likelihood of responding to a child involved in an event of weapons of mass destruction (WMD) is far less likely than responding on a sunny afternoon to a backyard for a child poisoned by one of the many household and commercial pesticide preparations containing organophosphates.

Summary of Toxicologic Management

Most children with toxic exposures do not require treatment of any kind in the field. Consider cancellation of EMS transport after consultation with medical control or the poison center only if the child is asymptomatic, has ingested a small amount of a single low-risk substance, and there are no "red flags" for child neglect or maltreatment. In other circumstances, when physical assessment and risk assessment together show physiologic instability or possible toxicity, treatment is indicated. After managing the ABCDEs, consider toxicologic management by decontamination or, in special situations, administering an antidote. Perform skin and eye decontamination when indicated. Attempt GI decontamination for serious or potentially fatal ingestions based on local protocol. Activated charcoal is a useful binding agent for many types of toxic ingestions, but can be safely administered only to a cooperative child. Sorbitol is contraindicated in children. Several antidotes carried by prehospital professionals may be diagnostic, therapeutic, and even lifesaving. More advanced antidote therapies are best performed in the ED or hospital setting. Remember to educate the family or caregiver on poisoning prevention if circumstances allow, as discussed in Chapter 1.

Medicolegal Issues

There are several scenarios where medicolegal issues play an important role in the management of toxicologic emergencies in children. If the caregiver refuses therapy and transport to the hospital, ask medical control to talk to him or her over the telephone. If this strategy does not work, then request assistance from law enforcement personnel.

The adolescent who makes any suicide attempt or gesture must be transported to the ED. An individual who has attempted suicide is legally incompetent to make treatment decisions and cannot refuse transport. In some cases, law enforcement must become involved in scene management. Place the patient in temporary protective custody and transport to the hospital (see Chapter 14).

The adolescent can also present legal problems because of such issues as the ability of a dependent minor to consent for care, and illegal use of alcohol or recreational drugs. If an adolescent has taken a potentially toxic dose of medication, or has life-threatening complications of drug use or overdose, treat based on the emergency exception rule (the doctrine of implied consent), as explained in Chapter 14. Leave the legal issues of alcohol or drug use to law enforcement officials.

Case Study 3

You respond to a call about an unconscious female. On arrival, you find a group of high-school students surrounding one of their friends who "passed out" at a party. The patient is a 17-year-old girl who is lying on a couch, is unresponsive to voice, and is not moving. Work of breathing is normal, but her skin is pale. Her respiratory rate is 8 breaths/min and shallow, heart rate is 50 beats/min, and blood pressure is 110/70 mm Hg. Her pupils are 3 mm and sluggishly reactive. There is no evidence of head trauma. The remainder of her examination is negative. There is an empty vodka bottle on the kitchen counter.

1. What are your initial management priorities?
2. Can you treat and transport this patient without parental consent?

CASE STUDY ANSWERS

Case Study 1 — page 160

The sudden onset of mucous membrane changes in a previously healthy toddler is concerning for a caustic (alkali or acid) ingestion. Laundry detergents and bleach are caustics, and although most household-strength products cause irritation with a swallow, industrial-strength products with alkaline pH values can cause severe tissue damage and swelling of the lining of the mouth, pharynx, and esophagus when ingested. Given the circumstances of this event, and the tell-tale odor on the child's breath, a bleach ingestion is most likely. Undertake skin and eye decontamination if indicated, and protect yourself with gloves and goggles.

Rapidly transport this child to the hospital, frequently reassessing his airway. Bring the bottle to the ED. Allow the child to sit upright in a position of comfort. Administer blow-by oxygen, because a face mask will not likely be tolerated. Contact with medical control or the regional poison center can provide information on potential complications to anticipate in transport, such as airway edema, stridor, or wheezing. Do not give anything by mouth, including charcoal or fluids to dilute the bleach, because this increases the risk of vomiting with the potential to further damage the esophagus as the stomach contents are regurgitated.

Bleach is a strong alkali whose corrosiveness depends on the pH (>12.5 is very corrosive). Most household detergents and bleaches (pH 11.0–12.0) are not as problematic as industrial-strength cleaners. Because the exact nature of this product is unknown, it should be assumed to be highly corrosive. Given the oral mucous membrane findings, this child may undergo esophagoscopy and bronchoscopy (fiberoptic inspection of the esophagus and airways while under anesthesia) in the operating room to assess the degree of damage and need for further treatment.

Case Study 2 — page 165

Although this child appears well, this is a potentially dangerous ingestion. Iron is one of the most common fatal ingestions in children. There are four phases to an iron ingestion. The initial phase begins with the ingestion and lasts 6 hours. Common signs and symptoms in mild ingestion include nausea and vomiting. Stage 2 (at 6–24 hours) is the quiet phase during which the child appears well. It is not until stage 3 that the child begins to show signs of toxicity, including GI hemorrhage, hypotension, AMS, and renal and hepatic failure. Stage 4 is the postrecovery phase, during which GI strictures can still occur. Because the extent of toxicity cannot be predicted from early symptoms, a cautious approach is warranted. Transport any child who has ingested iron-containing pills to the hospital for further evaluation unless the regional poison center has been contacted and has determined that this is a nontoxic ingestion based on the nature and number of pills taken. This is commonly the case with ingestion of children's multivitamins, where the concentration of iron is low; however because children's vitamins are often manufactured to look and taste a lot like candy, it is not unheard of for a toddler to ingest a full bottle of 60 colorful character vitamins, many of which can contain up to 17 mg of iron each. The ingestion of prenatal vitamins, however, can be very serious, especially now that the more palatable fruit-flavored chewables are becoming more and more popular for women with morning sickness and who are unable to swallow the larger traditional prenatal vitamins with iron. Bring any pill bottles to the ED to ensure proper identification and risk assessment. Because iron is not absorbed by activated charcoal, do not attempt GI decontamination.

Case Study 3 — page 171

The first priority is to establish an effective airway and begin bag-mask ventilation with 100% oxygen, because respiratory failure is present based on rate and depth of respirations.

Some questions to ask her friends include a SAMPLE history:

- Signs and symptoms: Did anyone see her before she passed out? Was she acting normally?
- Allergies: Any known drugs reactions or other allergies?
- Medications: Does she take any medications? Was she drinking any alcohol? Does she use illicit drugs? Did anyone see other drugs being passed around?
- Past medical problems: Does she have any medical problems?
- Last food or liquid: When was the last time anyone saw her with something to eat or drink?
- Events: Did anyone see her fall? When she passed out, did she hit her head?

The triad of respiratory depression, decreased level of consciousness, and pinpoint pupils is typical of an opiate ingestion. This can also be a mixed overdose, because there is evidence of alcohol on the scene. Consider naloxone, and transport the patient to the ED, supporting airway, breathing, and circulation as needed based on frequent reassessments.

Even without the girl's assent or her parents' consent, you are legally bound to treat and transport this patient, because she has a life-threatening condition.

SUGGESTED READINGS

Textbooks

American Academy of Pediatrics and the American College of Emergency Physicians. *APLS: The Pediatric Emergency Medicine Resource*, 5th ed. Burlington, MA, Jones and Bartlett Learning, 2012.

Dieckmann R: Toxic Exposures. In: Seidel J, Henderson D. *Prehospital Care of Pediatric Emergencies*, 2nd ed. Burlington, MA, Jones and Bartlett Learning, 1997:122–129.

Olson K. *Poisoning & Drug Overdose*, 4th ed. McGraw-Hill Professional, 2003.

References

American Academy of Pediatrics: *Acetaminophen toxicity in children*. http://aappolicy.aappublications.org/cgi/content/full/pediatrics;108/4/1020. Accessed September 12, 2012.

Clinical Toxicology. 2010. Informa Healthcare USA, Inc. ISSN 1556-3650 print/ISSN 1556-9519 online. DOI: 10.3109/15563650.2010.543906. 2010; 48:979–1178.

Collins D. 'Huffing' can kill your child—teens get high from fumes of common household products. CBS News Stories, New York, June 1, 2004. CBS News web site. http://www.cbsnews.com/stories/2004/06/01/eveningnews/main620528.shtml .Accessed September 12, 2012.

Dire DJ. Disk battery ingestion. WebMD, Medscape. emedicine.medscape.com/article/7748. Accessed May 4, 2011.

Jaffe, A. Early drug use problems: kids, inhalants, and huffing. Inhalants are often the first drugs that children try. Do you know enough? 20 January 2010. Psychology Today web site. http://www.psychologytoday.com/blog/all-about-addiction/201001/early-drug-use-problems-kids-inhalants-and-huffing. Accessed September 12, 2012.

McCarron MM, Challoner KR, Diphenoxylate-atropine (Lomotil) overdose in children: an update (report of eight cases and review of the literature). *Pediatrics*, 1991 May; 87(5)694-700. Accessed through PubMed online, U.S. National Library of Medicine, National Institutes of Health.

Merck Manual. 2009–2010. Iron Poisoning. 2009–2010 Merck Sharp & Dohme Corp.

Mowry JB, Spyker DA, Cantilena LR, et al. *2013 Annual Report of the American Association of Poison Control Centers' National Poison Data System (NPDS): 31st Annual Report,* Clinical Toxicology (2014), 52,1032–1283.

New York State Department of Health. SEMSCO protocol guidelines; SLUDGEM+respiratory distress+agitation. National Registry EMT protocols.

New York State Department of Health. Statewide Basic Life Support; Adult & Pediatric Treatment Protocols EMT-B and AEMT. Susquehanna Regional E.M.S. Program web site. http//srems.com/site/protocols/BLS_Protocols.pdf. Accessed September 12, 2012.

Nicotine Gum, NY Times. http://health.nytimes.com/health/guides/poison/nicotine/overview.html. Accessed May 4, 2011.

Nicotine gum toxicity. http://www.ncbi.nlm.nih.gov/pubmed/3346035. Accessed May 4, 2011.

The American Association of Poison Control Centers. Press Release re: Fake marijuana spurs more than 750 calls to U.S. Poison Centers this year alone" http://www.aapcc.org. Accessed May 4, 2011.

The American Association of Poison Control Centers. Press Release re: Toxic substances marketed as "bath salts." http://www.aapcc.org/dnn/Portals/0/prrel/BathSalts11811.pdf. Accessed May 4, 2011.

The Poison Post: National Capital Poison Center eNewsletter. *Cough and Cold Medicine No Longer Recommended for Children Younger than Four.* Winter 2008 edition. www.poison.org/poisonpost. Accessed September 12, 2012.

U.S. Department of Health and Human Services. 2007. 1.1 million kids huffed household products even though it can be fatal. Substance Abuse & Mental Health Services Administration (SAMHSA), U.S. Department of Health and Human Services. 15 March 2007. http://www.samhsa.gov/newsroom/advisories/0703143149.aspx. Accessed September 12, 2012.

U.S. Environmental Protection Agency: *Pool Chemical Alert: Safe Storage and Handling of Swimming Pool Chemicals.* U.S. Environmental Protection Agency, Office of Solid Waste and Emergency Response web site. http://www.epa.gov/osweroe1/docs/chem/spalert.pdf. Accessed September 12, 2012.

Waseem M. 2010. Pediatric Salicylate Toxicity. http://emedicine.medscape.com/article/1009987-overview. Accessed March 11, 2010.

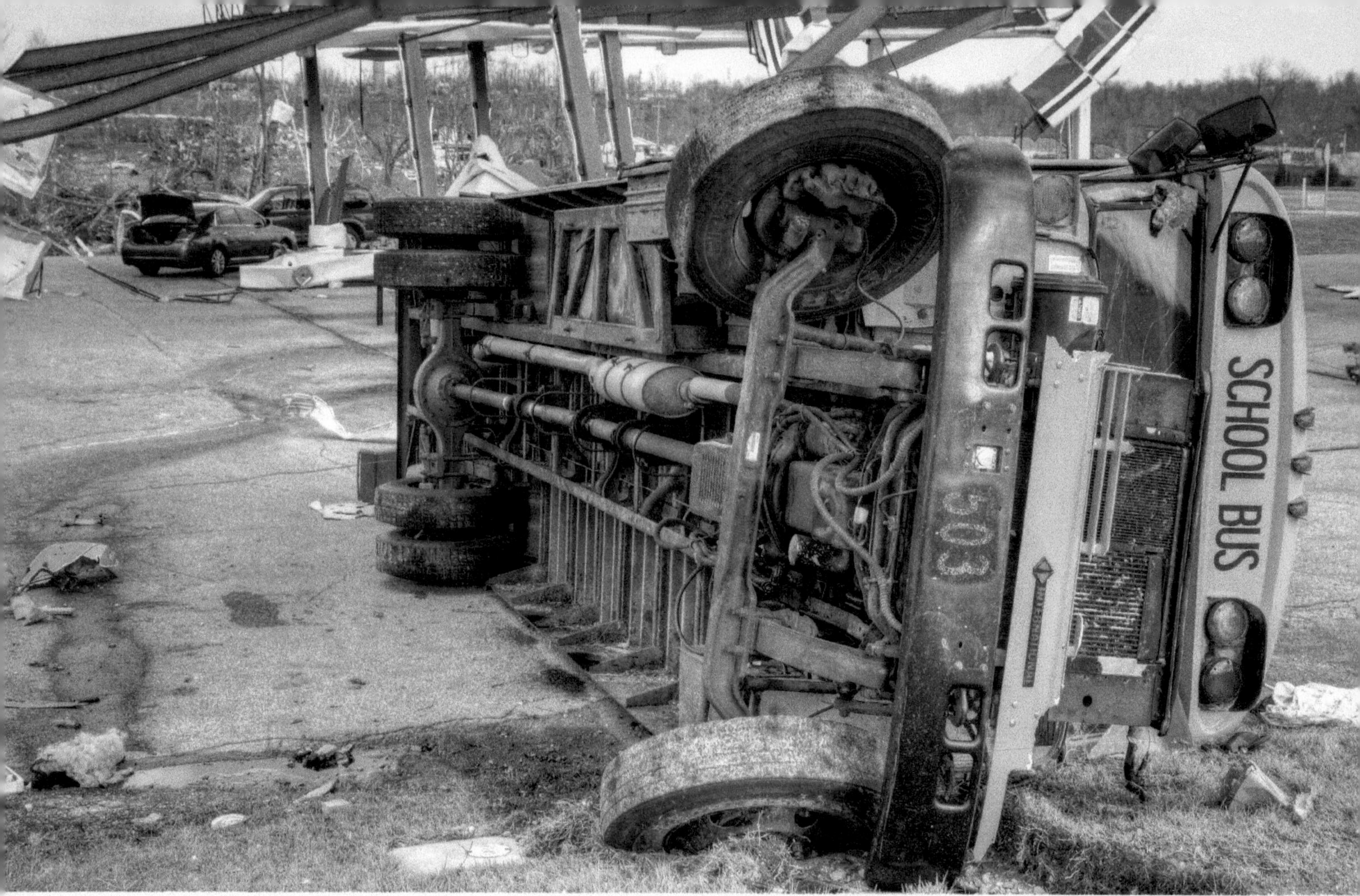

Learning Objectives

1. Define disaster and mass-casualty incident, providing examples of specific pediatric considerations in each.
2. Discuss the modifications required by prehospital professionals to accommodate the special needs of children during disasters and mass-casualty incidents.
3. Recognize the anatomic, physiologic, and psychologic features specific to children that increase their vulnerability and place them at special risk when disasters occur.
4. Differentiate the unique effects that chemical, biologic, radiologic, nuclear, and explosive events may have on children.
5. Discuss pediatric issues related to the assessment and management of specific types of toxic exposures.

Children in Disasters

Chapter 9

Children in Disasters

Disasters have always been a dramatic part of human history, and community responses to disasters are a highly visible feature of modern emergency care systems. Indeed, catastrophic events have afforded a good deal of affirmation about the essential role of the emergency medical services (EMS) system, as well as highlighting its limitations. Disasters present unique difficulties to prehospital professionals, and children present additional complex challenges because of their special anatomic, physiologic, psychologic, and transportation needs. There are limited data on the types and frequencies of children's injuries and illnesses during disasters, and additionally there are limited national guidelines on disaster triage, treatment, and transport of children. However, in such uncommon circumstances, chaos and an overwhelmed operating system are common, so planning and preparation are imperative. Hence, all prehospital professionals must have a basic understanding of the unique pediatric issues in disasters, and EMS agencies must possess a thorough, well-rehearsed disaster response plan that addresses children. Some disasters, such as school mayhem, may primarily victimize children; the horrific idea of prehospital professionals responding to a scene that involves their own children, or children in the community whom they know, is also a distinct possibility. Postevent critical incident stress management (CISM) has become an integral part of long-term disaster response.

What Is a Disaster?

Disasters pose a significant local impact but may often also have a county-wide, state-wide, or regional impact. The definition of a disaster varies by the size and location of the event. For example, a bus crash in a large city will not have much of an impact on that EMS system, but the same incident in a small rural town may exceed the community's response capabilities. Therefore, a **disaster** is an event or series of events that overwhelms the capabilities of the local emergency system and its mutual aid agreements.

Disasters are community emergencies that disrupt normal function and threaten the safety of citizens. Because the US emergency care system is designed primarily around the care of adults, the infrastructure for the care of children in a disaster in most communities is likely to be inadequate, with fewer hospital beds, fewer specialists, and less experience with pediatric critical illness or injury.

A **mass-casualty incident (MCI)** is an event that generates more patients than available resources to care for them using routine procedures. An MCI may require multiple ambulances and additional help from another EMS provider agency. In some circumstances, an MCI may have an enormous impact on the EMS system.

Case Study 1

Your town has been subjected to torrential rains for 4 days. Minor flooding has occurred, but it has been controlled thus far. You are dispatched to an elementary school where wind gusts have blown out windows and, reportedly, 12 children have been injured. While en route, you are notified that a nearby canal dam has just broken; the canal is one block away from the school, and tens of thousands of gallons of water are pouring into the surrounding neighborhoods each minute. Your agency has a total of three ambulances, and one of those is already out of town on a routine transfer.

1. What are your EMS and incident management priorities?
2. What are your specific concerns for the pediatric patients?

A Level I MCI occurs when local medical resources are available and adequate, and regional backup resources may be put on alert. A Level II MCI requires multi-jurisdictional medical mutual aid. Mutual aid agreements should be in place to provide backup for jurisdictions stripped of their local resources. A Level III MCI involves activation of the state disaster plan. Requests for federal assistance may be necessary.

There are two basic types of disasters: natural and man-made. **Table 9-1** lists common examples. Natural disasters are events caused by environmental perturbations, such as earthquakes, severe storms, flooding, wildfires, and natural epidemic disease outbreaks. Man-made disasters result from human errors, such as toxic spills, structural collapses, or malevolent intent, such as terrorism or mass shootings. Regardless of origin, disasters typically cause a significant increase in the incidence of pediatric injuries and illnesses.

Specific pediatric considerations in disasters and MCIs include the current lack of a universally accepted routine pediatric response and management plan, let alone a disaster response plan. States and territories have regional oversight of EMS activities, and there exists an overall diversity in the daily operating procedures for the coordination among first responders, recommendations for online or offline pediatric management protocols, and interfacility transfer guidelines and agreements. Additionally, there is an overall lack of essential pediatric equipment on ambulances and first responder units and a lack of pediatric training requirements for emergency medical personnel. Performance measures for Emergency Medical Services for Children (EMSC) can be found on the Health Resources and Services Administration website.

Table 9-1 Common Natural and Man-Made Disasters

Natural	Man-Made
Earthquake	Hazardous material spill
Hurricane	Structural fire
Tornado	Biologic exposure
Flood	Chemical exposure
Blizzard	Nuclear exposure
Wildland fire	Structural failure
Disease epidemic	Terrorism

EMSC is a federally funded program with the goal of ensuring that children receive state-of-the-art care in an emergency through the training of emergency medical personnel, both prehospital and in-hospital, developing pediatric protocols, guidelines, policy statements, and educational resources for the triage and treatment of children.

Roles of the Prehospital Professional in a Disaster

Predisaster Planning

EMS is a vital resource in predisaster preparedness and response. Prehospital professionals might be called on before a disaster to assist in evacuating hospitals, nursing homes, and other specific skilled care facilities and to provide medical staffing for evacuation shelters. After an MCI, EMS providers are responsible for performing search and rescue, providing medical care, and distributing information to the public.

Planning and preparation for such events are indispensable to the successful functioning of EMS before, during, and after a disaster. The most effective plans are often those that closely match an agency's daily activities. Unfortunately, because children are an infrequent part of an EMS provider's daily encounters, the child's needs are often only a small consideration in most EMS predisaster plans. Therefore, it is essential to include hospital-based pediatricians, nurses, and other personnel with expertise in pediatric illness and injury in the development process for EMS predisaster planning.

Phases of Disaster Response

Disaster response can be subdivided into three phases. The first phase is the activation phase. This occurs at the time of notification and initial response, and includes initiation of the Incident Management System and scene assessment. This is followed by the implementation phase, during which there is search and rescue, victim triage, initial stabilization and transport of the injured, and definitive management of scene hazards and victims. Finally, the recovery phase occurs at the time of scene withdrawal, with return to normal operations and postincident debriefing.

Overall Response Strategy

Disasters often overwhelm prehospital professionals and the EMS system. Prehospital professionals must recognize that the incident will probably exceed their individual capabilities and should immediately activate an appropriate response plan with a preestablished unified command and management structure. The National Incident Management System (NIMS) provides a scalable framework for this collaborated response. With the activation of an Incident Command System and an Incident Commander, a coordinated response can occur among various agencies and jurisdictions, with integration of facilities, personnel, and communication, all within a common organizational structure. This system provides structure and continuity for efficient management of the event. The goal in a disaster response is to do the most good for the most victims, and these actions allow optimal organization of the response.

Prehospital professionals must refrain from rushing into the scene and becoming victims themselves. This task is even more daunting when the victims are children and the impulse to help is powerful. *Remember that you cannot help if you become ill or injured.* Use appropriate safety gear and personal protective equipment (PPE) on every call when there is a potential that the rescuer may come in contact with contaminated patients. Chemical, biologic, and radiologic incidents require specific and specialized equipment. Therefore, before entering any scene, be sure it has been cleared by the appropriate authorities (e.g., law enforcement, fire, and HazMat). Level C respiratory protection (a facemask with a canister filtration system) may be adequate for most conventional disasters; however, higher levels of protection may be required to meet the needs of the incident.

Prehospital professionals must also exercise the highest vigilance in securing communications between victims and families. This is especially important for children during disaster triage, treatment, and transport.

Prehospital professionals must refrain from rushing into the scene and becoming victims themselves. Injured and dead rescuers are not able to save anyone.

Pediatric Response Considerations

After initial recognition and general response to a disaster, the subsequent organization consists of four specific components: (1) staging, (2) triage, (3) treatment, and (4) transport, with attention to predisaster planning as an essential component to an organized response.

Planning

Before a disaster occurs, having the appropriate resources and training to treat pediatric patients is essential. Response vehicles should have pediatric supplies, including a range of pediatric airway equipment, pediatric-sized cervical collars, intraosseous needles, smaller gauge intravenous (IV) catheters, and methods to control hypothermia. In addition, having a system in place for patient tracking and reunification is essential, given the likelihood of family separation.

Case Study 2

You are the first to arrive on the scene of a reported shooting at a local middle school. The dispatch information conveyed that at least four people had been shot, and the perpetrators had been apprehended. When you arrive on the scene, law enforcement has secured the area. Three students in the cafeteria and one adult on the second floor in the principal's office are seriously injured.

1. As you and your partner park and begin to pull your gear from the ambulance, what are your first considerations?
2. What pediatric issues are important to consider?

Staging

Staging occurs when ambulances and personnel arrive on the scene of a recognized disaster. Prehospital professionals should meet in an assigned location and await instructions from the staging officer. This ensures a quick and systematic deployment. Providers assigned to staging must remain close to their ambulances and equipment. For the incident management system to function properly, all prehospital professionals need to coordinate their efforts to ensure appropriate and timely patient care. Pediatric-equipped ambulances should be identified by the staging officer.

Triage

Triage is the process of prioritizing patients based on the severity of their injuries and available resources. The goal of triage in the disaster setting is to make a daunting task manageable. The pediatric population can be challenging, because many patients are nonverbal, frightened, and separated from family members, and they may have injuries with which rescuers are unfamiliar (e.g., crush injuries, bomb blasts, chemical or radiologic exposures). Proper triaging of pediatric patients requires standardized triage algorithms.

The Simple Triage and Rapid Treatment (START) triage system is one recognized method for triage of adult disaster patients. The START triage system categorizes patients by color and allows the prehospital professional to quickly classify each patient according to physiologic status and urgency for treatment. It is difficult to apply the START concept to young children because this system uses adult vital sign measurements and requires that victims have the ability to verbally communicate and ambulate.

The JumpSTART triage system was devised as a modification of the START triage system for use in children younger than 8 years of age or less than 100 pounds. This triage system uses important assessment characteristics of infants and children to distinguish them from older patients. JumpSTART uses breathing as the cornerstone for triage decisions (**Figure 9-1**).

As in the START triage system, there are four triage categories in the JumpSTART system, designated by colors corresponding to different levels of urgency for treatment. Decision points include: ability to walk (except infants), presence of spontaneous breathing, respirations less than 15 or greater than 45 breaths/min, palpable peripheral pulse, and appropriate response to painful stimuli on the alert-verbal-painful-unresponsive (AVPU) scale.

Patients who are able to walk should be assigned to the green category for "minor" and are not in immediate need of treatment. Those breathing spontaneously, with a peripheral pulse and an appropriate response to painful stimuli, should be assigned to the yellow category for "delayed" treatment. Children who have apnea responsive to positioning or rescue breathing, have respiratory failure, are breathing but do not have a palpable pulse, or have an inappropriate pain response should be assigned to the red category for "immediate" intervention. Children who are apneic and without a pulse, or apneic and unresponsive to rescue breathing, should be assigned to the black category and considered deceased or expectant deceased.

Another more recently developed triage system currently in use is the Sort, Assess, Lifesaving interventions,

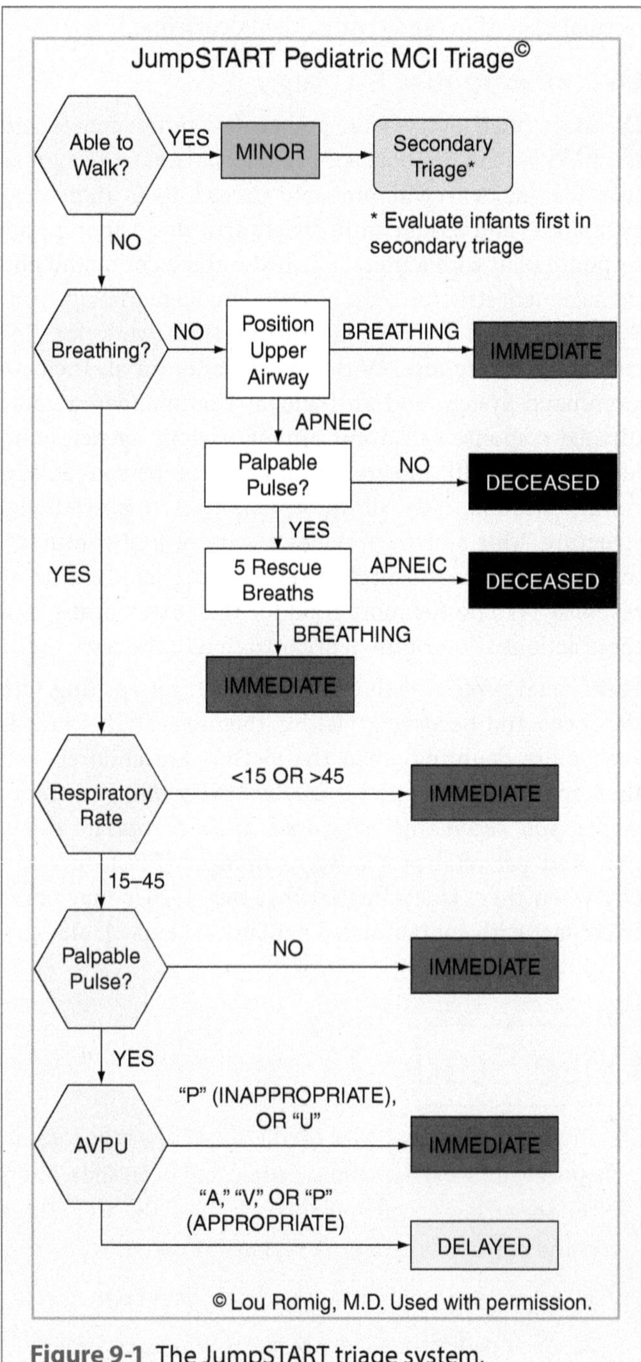

Figure 9-1 The JumpSTART triage system.

and Treatment and/or transport (SALT) triage system (**Figure 9-2**). This guideline has the advantage of being applicable in adults and children. It describes four sequential activities that take place. (1) Global sorting of patients using voice commands often works for older children who can understand and follow a command to move to another

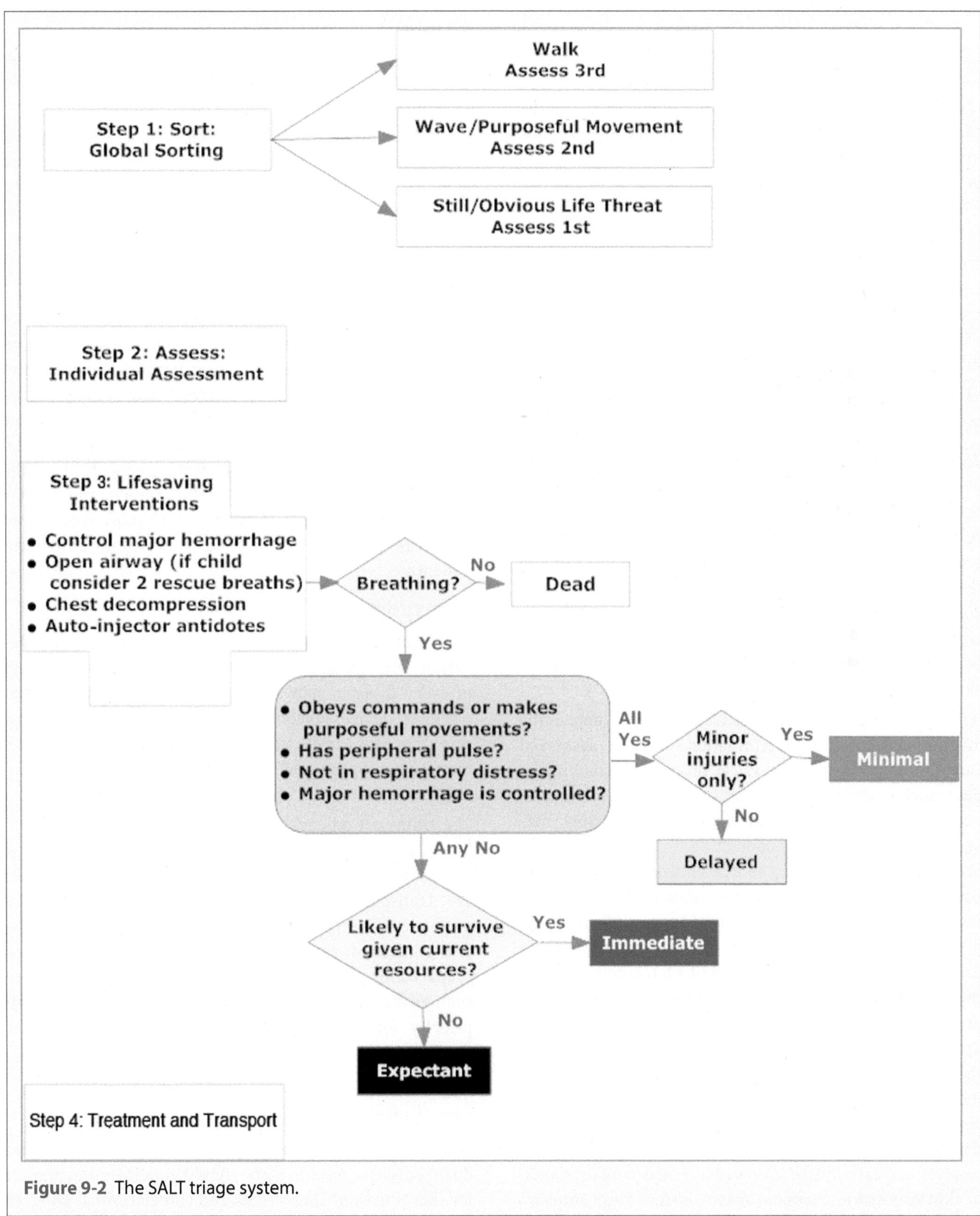

Figure 9-2 The SALT triage system.

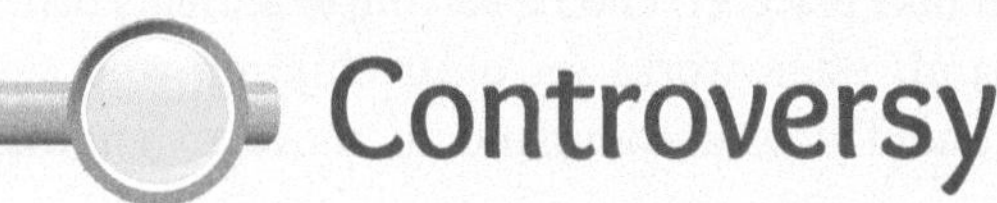

The JumpSTART system has not been clinically validated.

location, but young children may not be able to respond. (2) Individual assessment and assignment of a priority category follows, starting with the individuals who were unable to respond first. (3) Lifesaving interventions that can be quickly applied may include rescue breaths for children who do not respond to positioning of the airway. (4) Finally, provision of treatment or transport completes the process.

There are a variety of triage algorithms available, and no current recommended pediatric standard. All prehospital professionals within an EMS system should be familiar with the method used by their EMS system, and trained in its use. This system optimally should account for children in a disaster.

Treatment

Treatment of pediatric patients in disaster situations varies greatly depending on the specifics of the disaster, the exposure of the patient, and the availability of resources of the responding agencies. Treatment should always include removing the patient from the source of the threat or agent as immediately as possible, with due consideration to hot zone (contaminated area), warm zone (where full decontamination occurs), and cold zone (safe area); secondary threats; and the prehospital professional's safety.

After the patient is moved to safety, depending on the exposure, decontamination may be necessary. **Decontamination** is the physical process of removing or neutralizing potentially harmful substances from patients, personnel, equipment, and supplies. A person may become contaminated by contacting vapors, mists, solids, or liquids from a specific source or from others already contaminated. *Decontamination should be performed whenever an individual is actually or potentially contaminated with a hazardous substance.* Decontamination is designed to minimize the amount of a hazardous material that is available for absorption through a victim's skin and prevent contamination of the rescuers. Because of children's proportionally greater body surface area, and skin that is less keratinized and more permeable, they have an increased likelihood of systemic toxicity from agents that contact their skin; this underlies the importance of rapid decontamination in the pediatric population. Therefore, time is a critical consideration in effective decontamination of skin exposed to chemical agents. Even if large amounts of time have elapsed since the initial exposure, perform decontamination on the patient to eliminate any remaining agent and mitigate the risk of exposure to others.

Families are likely to be kept together during this process. However, lack of adequate protocols or preplanning may require that other adults or older children be recruited to assist in decontaminating younger children. Keeping families together reduces the risk of secondary contamination to responding health care providers and public safety personnel.

Because children lose body heat faster than adults, special care is indicated during decontamination because they are at an increased risk for hypothermia when exposed to the environment. Appropriate planning can ensure that there is warm water, warming equipment, and pediatric-sized clothing and blankets available after decontamination is complete.

When the number of patients exceeds the number of ambulances available for transport, designate and assign treatment areas and attempt to keep families together. After these patients have arrived at the treatment area, conduct a secondary triage to determine if the patient's initial triage status has changed. Essential medical equipment is vital to maintaining a functional treatment area. Each of the different triage divisions—red, yellow, green, and black—should have its own treatment area. The most experienced providers should treat the red and yellow designated patients.

Transport and Tracking

Early identification of patients by first responders in combination with patient tracking technology should be part of every disaster plan and drill. There are many patient tracking devices available. Coordination with regional resources (e.g., EMS agencies, hospitals, and emergency management personnel) is critical to ensuring compatibility and access.

The transport officer's duty is to get patients into ambulances and routed to appropriate hospitals. The transport officer must be flexible to ensure that the proper patients are transported to the proper facilities. Prehospital professionals must be cognizant of destination policies and guidelines, so that children go to the hospitals best prepared for pediatric emergencies or for specific injuries, such as trauma and burns. Do not give pediatric patients priority for transport just because they are children. Assign transport priority based on the specific patient's condition.

Family Reunification

Although child and parent separation should be minimized during disaster response, one should anticipate and prepare for this situation. The parents and caregivers that children depend on may also be injured and incapacitated. For those pediatric victims and caregivers who require transport, it is necessary to track patients to ensure reunification.

Natural Disasters

Earthquakes

North America is situated atop multiple seismically active fault lines. Faults are seams in the earth's crust along which geologic plates slide. An earthquake is a sudden, rapid shaking of the earth caused by the breaking and shifting of rock beneath the earth's surface along these fault lines. This shaking can cause buildings and bridges to collapse; disrupt gas, electric, and telephone service; and sometimes trigger landslides, avalanches, flash floods, fires, and huge destructive ocean waves (tsunamis). Ground movement during an earthquake is seldom the direct cause of death or injury. Most earthquake-related injuries result from collapsing walls, flying glass, and falling objects.

Damage from earthquakes can be extensive, and multiple types of injuries may occur. These injuries usually include blunt and multisystem trauma. *Seismic events have been known to also trigger illnesses, especially asthma.* The lack of appropriate shelter exposes children to environmental elements, such as stray animals, insects, hazardous chemicals, and exposed building materials. The additional psychologic stress caused by earthquakes may also contribute to increases in domestic violence and child abuse.

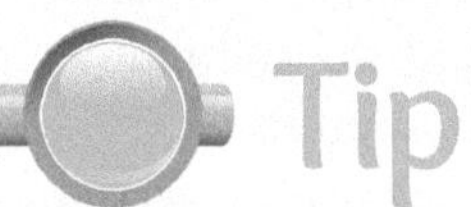

Tip

A natural disaster and environmental disturbance, such as an earthquake, often causes a major increase in pediatric respiratory ailments, especially asthma.

Floods

Several environmental events can cause flooding, including heavy rains, rapid snow melt, and coastal storm surges (**Figure 9-3**). Unlike earthquakes, flooding is usually somewhat predictable, and typically has a more gradual development. Therefore, family dislocation can be anticipated and plans can be implemented so that families are not separated unexpectedly. However, separation can occur during flash flooding. An additional public health consequence of flooding is contamination of drinking water and outbreaks of disease. Because of their small size and relatively low fluid reserve, children are at a greater risk of dehydration from vomiting and diarrhea associated with drinking contaminated water.

Hurricanes, Tornados, and Severe Storms

Severe storms differ from one geographic region to another. Coastal areas are subject to hurricanes, whereas inland regions often experience more tornado activity (**Figure 9-4**). Much of the continent is at risk from blizzards, heavy rains, and high winds, and these often wreak havoc on communities. Prehospital professionals must be aware of the potential for pediatric patients to experience cold-related emergencies during severe storms, because infants and young children have a higher body surface area-to-weight ratio and lose heat more quickly than adults when their skin is wet or cold.

Hurricanes, tornados, and severe storms can lead to structural damage, loss of power, communication outages, and isolation. Floods may result. EMS providers must coordinate efforts with other local agencies, such as search and rescue, to help the victims. These events place children and the elderly at high risk of injury from environmental conditions and structural damage. There are also the added problems of asthma exacerbations, respiratory ailments, gastroenteritis, and emotional crises over family separation.

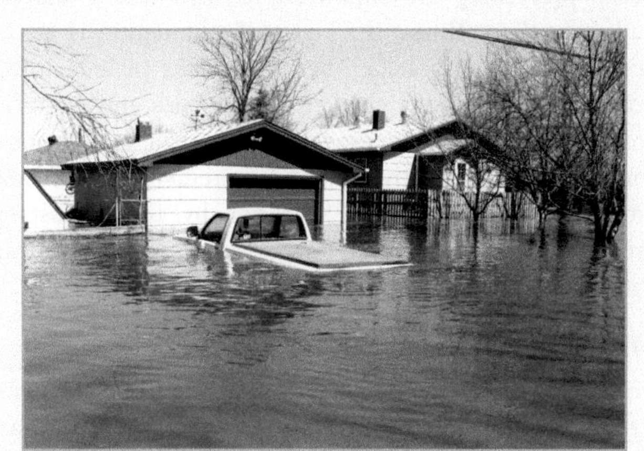

Figure 9-3 Flooding is a yearly concern in many areas of the country.

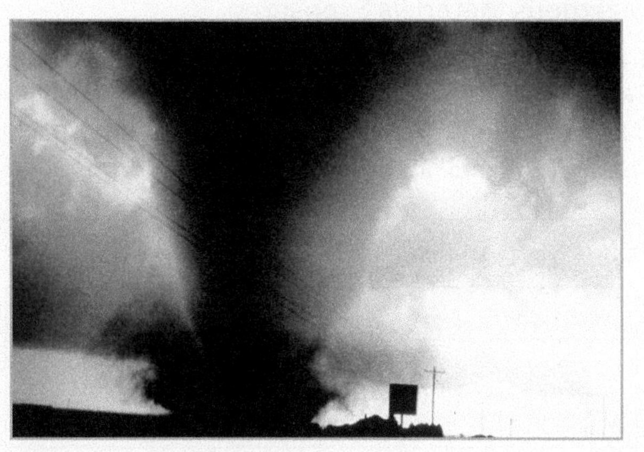

Figure 9-4 Inland regions experience tornados.

Depending on the time of day the event occurs, there may be heavy concentrations of children in schools, child care facilities, and other locations. Younger children will have little understanding of the events, and they may be primarily focused on separation from loved ones. Being separated from their caregivers, and not comprehending the current events, make the management of their emotional needs difficult. *EMS systems must anticipate these emotional crises and have a plan in place to establish communications and restore unity of families as quickly as possible.*

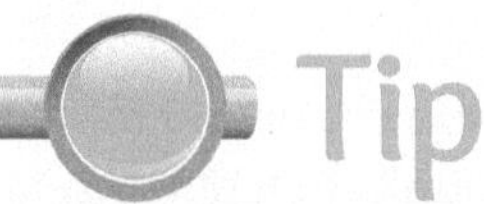

EMS systems must anticipate emotional crises in children who are separated from their families during a disaster and have a plan in place to establish communications and restore unity of families as quickly as possible.

Disease Epidemics

Every year there are significant communicable disease outbreaks. Sometimes, the pediatric population is at the heart of these outbreaks. These outbreaks include infections, such as influenza, chicken pox, measles, and hepatitis. Sometimes new viruses, especially influenza, may attack a community and greatly elevate requirements for prehospital and hospital services. Occasionally, the prehospital professional may be at risk for disease transmission from contact with an infected patient.

Man-Made Disasters

Man-made disasters include hazardous material incidents; structure failures; and criminal activities such as mass shootings or other acts of terrorism. These events can have an extensive impact on children, including those not directly involved in the disaster suffering from posttraumatic stress disorder (PTSD), separation anxiety, and agoraphobia.

Hazardous Materials Exposures

In daily life, hazardous materials are everywhere (**Table 9-2**). Examples of these hazards include chemicals used in cleaning, refrigeration, swimming pool maintenance, fuels, and agricultural products. Many of these materials are present in schools and other public facilities, and in homes. Additionally, illegal activities, such as methamphetamine laboratories, use materials that are highly explosive and toxic, which may cause burns and serious injuries to bystanders including children.

Table 9-2 Examples of Common Hazardous Materials

Diesel fuels	Insecticides
Gasoline	Fertilizers
Motor oil	Propane
Herbicides	Natural gas

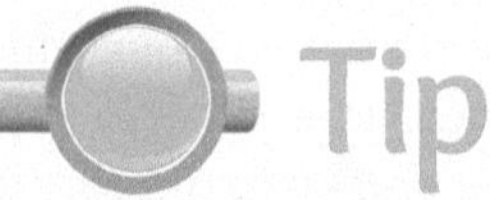

Children have a proportionally greater body surface area and thin skin, which make them more susceptible to injury from burns, chemicals, and absorbable toxins.

Structural Failures

Buildings, bridges, and platforms sometimes fail. These collapses typically cause multiple injuries. Victims may be hysterical and confused, and individuals may be buried under other victims. Children can be the primary victims, especially when structural failures involve schools or recreational facilities.

Criminal Activity and Terrorism

A troubling trend is the targeting of children by their peers for criminal acts. These disasters may generate horrific mass casualties. School shootings are the most publicized of these types of disasters. School shootings pose many unique difficulties because of safety issues for prehospital professionals, communication requirements, emotional responses of victims, providers, and the community, and gross overextension of emergency resources.

Terrorism is an emerging threat in all regions of the world. Children are frequent targets, sometimes precisely because of the psychologic impact of death and injury of vulnerable victims by the perpetrators (**Figure 9-5**).

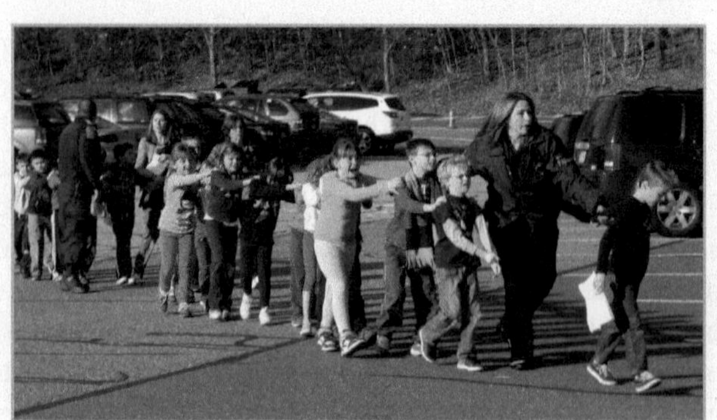

Figure 9-5 Evacuating children during a school terrorist attack.

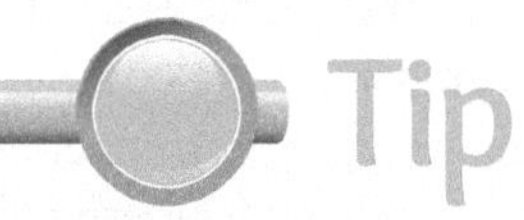

A new and troubling trend is the targeting of children, sometimes by their peers, for school shootings and terrorism.

Vulnerable Pediatric Physiologic and Psychologic Characteristics in Disasters

Because of their unique anatomy and physiology, children are especially vulnerable to the effects of disasters. In addition, their immature behavioral and psychologic characteristics place them at higher risk for immediate injury and longer-term effects. **Table 9-3** summarizes vulnerable physiologic and psychologic characteristics of children that place them at high risk during disasters.

Physiologic Considerations

Children have a higher respiratory rate compared to adults, which makes them more vulnerable to large quantities of inhaled chemical or biologic agents. Additionally, their shorter stature lowers their "breathing zone," potentially making them more susceptible to inhalation injuries from chemicals or fires where the materials are denser than air. Their increased respiratory rate also increases insensible fluid loss, further placing them at risk for dehydration. The characteristics of a pediatric patient's airway make them more susceptible to compromise. These features include a smaller-diameter airway that may easily become occluded with mucus, edema, or secretions.

Compared to adults, children have less fluid reserve and smaller circulating blood volumes, making them more prone to dehydration. Causes of dehydration include heat exposure, burns, vomiting, and diarrhea. An increased metabolism, compared to that of adults, often causes children to metabolize medications differently; this characteristic may require the prehospital professional to adjust medications and dosages when administering antidotes.

Children with special health care needs (CSHCN) include children who may have chronic physical, developmental, behavioral, or emotional conditions that require health-related services beyond those required by children generally. In a disaster, these children may be at an increased risk for suboptimal outcomes. An emergency information form (EIF), summarizing the child's critical medical information required for optimal care and support, may be available in these circumstances. See Chapter 11 for more information on CSHCN.

Emotional Responses of Children

Response to a disaster or MCI must include an assessment of the emotional state of a child and the child's caregivers. The mental health needs of children also must be recognized in the incident management system and when planning for disasters. *Appropriate mental health personnel with pediatric expertise have an important role in the aftermath of disasters, to help ensure adequate stress management and counseling services.* Reuniting children with their caregivers is key to child-family–centered care. Child and caregivers' emotional responses may range from fear and anxiety to depression, grief, and symptoms of posttraumatic stress. Children may be especially vulnerable to posttraumatic stress reactions. Pediatric aspects of shelter management need to be considered if children are separated from their caregivers. Each child will respond differently to a disaster, depending on his or her age, maturity, previous experience, and cultural background. However, children of all ages experience anxiety from disasters. Younger children may interpret the disaster as a personal danger to themselves and those about whom they care.

Table 9-3 Vulnerable Pediatric Characteristics

Pediatric Characteristic	Special Risk During Disaster
Respiratory	Higher minute volume increases risk from exposure to inhaled agents. Nuclear fallout and heavier gases settle lower to the ground and may affect children more severely.
Gastrointestinal	May be more at risk for dehydration from vomiting and diarrhea after exposure to contamination.
Skin	Proportionally greater body surface area and thinner skin make them more susceptible to injury from burns, chemicals, and absorbable toxins. Also, hypothermia is more likely.
Endocrine	Increased risk of thyroid cancer from radiation exposure.
Thermoregulation	Less able to cope with temperature problems with higher risk of hypothermia.
Developmental	Less ability to escape environmental dangers or anticipate hazards.
Psychologic	Prolonged stress from critical incidents. Susceptible to separation anxiety.

Effects of Chemical, Biologic, Radiation, Nuclear, and Explosive Disasters on Children

Chemicals

Millions of different chemicals in the world are potentially detrimental to human health (**Table 9-4**). Chemicals are transported throughout the country daily by trucks, trains, and planes with a potential for unintentional or deliberate population exposure. Additionally, chemical weapons are an important consideration for the prehospital provider, causing injury, death, and disease.

When chemical spills are identified, officials trained to work with hazardous materials (HazMat) are a key resource for identification of the toxicity, relative risk, decontamination procedures, and specific treatments required.

Assessment and Treatment of Specific Chemical Agents

Nerve Agents

Nerve agents are extremely toxic and have very rapid effects. Common agents include tabun, sarin, soman, VX, and organophosphates. The nerve agent, either as a gas, aerosol, or liquid, enters the body through inhalation or through the skin (transdermally). These two characteristics have a greater effect on children because of their faster respiratory rates and larger skin surface area-to-mass ratio. Poisoning may also occur through consumption of liquids or foods contaminated with nerve agents. All nerve agents produce toxic effects by preventing the proper operation of the chemical that acts as the body's "off switch" for glands and muscles. Without an "off switch," the glands and muscles are constantly being stimulated, causing the victim to tire and no longer be able to sustain breathing. Because of the extremely rapid onset of symptoms, it is likely that children exposed to these agents will develop symptoms before adults who are exposed to the same event.

Table 9-4 Common Chemicals Detrimental to Human Health

Alcohols, including antifreeze and windshield washer fluid	Laundry pod
Ammonia	Laundry soap
Asbestos	Pesticides
Bleach (laundry)	Rodenticides
Chlorine	Sulfuric acid
Drain and oven cleaners	Toilet bowl cleaner
Hydrocarbons, including furniture polish, gasoline, lighter fluid, and paint thinner	

The initial signs and symptoms of a nerve agent exposure include frontal headache, eye pain, miosis (pupil constriction), runny nose, anorexia (loss of appetite), nausea, excessive sweating, tightness in the chest, and heartburn. If the patient is exposed to large amounts of a nerve agent, abdominal cramps, vomiting, profuse sweating, dyspnea (shortness of breath), diarrhea, drooling and tearing, increased urinary frequency, involuntary urination or defecation, or excessive bronchial secretions with bronchospasm may occur. Children are more prone to dehydration because of gastrointestinal fluid losses, further complicating their management. Additionally, apnea, seizures, paralysis, and coma may ensue. Bradycardia is typical (although tachycardia may occur).

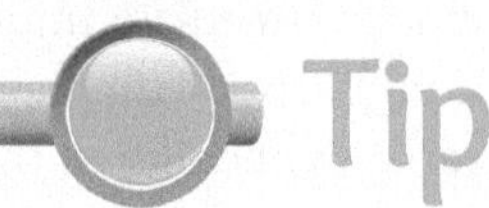

Symptoms of nerve gas exposure are often remembered as the mnemonic "DUMBELS:" diarrhea, diaphoresis, urination, miosis, bradycardia, bronchorrhea, bronchospasm, emesis, lacrimation, salivation.

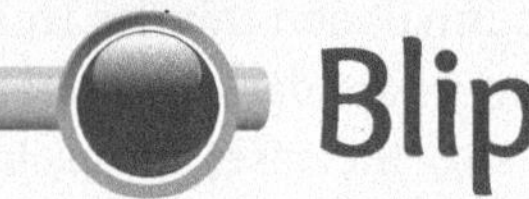

Inhalation of nerve gas may occur without the knowledge of the victim.

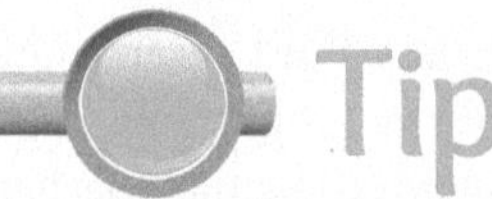

Children may be more susceptible to nerve gas because of their faster respiratory rates and larger skin surface area-to-mass ratio.

Treatment for nerve agents includes decontamination and use of atropine, pralidoxime (2-PAM), and benzodiazepines. These can all be given intramuscularly (IM) with effective absorption. Use antidotes only for severe exposures exhibiting the signs and symptoms listed previously. Treat skin contact by undressing and decontaminating the patient with copious amounts of water. Atropine dosing is 0.05–0.1 mg/kg IV or IM (with a maximum initial dose of 2 mg) repeated every 2–5 minutes as needed until there is drying of marked secretions and reversal of bronchospasm or seizures. Pralidoxime dosing is 25–50 mg/kg over 5–30 minutes, with a maximum dose of 1 g

IV, or 2 g IM, repeated as needed in 30–60 minutes for persistent weakness. Most packaging of 2-PAM is accessible to prehospital professionals in auto-injector form. To manipulate the dosing for children, discharge the auto-injector into a sterile vial and then draw up what is needed for administration. Personnel who are wearing PPE may find children challenging to care for, because it is difficult for rescuers to perform procedures while simultaneously having to battle their own environmental conditions. In addition, prehospital personnel wearing PPE may frighten children and render the assessment more complicated.

Cyanide

Cyanide is a rapidly acting, potentially deadly chemical that can exist in various forms. Cyanide can be a colorless gas or may be found in a crystallized form. Cyanide sometimes is described as having a "bitter almond" smell, but it does not always give off an odor; if it does, it has been found that not everyone can detect this odor. Cyanide is released from natural substances in some foods and in certain plants. It is in cigarette smoke and the combustion products of synthetic materials, such as plastics (e.g., in house fires). Patients may be exposed to cyanide by breathing air, drinking water, eating food, or touching soil that contains cyanide. The extent of poisoning caused by cyanide depends on the amount of cyanide a patient is exposed to, the route of exposure, and the length of time that a patient is exposed.

Breathing cyanide gas causes the most harm, but ingesting cyanide can be toxic as well. Cyanide prevents the cells of the body from using oxygen. When this happens, the cells die. Cyanide is more harmful to the heart and brain than to other organs, because the heart and brain require more oxygen compared to other areas. Children exposed to a small amount of cyanide by breathing it, absorbing it through their skin, or eating foods that contain it may have some or all of the following symptoms within minutes: tachypnea, restlessness, dizziness, weakness, headache, nausea and vomiting, and tachycardia. Exposure to a large amount of cyanide by any route may cause convulsions, hypotension, bradycardia, loss of consciousness, lung injury, and respiratory failure leading to death.

Cyanide is highly volatile, and removing the patient from the environment is often all that is needed to decontaminate them. If the child is soaked from a spill, remove the clothing and wash the child with soap and warm water. Even though cyanide inhibits cellular oxygen usage, administration of 100% oxygen is still useful and should be employed. Most cases of cyanide poisoning respond to these simple steps.

The newer cyanide antidote, hydroxocobalamin, has a lower risk of toxicity than the old three-component kit. Hydroxocobalamin works by exchanging the hydroxyl group for cyanide, creating cyanocobalamin (vitamin B_{12}, a water-soluble vitamin excreted by the kidneys). The initial dose for adults is 5 g, and the pediatric dose is 70 mg/kg, IV over 15 minutes. A second dose may be given at the same initial dosage, or half the initial dosage (depending on patient's toxicity), with the second infusion rate ranging from 15 minutes to 2 hours after the first dose. Hypertension and reddening of the skin, mucosa, and urine are side effects of this antidote.

An important distinction by the prehospital provider is determining if the exposure in question was from a nerve agent or from cyanide, given the different immediate antidotes required in each scenario. One important distinction is that patients exposed to nerve agents are more likely to have cyanosis, altered vision with miosis, copious secretions, and bronchospasm.

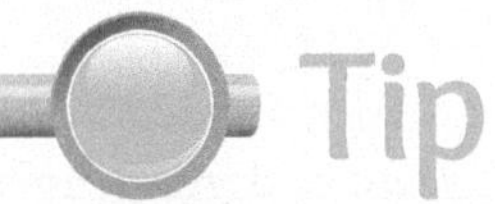

Tip

Patients exposed to a small amount of cyanide by breathing it, absorbing it through their skin, or eating foods that contain it may have symptoms within minutes.

Pulmonary Intoxicants

Pulmonary intoxicants produce pulmonary edema. The most widely known agents are phosgene and chlorine. Patients typically exhibit eye and airway irritation, dyspnea, and chest tightness. In most cases, patients have shortness of breath caused by pulmonary edema hours after the exposure. Without supportive treatment, including decontamination and advanced airway management with intubation if necessary, patients may progress to respiratory failure.

Vesicants

Vesicants are chemicals that cause blistering of the skin, irritation and inflammation of the eyes and airways, and vomiting and diarrhea. Exposure to vesicants can be through inhalation, absorption, or ingestion. The most common vesicants are sulfur mustard (mustard gas) and lewisite. Blistering usually occurs hours after contact. Mustard gas has no immediate effects, while lewisite causes immediate irritation to the eyes, skin, and upper airways. Within seconds, lewisite liquid causes pain and burning on any surface with which it comes in contact.

Treatment for these chemicals includes decontamination with large volumes of warm soapy water at low pressure, eye irrigation, airway control, and oxygen administration. Bandage wounds with dry dressings. Providers may consider administration of British anti-lewisite (BAL) as an antidote for lewisite at a dose of 3 mg/kg. However, there is little experience with this antidote when used in children.

Biologic Agents

There are many different biologic agents that can pose a threat to humans (**Table 9-5**). They can be as common as influenza or as lethal as plague. Biologic weapons used by terrorists can cause widespread disease and death. Typical agents that may be weaponized include anthrax, smallpox, botulism, and plague. Terrorists could use these agents because they are fairly easy to purchase or formulate. An added incentive is that some of the agents are extremely contagious and can be spread to a large number of people, which very often includes children in schools and child care facilities.

Assessment and Treatment of Specific Biologic Agents

Biologic Pathogens

Biologic pathogens, released intentionally, accidentally, or naturally occurring, can result in disease or death. Human exposure to these agents may occur through inhalation, cutaneous exposure, or ingestion of contaminated food or water. After exposure, physical symptoms may be delayed and are sometimes confused with naturally occurring illnesses. Biologic agents may persist in the environment and cause problems sometime after their release.

Smallpox

Because of the global eradication of smallpox, with the last endemic case in 1977, and the subsequent discontinued use of the vaccine, a large segment of the population remains unvaccinated. This population at risk includes children and young adults. Smallpox is caused by the variola virus. The incubation period is about 12 days (range, 7–17 days) after exposure. Initial symptoms include high fever, fatigue, and head and back aches. A characteristic rash, most prominent on the face, arms, and legs, follows in 2–3 days (**Figure 9-6**). The rash starts with flat red lesions that evolve at the same rate. Lesions become pus-filled and begin to crust early in the second week. Scabs develop, then separate and fall off after about 3–4 weeks. The majority of patients with smallpox recover, but death occurs in up to 30% of cases. Smallpox is spread from one person to another by infected saliva droplets; this exposure is usually through a susceptible person having face-to-face contact with the ill person. Persons with smallpox are most infectious during the first week of illness, because that is when the largest amount of virus is present in the saliva. Airborne, droplet, and contact precautions (**Table 9-6**) are essential and should be initiated immediately, wearing gowns, gloves, N-95 respirators, and eye protection. Exposed lesions should be covered with a sheet, and the patient should wear a mask. For exposed individuals, vaccination with vaccinia within 4 days from exposure may prevent development of the disease. Those who have come in contact should be observed for 17 days after the last exposure, with fever being the criterion for isolation in a negative-pressure room.

Table 9-5 Biologic Agents That Pose a Threat to Humans

Anthrax	Plague
Botulism	Ricin
Cholera	Smallpox
Influenza	Tularemia

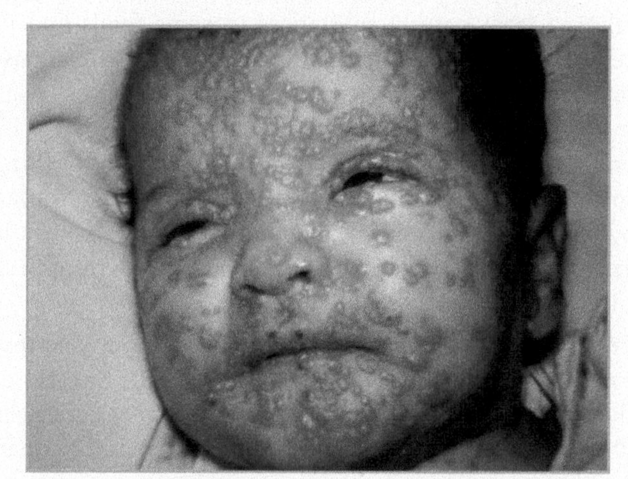

Figure 9-6 Smallpox.

Anthrax

Anthrax is an acute infectious disease caused by the spore-forming bacterium *Bacillus anthracis*. Anthrax most commonly occurs in hoofed mammals but can also infect humans. Symptoms of disease vary depending on how the disease was contracted, but usually occur within 7 days after exposure. The serious forms of human anthrax are inhalation anthrax, cutaneous anthrax, and intestinal anthrax. Initial symptoms of inhalation anthrax infection may resemble a common cold. After several days, the symptoms may progress to severe breathing problems and shock. Inhalation anthrax is often fatal. The intestinal disease form of anthrax may follow the consumption of contaminated food and is characterized by an acute inflammation of the intestinal tract. Initial signs of nausea, loss of appetite, vomiting, and fever are usually followed by abdominal pain,

Table 9-6 Recommendations for Transmission-Based Precautions for Hospitalized Patients

Category of Precautions	Hand Washing for Patient Contact	Single Room	Masks	Gowns	Gloves
Airborne	Yes	Yes, with negative-pressure ventilation	Yes	No	No
Droplet	Yes	Yes*	Yes, for those close to patient	No	No
Contact	Yes	Yes*	No	Yes	Yes

*Preferred but not required for crib-confined patients. Cohorting of children infected with the same pathogen is acceptable.

Source: American Academy of Pediatrics. The revised CDC guidelines for isolation precautions in hospitals: implications for pediatrics. http://pediatrics.aappublications.org/content/101/3/e13/T3.expansion.html. Accessed August 8, 2012.

vomiting of blood, and severe diarrhea. For inhalational and gastrointestinal anthrax, direct person-to-person spread of anthrax is extremely unlikely; however, with cutaneous anthrax, contact precautions should be employed. The use of gloves when in contact with skin lesions, hand washing, and cleaning and sterilizing equipment is required. In situations where risk of exposure to spores exists, decontamination of patients is recommended with providers wearing gloves, gown, and mask when handling contaminated clothing or other fomites.

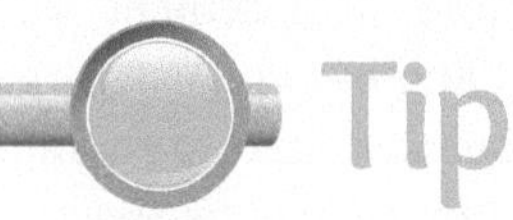

The serious forms of human anthrax are inhalation anthrax, cutaneous anthrax, and intestinal anthrax.

Plague

Plague is an infectious disease of animals and humans caused by the bacterium *Yersinia pestis*. *Y. pestis* is found in rodents and the fleas that feed on them in many areas around the world. Pneumonic plague occurs when *Y. pestis* infects the lungs. The first signs of illness in pneumonic plague are fever, headache, weakness, and a cough productive of bloody or watery sputum. The pneumonia progresses over 2–4 days and may cause septic shock and, without early treatment, death. Person-to-person transmission of pneumonic plague occurs through respiratory droplets, which can infect those who have face-to-face contact with the ill patient; therefore, droplet precautions must be used.

Ricin

Ricin is a potent protein synthesis inhibitor derived from the beans of the castor plant (*Ricinus communis*). The beans are

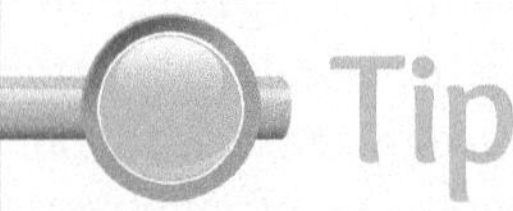

Plague is an infectious disease carried by rodents and their fleas in many areas around the world.

available worldwide, and the toxin is fairly easily produced. When inhaled as a small particle aerosol, this toxin may produce pathologic changes within 8 hours and have severe respiratory symptoms (chest tightness, shortness of breath, cough), fever, and myalgias. Within 36–72 hours, cyanosis with pulmonary edema and respiratory failure occurs. When ingested, ricin causes severe gastrointestinal symptoms with vomiting and bloody diarrhea. Ingested ricin exposure may eventually lead to hallucinations, seizures, and low blood pressure, followed by vascular collapse and death. Treatment is supportive depending on the symptoms, and early diagnosis may be difficult. Decontamination should occur at the site of release before transport in the warm zone with a full chemical-resistant suit, gloves, surgical mask, and eye and face protection, such as a face shield and goggles. Clothing that has to be pulled over the head should be cut and double-bagged, and there should be soap and water decontamination of the skin, and irrigation to the eyes for 10–15 minutes with disposal of contact lenses. Once decontaminated, ricin cannot be transmitted from person to person; therefore, standard precautions should be used.

Botulism

Botulinum toxins are created by *Clostridium botulinum*, an anaerobic bacterium found commonly in soil. Botulism is the result of exposure to these toxins and can occur naturally through the ingestion of contaminated food or through bioterrorism exposure. The toxins act primarily at the neuromuscular junction, preventing the release of acetylcholine and ultimately leading to flaccid paralysis. The toxin effects can take from 24 hours to several days to manifest, and patients exhibit eyelid droop, dilated pupils, blurry vision, slurred speech, difficulty swallowing, dry oral mucosa, flaccid paralysis, and respiratory failure. The distinguishing factors from nerve agent exposure are the lack of initial muscle fasciculations, the dilation of the pupils, dry mucus membranes, and the period from exposure to onset of symptoms.

Infants are particularly susceptible to botulism because of the potential for colonization of their gastrointestinal tract with the bacteria. This spore-forming bacterium can be introduced through environmental dust or by honey products. Therefore, it is recommended to avoid giving honey to children under 1 year of age. Treatment for this exposure is primarily supportive care with ventilator support. However, there may be benefit in using botulinum antitoxin, which is best given during the latent period after exposure. After the symptoms are recognized, this therapy may only reduce the further progression of symptoms. Botulism is not contagious, and standard precautions should be used for patient care.

Specific Treatment of Biologic Disease

Radiation

Radiation disasters, although rare, can occur wherever radioactive materials are used, stored, or transported. Nuclear power plants, hospitals, universities, research laboratories, industries, major highways, railroads, and shipping yards are all possible sites. Radioactive materials are dangerous because of the harmful effect certain types of radiation have on the cells of the body. The longer a person is exposed to radiation, the greater the risk. Children are more susceptible to radiation injury because of their rapidly reproducing cells. Radiation weapons include nuclear and "dirty" bombs. Radiation cannot be detected by sight, smell, or any other sense.

Nuclear

A **dirty bomb**, also known as a radiologic dispersal device (RDD), consists of a conventional explosive, such as dynamite packaged with radioactive material that is meant to scatter when the bomb explodes. A dirty bomb can kill or injure by means of the initial blast of the conventional explosive or by airborne radiation and contamination (hence the term "dirty").

A **nuclear bomb** uses the power of nuclear fission or fusion to produce an intense pulse or wave of heat, light, air pressure, and radiation. In a nuclear blast, injury or death may occur as a result of the blast itself or as a result of debris thrown from the blast. Victims may experience moderate to severe skin burns, depending on their distance from the blast site. Those who look directly at the blast may experience eye damage, ranging from temporary blindness to severe burns on the retina. Individuals near the blast site may be exposed to high levels of radiation and develop symptoms of radiation sickness.

There are two types of exposure from radioactive materials from a nuclear blast: external exposure and internal exposure. External exposure occurs when patients are exposed to radiation outside of their body from the blast or its fallout. Internal exposure occurs when patients eat food or breathe air that is contaminated with radioactive fallout. Both internal and external exposure from fallout can occur miles away from the blast site.

Protection from radiation exposure can be attained by using a shield, minimizing exposure time, and maximizing the distance from the source. Depending on the type of radiation emitted, different shielding may be required, with alpha particles being stopped by a sheet of paper, beta particles by a layer of clothing or less than an inch of substance, and gamma rays by less than an inch of lead. Because PPE cannot protect against high energy, highly penetrating forms of radiation associated with most radiation emergencies, first responders should wear direct-reading personal radiation dosimeters to monitor radiation doses and stay within recommended dose limits for radiation workers. External decontamination of radioactive particulate can be accomplished by removal of all clothing, warm soap water irrigation, wound debridement with foreign body removal, oral rinsing, and eye and ear irrigation. A radiation survey meter should be used to monitor the decontamination progress, and there may be the need to clip hair if washing was insufficient to remove the radioactive particulates. The goal is to reduce radiation level to no more than two times background radiation level.

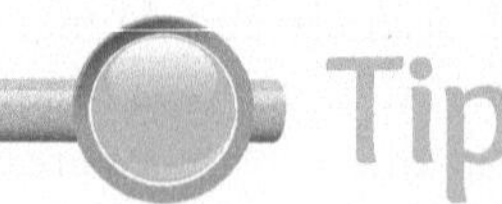

Perform decontamination whenever an individual is possibly contaminated with a hazardous substance.

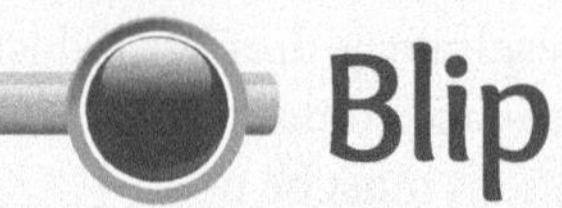

Be sure children do not get hypothermic after decontamination. Immediately dry them and give them warm clothes.

Care should be made to avoid the contamination of vehicles and equipment through onsite decontamination, and hospitals should not be used as decontamination centers. The management of internal radiation exposure varies by the radioactive element involved. Because radioactive fallout does enter the ecosystem and the foods that are consumed, radioactive iodine is a concern. In these cases, prophylactic treatment with potassium iodide prevents the radioactive form of the element from being absorbed into the thyroid gland, because children are vulnerable to late carcinogenic effects, especially of the thyroid.

Explosives

Explosive devices are frequently used for terrorism. Children are at risk for blast injury because of their size and susceptibility to head and abdominal injuries. The blast wave, flying debris, and injuries from being thrown may have deadly results.

Critical Incident Stress Management

A critical incident stress management (CISM) team can provide support and counseling for prehospital professionals who have been exposed to stressful incidents in the course of providing EMS. The need for this may be especially acute after dealing with pediatric patients in disasters. A mental health professional is often part of the CISM team. The debriefing process is intended to be educational; CISM is not psychotherapy. The effectiveness of CISM after disasters for prehospital professionals and for children is not known.

Summary

Disasters are fortunately a rare occurrence, but when they happen they will likely involve children, either directly or indirectly. Preparation is the key to providing the best care possible. Using the National Incident Management System (NIMS) framework and the Incident Command System (ICS) will enable the responding team to acquire appropriate resources, personnel, and communication, and to organize assistance from additional responding agencies. When children are triaged in a disaster scenario, there are several different triage methods used, which vary regionally. The JumpSTART triage system is one standardized method that takes into consideration the distinctive features of young children. Another recognized triage approach is the SALT triage system. However, these systems have not been validated; therefore, there is no nationally recognized recommendation.

Because of their physiologic, anatomic, and psychologic differences, children present a unique challenge to the prehospital professional. Natural and man-made disasters necessitate that EMS preplan their response and rehearse their roles in an ever-changing world.

Case Study 3

You are dispatched to a large downtown hotel at 7:00 AM. On arrival, you find two adult and three pediatric patients, all tourists from a neighboring state. They all have some level of respiratory distress, chest tightness, and coughing. The adults complain of weakness and joint pain; two of the children and one adult are cyanotic, especially around their lips. They state the only thing they can relate this to is being sprayed with an aerosol can in the subway at 10:00 PM last night by a group of protesters. The patients state they thought it was just air in the aerosol can. There was no odor or color. They also state that there are 36 of them traveling together, but the others have not shown up for breakfast as planned.

1. Would you suspect a biologic or chemical agent in this case?
2. How would you treat and transport these patients?

CASE STUDY ANSWERS

Case Study 1 — page 178

Your first action should be to confirm your position is safe and to identify all other potential initial responders. Ask for an official determination about whether the school is in a flood zone, and consider the necessity of an evacuation order. Initiate the Incident Management System and identify a casualty collection point at the nearest safe location. Begin rescue and evacuation operations. Implement your disaster operations plan and activate your mutual aid agreements as necessary. Have dispatch notify local medical facilities of the MCI/disaster, and ensure the necessary notifications are made to emergency relief agencies.

During your assessment of the children, determine the severity of injuries and triage them using an appropriate standardized technique, such as the JumpSTART triage system. Provide psychologic support to the children by remaining calm, and attempt to reunite families when possible. Pediatric patients require additional care to maintain thermal balance during a weather-related emergency. Providing blankets and protection from the wind and rain is an important aspect of caring for these patients.

Case Study 2 — page 179

Scene safety must be your primary consideration. Law enforcement should provide verification of a safe scene and provide clear access to the patients. Establish Incident Command if it has not already been established by the initial officers on scene, and determine staging and triage areas. Request appropriate response of other providers (ALS/BLS), and ensure transportation or additional resources, such as an aeromedical team.

Determine the amount of pediatric equipment that is available and the level of care that may be needed; then request any additional resources you may need. Decide which hospitals in your area have pediatric trauma capability and how you will transport the patients. Don't forget to consider how best to plan for family reunification.

Case Study 3 — page 192

These patients may have been exposed to a toxic agent, dispersed in the aerosol spray. Most likely it is a toxin (e.g., ricin), because many chemical agents work within minutes of contact, and biologic agents require time to incubate. Ricin is a midspectrum toxic agent derived from a biologic organism, which causes a chemical poisoning.

Begin by donning PPE including gowns, gloves, and masks. Treatment should commence by first securing the scene to contain the spread of the potential disease. Have someone trustworthy attempt to make contact with the other guests from the group and determine if additional concerns exist. Contact medical control to determine the best location for transport of the patients. Make sure to notify law enforcement authorities, because events of terrorism are first and foremost a crime scene. Determine if additional notifications must be made to the health department or other governmental agency.

SUGGESTED READINGS

Textbooks

Bledsoe B, Porter R, Cherry R. *Essentials of Paramedic Care.* Upper Saddle River, NJ: Prentice Hall; 2003.

Fleisher GR, Ludwig S. *Textbook of Pediatric Emergency Medicine.* 6th ed. Philadelphia, PA: Wolters Kluwer Lippincott Williams & Wilkins; 2010.

Hogan D, Burstein J. *Disaster Medicine.* Philadelphia, PA: Lippincott Williams & Wilkins; 2002.

Articles

American Academy of Pediatrics, Committee on Environmental Health and Committee on Infectious Diseases. Policy statement. Chemical-biological terrorism and its impact on children. *Pediatrics.* 2006;118(3):1267–1278.

American Academy of Pediatrics, Committee on Pediatric Emergency Medicine and Council on Clinical Information Technology, American College of Emergency Physicians, Pediatric Emergency Medicine Committee. Policy statement. Emergency information forms and emergency preparedness for children with special health care needs. *Pediatrics.* 2010;125(4):829–837.

Ball J, Allen K. Consensus recommendations for responding to children's emergencies in disasters. *Natl Acad Pract Forum.* 2000;2:253–257.

Ginter PM, Wingate MS, Rucks AC, et al. Creating a regional pediatric medical disaster preparedness network: imperative and issues. *Maternal Child Health J.* 2006;10(4):391–396.

Holbrook PR. Pediatric disaster medicine. *Crit Care Clin.* 1991;7:463–470.

Lerner EB, Cone DC, Weinstein ES, et al. Mass casualty triage: an evaluation of the science and refinement of a national guideline. *Disaster Med Public Health Prep.* 2011;5(2):129–137.

Lerner EB, Schwartz RB, Coule PL, et al. Use of SALT triage in a simulated mass-casualty incident. *Prehosp Emerg Care.* 2010;14(1):21–25.

Lerner EB, Schwartz RB, Coule PL, et al. Mass casualty triage: an evaluation of the data and development of a proposed national guideline. *Disaster Med Public Health Prep.* 2008; 2(Suppl 1):S25–S34.

Lovejoy J. Disaster medicine: initial approach to patient management after large-scale disasters. *Clin Ped Emerg Med.* 2002;3(4):217–223.

Markenson D, Redlener I. Executive summary. *Pediatric Preparedness for Disasters and Terrorism: National Consensus Conference.* 2006; 12.

Waeckerle JF, Seamans S, Whiteside M, et al. Executive summary. Developing objectives, content, and competencies for the training of emergency medical technicians, emergency physicians, and emergency nurses to care for casualties resulting from nuclear, biological, or chemical (NBC) incidents. *Ann Emerg Med.* 2001;37:587–601.

Wallis LA, Carley S. Comparison of paediatric major incident primary triage tools. *Emerg Med J.* 2006;23(6):475–478.

Other Resources

American Academy of Pediatrics. Pediatric disaster preparedness & emergency medical services for children. http://www2.aap.org/disasters/pdf/Children-and-Disasters-One-Pager.pdf. Accessed August 7, 2012.

American Academy of Pediatrics. The revised CDC guidelines for isolation precautions in hospitals: implications for pediatrics. http://pediatrics.aappublications.org/content/101/3/e13/T3.expansion.html. Accessed August 8, 2012.

Centers for Disease Control and Prevention. Emergency preparedness and response. http://www.bt.cdc.gov/agent/ricin/clinicians/control.asp. Accessed August 8, 2012.

Centers for Disease Control and Prevention. Emergency preparedness and response: bioterrorism. http://www.bt.cdc.gov/bioterrorism. Accessed December 10, 2012.

Centers for Disease Control and Prevention. Healthcare-associated infections (HAI). http://www.cdc.gov/ncidod/dhqp/pdf/bt/13apr99APIC-CDCBioterrorism.pdf. Accessed August 8, 2012.

Curtis T, Miller BC, Berry EH. Changes in reports and incidence of child abuse following natural disasters. *Child Abuse Negl.* 2000;24(9):1151–1162.

Food and Drug Administration. Emergency preparedness, bioterrorism and drug preparedness. http://www.fda.gov/Drugs/EmergencyPreparedness/BioterrorismandDrugPreparedness/defult.htm. Accessed December 10, 2012.

Freyberg C, Arquilla B, Fertel B, et al. Disaster preparedness: hospital decontamination and the pediatric patient: guidelines for hospitals and emergency planners. *Prehosp and Disaster Med.* 2008;23(2):166–173.

Gausche-Hill M. Pediatric disaster preparedness: are we really prepared? *J Trauma.* 2009;67(suppl 2):S73–S76.

Hoven CW, Duarte CS, Lucas CP, et al. Psychopathology among New York City public school children 6 months after September 11. *Arch Gen Psychiatry.* 2005;62(5):545–552.

Lindell M, Prater C, Perry R. Fundamentals of emergency management. 2006. http://training.fema.gov/EMIWeb/edu/fem.asp. Accessed April 14, 2011.

Newport Beach Fire Department. Simple triage and rapid transport. http://www.start-triage.com. Accessed December 10, 2012.

Romig L. *JumpSTART Pediatric MCI Triage Tools.* Team Life Support. 2011. http://www.jumpstarttriage.com. Accessed December 10, 2012.

U.S. Department of Health and Human Services. Decontamination procedures. http://www.remm.nlm.gov/ext_contamination.htm. Accessed August 8, 2012.

U.S. Department of Health and Human Services. Emergency medical services and pediatric transport. http://archive.ahrq.gov/prep/nccdreport/nccdrpt4.htm. Accessed August 7, 2012.

U.S. Department of Health and Human Services. Emergency worker exposure guidelines in the early phase. http://www.remm.nlm.gov/pag.htm. Accessed August 8, 2012.

U.S. Department of Health and Human Services. Personal protective equipment (PPE) in a radiation emergency. http://www.remm.nlm.gov/radiation_ppe.htm. Accessed August 8, 2012.

U.S. Department of Health and Human Services. Types of ionizing radiation and shielding required. http://www.remm.nlm.gov/ionizingrads.htm. Accessed August 8, 2012.

World Health Organization. *Psychosocial Consequences of Disasters—Prevention and Management.* Geneva: WHO, Division of Mental Health; 2002.

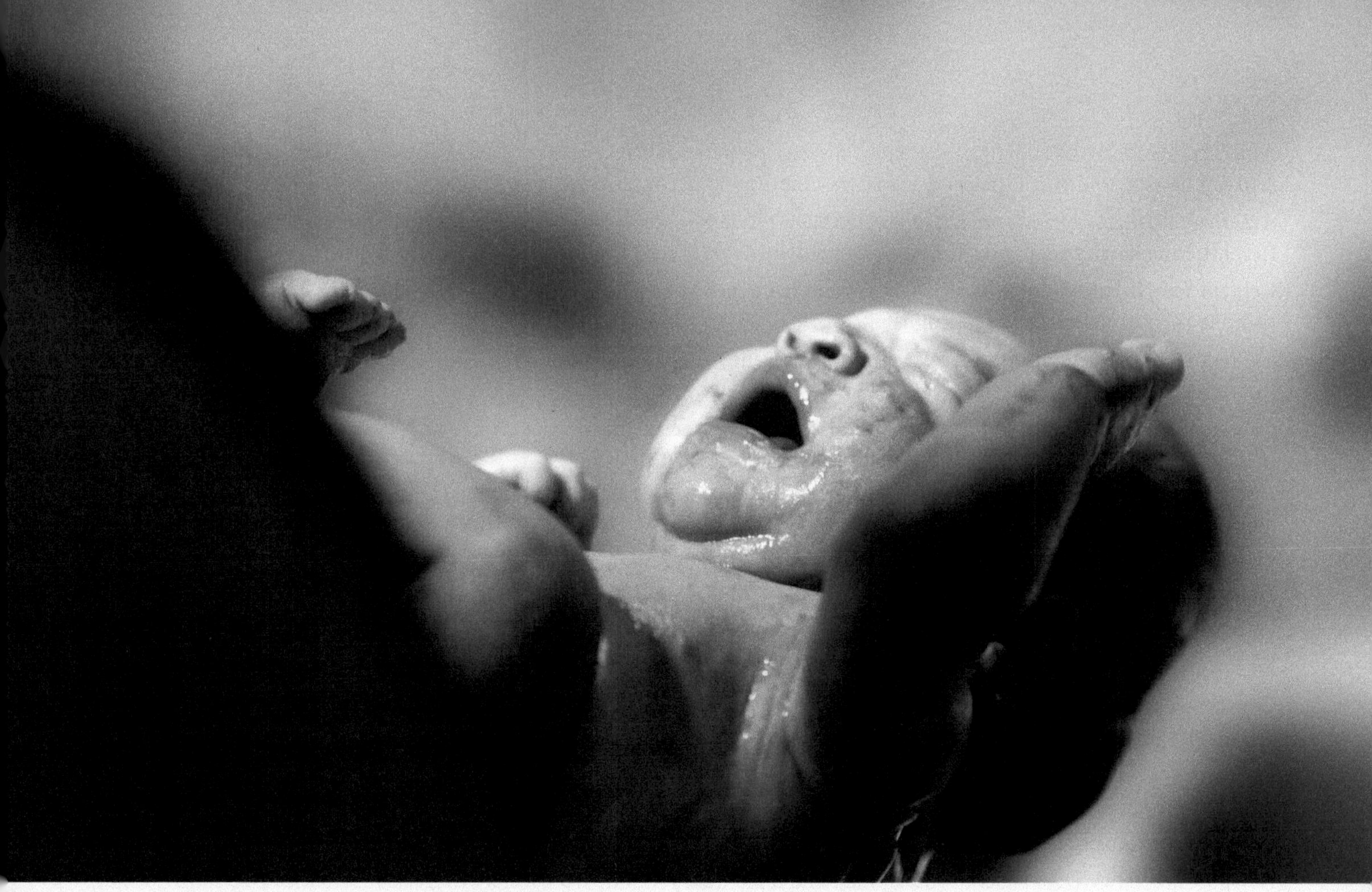

Learning Objectives

1. Describe the components of the patient history and physical exam that would identify pregnant patients at risk for emergent delivery of a newborn outside of a hospital setting.
2. List potential maternal, fetal, and newborn risk factors that may adversely affect the health of the mother or child during or immediately after delivery.
3. Compare and contrast when it is appropriate to initiate transport of a pregnant patient to a hospital for delivery of a newborn versus when it is appropriate to prepare for imminent delivery of a newborn in the prehospital setting.
4. Describe how to prepare for a delivery, perform a delivery, and provide postdelivery care to the mother and newborn.
5. Recognize the conditions and identify the correct interventions when complications jeopardize the health of the mother or newborn child during childbirth.
6. Explain the indications and technique for assisting ventilations in a newborn infant.
7. Identify situations in which a newborn infant might require vascular access for drug and fluid administration.

Emergency Delivery and Newborn Stabilization

Chapter 10

Introduction

Emergency medical services (EMS) providers may be called to assess a patient in labor or assist with childbirth in the prehospital setting. In early American history, childbirth occurred in the home, often without the presence of trained medical personnel. Gradually, it has evolved into a highly specialized area of medicine, using technology and hospitalization for care of the mother and delivery of the child. Despite the overwhelming trend toward childbirth in a health care setting, a significant number of parents choose to deliver a child at home. Almost 1% of childbirths occur each year outside the hospital setting.

Less than two-thirds of home births involve a certified nurse midwife or lay midwife. For these patients, EMS providers may become the only trained option when complications develop for the mother or newborn child. EMS personnel may encounter pregnant patients, with active labor, in a vast array of clinical settings or locations. EMS may be called to assist with transport of childbirth when labor or pregnancy are unrecognized or concealed, when a transportation misadventure prevents a patient in labor from reaching a hospital in time, when unexpected complications develop during a planned out-of-hospital delivery, or when labor or precipitous delivery occurs in another prehospital setting.

Obstetric Delivery in the Prehospital Setting

EMS Capabilities, Scope of Practice, and Legal Pitfalls

Delivery of an infant is not a common procedure in the out-of-hospital setting, so the level of anxiety for both the laboring patient and the prehospital professional is often high. Most newborns require only minimal assistance to make the transition to life outside the uterus. EMS providers should remain aware that although most obstetric deliveries require minimal resuscitative efforts, complications during delivery have the potential to cause devastating, lifelong neurologic impairment or even death for the child. Limited training, equipment, scope of practice, and experience may prevent EMS providers from recognizing serious complications of pregnancy or delivery until it is too late to prevent injury to the mother or child. Although uncomplicated childbirth is arguably a basic life support (BLS) level skill, many neonatal or maternal complications outlined in this chapter require advanced life support (ALS) interventions. The highest level of prehospital care available should be requested when prehospital childbirth is imminent.

Case Study 1

EMS is requested to respond to a local residence for a 22-year-old patient reported to be in labor. The patient reports that this is her second pregnancy and she has been having contractions for 4 hours, which are now becoming more frequent and intense. She states she was in labor for 5 hours with her first child, and she thinks it is almost time. She also states that her "bag of water has ruptured." The patient tells you that she has taken time to clean up after her water broke, but now thinks it may be too late.

1. What questions will help you decide whether to transport immediately or perform a delivery at the scene?
2. What physical findings would tell you to prepare to deliver on scene?

Ethical Considerations and EMS Professionalism

The goal of every obstetric delivery is a healthy mother and child. Not every childbirth performed by EMS providers produces a viable, healthy newborn. For example, extreme fetal prematurity is a situation where full resuscitative efforts may not be appropriate. EMS providers periodically encounter these situations without the benefit of prior diagnosis and often without the opportunity to discuss resuscitation decisions with the child's parents in a controlled environment. When faced with this situation, EMS providers should contact medical control and delicately balance ethical responsibilities to the patient with the professional requirement to adhere to EMS laws and regulations pertaining to initiation and termination of resuscitation.

Complications During Pregnancy

A wide variety of conditions can adversely impact the health of the mother and fetus during pregnancy. These conditions have the potential to create complications for the mother or newborn during or after delivery. EMS providers should consider these conditions when weighing the risks and benefits of performing a delivery in the prehospital setting versus initiating prompt transport to a health care facility for delivery. Many complications, such as breech presentations or placenta previa, simply cannot be managed in the prehospital setting. When known complications exist that are definitely beyond the ability of EMS personnel, it is often better to begin transportation immediately.

Preterm Labor

Preterm labor refers to labor beginning before the 37th week of gestation. Technologic advances allow newborns as young as 22–24 weeks to survive, although often with severe, lifelong complications. Between 24 and 37 weeks, each additional week of gestation reduces the impact or severity of complications on a newborn. EMS providers may encounter patients in labor with a gestational age less than 22–23 weeks; in many instances, the infant will not survive an out-of-hospital delivery. Older preterm infants require immediate assistance from health care providers who specialize in newborn resuscitation. Treatment of a patient in preterm labor is largely supportive until definitive care can be reached. If an infant is delivered before 37 weeks, EMS providers should expect a vast array of complications roughly proportional to the degree of prematurity.

Postterm Pregnancy

The normal gestational period lasts from 37 to 42 weeks. As a fetus remains in the uterus past 42 weeks, the uterus and placenta are unable to support the physiologic and environmental needs of the growing fetus. Meconium may be released into the amniotic fluid. EMS providers should provide supportive care to the mother and expect a difficult labor and delivery, and a newborn with potential complications.

Multiple Gestations

Most multifetal (more than one fetus) pregnancies are diagnosed during prenatal care. Every maternal assessment should include questions about the possibility of multiple gestations, especially if delivery is believed to be imminent. EMS providers should consider every multifetal pregnancy a high-risk pregnancy. Breech presentation, umbilical cord prolapse, premature labor, and a variety of other maternal and fetal conditions are more common when more than one fetus is present.

Placenta Previa

During gestation, the placenta may become implanted either partially or completely over the cervical os (opening) at the base of the uterus. This is placenta previa (**Figure 10-1**).

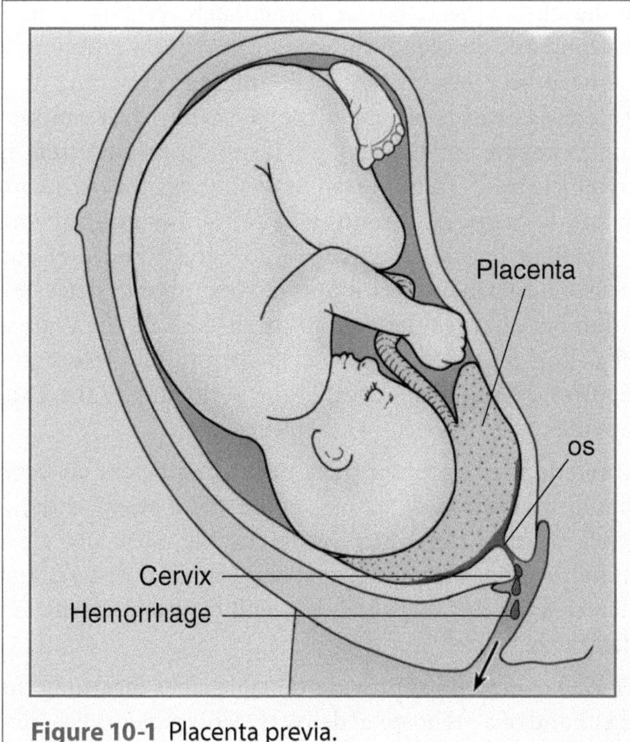

Figure 10-1 Placenta previa.

If placental rupture occurs, either from cervical dilation or mechanical perforation, bleeding can be massive and is usually painless. Patients with a placenta over or close to the cervical os (opening) require a cesarean section for delivery. Profound hemorrhage can be fatal for mother and fetus. These patients cannot safely have childbirth by EMS in the field. Prompt transport of patients in labor should begin immediately.

Known Breech Presentation

During childbirth, the fetus is designed to move headfirst, facing posterior as it passes through the cervix, into the vaginal canal. Some presentations require minimal manipulation as the fetus is delivered. Other presentations, such as a transverse breech, require a cesarean section or extensive manipulation by a trained physician to allow a vaginal delivery. Breech deliveries occur more frequently during preterm labor, multiple gestations, and when fetal abnormalities are present. EMS providers should begin transport immediately when a breech delivery is known or suspected.

Triage of a Patient in Labor

EMS providers must be capable of deciding whether a patient can safely be transported to a hospital for childbirth or when it is more prudent to prepare for an imminent delivery outside the hospital. The goal of every EMS response should be to transport the patient in labor to a hospital before childbirth occurs. Physicians and nurses experienced in labor and delivery have the training, diagnostic equipment, and procedural skills necessary to intervene in many situations that cannot be adequately managed in the prehospital setting. In instances when labor has progressed or delivery is imminent, EMS providers may be forced to assist with childbirth outside the hospital. Transport time, type of health care facilities available, EMS capabilities, anticipated complications, and ultimately the patient presentation guide the decision regarding whether to transport or assist with childbirth on scene.

Maternal History

EMS providers should obtain a brief, focused patient history when assessing a patient suspected to be in labor. Many factors help determine whether delivery is likely or if complications should be expected. Ultimately, the answer to three questions helps determine whether EMS should anticipate a prehospital delivery (**Table 10-1**):

1. How many times has the patient given birth? Typically, the time in active labor is longer for first-time mothers (primiparas) than for women who have had prior deliveries (multiparas). If this is not a first-time delivery, ask the woman the length of her previous labors. A history of short labor with prior pregnancies may repeat itself. Unless there is a long period between pregnancies, expect each successive labor to be shorter than the previous.
2. Does the patient feel the need to push? Most pregnant patients experience this sensation as delivery becomes imminent, usually within 30 minutes, often sooner. Patients with the urge to push require immediate inspection of the perineum and preparation for delivery of the newborn.
3. Do anatomic conditions allow for a successful prehospital delivery? Such conditions as placenta previa or transverse breech presentation cannot be safely delivered in the prehospital setting. Transportation should begin immediately.

Table 10-1 Determining if Delivery Is Imminent

Questions
Is this your first delivery?
If you have delivered before, how long was the labor?
Do you feel the "urge to push"?
Physical Findings
Is the child's head crowning?
Is the head or scalp visible at the perineum during contractions?

As time permits, prehospital providers should inquire about maternal medical history (including medications and allergies), whether abnormalities were identified during prenatal care, previous complications during delivery, and gestational age of the fetus. The gestational age or the due date may be calculated from the last menstrual period or the expected date of conception. Other factors, such as rupture of membranes, the possibility of multiple gestation, and prior newborn anomalies, should also be included when obtaining a patient history. History may be obtained while simultaneously performing a physical examination or preparing the ambulance and equipment for delivery.

Maternal Physical Assessment

Every patient encountered by EMS requires a primary assessment to identify any immediate threats to life. This assessment includes airway patency, the quality of respirations and perfusion, and an assessment of level of consciousness. In many instances, immediate threats to life can be excluded if a patient is awake, speaking appropriately in full sentences, while demonstrating good skin color and strong pulses. Any deviation from these findings suggests a potential threat to life and must be further evaluated before proceeding to a more focused assessment related to the pregnancy.

The prehospital provider needs to perform a brief physical assessment of the perineum if an imminent delivery is suspected. Look for crowning—the visible appearance of the fetal head at the vaginal introitus (**Figure 10-2**). Crowning is a sign that delivery is near.

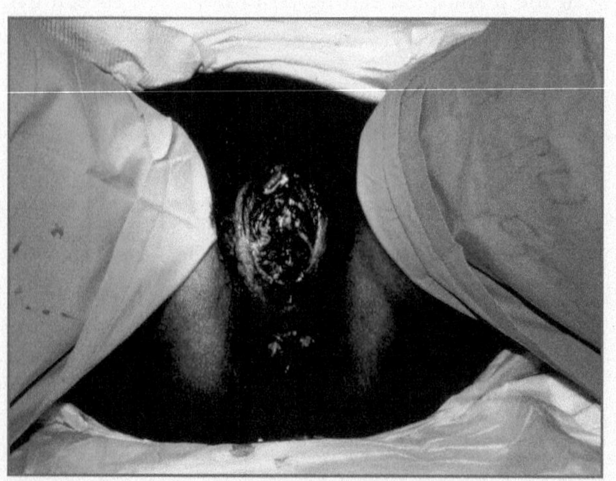

Figure 10-2 Use the presence or absence of crowning to help decide whether to transport or prepare for delivery.

If the child's head is not immediately visible, inspect the mother's perineum during a contraction and note if the head becomes visible. If the infant is crowning or if the baby's head is visible at the perineum with contractions, prepare for delivery unless the transport time is extremely brief (<5 minutes). Assessment of the perineum should be deferred if imminent delivery is unlikely and the patient is able to reliably report the absence of any pressure, unusual sensation (including urge to defecate), or fluid discharge (blood or amniotic fluid) in the vaginal area. The presence or suspicion of any of these items requires a visual inspection of the perineum by the EMS provider.

Amniotic fluid, released from the vagina before delivery, should be examined for meconium (fetal stool), a dark-green viscous substance visible in the normally clear amniotic fluid. Meconium may indicate fetal distress and increases the risk that the infant will require resuscitation after birth.

Uterine contractions provide valuable clues regarding the likelihood of a prehospital delivery. Most patients in active labor demonstrate obvious contractions readily identifiable through simple visual observation of a patient. The patient may show periods of discomfort, panting respirations, and often verbalize that a contraction is occurring. Gentle palpation of the abdomen reveals a uterus that becomes noticeably firm during a contraction and relaxes between contractions. When contractions increase in intensity and duration, while becoming closer together (<2 minutes from the start of one until the start of the next), delivery of the newborn is expected within a short period of time. It is always possible for patients to present with subtle contractions, occasionally described as back pain, urge to defecate, or even abdominal or menstrual cramping. The absence of classic, obvious uterine contractions does not exclude the potential for imminent prehospital delivery.

Breech Deliveries

Four percent of term deliveries are breech deliveries (**Figure 10-3**). Inspection of the perineum does not show a head crowning, but another anatomic part, such as the feet or buttocks, might be visible. In this situation, transport immediately to the nearest emergency department with labor and delivery capabilities. Given the risk of complications and the potential need for an emergency cesarean section to safely deliver the baby, initiate transport to the hospital as soon as a breech presentation is identified, even if delivery seems imminent.

Additional Complications

Many of the conditions identified during the prenatal period or through the maternal history and physical

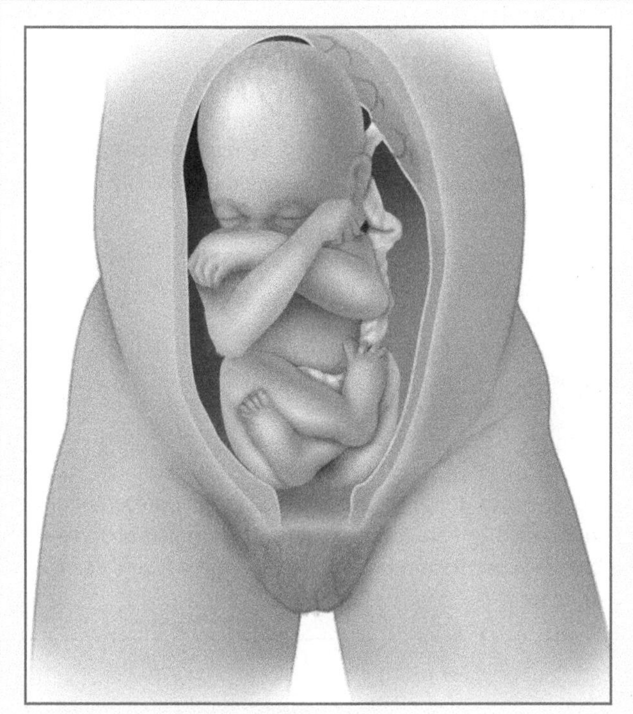

Figure 10-3 Breech birth.

examination prompt EMS providers to anticipate complications. Some complications can be mitigated by the skills and experience of EMS providers, but many complications require specialized care, techniques, and equipment not available in the prehospital setting. When potential or certain complications are identified, EMS providers must carefully consider whether the risks and benefits of delivering a newborn on scene (**Table 10-2**) exceed the risks and benefits of initiating prompt transportation (**Table 10-3**).

Transport Considerations for the Patient in Labor

Patients in labor, who have not delivered before transport, may require a wide range of services at the destination hospital. This is also true when a newborn has been delivered and complications are present. The destination decision for EMS providers is based on a combination of

Table 10-2 Risks and Benefits of Delivery on Scene

Benefits	Risks
• At least one additional EMS provider to assist with delivery • Nobody is needed to drive the transport vehicle at this time	• No progress toward definitive care if complications develop or additional trained personnel or equipment are needed
• Possible helpful assistance from patient's family or bystanders	• Bystanders or patient's family may interfere with patient care, disrupt privacy, or otherwise distract EMS providers from providing optimal care
• No vehicle movement, noise, or road hazards to undermine patient care	• The scene may pose safety hazards to EMS personnel or patient; may not have adequate climate control for newborn care
• Possibly more room to assess patient and deliver newborn	• Scene may have less room, more obstacles, or poor lighting, which make assessment and newborn delivery more difficult

Table 10-3 Risks and Benefits of Initiating Prompt Transportation

Benefits	Risks
• Movement toward definitive patient care where trained personnel, specialized equipment, and a controlled environment are available	• One less EMS provider to assist with patient care (this may be mitigated in certain situations if an alternate trained driver is available)
• Patient may have increased privacy in the transport vehicle, without detrimental interference from bystanders or family members	• Limited or no assistance available from family or bystanders
• May avoid safety risks and uncontrolled environmental temperature that may have been present on scene	• Vehicle movement, noise, and road hazards may undermine patient care efforts
• May have more room to assess patient and deliver the newborn than was available on scene • May have better lighting; resuscitation equipment immediately available	• May have less room or less access to the patient for assessment and newborn delivery

patient preference, geographic location, and the type of services required by the mother and child. When complications are expected and delivery is not imminent, it may be much better to bypass a smaller community hospital and transport the patient to a health care facility with high-risk obstetric services or neonatal intensive care unit capabilities. Conversely, it may be in the patient's best interest to transport directly to the closest available facility where the mother or child can be stabilized before a longer transport to a tertiary care center. EMS providers should consult with online medical control when required by protocol or when the appropriate destination choice is not clear. Providers should also make efforts to understand the obstetric capabilities of the various destination hospitals within their coverage area. Not every hospital has labor and delivery services. In many locations obstetric physicians are not always in the hospital. Early notification provides hospitals the opportunity to activate essential resources when they are not immediately available 24 hours, 7 days a week.

Routine care for patients in labor includes skills frequently performed by EMS. Patients in labor should receive supplemental oxygen to prevent or limit the severity of unrecognized fetal hypoxia. Intravenous (IV) fluids should be administered to patients in active labor to prevent dehydration or hemoconcentration and maintain a favorable fluid–volume status.

Vital signs remain a valuable part of any prehospital patient assessment and should be monitored at appropriate intervals during patient care. Patients in active labor may have vital signs temporarily deferred if delivery is imminent, personnel are limited, or the primary assessment does not suggest any likelihood of abnormality.

Because of the position of the vena cava, pregnant patients are at risk of hypotension when placed in a supine position. In the supine position, the uterus can compress the inferior vena cava, which can result in decreased cardiac output. This is primarily a complication during the third trimester. Whether placed on an ambulance stretcher or backboard, the pregnant patient should be positioned on an angle to one side or the other to displace the uterus off of her inferior vena cava and promote optimal blood return to her heart. The exception to this is when a supine position is absolutely necessary for spinal immobilization purposes. The left lateral recumbent position is preferred, but this may not be possible in certain transport vehicles when continuous airway monitoring is needed. Stretcher and backboard straps should not be placed over the pregnant patient's gravid abdomen. Place straps or seat belts above and below the patient's abdomen instead during transport.

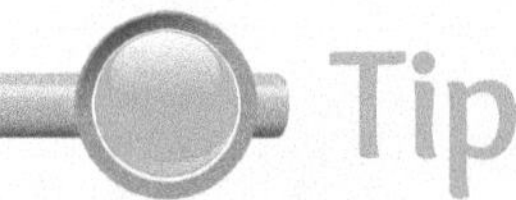

The "urge to push" experienced by most women at the end of labor is a sign that delivery is near, usually within 30–60 minutes.

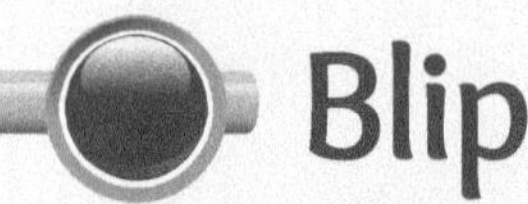

Never try to deliver a baby with a breech presentation in the field. Initiate transport to the hospital as soon as a breech presentation is identified, even if delivery seems imminent.

Summary of Triage of Patient in Labor

The responses to the three previously asked questions (**Table 10-1**), along with visual assessment of the perineum, provide the essential information to triage a laboring woman in the field. Known breech births and patients diagnosed with placenta previa require immediate transport, regardless of whether or not delivery is imminent. Other findings obtained from the maternal history and physical examination influence the decision whether to initiate transport or prepare for delivery on scene.

Preparation for Delivery

Resuscitation-Oriented History

Many factors in the mother's medical history affect the outcome of the baby and help predict the need for resuscitation of the newly born. However, once the decision has been made to deliver on scene, only three questions are pertinent for the immediate safety of the baby (**Table 10-4**).

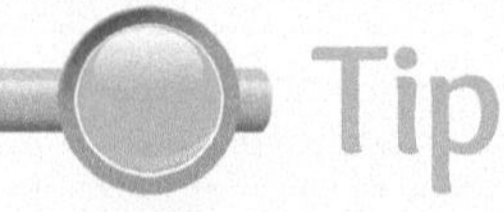

A large number of out-of-hospital deliveries are preterm, and the need for resuscitative efforts rises with the number of weeks of prematurity.

Case Study 2

You are called to a residence by a woman in labor who has no transportation to the hospital. On arrival you find the woman lying on the floor screaming, "It's time!" She tells you that this is her sixth baby and the last one came "real quick." Her water broke 30 minutes ago and it was clear. Your examination shows the baby is crowning and the mother has an urge to push.

1. What three questions are most appropriate to ask at this time to best prepare for delivery?
2. What equipment should be prepared for delivery?

Table 10-4 Resuscitation-Oriented History: Three Essential Questions

1. Do you have twins or multiple fetuses?
2. When are you due to deliver?
3. What color is the amniotic fluid?

1. Is there more than one fetus present? If twins or multiple newborns are expected, prepare for more than one delivery. This may mean finding extra equipment, preparing an additional warm environment, and planning the management of the first baby while delivering the second. This usually requires calling for a second ambulance. In tiered EMS systems, an ALS ambulance should be requested.
2. When are you due to deliver? A significant number of out-of-hospital deliveries are preterm (less than 37 weeks, gestation), and the further from the expected delivery date, the greater the chances of delivering a depressed newborn. Knowing the due date is important for preparing the right resuscitation equipment for airway management and breathing support. Make sure there are masks sized for preterm newborns less than 30 weeks, gestation. Have ready a size 0 laryngoscope blade and endotracheal tubes in sizes to fit the expected size of the newborn (**Figure 10-4**).
3. What color is the amniotic fluid? Greenish color in the amniotic fluid is a sign of passage of meconium, which is fetal stool. Meconium is released by the fetus during periods of intrauterine stress, especially hypoxia. If meconium is observed, be prepared to deal with a depressed baby or airway obstruction.

Assembling Equipment

If the triage decision is to deliver on scene, get the appropriate equipment ready. **Table 10-5** lists the essential ambulance equipment, best organized in a portable obstetric pack (**Figure 10-5**).

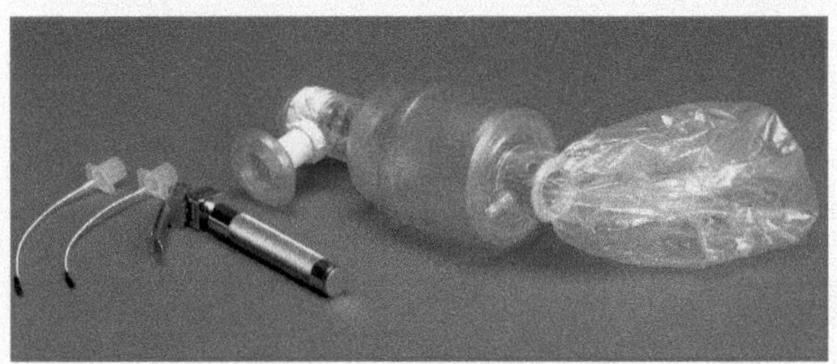

Figure 10-4 Special equipment for premature infant resuscitation: bag-mask device with small mask, size 0 laryngoscope blade, and endotracheal tubes sizes 2.5 and 3.0.

Table 10-5 Contents of a Portable Obstetric Pack for Vaginal Delivery

Number	Item
1	Sterile disposable scalpel or scissors
3	Disposable towels
1	Receiving blanket
1	Sterile disposable bulb syringe
2	Sterile umbilical clamps or ties
1	Large plastic bag with twist tie (to store the placenta)
2	Plastic-lined underpads
1	Disposable plastic apron, mask, and protective eyewear

Warming the Environment

Avoiding hypothermia is an important part of newly born patient care. Before delivery, make the room or

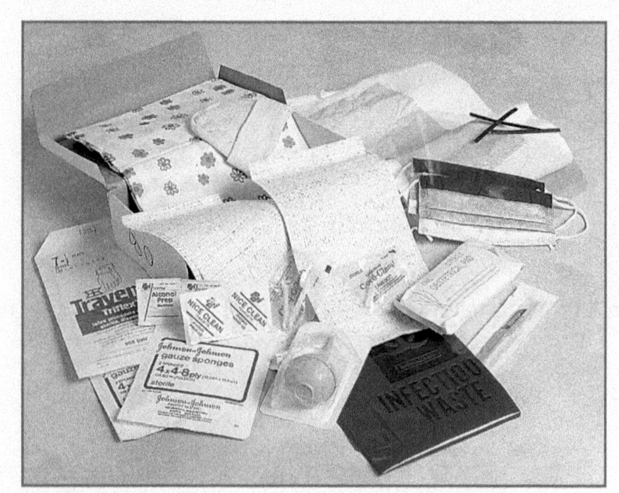

Figure 10-5 Obstetric pack.

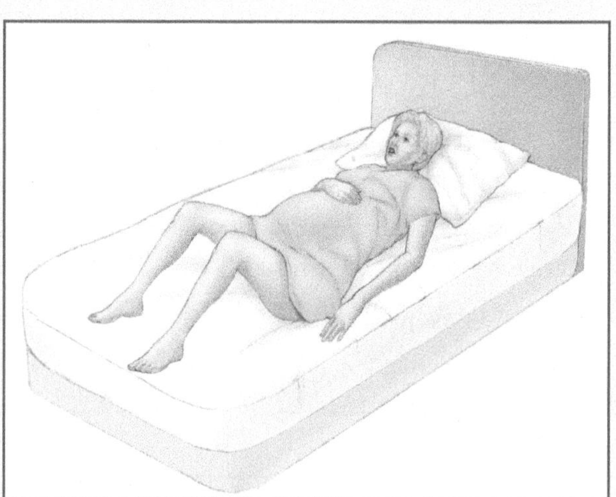

Figure 10-6 A safe position for delivery is with the mother lying supine towards the back of a bed, allowing her to deliver the baby onto the bed with minimal handling.

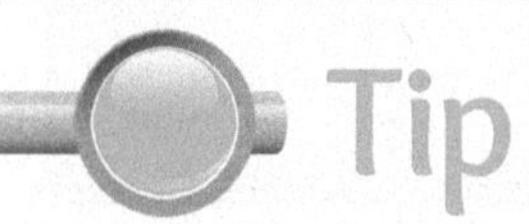

Tip

The presence of meconium increases the risk of resuscitation needs in the newly born.

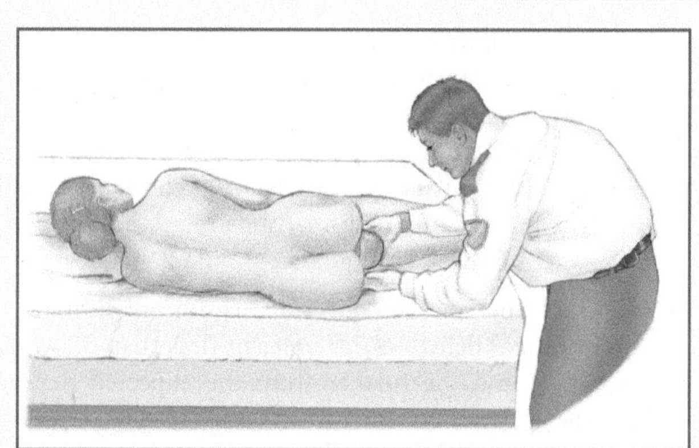

Figure 10-7 The Sims position has the mother on her side with her back toward the attendant and her knees drawn toward her chest.

ambulance as warm as possible. Turn up the heat until it is uncomfortable for an adult. Air blowing across the newly born can lead to heat loss, so turn off all fans. If the setting allows, consider having a family member warm towels in the dryer in anticipation of the delivery.

Positioning the Mother

Although it is a medical emergency for the patient and the family, the delivery of a baby is also a highly personal and emotional event. Establish a plan for positioning for delivery with the mother, but let her stay in a comfortable position and covered before delivery.

A safe maternal position for the delivery is lying supine (on her back) towards the back of a bed. Allow her to deliver the baby onto the bed with minimal handling (**Figure 10-6**). Suctioning the baby's mouth and nose, if necessary, before delivery of the body is difficult with the mother in this position because most infants are born face down. Another technique involves raising the mother's buttocks with a stack of folded towels to allow oropharyngeal suctioning of the baby, if necessary, after the head has been delivered.

Another safe position is the Sims position, in which the mother lies on her side with her back toward the attendant and her knees drawn toward her chest (**Figure 10-7**). In this position, the infant's head is easy to reach for suctioning if necessary. In this position, the mother's perineum is still over the bed, so delivery onto the bed with minimal handling is still possible.

A third position to consider is with the woman lying supine and positioned sideways on the bed, with each foot on a separate chair and her perineum at the edge of the bed (**Figure 10-8**). After the baby's head is delivered, this position provides enough space to suction the mouth and nose if necessary before delivering the body. The disadvantage of this position is the lack of a supportive surface under the perineum, so that the prehospital professional must actually "catch" the baby.

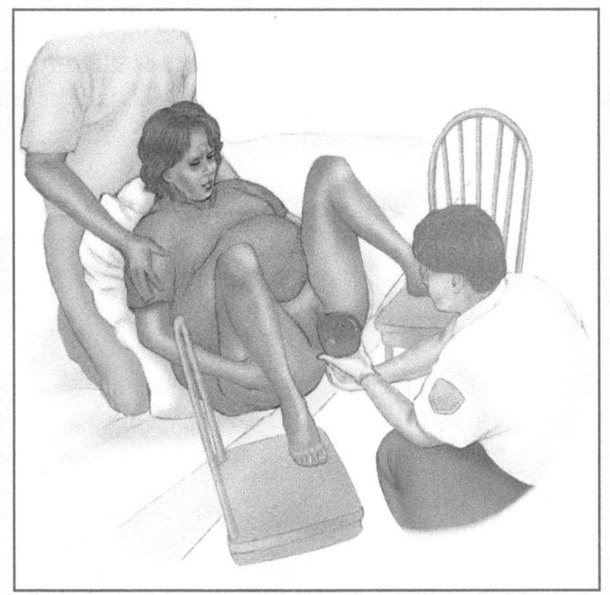

Figure 10-8 Alternate delivery position. The woman is perpendicular to the bed with each foot on a separate chair and her perineum at the edge of the bed.

Selecting a Clean Delivery Surface

Select a surface that is as clean as possible to conduct the immediate care of the child. Make sure everyone involved in the child's care has washed their hands and has several pairs of gloves.

Performing the Delivery

Most babies deliver themselves without assistance, especially if the laboring mother is lying supine or in the Sims position in bed. Although the prehospital professional may attempt to control the delivery as described next, only minimal interference with this natural process is necessary in most cases.

Use the following sequence for all deliveries:

1. Allow the mother to push the head out of the vaginal opening.
2. Next, with one finger, feel the infant's neck for the umbilical cord (**Figure 10-9**). If it is there, gently lift it over the baby's head. Do not pull hard on the cord because it may lead to avulsion of the cord with severe hemorrhage.
3. If the woman is delivering in bed, let the delivery proceed without intervention. Place one hand around the infant's neck posteriorly and one hand underneath the infant to help support the delivery (**Figure 10-10**). On occasion, the infant's anterior shoulder needs to be gently moved posteriorly to clear the mother's symphysis pubis. Place a hand on either side of the infant's head and gently pull downward (**Figure 10-11**).
4. Keep the infant lying on the bed at the level of the vaginal introitus until the umbilical cord is clamped or tied. Do not hold the baby higher than the uterus or womb before clamping the cord because this may lead to transfusion of blood from the baby to the placenta (fetal-placental transfusion), hypovolemia, and anemia. Alternatively, holding the baby with an unclamped cord below the level of the uterus can lead to transfusion of blood from the placenta to the baby, leading to a dangerously high hematocrit.
5. Tie or clamp the cord in two places, approximately 3 inches to 4 inches from its connection to the baby. Cut the cord between the two ties (**Figure 10-12**).

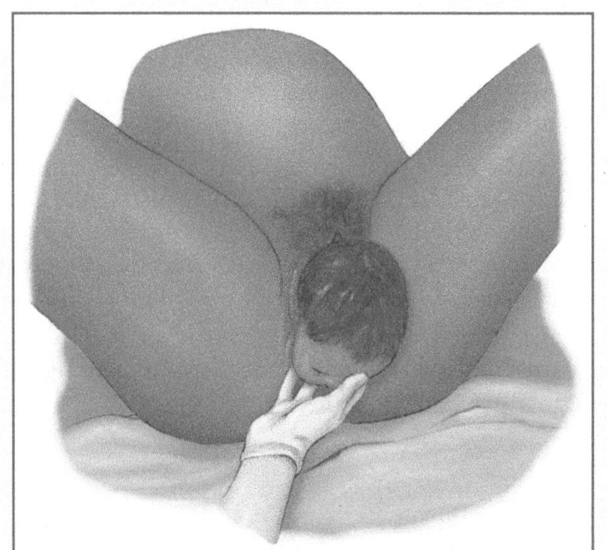

Figure 10-9 Ensure the umbilical cord is not wrapped around the baby's neck.

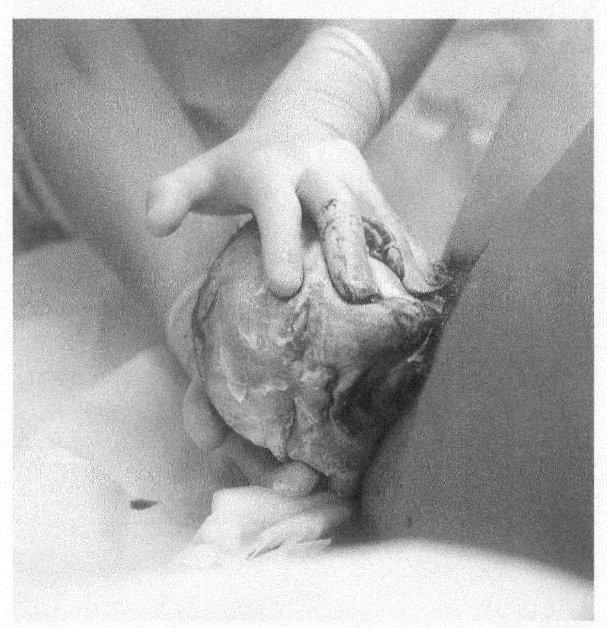

Figure 10-10 Place a hand around the neck posteriorly and one underneath the infant to help control the delivery.

6. Dry and warm the baby with clean, warm towels. Clear secretions if needed. This removes amniotic fluid, prevents heat loss, and stimulates the newborn to breathe. Remove damp towels or blankets from around the baby and replace them with clean, dry ones.
7. The last step in the delivery process is the delivery of the placenta. This generally occurs spontaneously 10–15 minutes after birth. Delivery of the placenta is not an emergency procedure and must not delay the transport of the mother and infant. Do not pull on the umbilical cord to hurry the process.

Separation of the placenta from the uterus is often signaled by a "gush of blood" from the vagina. After the placenta has separated from the uterine wall, gentle pulling on the cord removes it from the vagina. Too much pulling before it has separated naturally may lead to avulsion of the cord and bleeding. Place the placenta in a plastic bag and transport it with the patient for pathologic evaluation.

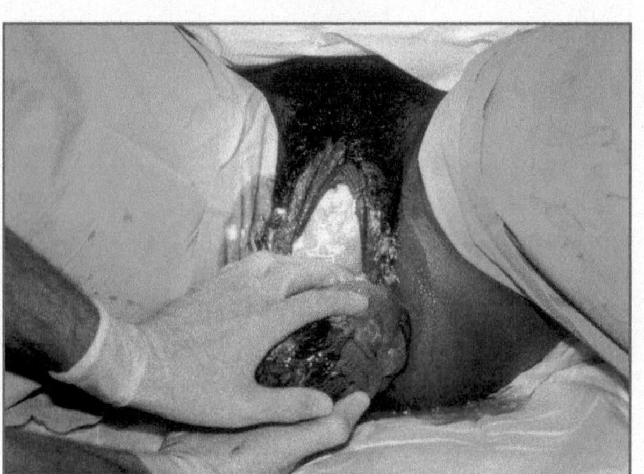

Figure 10-11 On occasion, the infant's anterior shoulder may need to be pulled posteriorly to clear the mother's symphysis pubis. This can be accomplished by placing a hand on either side of the infant's head and gently pulling downward.

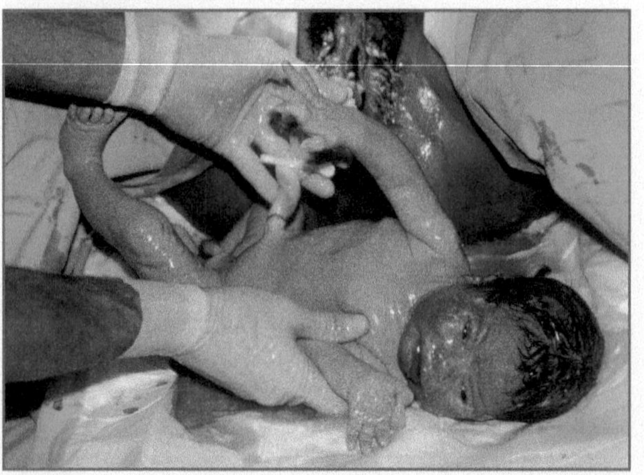

Figure 10-12 Tie or clamp the cord in two places (approximately 3 and 4 inches from its insertion into the baby). Cut the cord between the two ties or clamps.

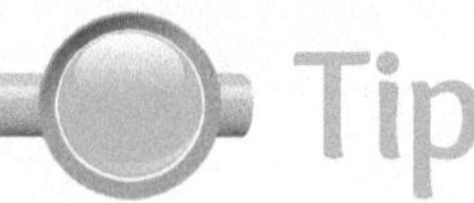

Tip

Delivery of the placenta is a natural act that requires no assistance in the field.

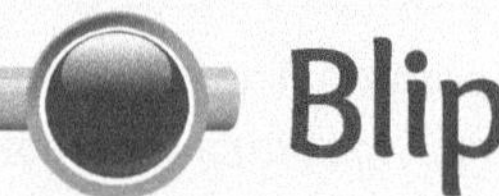

Blip

Do not hold the baby higher than the womb before clamping the cord, because this may lead to hypovolemia and anemia from transfusion of the baby's blood back to the placenta.

Maternal and Newborn Complications During Vaginal Delivery

Umbilical Cord Prolapse

Disruption of the oxygen and nutrients supplied to the fetus through the umbilical cord can cause devastating injury to the fetus, including fetal death. On rare occasions, the umbilical cord may enter the vaginal cavity before or simultaneously with a delivering fetus. The umbilical cord becomes compressed and the fetal blood supply is compromised. During assessment the umbilical cord will be visible at the vaginal opening. When recognized in the prehospital setting, only one treatment option is available. The patient is placed into a knee-chest position (**Figure 10-13**) and the EMS provider inserts two fingers from a gloved hand into the vaginal cavity to prevent the presenting fetal body part from compressing the umbilical cord. One finger should be placed on either side of the cord to release pressure and allow blood to continue to flow through the cord. Transportation should commence immediately to a facility capable of performing an emergency cesarean section. Umbilical cord prolapse is more common in patients with premature rupture of membranes, premature delivery, multiple gestation, multiparity, and fetal breech presentations.

Nuchal Umbilical Cord

During the delivery, EMS providers should assess for the presence of a nuchal cord, which is the umbilical cord wrapped around the neck of a newly born as it delivers. Although it is more common to have the umbilical cord wrapped around the newborn's neck only once, it is possible for the umbilical cord to wrap around the neck more than once. To reduce a single-wrapped nuchal cord, simply slide the umbilical cord from around the newborn's neck. When the cord is wrapped too tightly or around the neck multiple times, EMS providers should apply two clamps across the cord then cut the umbilical cord between the clamps. Multiple gestation pregnancies create a noteworthy hazard regarding nuchal umbilical cords. It is possible for the umbilical cord of one fetus to strangle another fetus. Use extreme caution when considering whether to clamp and cut a nuchal cord when multiple gestation has not been excluded.

Meconium

Meconium is fetal stool passed in the uterus. It can be thin and watery or thick and sticky. If the newly born is vigorous (normal respiratory effort, muscle tone, and a heart rate >100 beats/min), simply use a bulb syringe or large-bore suction catheter (12F or 14F catheter) to clear the secretions and any meconium from the mouth and nose if necessary.

Shoulder Dystocia/Cephalopelvic Disproportion

Shoulder dystocia is the mechanical entrapment of a fetus in the birth canal after the fetal head has successfully emerged from the vaginal introitus (**Figure 10-14**). A relatively large or disproportioned fetus may not deliver through the vaginal canal without assistance from EMS providers. One or both fetal shoulders may become stuck within the maternal pelvis, typically against the symphysis pubis. The initial treatment is the McRoberts maneuver (**Figure 10-15**), which has two assistants hyperflex the maternal thighs against the patient's abdomen rotating the pelvis anteriorly. This position resolves many episodes of shoulder dystocia. Cephalopelvic disproportion is a similar condition, where the fetal head is too large to pass through the pelvic opening. In true cases of cephalopelvic disproportion, a cesarean section is the only method available for successful delivery.

Postpartum Hemorrhage

The most common postpartum maternal complication and leading cause of maternal death is excessive bleeding after delivery. Usually, pregnant women lose 500 mL of blood with a vaginal delivery. Symptoms such as tachycardia and orthostatic hypotension begin to appear in the mother with 1,200–1,500 mL of blood loss. Because estimating blood loss is difficult, one must monitor the postpartum mother's vital signs carefully.

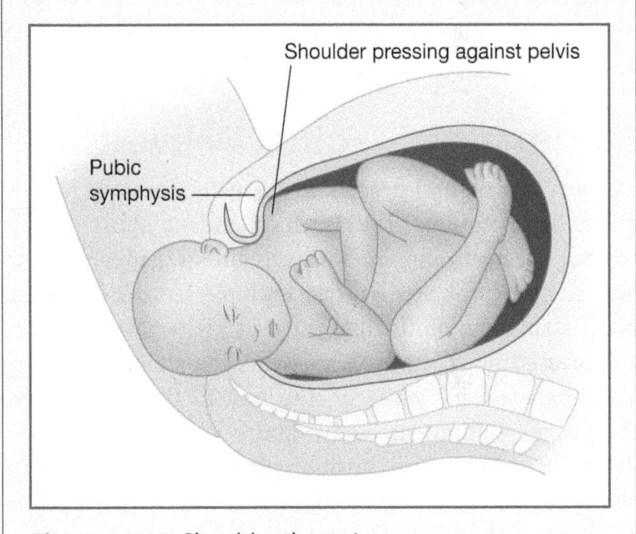

Figure 10-14 Shoulder dystocia.

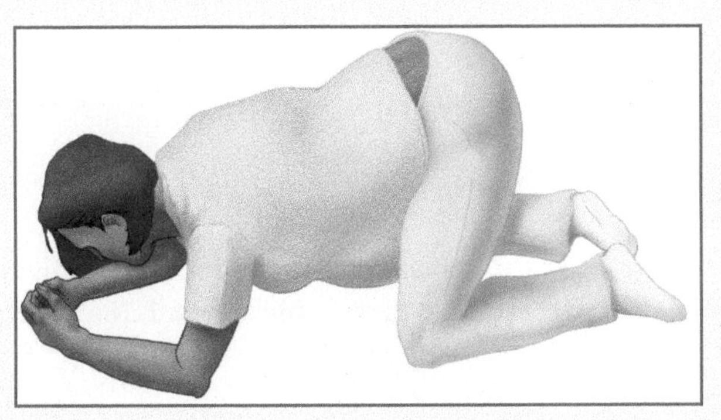

Figure 10-13 The knee-chest position.

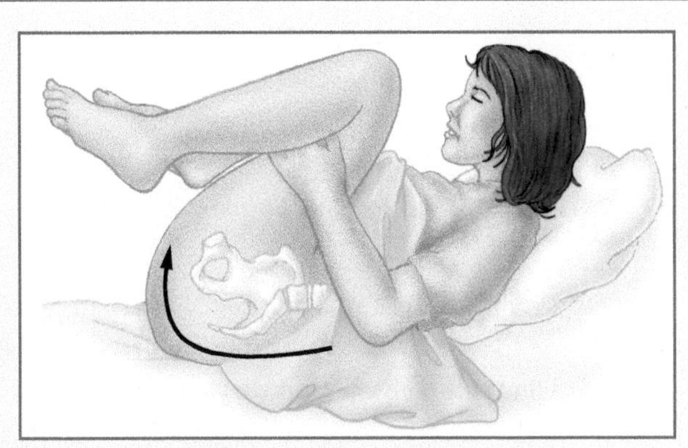

Figure 10-15 The McRoberts maneuver.

If a postpartum mother has excessive vaginal blood loss, perform uterine massage (**Figure 10-16**). To massage the uterus, place one hand with fingers fully extended just above the mother's pubic bone and use the other hand to press down into the lower abdomen and gently massage the uterus until it becomes firm. This should take from 3 to 5 minutes. As the uterus firms up, it should feel about the size of a softball or large grapefruit. If the infant is stable, encourage breastfeeding to increase uterine tone and to slow uterine bleeding.

ALS

Treatment of Postpartum Hemorrhage. Begin volume resuscitation with crystalloid fluid in the mother who continues to bleed after the placenta is delivered and has dizziness, pallor, tachycardia, or low blood pressure. Administer IV lactated Ringer's or normal saline solution during transport while continuing to monitor vital signs and clinical presentation of the patient. Maternal stability determines the rate and amount of IV fluids needed. In severe situations, massive amounts of IV fluids and blood products may be required. Persistent hemorrhage requires uterine exploration, surgical intervention, or uterotonic medications not generally available to EMS providers.

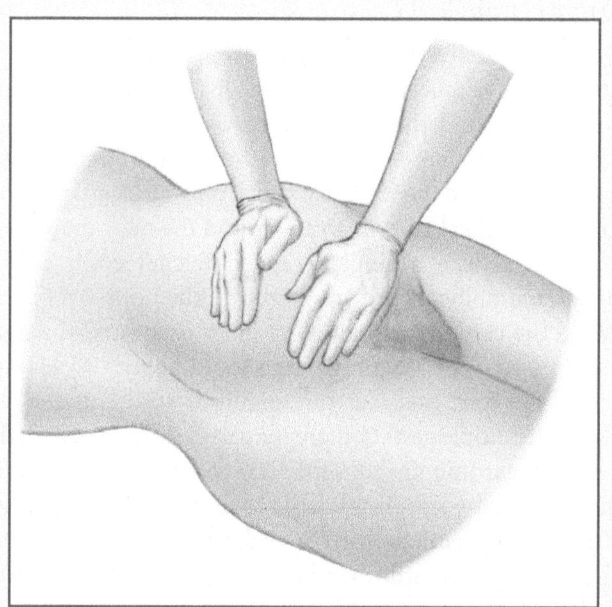

Figure 10-16 To massage the uterus, place one hand with fingers fully extended just above the mother's pubic bone, and use your other hand to press down into the lower abdomen and gently massage the uterus until it becomes firm.

Summary of Vaginal Delivery

Delivery is a natural process that usually does not require much intervention. The birth attendant must simply control the environment to avoid things happening too fast. A history of prematurity, multiple fetuses, or meconium-stained amniotic fluid suggests higher probability of a depressed newly born. Review the steps for performing a vaginal delivery while on the way to the scene. Have the proper equipment ready, control the temperature of the environment, and position the mother to facilitate childbirth and care of the newly born. Control postpartum bleeding with uterine massage and encouragement of breastfeeding.

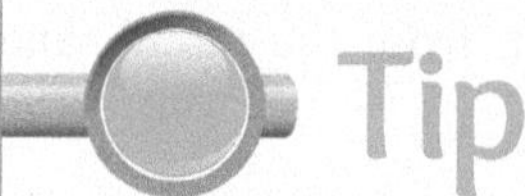

Tip

Encourage the mother to breastfeed the active, vigorous infant.

Immediate Care of the Newly Born

A well-organized plan guides prehospital providers through the optimal care of the newly born infant. **Table 10-6** lists the five essential steps to care for every newly born in every setting. EMS providers should keep

Case Study 3

On arriving at the home of a family who had called 9-1-1 for labor, you find a woman lying on the floor who has just delivered an apparently term female. The infant is lying on the floor, still attached to the umbilical cord. The newly born infant is blue and is not crying or moving.

1. What are the steps in the resuscitation of this newborn?
2. What is the role of vascular access?

Table 10-6 Organized Approach to Assessment and Care of the Newly Born

Dry and warm the baby
Clear the airway, if needed
Assess breathing
Assess heart rate
Assess color

every infant warm and dry, maintain a patent airway, and support newborn respiratory and circulatory function when indicated. Most term newly borns do not require any ALS interventions.

Vigor is an immediate assessment of a newborn infant's appearance. This determination is based on the quality of respirations or crying, skin color, and muscle tone. This rapid visual assessment gives providers an immediate indication of the clinical status of a newborn infant and guides the approach to resuscitation when meconium is present. The APGAR score (**Table 10-7**) is a numerical representation of vigor obtained at 1 minute and again at 5 minutes after delivery, after initiating supportive and resuscitation measures. EMS providers must not interrupt critical resuscitation procedures to obtain or calculate an APGAR score on an unstable newborn.

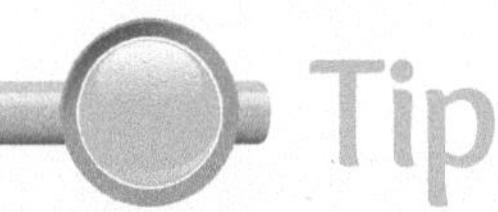

Tip

Perform the initial steps of drying, warming, and positioning on all newborns, whether active or depressed.

Dry and Warm the Baby

At birth the baby is covered in amniotic fluid and can lose a lot of heat through evaporation unless immediately dried. Heat loss drastically increases the metabolic demand and oxygen consumption. Remove wet towels or blankets from around the baby after drying and replace them with clean, warm, dry towels. This should take no more than 5–10 seconds.

Clear the Airway

Clear the airway if needed. Use of a bulb syringe or suction catheter may be considered only if the airway appears obstructed or the infant will require positive pressure ventilation. When necessary, gently suction the mouth then nose. Care should be taken when suctioning as suctioning of the nasopharynx may cause an exaggerated vagal response.

A newborn's head is larger than an older child's or an adult's compared to its overall body size, which leads to flexion of the neck in a supine position. This may cause airway occlusion. Extend the head slightly and place a towel under the infant's shoulders to place the airway in a neutral position.

Assess Breathing

Most babies will be crying, indicating adequate respiratory effort. Breathing effort may be slightly irregular in normal newly borns. Grunting is a sign of increased work of breathing. Gasping occurs pre-arrest and indicates the need for assisted ventilation.

An apneic baby, with no visible respiratory effort, requires immediate treatment. Most apneic newborns start breathing simply with tactile stimulation. If the baby is completely apneic or only has gasping respiration after drying and suctioning, further stimulation is not likely to improve respiratory effort. Begin positive pressure ventilation with a bag and mask at a rate of 40–60 breaths/min. The American Academy of Pediatrics has recently updated their guidelines for the routine use of supplemental oxygen

Table 10-7 APGAR Scoring

Sign	0	1	2
Appearance: Color	Blue or pale	Acrocyanotic	Completely pink
Pulse: Heart rate	Absent	<100 bpm	>100 bpm
Grimace: Reflex irritability	No response	Grimace	Cry or active withdrawal
Activity: Muscle tone	Limp	Some flexion	Active motion
Respiration	Absent	Weak cry; hypoventilation	Good; crying

in neonatal resuscitation. Initial resuscitation should be started without supplemental oxygen attached to the bag-mask device. This represents a huge paradigm shift from decades of resuscitation procedures. Supplementary oxygen, if needed, should be titrated to achieve a preductal oxygen saturation (see table in Neonatal Resuscitation algorithm). EMS providers need to follow local protocols and medical direction pertaining to the use of supplemental oxygen in neonatal resuscitation.

Treatment of an Infant Born to a Mother on Opiates. A special situation occurs when the prehospital professional encounters a newly born with respiratory depression after delivery by a narcotic-addicted mother. Do not give naloxone (Narcan) to the baby if the mother is addicted to narcotics. Reversal of narcotics may precipitate acute withdrawal symptoms and seizure activity. Assist ventilation with bag-mask and follow the guidelines for care of a depressed newly born. Consider endotracheal intubation if the infant requires prolonged ventilation or continued resuscitation measures.

Assess Heart Rate

Bradycardia in a newly born is usually caused by hypoxia, not primary cardiac disease. The crying, active baby usually has an adequate heart rate. Assess heart rate carefully in a baby who is not active or who requires assisted ventilation. This is most easily accomplished by palpating a pulse at the base of the umbilical cord (**Figure 10-17**). Count the number of beats over 6 seconds and multiply this number by 10. This rapid assessment of heart rate is needed to assist decision making. Sometimes the umbilical vessels are constricted so that the pulse is not palpable. If a pulse cannot be felt, listen for the heartbeat over the left side of the chest using a stethoscope.

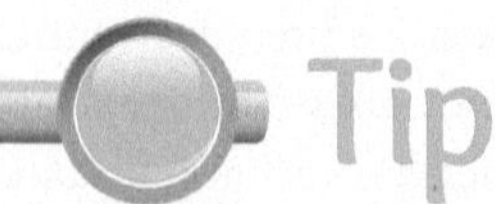

Tip

You may encounter pregnant women who have not received prenatal care, or who are addicted to drugs. If the pregnant woman is "high," so is her baby. With such patients, it can be difficult to determine how long the woman has been in labor and what complications she has in addition to her drug addiction. Be prepared for anything.

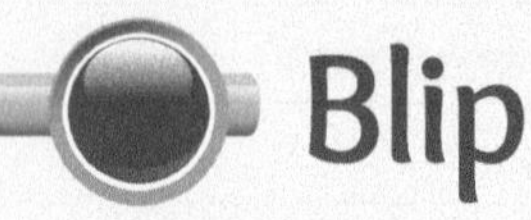

Blip

Do not give naloxone to the newly born if the mother is addicted to narcotics.

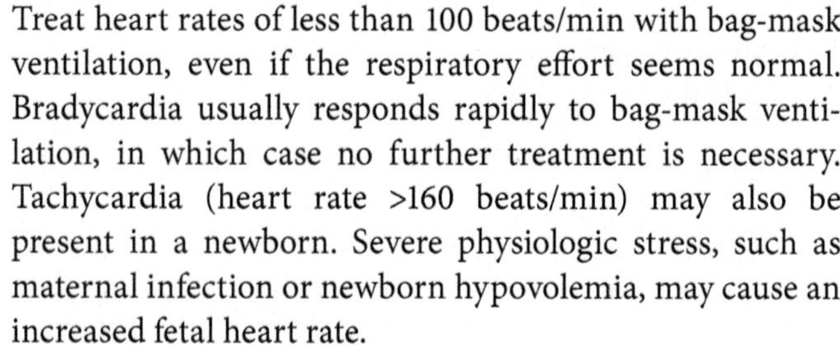

Treat heart rates of less than 100 beats/min with bag-mask ventilation, even if the respiratory effort seems normal. Bradycardia usually responds rapidly to bag-mask ventilation, in which case no further treatment is necessary. Tachycardia (heart rate >160 beats/min) may also be present in a newborn. Severe physiologic stress, such as maternal infection or newborn hypovolemia, may cause an increased fetal heart rate.

Assess Color

Skin color assessment in newly borns has several unique features. In utero, the fetus depends on placental delivery of oxygen, and blood oxygen concentrations are very low compared to conditions after birth. Therefore, before the initiation of respiration after delivery, the infant appears cyanotic.

If the cyanotic newly born is apneic, immediately begin positive-pressure ventilation and bag-mask ventilation. If the baby is breathing, but appears blue, determine if the cyanosis is central (on the trunk and face) or peripheral (limited to the hands and feet). This difference helps with decision making and therapy. If central cyanosis is present, a pulse oximeter with an infant probe should be applied to confirm hypoxia. When hypoxia is present, administer supplemental oxygen by a mask held loosely over the baby's face and titrate to preductal SpO_2.

Peripheral cyanosis, bluish skin color present only in the extremities, is also termed acrocyanosis. This is a common

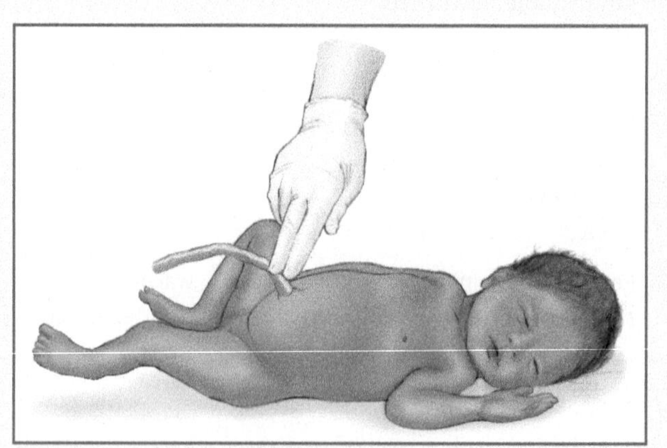

Figure 10-17 Feel for a pulse at the base of the umbilical cord.

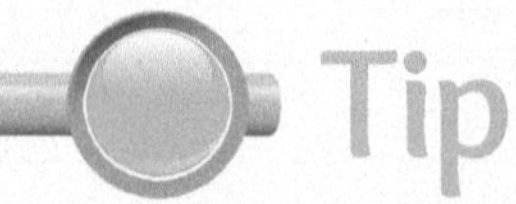

Tip

Assist ventilation in an infant with a heart rate less than 100 beats/min with bag-mask ventilation. Bradycardia usually reflects inadequate respiratory effort.

finding in newborns through the first 24–48 hours of life and requires no therapy.

Infant color and pulse quality provide an indication of overall perfusion status. Hypovolemia, shock, and congenital cardiovascular defects may present with central cyanosis, poor overall skin color, delayed capillary refill, or absent peripheral pulses. Persistent infant bradycardia, tachycardia, or alterations in perfusion may represent a severe condition requiring ALS intervention and transport to a specialty care center.

General Principles of Newborn Resuscitation

Newborn resuscitation includes a series of interventions designed to treat a variety of airway, respiratory, or cardiovascular problems after delivery in the prehospital setting. Most do not require the complex interventions discussed next. The initial steps of resuscitation are completed on every newly born. They include:

1. Dry the infant, remove all wet items, and place the newly born in the supine position in a warm environment.
2. Position the head in slight extension.
3. Suction the mouth then nose if needed.

When the baby remains depressed after initial drying, warming, and clearing of the airway, begin resuscitation. Use the following sequence:

1. Assess heart rate and breathing. If less than 100 beats/min, or if respiratory effort is absent or gasping, start bag-mask ventilation at 40–60 breaths/min (**Figure 10-18**).
2. Assess heart rate after 60 seconds of adequate ventilation. If less than 60 beats/min, begin chest compressions. Compressions should be delivered a depth of one-third the anteroposterior diameter of the chest. The "two thumb encircling hand" technique is recommended (compressions using two thumbs with fingers encircling the chest and supporting the back). Deliver 90 compressions and 30 ventilations (120 events) per minute with a 3:1 compression to ventilation ratio (**Figure 10-19**).
3. Reassess heart rate after 30 seconds. Continue compressions and positive-pressure ventilation until heart rate is more than 60 beats/min. Positive-pressure ventilations should be continued until the heart rate is more than 100 beats/min.

ALS

Endotracheal Intubation and Epinephrine Administration. Check the heart rate after 60 seconds of compressions. If less than 60 beats/min, prepare for endotracheal intubation and administration of epinephrine 0.01–0.03 mg/kg of the 0.1 mg/mL concentration. The endotracheal route may be associated with lower blood levels of the drug. IV or intraosseous (IO) access should be obtained as soon as possible. The recommended dose is 0.01-0.03 mg/kg of the 0.1 mg/mL concentration, the same as the endotracheal intubation dose.

Continue chest compressions and give repeated doses of epinephrine every 3–5 minutes until heart rate is more than 60 beats/min.

Monitor blood glucose concentrations, especially if the infant has received prolonged or aggressive resuscitation measures. If a serum glucose of less than 40 mg/dL is documented in a depressed newly born, and an IV or IO line can be established during transport, give 10% dextrose in a 2 mL/kg bolus. Initiate prompt transport to a health care facility capable of neonatal stabilization.

The Inverted Pyramid. The inverted pyramid (**Figure 10-20**) illustrates the relative need for interventions in depressed newborns.

BLS is usually all that is required during deliveries and therefore comprises the largest area at the top of the inverted pyramid. In contrast, chest compressions and ALS interventions, such as intubation, and medication administration are rarely required, and comprise the smallest area at the bottom of the inverted pyramid.

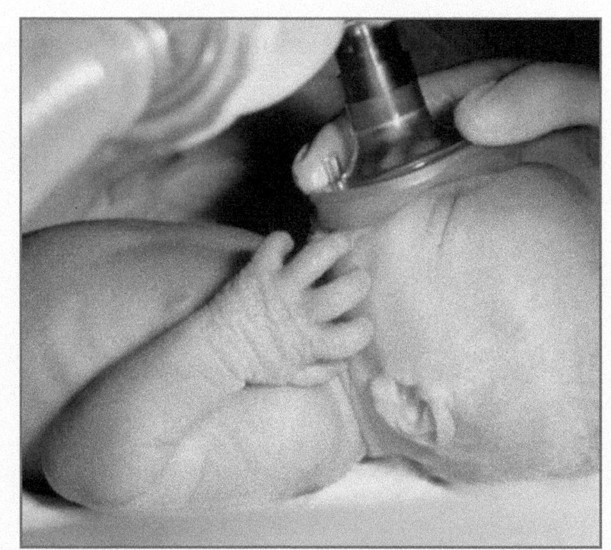

Figure 10-18 Using a bag-mask device on a newborn.

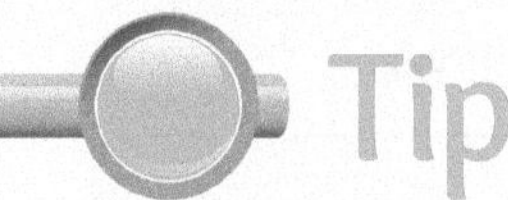

Tip

Good ventilation usually reverses bradycardia.

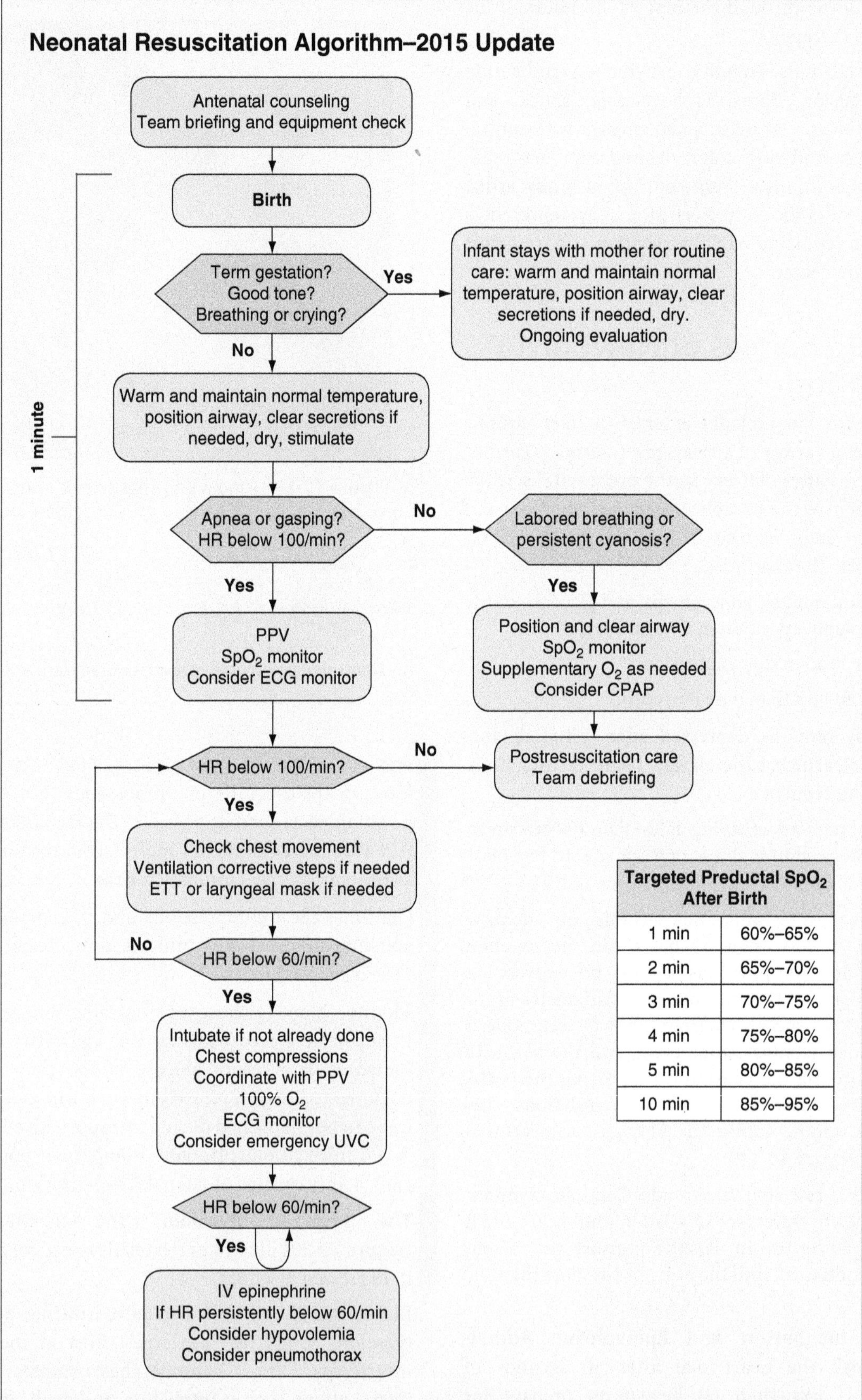

Targeted Preductal SpO_2 After Birth	
1 min	60%–65%
2 min	65%–70%
3 min	70%–75%
4 min	75%–80%
5 min	80%–85%
10 min	85%–95%

Figure 10-19 2015 AHA Guidelines criteria showing the Neonatal Resuscitation Algorithm.

Reproduced from Wyckoff, MH, et al. Part 13: neonatal resuscitation: 2015 American Heart Association Guidelines Update for Cardiopulmonary Resuscitation and Emergency Cardiovascular Care. *Circulation.* 2015;132(suppl 2):S543–S560

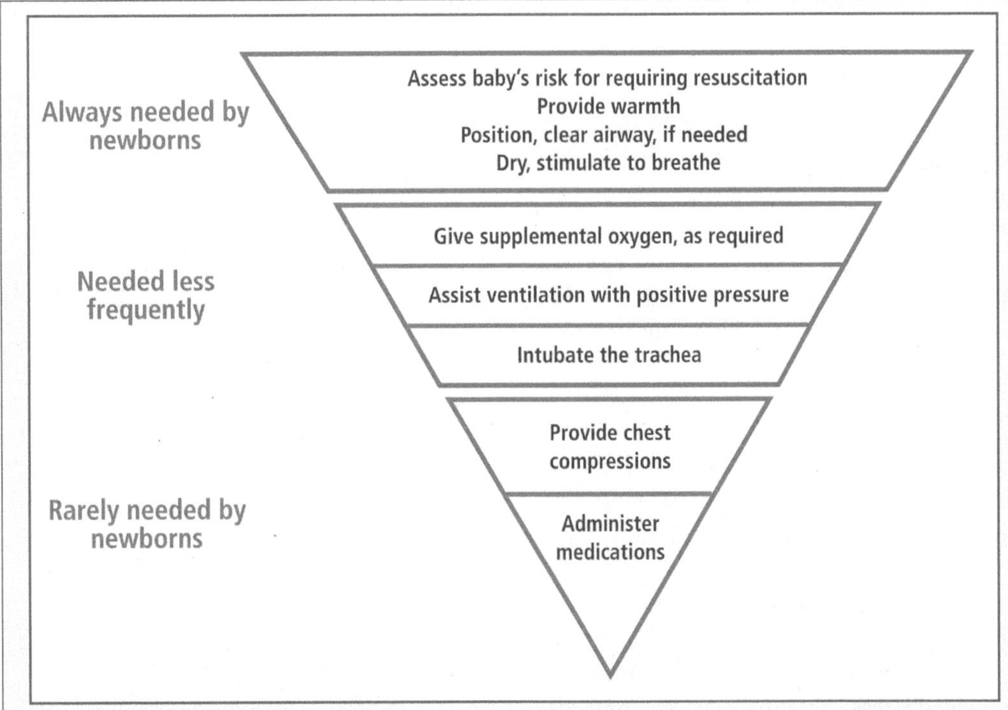

Figure 10-20 The relationship between resuscitation procedures and the number of newly born babies who need them.

Figure from: Kattwinkel J, ed. *Textbook of Neonatal Resuscitation.* 6th ed. Elk Grove, IL: American Academy of Pediatrics and American Heart Association; 2011: 3.

Specific Newborn Complications

Meconium Aspiration

A child born with meconium-stained amniotic fluid, who appears active and without respiratory distress, needs only oral then nasal suctioning as needed along with standard care of the newly born. Provide adequate suctioning to remove meconium from the upper airway, but do not allow prolonged suctioning to delay assisted ventilation or other critical resuscitation measures. Overly aggressive suctioning may cause vagal stimulation and lead to bradycardia.

ALS

Treatment of Meconium Aspiration in a Nonvigorous Newborn. If meconium is present and a newborn is not considered vigorous, initial steps of resuscitation should occur. Positive-pressure ventilation should be initiated if the infant has a heart rate less than 100 beats/min or is not breathing. Routine intubation for tracheal suctioning is no longer required.

Preterm Infants

Premature infants are at risk for a vast array of complications, which increase in likelihood and severity as the degree of prematurity increases. Many of these complications, such as acute respiratory distress syndrome, bronchopulmonary dysplasia, or intraventricular hemorrhage, cannot be adequately managed in the prehospital or transport setting because of the medications or procedures required. EMS providers need to provide the warmest environment possible during resuscitation and transport. Support ventilations as needed with bag-mask ventilation for those with apnea, labored breathing, cyanosis, or heart rate less than 100 beats/min.

Congenital Disorders

Choanal Atresia

Infants are occasionally born with a complete nasal obstruction. In severe, untreated cases, this condition may cause newborn death from hypoxia. Unless crying, newly born infants breathe exclusively through their nasal passages. Patients with choanal atresia may present with profound respiratory distress that resolves during crying episodes. If EMS providers suspect this condition, place an oral airway or endotracheal tube into the posterior pharynx (does not need to enter the trachea). The respiratory distress should improve. A more presumptive diagnosis may be made in EMS systems that carry small suction catheters, capable of being placed into the infant's nose. If the catheter cannot pass through either nasal passage into the posterior pharynx, choanal atresia is presumed (**Figure 10-21**). Do not use excessive force to try to pass a nasal suction catheter.

Pierre Robin Syndrome

Pierre Robin syndrome is another potential cause of airway obstruction in newborn infants (**Figure 10-22**). An underdeveloped mandible causes the tongue to obstruct the posterior pharynx. This can usually be treated in the prehospital setting by turning the infant onto his or her stomach (prone). If this proves unsuccessful, a suction catheter (12 F) or endotracheal tube (2.5 mm) can be inserted through the baby's nose, with its tip located in the posterior pharynx, past the base of the tongue, but not into the trachea.

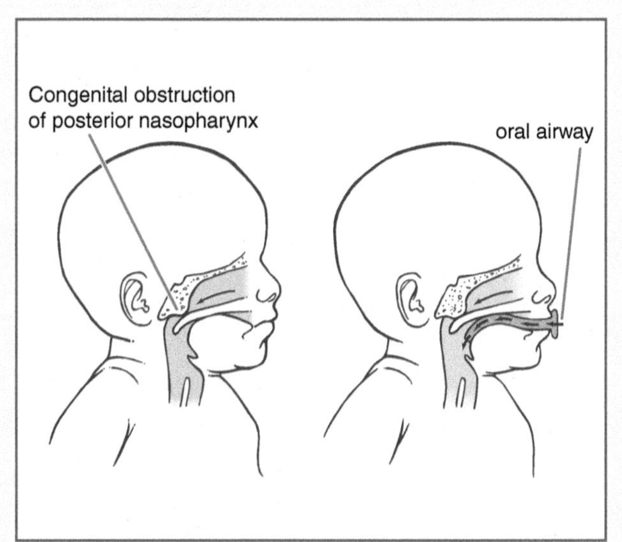

Figure 10-21 Choanal atresia.

Figure from: Kattwinkel J, ed. *Textbook of Neonatal Resuscitation.* 6th ed. Elk Grove, IL: American Academy of Pediatrics and American Heart Association; 2011: 240.

Congenital Diaphragmatic Hernia

It is possible for infants to be born without a completely intact diaphragm. The stomach or intestines may migrate into the chest cavity, collapsing lungs or inhibiting ventilation. EMS providers should suspect congenital diaphragmatic hernia when an infant presents with a flat (scaphoid) abdomen and respiratory distress (**Figure 10-23**). Prolonged bag-mask ventilations force additional air into the infant's stomach, worsening respiratory distress. Treatment in the prehospital setting requires prompt endotracheal intubation and decompression of the stomach with a gastric tube if available. Prompt transport and cautious bag-mask technique may be the only intervention available to BLS prehospital providers.

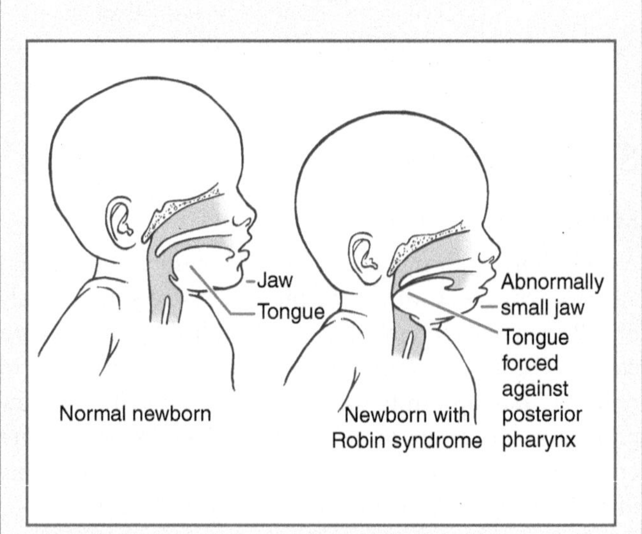

Figure 10-22 Pierre Robin syndrome.

Figure from: Kattwinkel J, ed. *Textbook of Neonatal Resuscitation.* 6th ed. Elk Grove, IL: American Academy of Pediatrics and American Heart Association; 2011: 241.

Congenital Cardiovascular Defects

Approximately 1% of infants are born with a congenital cardiovascular defect. Defects may involve several different parts of the heart and one or more of the great vessels in the chest. Diagnosis is often impossible without the assistance of a pediatric cardiologist or similar specialist, but certain cues may alert EMS providers to infants with these conditions. Cyanosis, shock, pulmonary edema, and altered peripheral pulses occur in infants with cardiovascular defects and may present across the full spectrum of severity. EMS providers should initiate immediate transport to a facility capable of neonatal stabilization whenever a congenital cardiovascular defect is suspected. Many types of defects present with persistent cyanosis that cannot be corrected in the prehospital setting, even with optimal resuscitation measures. Conversely, resuscitation with high concentrations of oxygen may actually worsen many of these conditions by altering the pulmonary circulation and vascular resistance. EMS providers are often limited to basic supportive care and prompt transport of infants with suspected cardiovascular defects.

Shock

Shock at birth is most commonly caused by asphyxia (severe hypoxia in the uterus or during delivery) and acidosis. Blood loss during delivery caused by umbilical cord avulsion or fetal-placental transfusion is an uncommon cause of shock in the newly born. Signs and symptoms of shock, whatever the cause, include abnormal appearance (lethargy, hypotonia), abnormal color (pallor, mottling), tachycardia, and prolonged capillary refill time. Hypothermia may also mimic these findings.

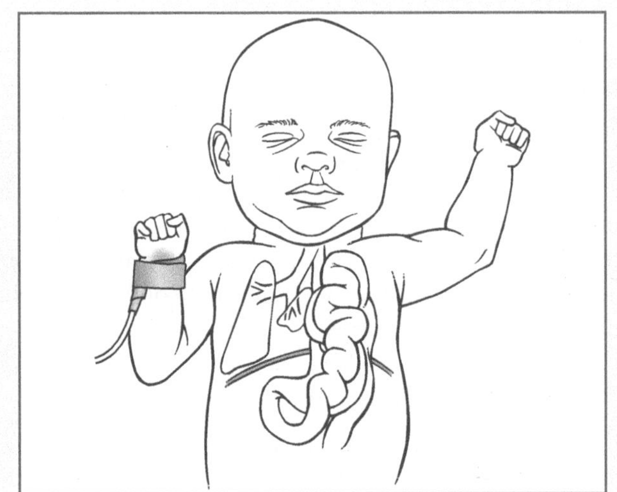

Figure 10-23 Congenital diaphragmatic hernia.

Figure from: Kattwinkel J, ed. *Textbook of Neonatal Resuscitation.* 6th ed. Elk Grove, IL: American Academy of Pediatrics and American Heart Association; 2011: 245.

ALS

Treatment of Shock. Because intrauterine or perinatal asphyxia is the most common cause of depression in the newly born, initial resuscitative efforts should ensure adequate oxygenation and ventilation. Volume resuscitation is rarely needed. In exceptional circumstances where hypovolemic shock is suspected, consider placing an IV or IO line. Isotonic crystalloid is recommended at a dose of 10 mL/kg. Fluid resuscitation should be limited in premature infants, because giving volume expanders too rapidly has been associated with intraventricular hemorrhage.

Vascular Access. Vascular access is rarely needed in newborn infants in the field because resuscitation is largely focused on airway management and breathing. In reality, establishing vascular access is challenging in infants and its benefits must be carefully weighed against prolonged on-scene time and potential complications. IV access may be attempted in the **antecubital fossa** or the **saphenous vein** at the ankle. IO infusion is an alternative.

Newborn Hypoglycemia. The depressed newborn or prematurely delivered baby is at risk for hypoglycemia, but this complication is unlikely to develop in the first 30 minutes of life. If transport times are longer, measure a bedside glucose level at approximately 30 minutes after birth, or immediately in any baby who has a drastic change in responsiveness or perfusion. If a serum glucose of less than 40 mg/dL is documented in a depressed newly born, and an IV or IO line can be established in transport, give 10% dextrose in a 2 mL/kg bolus. Recheck serum glucose every 30 minutes during long transports. If the infant has documented hypoglycemia but is active, is in no respiratory distress, and has a suck reflex, allow the infant to breastfeed or offer the infant 20–30 mL of 5% dextrose by bottle.

ALS

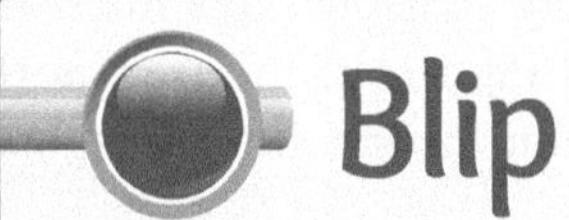

Umbilical catheterization in the field is a controversial procedure. Although this route of vascular access is widely used in the neonatal intensive care unit, there are very few opportunities for the prehospital professional to practice and maintain this skill, and serious complications can occur.

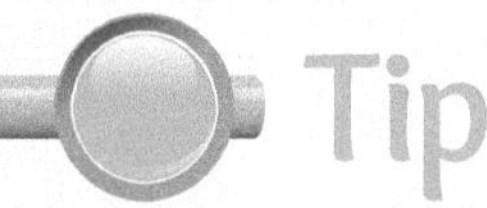

IO infusion may be preferable if vascular access is clearly necessary for resuscitation, and a peripheral IV cannot be placed.

When there is no IV or IO access, give resuscitation medications, such as epinephrine, through the endotracheal tube. Do not give other solutions, such as dextrose, through the endotracheal tube.

Summary of Resuscitation of the Newly Born

A variety of newborn conditions present with airway, respiratory, or cardiovascular compromise. The primary treatment of the depressed newborn involves reversal of hypoxia with immediate bag-mask ventilation. Follow local protocols regarding when to initiate oxygen administration during newborn resuscitation. If the child does not improve, begin chest compressions and perform endotracheal intubation on the scene before transport. Shock is rare, and is most commonly the result of asphyxia. Hypovolemia is an uncommon cause of shock in the newly born. If hypovolemic shock is suspected, transport immediately and initiate volume resuscitation by IV or IO line on the way to the hospital.

Transport Considerations

EMS providers may need to transport healthy infants who have had an uncomplicated delivery in the prehospital setting or critical infants in continued cardiopulmonary arrest. The degree of monitoring and ongoing intervention depends entirely on the clinical status of the patient. All infants require a warm environment. Every infant needs to be secured during transport in a manner that will not cause devastating injuries if the transport vehicle is involved in a collision during the transport (see Chapter 15).

Healthy Infant

The active, term infant requires no intervention or electronic monitoring during transport. Be sure the child is restrained as per local EMS system policy. Encourage the mother to breastfeed the active infant if possible. This may prevent hypoglycemia and promote maternal-infant bonding, uterine contraction, and decreased uterine bleeding.

Newborn With Complications

Oxygen Therapy

It is not appropriate to give supplemental oxygen to all infants. Infants with congenital cardiovascular defects and preterm infants should receive only limited amounts of oxygen during transport. Most infant conditions do not require any supplemental oxygen, provided that the infant's heart rate and oxygen saturation can be continuously monitored and remain stable. In the event that a newborn is having respiratory distress, carefully monitor the patient's condition and provide only the oxygen necessary.

Monitoring

After resuscitation, reassess the status of the infant throughout transport. Place cardiac leads in the same position as in an adult. A heart rate between 120 and 160 beats/min is normal in a newly born. If heart rate decreases or increases unexpectedly, search for possible causes, which often include airway or respiratory compromise.

Attach an infant pulse oximetry probe on a finger or toe. If unable to get an accurate reading, the probe may have to be placed around the hand or the foot. Saturations between 85% and 95% are normal after the first 10 minutes. Although there are negative effects of hyperoxia (high oxygen saturation) in the newly born infant, if the baby is distressed, the goal in the field should be to ensure adequate oxygenation through administration of supplemental oxygen and assisted ventilation when needed.

Hypothermia

Hypothermia develops quickly in newly born infants. Oxygen demand triples when skin temperature drops by 1 degree. Signs of hypothermia are similar to those of shock. Keep the baby warm during transport. Have a small knit cap available to cover the infant's head. Turn the heat on in the ambulance even at the risk of discomfort to the mother and crew. Prior to transport, place the baby on the mother's bare chest (skin-to-skin contact) and cover both of them to maintain the infant's temperature.

Transport Destination

It is impossible to account for all potential variables when discussing transport destination. When choosing a receiving hospital, EMS providers should consider the condition of the mother and newborn, patient preference, transport times, and the obstetric and neonatal capabilities of the potential receiving hospitals. In many situations it is appropriate to bypass a smaller community hospital to take the infant to a larger tertiary care center where specialty services are immediately available. In other instances, EMS providers should transport to the closest facility available where the newborn can be stabilized for later transport. Contact online medical control when required by protocol or when the destination choice is not entirely clear.

Specialty Care Teams

Many regions of the country have specialty high-risk obstetric or neonatal transport teams, often comprising a physician, nurse, respiratory therapist, or specially trained paramedics. Consider activating these resources early when maternal, fetal, or newborn complications are present or expected. Prompt access to specialty care dramatically improves the outcome for many critical maternal or newborn patients.

Summary

EMS providers are in the unique position to provide assistance to patients in labor outside the hospital setting, assist with delivery, and provide immediate lifesaving care to compromised newborns. Decisions and interventions performed by EMS providers have a potential to impact the health and lives of a pregnant mother and her child.

CASE STUDY ANSWERS

Case Study 1 — page 198

First decide whether to transport the mother to the nearest hospital or to prepare for delivery of the newly born infant. Ask if this is a first pregnancy. If the mother has delivered before, how long was the labor? Does the mother feel the urge to push? If the mother feels the urge to push, then examine for the presence of crowning. If crowning is not visible, wait and examine again during the next contraction.

If you decide to deliver at the scene, obtain a resuscitation-oriented history. Are twins present? What is the due date? What color was the amniotic fluid when the membranes ruptured? These questions assist you in preparation.

If the child is crowning at the perineum, prepare the obstetric delivery pack, familiarize yourself with the contents, and make sure all necessary equipment is present. Warm the environment and get clean towels to dry the baby. Get or make a cap to place over the child's scalp to reduce heat loss from the head once delivered and dried. Find a clean delivery surface for the baby.

Case Study 2 — page 203

If time allows, review the procedure for a vaginal delivery while on the way to the scene. On arrival, first plan for appropriate positioning of the mother. Discuss the position with the patient ahead of time so that she understands the plan for delivery. The woman should be lying supine with an object (e.g., stack of towels or a phone book) under her hips to allow for suctioning the mouth and nose if necessary. Alternatively, she can lie on her side facing away from you with her knees drawn toward the chest (Sims position).

Obtain resuscitation-oriented history. Are twins present? What is the due date? What color was the amniotic fluid when the membranes ruptured?

Clear amniotic fluid implies there is no meconium. Meconium is released by the fetus in conditions of stress. Although the presence of clear fluid does not rule out the possibility of a depressed newly born, it is a reassuring sign and increases the chances of an active child who will need only the initial steps of standard newly born care.

Equipment prepared should include the obstetric delivery pack. Neonatal resuscitation equipment should be readily available.

Case Study 3 — page 208

The baby is in acute distress and needs immediate intervention. Thoroughly dry the baby, position her on her back, and suction the mouth then nose if needed. Tie or clamp the umbilical cord at 3 inches and 4 inches from the baby and cut it. At this point, if the infant is still not breathing, begin bag-mask ventilation at 40–60 breaths/min and observe for chest rise. After 30 seconds of adequate assisted ventilation, assess the heart rate. If the heart rate is less than 60 beats/min, begin chest compressions at 90 compressions and 30 breaths/min. Administer three compressions followed by one bag-mask ventilation.

ALS

If the infant does not respond to these efforts with improvement in tone, color, and heart rate within 45–60 seconds, have one member of the team prepare for intubation and administration of epinephrine. Optimal cardiopulmonary resuscitation requires three individuals: one to assist ventilation, one to administer chest compressions, and one to prepare for intubation and possible administration of epinephrine. If only two prehospital professionals are present, as is frequently the case, get help from another adult to perform chest compressions if possible.

ALS

Epinephrine 1:10,000 can be administered at a dose of 0.01–0.03 mg/kg (0.1–0.3 mL/kg) via endotracheal tube, IV, or IO. Chest compressions and ventilations should be continued, with epinephrine given every 3–5 minutes until the heart rate is more than 60 beats/min.

Although vascular access is not usually needed for newly born resuscitation, this baby is also at high risk for hypoglycemia and hypotension during transport and may benefit from IV access. Attempt an IV or IO line in transport. Check the serum glucose at 30 minutes of life and treat for a level of less than 40 mg/dL. Because further resuscitation may be necessary, secure the infant to the stretcher and transport with continuous electrocardiogram and oxygen saturation monitoring. Consider transport to a facility with a neonatal intensive care unit, because this baby is likely to need ongoing critical care.

SUGGESTED READINGS

Textbooks

American Academy of Orthopaedic Surgeons. *Emergency Care and Transportation of the Sick and Injured*. 10th ed. Burlington, MA: Jones and Bartlett Learning; 2011.

American Academy of Orthopaedic Surgeons. *Emergency Care in the Streets*. 7th ed. Burlington, MA: Jones and Bartlett Learning; 2013.

Wyckoff MH, Aziz K, Escobedo MB, et al. Part 13: Neonatal Resuscitation: 2015 American Heart Association Guidelines Update for Cardiopulmonary Resuscitation and Emergency Cardiovascular Care. *Circulation*. 2015;132(suppl 2):S543–S560.

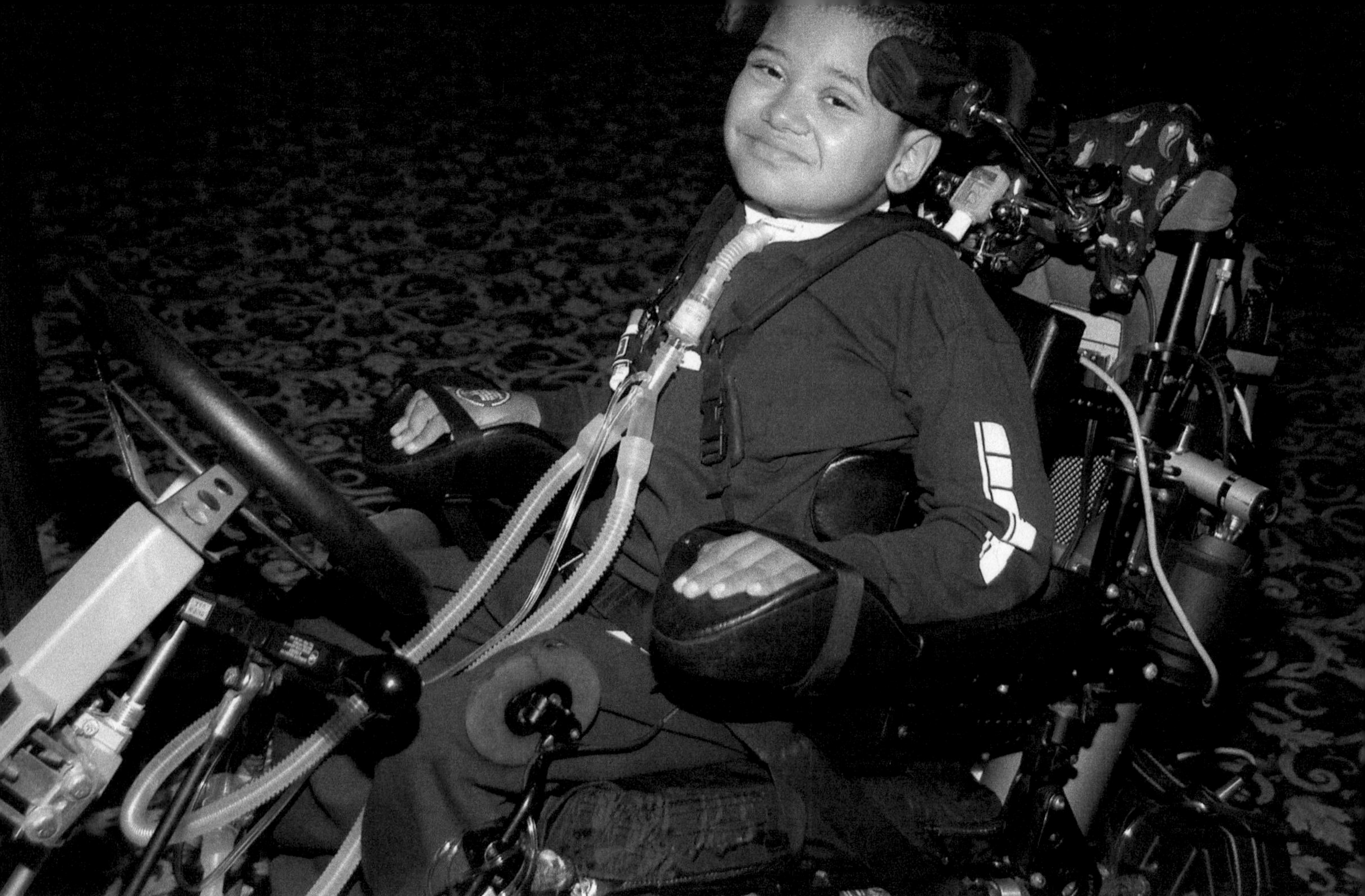

Learning Objectives

1. Define and describe two examples of cognitive disabilities, physical disabilities, and chronic conditions seen in children.
2. List important modifications of field assessment techniques for children with special health care needs (CSHCN).
3. Outline common transport considerations for CSHCN.
4. Describe the most common complications associated with assistive devices (tracheostomy tubes, central venous lines, gastrostomy tubes or gastric feeding tubes, cerebrospinal fluid [CSF] shunts, ostomies, implantable pacemakers and defibrillators) and the emergency management of those complications.
5. Discuss the management of behavioral emergencies in children.
6. Describe the use of health information technology (HIT) including an interoperable emergency information form (EIF) for CSHCN.

Children with Special Health Care Needs

Chapter 11

Introduction

According to an article by McPherson in *Pediatrics*, children with special health care needs (CSHCN) are defined as "those who have or are at an increased risk for a chronic physical, developmental, or emotional condition and who also require health and related services of a type or amount beyond that required by children generally."

The conditions can be either acquired or congenital. These children are a diverse group of patients who frequently need out-of-hospital emergency assessment and treatment. This high-user group includes but is not limited to children who were born prematurely; have suffered closed head injury and have central nervous system (CNS) injuries; or have chronic problems of the lungs, brain, or kidneys. Examples of acquired conditions include cerebral palsy or bronchopulmonary dysplasia. Examples of congenital problems are cyanotic heart disease or spina bifida.

Children assisted by or dependent on technology are a subgroup of CSHCN who need medical devices for their survival. Common devices include tracheostomy tubes, home ventilators, indwelling central venous lines, feeding tubes, pacemakers, and cerebral spinal fluid (CSF) shunts.

Today CSHCN are surviving longer and often live at home. They need emergency medical care more frequently than children without special health care needs. Because of their unique baseline status, CSHCN pose unique challenges in field assessment and treatment. Therefore, prehospital professionals should recognize common types of CSHCN, incorporate modifications during assessment, and understand management of frequent problems.

Cognitive and Physical Disabilities

According to the American Association on Intellectual and Developmental Disabilities, an intellectual disability is defined as a "disability characterized by significant limitations both in intellectual functioning (reasoning, learning, problem solving) and in adaptive behavior, which covers a range of everyday social and practical skills." The terms "intellectual disability" and "mental retardation" mean the same thing, yet intellectual disability is less offensive and is the preferred term.

Case Study 1

You are called to the scene of a 9-month-old girl with multiple underlying medical problems, including ventilator dependence through a tracheostomy tube.

On your arrival, her caregiver states that the girl has had difficulty breathing all day with fever and increased tracheostomy secretions. The child has cerebral palsy, with spasticity and a seizure disorder. She depends on a ventilator because of chronic lung disease as a result of prematurity at birth and respiratory distress syndrome. The child receives carbamazepine for her seizures and received her morning dose. Currently, she is receiving her feedings through her gastrostomy tube, which is connected to a pump.

Your assessment shows a child who is in bed and connected to a home ventilator. She does not engage visually and has subcostal retractions and nasal flaring. Her skin is pink. She has wheezing and crackles on lung examination. Her heart rate is 130 beats/min, despite a ventilator rate of 20 breaths/minute, she is breathing at an additional rate of 20 breaths/minute, blood pressure is 85 mm Hg/palp, and pulse oximetry is 90%. Her ventilator is set at 20 breaths/min.

1. What are the key principles in assessing this child?
2. Describe treatment and transport approaches.

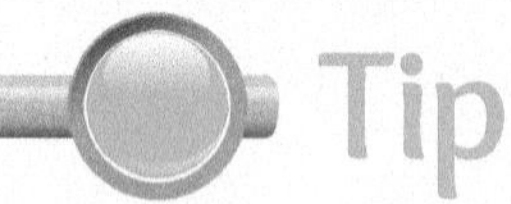

Intellectual disability is less offensive and is the preferred term when referring to those with cognitive disabilities.

Mental processes, such as judgment, reasoning, memory, and comprehension, are cognitive in nature and develop as the child acquires knowledge. Cognitive impairments are present when there is an alteration in the child's ability to think, reason, learn, and abstract. Several examples are outlined in **Table 11-1**.

Physical disabilities may alter the child's ability to be mobile or to accomplish activities of daily living independently. Medical and traumatic emergencies may occur that have nothing to do with the actual physical impairment. Several examples of physical conditions are outlined in **Table 11-2**.

Chronic conditions are present when the child receives ongoing treatment for an injury or illness. Even if the child seems to be healthy, he or she may be on maintenance medications or treatments to prevent complications. Examples of chronic conditions are listed in **Table 11-3**.

Assessment of CSHCN

Modifications

The most important resource for the prehospital provider is the child's caregiver. He or she usually knows how to care for the child's particular condition and understands the child's equipment. Often caregivers have forms or cards that outline the child's medical history, medications, and baseline general appearance, oxygen saturation, and vital signs.

Begin evaluation of CSHCN with emergency pediatric assessment techniques adjusted to the child's developmental level, rather than his or her chronologic age. Caregivers can usually provide the child's developmental age, weight, and baseline vital signs. *With children assisted by technology, do not become distracted by their specialized equipment.* Care for the child, not the machinery. Caregivers are often extremely helpful in figuring out the baseline status of CSHCN or in operating or troubleshooting the equipment. *Ask for assistance from the caregiver!*

The assessment of CSHCN has the following important modifications:

1. Baseline status: Ask the caregivers what is usual for the child. Most likely, they will know the child's baseline better than anyone.
2. Rely on the caregivers' opinions: What do they think is wrong? In what ways is the child "acting differently"?
3. If the child is physiologically stable, take a full history on scene. Caregivers usually know the child's medical history, health problems, medications, medical devices, and current complaints. They are also aware of what approaches work best.
4. The child may be slow to answer questions or may be unable to talk. Use a patient approach to the stable child and begin by talking directly to the child, rather than to their caregiver.

Table 11-1 Examples of Cognitive Disabilities

Disability	Definition	Behaviors
Attention-deficit/hyperactivity disorder (ADHD)	Hyperactivity, impulsivity, or periods of inattention	• Usually present before 7 years of age • Occur for at least 6 months • No identifiable cause • Children experience difficulty with impulse control, motor activity, and sustained attention
Autism	Pervasive, developmental disorder characterized by a lack of social interaction and a lack of communication skills	• Speech is affected. May repeat words spoken by others. May not speak at all. • Inability to maintain eye contact • Decreased number of play interests and activities • May exhibit repetitive behaviors (e.g., hand flapping, rocking, flipping a light switch, spinning in circles)
Intellectual disability	Limited mental function in two or more of the following areas: • Self-care • Social skills • Communication • Home living • Health and safety • Self-direction • Leisure • Functional academics • Community use	• Causes are many, and include disease, toxin exposure, genetic causes, metabolic disorders, and psychiatric conditions • Support and therapy are required to participate in activities of daily living

Adapted from Wertz E. *Emergency Care for Children*. Albany, NY: Delmar; 2002.

Table 11-2 Examples of Physical Disabilities

Disability	Definition	Characteristics
Cleft lip	The presence of one or more openings in the upper lip, caused by a genetic anomaly; openings may be an indent in one or both sides of the upper lip, or a deep, wide opening up to the nose.	• Infants may have difficulty sucking; creates difficulty feeding and therefore difficulty in receiving adequate nutrition • May affect the teeth, which may be absent or deformed
Cleft palate	An opening in the middle of the upper palate of the mouth, caused by a genetic anomaly; often exists concurrently with cleft lip. May occur in soft palate alone, or may extend through the hard palate into the nose.	• Creates difficulty feeding and therefore difficulty in receiving adequate nutrition • May cause choking, aspiration, vomiting • Ear infections and speech impairments are common
Hearing impairment	A condition in which the ear has a reduced response to pitch and loudness.	• Types: – Hard of hearing: person has impaired hearing ability – Deaf: person is born with inability to hear • Speaking ability can be affected • Potential solutions: hearing aid, cochlear implant, sign language, lip reading, or separate communication device
Visual impairment	A condition in which the eye has a reduced ability to see.	• Can be caused by obstruction that prevents light from reaching the retina • Degrees of visual impairment: – Partial sight: some visual impairment – Low vision: inability to read at usual viewing distance, even with eyeglasses or contact lenses – Legally blind: less than 20/200 vision in at least one eye or a very limited field of vision – Totally blind: no vision • Total blindness requires use of nonvisual media or reading by Braille

Adapted from Wertz E. *Emergency Care for Children*. Albany, NY: Delmar; 2002.

Table 11-3 Examples of Chronic Conditions

Condition	Definition	Characteristics
Asthma (reactive airway disease)	A disease caused by increased responsiveness of the tracheobronchial tree to various stimuli, resulting in inflammation, bronchoconstriction, mucosal edema, profuse secretions, and ultimately severe airflow obstruction	• Most common chronic disease of childhood; affects almost 5 million children in the United States • Possible causes of an asthma attack include upper respiratory infection, exercise, exposure to cold air, emotional stress, and passive exposure to smoke • Patient experiences tachypnea, tachycardia, increased work of breathing, and wheezing on exhalation
Bronchopulmonary dysplasia (BPD)	Chronic lung disease that develops in premature infants	• Potential causes: pneumonia, cyanotic heart disease, meconium aspiration, persistent pulmonary hypertension; also can occur in response to oxygen and positive pressure ventilation given after birth • Patient usually has respiratory distress • Long-term complications: – Hyperexpansion of lungs – Airway hyperreactivity – Infections – Gastroesophageal reflux – Cardiac conditions – Seizures – Poor growth and nutrition, failure to grow – Neurodevelopmental conditions – Visual problems – Overall decreased pulmonary function
Cancer	A pathologic lack of regulation of production of cells, leading to a neoplasm or tumor	• There are multiple types, determined by location, signs, and symptoms • Chemotherapy and radiation treatments are used; these can produce nausea, vomiting, hair loss, decreased appetite, fatigue, and burns to the skin
Cerebral palsy	A disorder of movement and posture that results from brain injury during fetal development or during delivery	• Symptoms: abnormal muscle tone, poor coordination, fixation and flexion of a joint, "scissoring" of the legs, exaggerated arching of the back, perceptual problems, intellectual involvement, language deficits • Patient may wear ankle-foot orthosis or braces to help prevent contractures • Patient may use a specialized wheelchair controlled by hand or head movements
Congenital heart disease (CHD)	Functional or structural defect of heart or great vessels formed in utero	• Major cause of death during first year of life • Cause unknown, suspected to be mother who is older than 40, has type I diabetes, is an active alcoholic, or who contracts rubella (measles) during pregnancy • Can be cyanotic or acyanotic • Signs and symptoms: tachycardia, tachypnea, dyspnea, costal retractions, edema, diaphoresis with exertion, distended neck and peripheral veins, mottled skin caused by poor perfusion, cold extremities, hypotension, slow capillary refill, clubbed toes and fingers
Cystic fibrosis	A condition in which mucus-producing or exocrine glands do not function properly	• Involves sweat and sebaceous glands • Progressive • Symptoms: thick mucous gland secretions, autonomic nervous system abnormalities, high sodium and chloride concentrations in sweat • Complications: pulmonary complications, drug-resistant infections, impaired digestion or absorption of nutrients

Adapted from Wertz E. *Emergency Care for Children*. Albany, NY: Delmar; 2002.

Table 11-3 Examples of Chronic Conditions (continued)

Condition	Definition	Characteristics
Down syndrome	A congenital disorder in which a person is born with three copies of chromosome 21; also called trisomy 21	• Patients have varying levels of cognitive delay • 50% have some form of congenital heart defect • Increased risk of medical complications: cardiovascular, endocrine, orthopedic, hematologic, neurologic, gastrointestinal
Hemophilia	A congenital condition in which the patient lacks one or more of the blood's normal clotting factors	• Prolonged bleeding can occur anywhere inside the body or from the body • Bleeding into joint cavities is most frequent, affecting range of motion • Children may receive in-home transfusions of the missing clotting factor
Human immunodeficiency virus (HIV)/Acquired immunodeficiency syndrome (AIDS)	HIV: a virus that is transmitted through direct contact with bodily fluids, and which causes AIDS AIDS: disease causing decreased immunity, which leads to opportunistic infections; debilitating with poor prognosis	• Present in children whose mothers were HIV positive • Symptoms include poor weight gain, opportunistic infections
Muscular dystrophy	Genetic, progressive, disabling muscle disorder in which muscle fibers gradually degenerate	• Multiple types occur • Symptoms: muscle weakness, muscle wasting, deformity, loss of strength, contractures • Psychologically, many children understand that they will eventually be completely dependent on someone else for their care and then die from the disease
Spina bifida	A congenital anomaly where the posterior elements of the vertebrae have failed to fuse together; the spinal cord and meninges may protrude	• Forms: – Myelomeningocele or meningomyelocele: sac on outside of body contains portion of spinal cord with nerves, spinal fluid, and meninges – Meningocele: sac-like cyst contains CSF and meninges – Encephalocele: meninges and brain herniate through defect in skull; sac present on back of neck – Most children have an Arnold-Chiari malformation (ACM) in which a portion of the brain herniates through an enlarged foramen magnum • Leads to neurologic impairment in the lower extremities • Surgery to repair the defect usually occurs soon after birth • Most children have hydrocephalus and have a shunt implanted to drain the extra CSF • Symptoms: decrease in skin sensation leading to pressure sores, loss of bladder or bowel control, and loss of voluntary muscle movement • Latex allergies are VERY common
Transplants	Performed in children because of defects in organ structure, organ failure, or disease	• Kidney, liver, and heart transplants are most common in children • Medications are given to lessen the potential for rejection of the transplanted organ • Complications: immunosuppression (most frequent), infections, organ rejection

Adapted from Wertz E. *Emergency Care for Children.* Albany, NY: Delmar; 2002.

5. Seemingly minor illnesses can be life-threatening in some CSHCN. An example is a cold in a child with chronic lung disease who is dependent on a ventilator. The child may have little reserve and may easily become hypoxic.
6. Communicate with the child using developmentally appropriate language, gestures, and techniques, as discussed in Chapter 2.
7. If a caregiver is not present, find out if the child has a form or card with information about his or her medical problem, normal vital signs, medications, and other important medical data. An emergency information form (EIF) is also available from the American Academy of Pediatrics (AAP) and the American College of Emergency Physicians (ACEP). Several states recommend that CSHCN carry

information cards, such as Wisconsin's Child Alert 10-33, New Mexico's Children's Updated Medical Summary (ChUMS), New Hampshire's Special Kids Information Program (SKIP), and the District of Columbia's EMS Outreach program.

8. Look for a bracelet or necklace that might describe the child's condition.
9. The usual baseline vital signs for a CSHCN may be "out of the normal range" compared to a child of the same age who does not have special health care needs. Standard vital signs may have limited value in assessment of these children. Pay more attention to the Pediatric Assessment Triangle (PAT) and observations from the caregiver.
10. Do not assume that a child with a physical disability is cognitively impaired. Many children with cerebral palsy, for example, have spasticity but do not have cognitive limitations. Discreetly ask the caregiver about the child's typical level of functioning, understanding, and interactions.
11. Be polite and professional. Listen to the caregiver and take his or her concerns seriously. Families of CSHCN often have had a lot of experience with the medical system. If most of their experience has been positive, they view the prehospital professional as an ally. However, if they have had bad experiences with the medical system, they may be suspicious or aggressive.
12. Keep in mind the amount of stress caregivers of a CSHCN may be experiencing.
13. Ask the caregivers what therapies or interventions have been already undertaken in response to their child's emergency.
14. If possible, try to transport CSHCN to their "medical home" facility. Always follow local protocol.

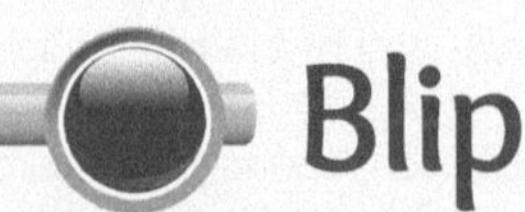

Do not become distracted by the specialized equipment used by children assisted by technology. Care for the child, not the machinery.

Pediatric Assessment Triangle

The PAT is a good way to look and listen for signs that help determine the type of physiologic problem and the urgency for treatment of a CSHCN. However, because CSHCN often have altered baseline physiology, there are several limitations and modifications to the PAT.

Appearance

Although the child's overall appearance reflects the adequacy of oxygenation, ventilation, perfusion, and CNS status, this is the part of the PAT that may differ the most

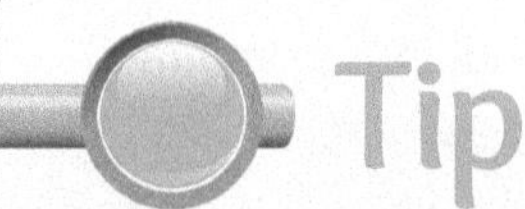

Approach the child with an intellectual disability using techniques appropriate to his or her developmental level, not age in years.

in CSHCN. The underlying medical problem may cause abnormal muscle tone, such as the increased tone and spasticity in a child with cerebral palsy or the decreased tone seen in children with Down syndrome. There may be decreased interactiveness, a common behavioral state in a child with brain damage or an intellectual disability. Look or gaze is helpful because many CSHCN can recognize their caregiver by looking or by hearing their voice. A CSHCN may be unable to speak, but the strength and quality of his or her cry or facial expressions may be a useful sign of health or distress. For example, a high-pitched cry in a child with a CSF shunt may mean obstruction.

Work of Breathing

Many CSHCN have respiratory problems. Children with chronic pulmonary disease, such as bronchopulmonary dysplasia (BPD), have rapid respiratory rates and increased work of breathing. When such children have a fever or

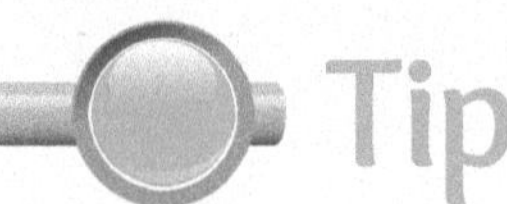

Assess appearance by asking the caregiver about the child's baseline.

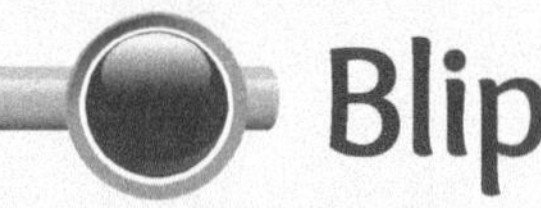

Do not assume that a child with a physical disability is mentally impaired. Many children with cerebral palsy, for example, have spasticity but not cognitive limitations.

experience an added respiratory illness or injury, such as pneumonia or chest trauma, they have less reserve. Therefore, work of breathing in these patients increases rapidly with any acute illness or injury.

Assess abnormal breath sounds (stridor, wheezing, or grunting) from across the room. Some "abnormal" airway sounds may be usual for a CSHCN. For example, a child with a tracheostomy tube usually has noisy breathing, and an infant with BPD may have slight expiratory wheezing. Children with BPD or congenital heart disease are much more likely to develop respiratory infections, especially from respiratory syncytial virus (RSV), in the winter. They can decompensate quickly. CSHCN who have an intellectual disability and neurologic problems are at high risk for aspiration, pneumonia, and respiratory failure.

Unusual positioning, such as tripoding and head bobbing, are important visual signs of increased work of breathing and hypoxia, and usually indicate serious breathing problems. For the child who usually has mild retractions, the degree or location of retractions provides clues to increased work of breathing. For example, the baseline retractions may be mild and only subcostal, but are now severe and also suprasternal. Nasal flaring is an indication of increased work of breathing, especially when associated with tachypnea, grunting, or retractions.

Circulation to Skin

The skin color may appear different in CSHCN, such as in infants with cyanotic congenital heart disease, chronic lung disease, cancer, or liver failure. A child with cyanotic congenital heart disease or chronic lung disease may have bluish lips and mucous membranes, nail beds, and extremities at baseline. A child with cancer may appear pale, whereas the skin of a child with liver disease may appear yellow. Ask a caregiver to describe the child's baseline color (**Figure 11-1**).

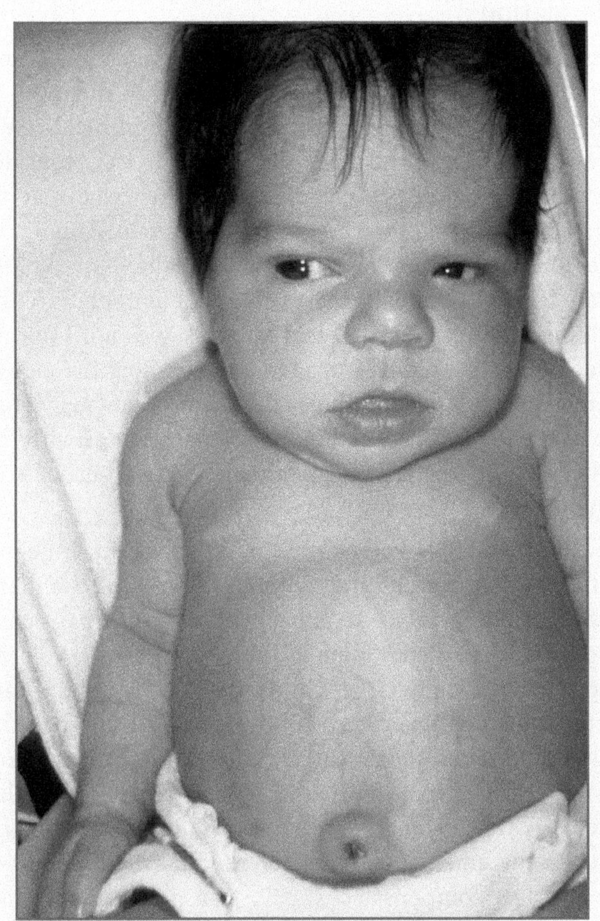

Figure 11-1 Ask a caregiver to describe the child's baseline color.

Adaptations in the Hands-on ABCDEs

After performing the PAT, complete the primary assessment by adjusting the evaluation of the ABCDEs to the child's baseline.

Airway

Open and maintain the airway. Keeping an open airway may be more difficult with the CSHCN. The child may have poor muscle tone and head control, or copious secretions. In children with Down syndrome, the large, protruding tongue may make airway procedures difficult. Getting, and then keeping, the right head position may require several maneuvers: a shoulder roll to correctly position the head in a neutral axis with the airway, and a chin lift or jaw thrust to open the airway. Always have suction available.

Many children with spina bifida have an Arnold-Chiari malformation (ACM) in which the base of the brain pushes down through a large foramen magnum. Do NOT hyperextend the neck of a child with spina bifida because any pressure on the herniated brain may cause the child to stop breathing. For these children, use in-line stabilization for any airway maneuvers even if no trauma is suspected.

ALS **Special Management in CSHCN: Tracheostomy Care.** A child with a tracheostomy has an artificial airway that is easily blocked by secretions or by dislodgment of the device. The tracheostomy section of this chapter addresses specific management techniques for these children.

Breathing

Count the respiratory rate. Listen to the lungs for bilateral air movement and abnormal chest sounds. Listening may not give accurate results in the CSHCN who cannot sit still or who has noisy breathing. Also, obtain pulse oximetry and compare to baseline. Keep the child in a position of comfort. Give supplemental oxygen to any CSHCN with increased work of breathing or increased respiratory rate by blow-by, face mask, or bag-mask device. If the caregiver knows the usual baseline oxygen saturation, only give oxygen to achieve baseline levels. Children with chronic lung disease or some forms of congenital heart disease can get worse if too much oxygen is given. For CSHCN, the caregiver may know the best way to give oxygen to the child. For infants or children already on home oxygen, increase the flow rate. For a patient with a tracheostomy tube, place the oxygen directly over the tube or stoma.

ALS **Special Management in CSHCN: Bronchodilator Administration.** If a CSHCN has a history of breathing problems or uses bronchodilators at home, give a nebulized bronchodilator when wheezing is present.

Circulation

Assess heart rate, pulse quality, skin temperature, and capillary refill time. These are not usually different in CSHCN and require no modifications in clinical interpretation. If the child's age is 3 years or less, consider obtaining a blood pressure. However, the value may be hard to obtain and interpret in this age group. Attempt to measure blood pressure at least once in all children older than 3 years of age. Tachycardia is a common baseline finding in some CSHCN, and by itself does not indicate shock. This is diagnosis-dependent, so asking the child's caregiver about the child's usual heart rate can be helpful. To evaluate heart rate and blood pressure, assess with the other key characteristics of circulation, as outlined in Chapter 3.

In some CSHCN, management of shock may be no different than for children without disabilities. Standard management includes oxygen, positioning, and bag-mask support as needed. Some CSHCN may need volume replacement, unless the child has a congenital heart defect and possible heart failure. The CSHCN has the same fluid requirements as any other child. If the patient is injured, transport immediately and attempt vascular access. Give 20-mL boluses of crystalloid fluid on the way to the emergency department (ED). If the child is ill and has compensated shock, transport and attempt access and fluid administration on the way. If the ill child has decompensated shock, make one attempt at vascular access on scene, if possible. In extreme cases, intraosseous access may be necessary. When a child has a vertical chest scar or a history of congenital heart disease, consider cardiogenic shock as an explanation for poor perfusion. Because a CSHCN may be more difficult to assess accurately, and because vascular access is often troublesome, always transport a child with suspected shock as soon as possible.

Some children with severe, uncontrolled epilepsy may be on the ketogenic diet. This regimen eliminates foods with glucose and keeps the child in a state of ketosis to control the seizures. For these children, do NOT use any fluids containing dextrose.

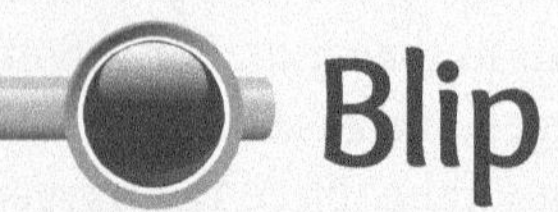

Blip

Do not give glucose or glucose-containing fluids to children on a ketogenic diet.

ALS

Special Management in CSHCN. Bradycardia is not usual for CSHCN. It is a sign of hypoxia or inadequate brain perfusion. Suspect hypoxia in a child with BPD or other chronic cardiopulmonary condition who has a heart rate below normal for chronologic age. Suspect increased intracranial pressure in a child with a CSF shunt.

Disability

Many CSHCN often have a compromised baseline neurologic status. Assess neurologic status by looking at appearance as part of the PAT, and establish level of consciousness with the Alert, Verbal, Painful, Unresponsive (AVPU) mnemonic. Compare the findings to the child's baseline. In the assessment of motor activity, assess purposeful movement, symmetrical movement of extremities, seizures, posturing, or flaccidity. Treat altered mental status if it is a change from baseline. The Glasgow Coma Scale may not be applicable for assessment of CSHCN because many CSHCN have baseline cognitive and physical challenges that would affect the score. It is better to describe the child as being different from baseline.

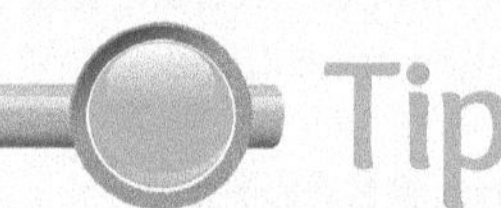

Tip

The usual baseline vital signs for a CSHCN may be different or "out of the normal range" for the child's chronologic age.

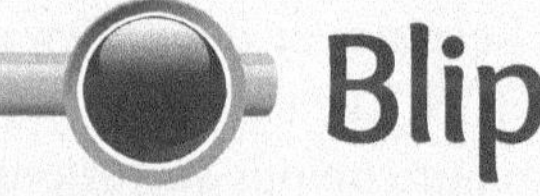

Blip

Bradycardia is not usual for CSHCN.

Exposure

Be sure to inspect the child's entire body, but respect his or her modesty. Do not allow the child to become cold. Many CSHCN have minimal body fat and can become hypothermic quickly.

Summary of Assessment of CSHCN

Listen carefully to the caregiver when assessing CSHCN. Ask about the child's baseline status. What is typical for this child? Such children may present a confusing picture, with unexpected behaviors, communication difficulties, extensive medical histories, and complicated equipment. The child's neurologic status is often compromised. If the caregiver is not present, look for sources of baseline information, such as a medical information form or a bracelet. Use standard assessment techniques and developmentally appropriate approaches modified by baseline comparisons to evaluate and manage acute problems. Transport early.

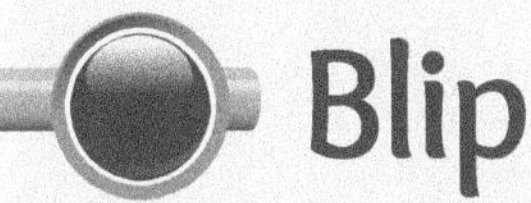

Blip

The Glasgow Coma Scale may not be applicable for assessment of CSHCN because many CSHCN have baseline cognitive and physical challenges that affect the score.

Transport

Table 11-4 lists key principles of transport of CSHCN. *Always restrain children in the ambulance.* The best type of restraint device and the best method for securing the device in the ambulance are controversial issues.

In general, if the child is critically ill or injured, restrain the child on his or her back secured on a gurney. Try to use a backboard for spinal stabilization if the child has suffered an injury to the head or has a spinal injury. Be careful if the child has any contractures or rigid posturing, such as scissoring of the legs or an exaggerated arching of the back seen in children with cerebral palsy. Pad any open areas and do not force the child to conform to the equipment. When immobilizing a small child, consider using a vest-type immobilization device, such as a Kendrick extrication device (KED), which can work very well. Check with the caregiver about positioning and availability of any special car seat. In some children, the supine position may compromise the airway because of an abundance of secretions, poor tone, or anatomic differences. The child's specially designed child restraint system or car seat may be the best option if it can be safely secured in the ambulance.

Many CSHCN have supplemental oxygen and oxygen delivery equipment. It is unsafe to transport liquid oxygen in an ambulance. Consider transporting nonliquid (or gaseous) oxygen and the child's personal devices or equipment to the ED.

Table 11-4 Principles of Transport of a CSHCN

1. Transport a CSHCN who is on home oxygen with the oxygen (except for liquid oxygen). If the child has no respiratory distress, continue the same rate of oxygen flow.
2. Transport a child on a home ventilator with the ventilator if there are no equipment problems. If there is a concern about the ventilator, provide assisted ventilation by bag-mask. Regardless of the method of ventilation, always secure the child's home ventilator in the ambulance and transport with the child, so that it can be assessed by hospital personnel for potential problems and appropriate settings.
3. If the child has poor muscle control, or increased muscle tone, immobilize the child as needed in a position that is comfortable for him or her. If the child has a special seat, wheelchair, or other equipment (e.g., feeding pump or suctioning device), transport these items to the ED if these items can be safely secured in the ambulance while still allowing enough room to safely care for the child during transport.
4. If the child has any contractures or rigid postures, such as scissoring of the legs or an arched back, pad around any open areas when the child is on the stretcher or during spinal immobilization. Do NOT force the child to conform to the equipment.

Summary of Transport

CSHCN often have special transport considerations. Make sure the child is safely restrained in the ambulance. This may require using a special seat. Address the issue of transport with the caregiver, and consider bringing supportive equipment to the ED if it can be safely secured in the ambulance.

Children Assisted by Technology

Children assisted by technology have devices that may malfunction at home. The most common devices are **tracheostomy tubes**, **cerebral spinal fluid (CSF) shunts**, **indwelling central venous catheters**, and **feeding tubes** (buttons). Equipment malfunction can cause a range of problems. Some malfunctioning may have minor or no immediate effects, such as loss of a feeding tube or clotting of an indwelling central venous catheter. Other malfunctioning may cause serious physiologic effects, such as respiratory distress from loss of a tracheostomy tube or intracranial pressure elevation from obstruction of a CSF shunt.

Tracheostomy Tubes

A tracheostomy is a surgical opening (stoma) in the front of the neck into the trachea. A tracheostomy tube (sometimes called a "trach tube") is an artificial airway passed through this opening that allows the child to breathe (**Figure 11-2**). Infants and children may have a tracheostomy for several reasons, as noted in **Table 11-5**.

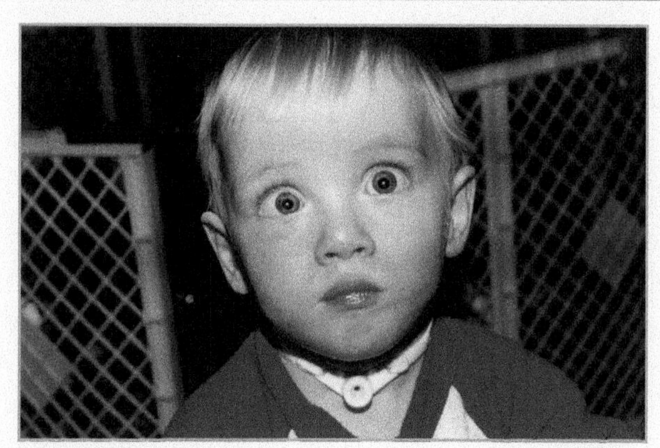

Figure 11-2 A tracheostomy.

Table 11-5 Indications for a Tracheostomy

1. To bypass an obstruction in the upper airway caused by trauma, surgery, or a birth defect
2. To allow clearance of secretions
3. To provide long-term mechanical ventilation of children with chronic respiratory problems, injuries to the lungs, major CNS deficits, or severe muscle weakness

There are several types of tracheostomy tubes, and they come in many sizes. The size is written on the wings or flanges of the tube. The size and name (indicating type of tube) are also on the box. The inner and outer diameters are often on the wings (**Figure 11-3**). The most common pediatric tube sizes are 2.5–10 mm (sizes 000–10). Tracheostomy tubes have a standard outer opening or hub outside the neck so a bag-mask device can be attached. For some tubes, an adapter may be needed to make this connection.

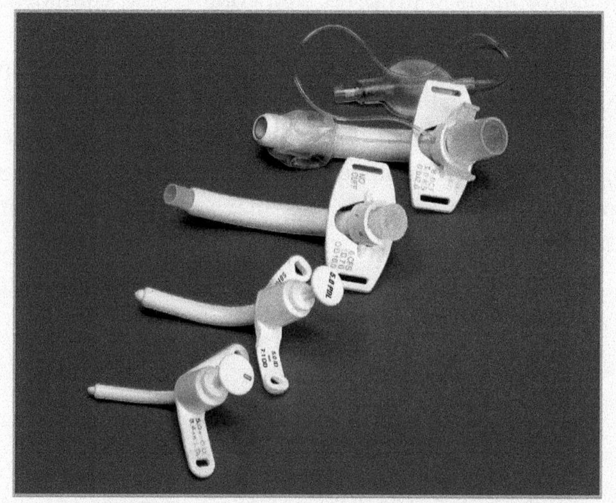

Figure 11-3 Sizes and inner and outer diameters are often written on the wings of tracheostomy tubes.

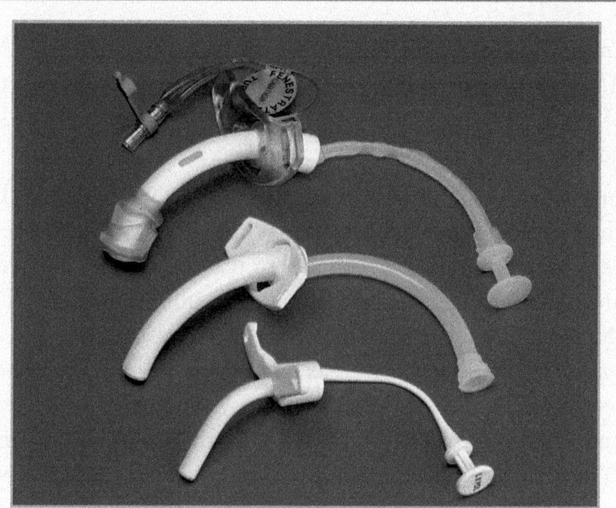

Figure 11-4 Fenestrated, double-lumen, and single-lumen tracheostomy tubes (top to bottom).

Types of Tracheostomy Tubes

The main types of tracheostomy tubes are fenestrated, double lumen, and single lumen (**Figure 11-4**). Tubes can also come with or without a cuff. These cuffs can be filled with air or foam. All tubes have an **obturator**, which is a solid plastic guide placed inside the tube to make insertion easier. Use the obturator to clear the tube of secretions in an emergency if a suction catheter is not available.

A single-lumen tracheostomy tube has one hollow tube or cannula for airflow and suctioning of secretions. Uncuffed, single-lumen tubes are usually used for neonates, infants, and young children. A double-lumen tube has a hollow outer cannula and a removable (also hollow) inner cannula. Remove the inner cannula for cleaning, and keep it in place to provide mechanical ventilation. Never remove the outer cannula unless the entire tube must be replaced.

A fenestrated tube has holes (fenestrations) for air to flow upward through the vocal cords and mouth. This structure lets the child talk and breathe naturally. Fenestrated tubes have a decannulation plug attached to the outer cannula

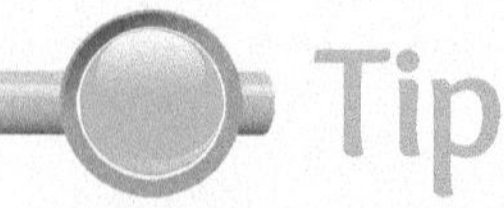

If the inner cannula of a double-lumen tracheostomy tube has been removed, a bag-mask device will not secure to the outer lumen of the tube. To ventilate a tracheostomy tube with the inner cannula removed, secure an infant face mask onto the bag, and then cover the tracheostomy tube's opening and seal the face mask on the neck.

that blocks airflow through the stoma. If the child cannot breathe through the nose or mouth, remove this plug so breathing is possible through the stoma. In addition, many fenestrated tubes also have a hollow inner cannula that must be in place for mechanical ventilation.

Oxygen Delivery and Assisted Ventilation Through a Tracheostomy Tube

A child with a functioning tracheostomy tube can receive oxygen from the blow-by method, by a face mask or tracheostomy mask placed directly over the tube opening, or by manual ventilation with a bag-mask device.

1. Provide blow-by oxygen. Place a stoma mask or pediatric face mask a short distance above the tracheostomy tube or stoma and give oxygen at 10–15 L/min.
2. Secure a face or tracheostomy mask directly over the tracheostomy tube opening and secure the straps around the neck.
3. Attach a bag-mask device to a tracheostomy tube adapter. Attach a bag-mask device directly to the outer end of the tracheostomy tube (**Figure 11-5**).

For a child who has a stoma (surgical opening in the neck) but no tracheostomy tube, or when a tube cannot be reinserted, apply a seal with a mask over the stoma and ventilate through the stoma; or cover the stoma with a sterile gauze, and ventilate with a mask to the mouth or mask to the mouth and nose technique. Begin bag-mask ventilation as needed.

Tracheostomy Complications: Obstruction

Obstruction of the tracheostomy tube is a life-threatening emergency. Obstruction can be caused by secretions, incorrect insertion (tube malposition), improper positioning of the child's head, or mechanical problems with the tube. Obstruction causes respiratory distress and failure.

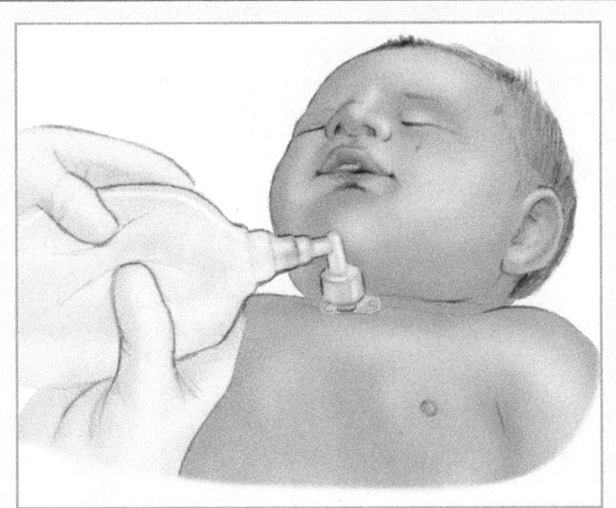

Figure 11-5 Bag-mask device attached directly to the external end of the tracheostomy tube.

Assessment. When a child has an obstructed tracheostomy tube, the chest is not rising and the child cannot breathe on his or her own. The PAT shows poor appearance, increased work of breathing, and cyanosis in cases of respiratory failure. The ABCDEs further indicate poor air movement and bradycardia.

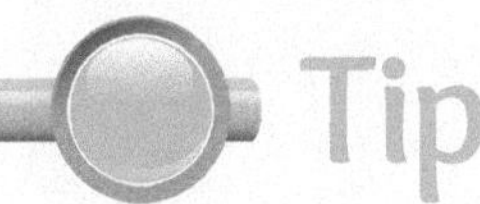

Tip

The most common complication of a child with a tracheostomy tube is respiratory distress caused by obstruction of the tube.

Treatment: Clearing an Obstructed Tube. To clear an obstructed tracheostomy tube, follow these steps:

1. Position the child's head with a towel roll under the shoulders. Ensure that the outer opening of the tube is clear.
2. Check that the tube is in the proper location. The wings or flange should be against the neck, and the obturator should not be in place.
3. If the child has a fenestrated tube, remove the decannulation plug.
4. If the child has a double-lumen tracheostomy tube, remove the inner lumen to clear secretions.
5. If none of these maneuvers work, suction the tube with a suction catheter.

Treatment: Suctioning a Tracheostomy Tube. If efforts to clear the obstruction are unsuccessful, suction the tracheostomy tube using the following procedure (**Figures 11-6** and **11-7**):

1. Ask the caregiver if he or she has suction catheters, equipment, and supplies. If so, use these. Otherwise, choose a suction catheter small enough to pass through the tube. (A size 1.0 [or 3.0-mm] tube will take a size 6 to 8 French catheter.) The caregiver may know the right size catheter. If equipment is not immediately available, insert the obturator to try to clear the obstruction.
2. If using a portable suction machine, set it to 100 mm Hg or less.
3. Give oxygen via a ventilation bag with a mask, and then loosen secretions by placing up to 1.0 to 2.0 mL of normal saline into the tube.
4. Insert the suction catheter approximately 2 inches (5 cm) into the tube. If the child begins to cough, the catheter is through the tube and into the trachea, and the depth of insertion is too deep. Do not use suction while inserting the catheter, and never force the catheter.

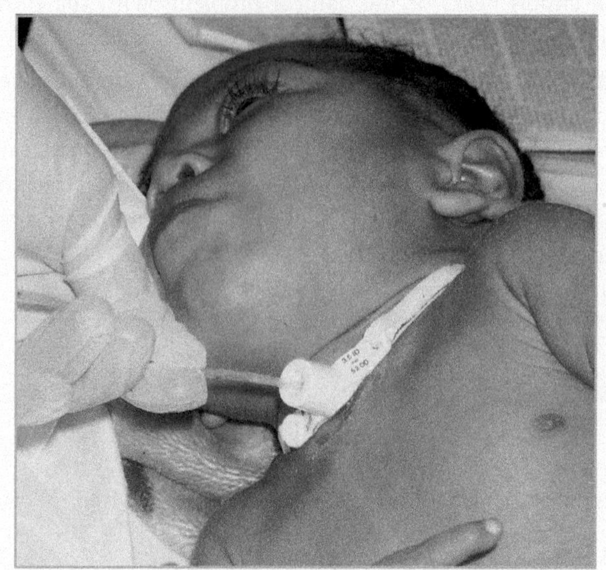

Figure 11-6 Suctioning a tracheostomy tube.

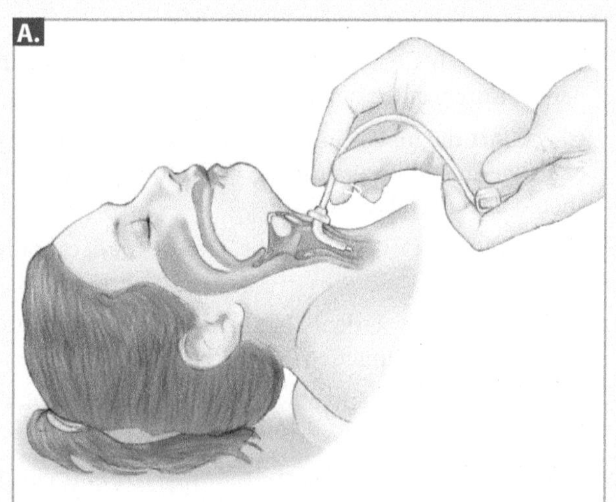

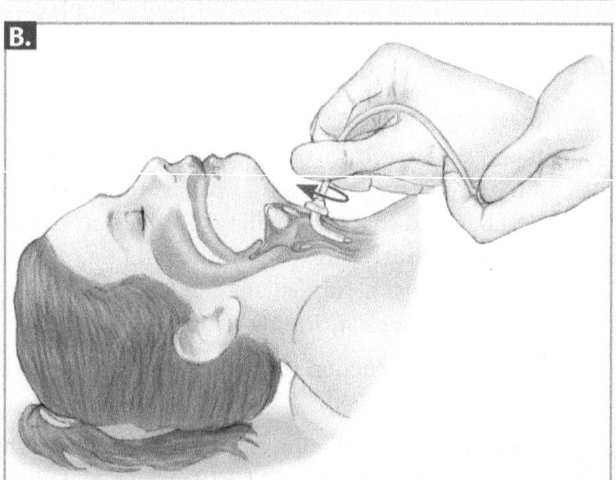

Figure 11-7 A. Insertion of suction catheter to proper depth; suction port remains open. B. Suctioning airway in circular motion as catheter is removed; suction port is closed.

5. Cover the suction port (hole on the tubing) and suction for 3 to 5 seconds, while slowly removing the catheter. Never suction for longer than 10 seconds. Always monitor the child's heart rate and color during this procedure. Stop suctioning immediately if the heart rate begins to drop or the child becomes blue.
6. If the obstruction is removed, and the child can breathe on his or her own, do not suction further. If additional suctioning is needed, apply oxygen (by blow-by or direct ventilation) and repeat steps 3–5.
7. Always provide supplemental oxygen after suctioning by using the blow-by method or with manual ventilations.

Replacing a Tracheostomy Tube

Treatment of a tracheostomy problem usually requires simple techniques to establish a patent airway, such as suctioning or removal of the old tracheostomy tube and replacement with a new tube (**Figure 11-8**). Occasionally, it is impossible to ventilate a child through an existing tracheostomy tube because of decannulation or complete obstruction. Under these conditions, the prehospital professional must place a new tracheostomy tube to save the child's life. For a step-by-step explanation of this procedure, see **Removing and Replacing a Tracheostomy Tube, Procedure 23.**

Central Venous Catheters

Many children receive nutritional support or medications at home through a central venous catheter. This includes children with poor weight gain caused by gastrointestinal or liver problems, children with cancer who require chemotherapy, and children with infections who are receiving antibiotics at home.

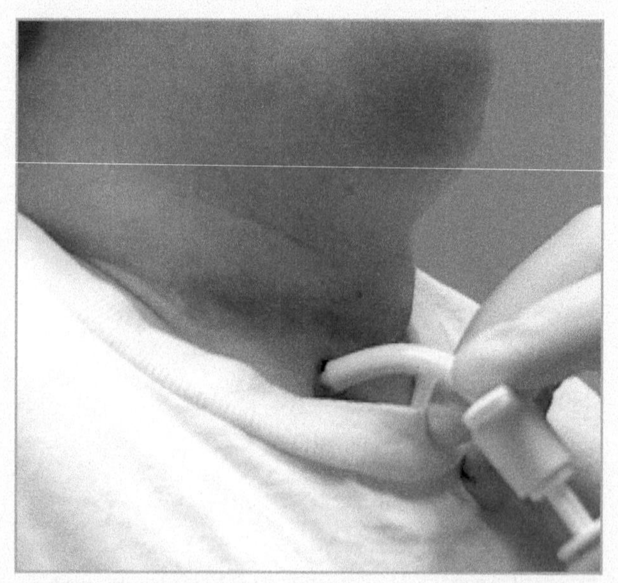

Figure 11-8 Replacing a tracheostomy tube.

Case Study 2

You are called to the home of a 6-year-old boy whose central venous catheter has bleeding around the insertion site. His mother panicked because it is a new catheter and she is not used to taking care of it. She tells you that he has a history of short-gut syndrome caused by an infarcted bowel sustained 6 months ago. He also has a gastrostomy tube through which he receives some medications, but he is totally reliant on his central venous catheter for his nutrition.

On arrival, you note a thin 6-year-old boy sitting quietly on the family's couch. His skin is yellowish. He has no increased work of breathing. His respiratory rate is 22 breaths/min, his heart rate is 95 beats/min, and his blood pressure is 90/50 mm Hg. Pulse oximetry is 98%. There is a tiny ooze of blood from the insertion site of the catheter in the right neck.

1. What are the key historical points?
2. Outline the assessment and management priorities.

Many central venous catheters require a surgical incision, but some can be placed percutaneously or through intact skin (often called PICC lines for percutaneously inserted central catheter). They can enter through the skin of the chest, neck, or arm, and the internal end usually lies in or near the superior vena cava or right atrium. Some are single-lumen lines. Others are double lumen, with two separate external openings, but only one internal opening or port.

Types of Catheters

Central venous catheters may be inserted into the femoral, internal jugular, and subclavian veins (**Figure 11-9**). The skin entry site for the catheter is usually on the chest or arm. This is called a peripherally implanted central catheter (PICC).

Totally implanted devices (mediport) are catheters attached to totally implanted injection ports or reservoirs. The catheter is in a central vein, such as the superior vena cava. Instead of coming out of the skin, as in partially implanted catheters, the end is attached to a reservoir (dome or port) that is in a subcutaneous pocket, usually on the chest. Therefore, there are no external parts visible, just a bulge or bump where the device rests.

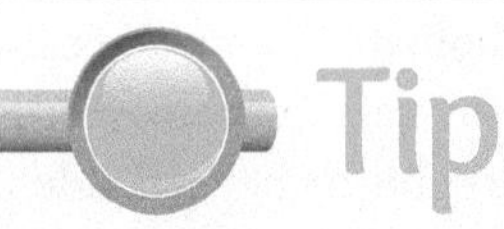

The most common complication in a child assisted by technology with a partially implanted central venous catheter is a broken or dislodged catheter. If the bleeding is from the catheter and the catheter is in place, inspect the catheter and its end. If a cap is missing, replace the cap, if possible.

Complications of Central Venous Catheters

Table 11-6 lists common complications of central venous catheters. The most common problem with partially implanted devices is a broken or dislodged catheter. Check the site for bleeding. If the catheter is in place, but there is bleeding from the entry site, apply direct pressure with sterile gauze. Likewise, if the catheter has been completely pulled out, and there is bleeding, apply direct pressure with sterile gauze.

ALS

Clamping a Leaking Central Venous Catheter. If the child is bleeding through a hole or cut in the catheter, clamp the exposed end. The caregiver usually has a clamp available, but if this has been misplaced, wrap the tips of a hemostat with gauze and apply to the catheter. If no hemostat is available, open the emergency delivery kit and use an umbilical clamp. If there has been bleeding, estimate the amount of blood loss.

Provide appropriate fluid therapy if there are signs of poor perfusion or shock. Do not use the central venous catheter.

Infection at Catheter Site. Infection can occur at the site where a partially implanted catheter enters the skin or in the pocket where a totally implanted device is placed. Signs of infection are redness, tenderness, swelling, warmth, or yellow discharge (pus) from the site.

The child can also have a blood infection with fever, chills, and shock. In this case, treat for septic shock, as described in Chapter 4. If the line is possibly infected, do not use it for vascular access.

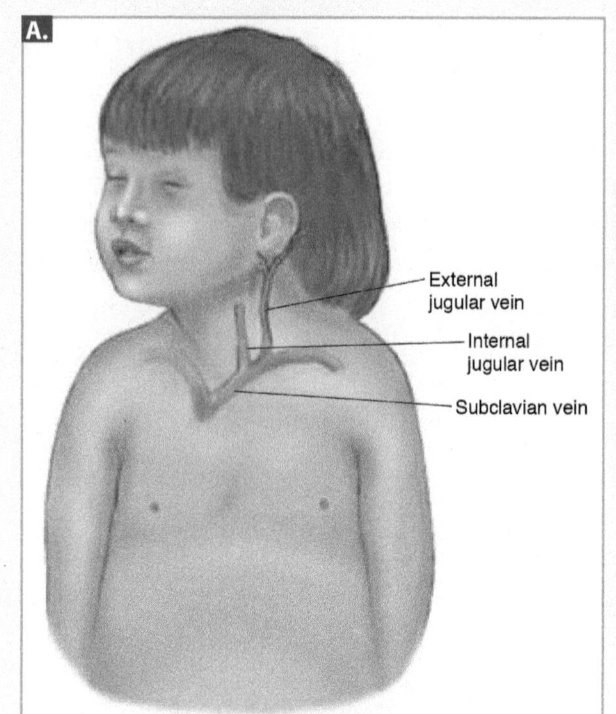

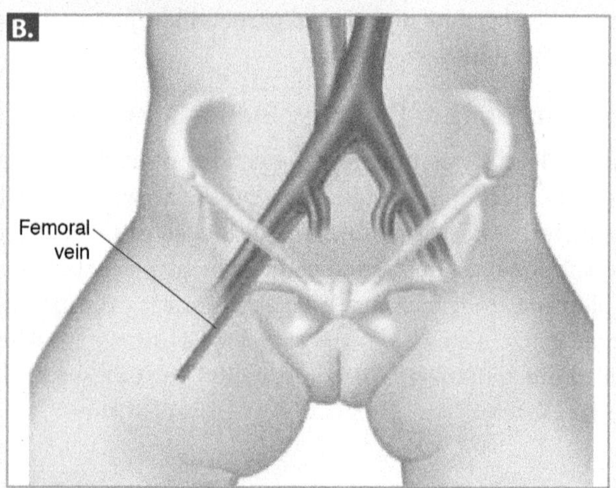

Figure 11-9 Possible insertion sites for a central venous catheter. **A.** Subclavian, internal jugular, and external jugular sites. **B.** Femoral vein locations.

Table 11-6 Common Central Venous Catheter Complications

Dislodged or broken catheter
Infection at catheter site
Problems with accessing or flushing the catheter (obstruction)
Air embolism
Medical problems related to **infusion**

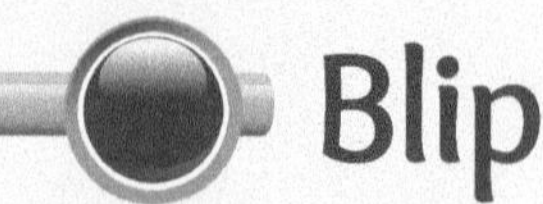

If the indwelling central venous catheter seems infected, do not use it for vascular access.

Obstruction. A problem with accessing or flushing the catheter usually means obstruction. This complication can occur with all types of catheters. All that is required is patient assessment and transport. The major concern is a child who depends on hyperalimentation (intravenous [IV] nutrition) for calories and glucose. If the line is malfunctioning, and the child has not received any nutrition, their blood glucose may be low.

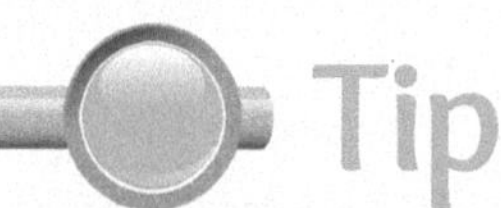

In a child who depends on hyperalimentation for calories and glucose, if the line is malfunctioning and the child has not received any nutrition, their blood glucose may be low.

Treatment of Hypoglycemia. Perform a quick fingerstick check of the blood sugar if there are signs or symptoms of hypoglycemia. For low blood sugar, basic life support (BLS) providers can give oral glucose per local protocol or advanced life support (ALS) providers can treat with IV dextrose or intramuscular (IM) glucagon as described in Chapter 6.

Air Embolism. This complication can occur if air accidentally gets into a central venous catheter when the line is being flushed or if the catheter breaks. Symptoms of air embolism include shortness of breath, chest pain, and coughing. Sometimes there is cardiovascular collapse and cardiopulmonary arrest.

ALS

Treatment of Suspected Air Embolism. Clamp the catheter or ask the caregiver to clamp the catheter, provide the child with oxygen, place the child on his or her left side in the head-down position, and transport to the ED.

Medical Problems Related to Infusion. Because of the various fluids and medications delivered through central venous catheters, several medical problems can develop, such as allergic reactions, abnormal heart rate or rhythms, or respiratory problems. Treat the appropriate problem, and bring the fluids that were being infused to the ED for analysis.

Feeding Devices

A feeding device provides an avenue for nutrition and medications to CSHCN who are unable to take food or fluids by mouth. This device allows the child to take in enough calories for adequate growth and nutrition and may be used to administer medications.

Types of Feeding Tubes

Some feeding tubes go through the nose (nasogastric [NG]) or, occasionally, through the mouth (orogastric [OG]) and into the stomach or small intestine (nasojejunal [NJ], orojejunal) (**Figure 11-10**). These tubes are usually long catheters that are taped in place on the child's face. Another type of feeding tube goes directly into the stomach from an external site on the abdomen (gastrostomy tube or G-tube).

Another example is a device called a percutaneous endoscopic gastrostomy (PEG) or button that is inserted into an opening in the stomach (**Figure 11-11**). It has a balloon on the end inserted into the stomach that is similar to the balloon on an intubation tube. It is inflated to keep the button in place. There is also a small cap with a valve on the outside to allow access. It can be replaced by the child's caregivers. Many caregivers prefer a button because there is no tube hanging from the abdomen that could be dislodged during physical activity.

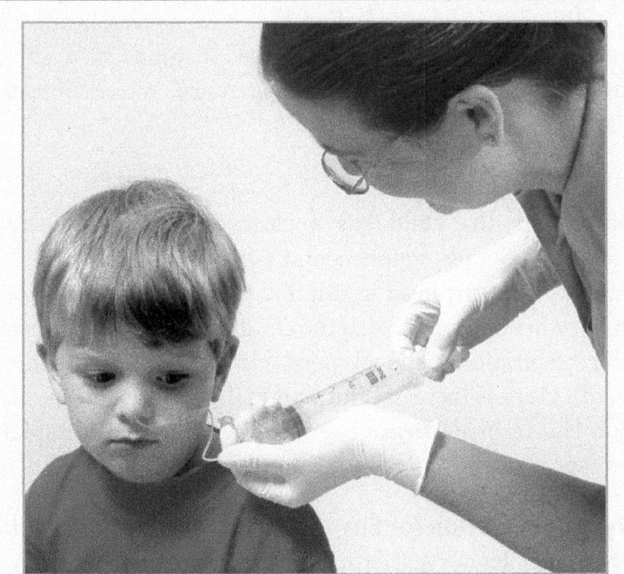

Figure 11-10 Nasojejunal catheter taped in place on the child's face.

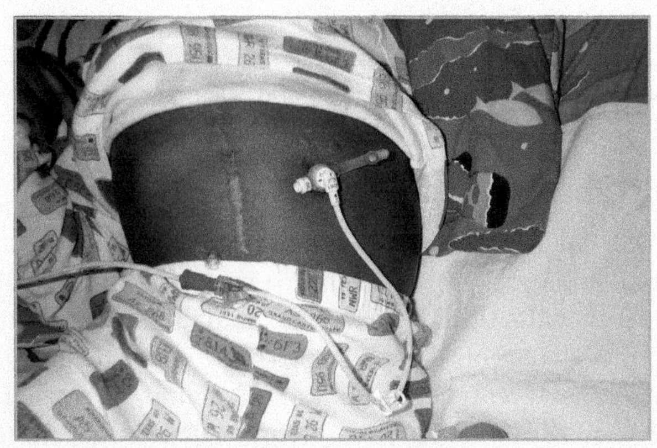

Figure 11-11 A percutaneous endoscopic gastrostomy, with connector attached.

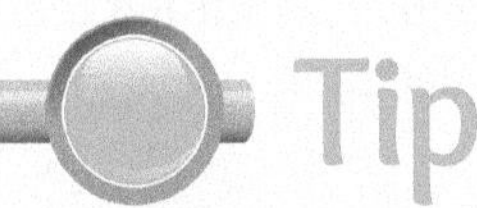

Tip

The main complication of feeding tubes is dislodgment.

Complications of Feeding Tubes

The main complication of a feeding tube is dislodgment. The child may have aspirated fluid if a nasal or oral feeding tube has come out. For tubes inserted into the abdomen, there may be bleeding or leakage of fluid. For a button, a replacement button may not fit into the stoma on the abdomen if it is the wrong size or there was a delay in replacing it. Perform an assessment, paying special attention to the work of breathing, chest auscultation, and pulse oximetry.

Treatment

If an implanted tube (G-tube) comes out, check the site for bleeding and apply direct pressure with a sterile dressing. If the insertion site around the implanted tube seems irritated or infected (the skin seems red, warm, or swollen), apply a sterile dressing to the site.

Whenever a tube dislodges or there is evidence of infection, transport the child to the ED. Ask the caregiver to bring the tube that fell out with the child to the hospital for sizing purposes. If the child was on an infusion of fluid or medication, ask the caregiver to disconnect the pump (infusion device) and transport it with the child. If the child has received fluid through a feeding catheter within 30 minutes of EMS arrival, consider transporting the child in a sitting position to prevent reflux, vomiting, and possible aspiration.

ALS

Removing a Feeding Tube. If the NG or OG tube seems to be in place but the child is having respiratory difficulty, ask the caregiver to check its position. If position cannot be confirmed, remove the tube.

CSF Shunts

A CSF shunt is a device that drains excess CSF from the brain. It is usually inserted from a ventricle (in the brain) under the skin, then down the neck into the peritoneum of the abdomen (ventriculoperitoneal or VP shunt), the pleura of the chest (ventriculopleural or VP shunt), or the heart (ventriculoatrial or VA shunt) (**Figure 11-12**). Its path (or track) can usually be felt on one side of the head and down the neck until the track reaches a scar on the chest wall or abdomen. A CSF shunt helps a child with hydrocephalus maintain normal brain pressure. The hydrocephalus may be caused by a congenital problem or by an acquired condition, such as bleeding, trauma, or infection.

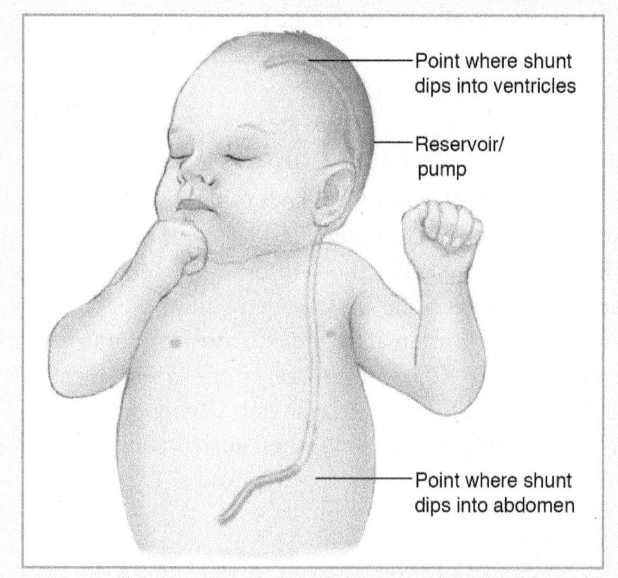

Figure 11-12 A CSF shunt directs CSF from a ventricle in the brain to either the abdomen or the heart.

Complications of CSF Shunts

The major complications with a CSF shunt are obstruction and infection. The most common complication is a shunt obstruction and malfunction. **Table 11-7** lists key questions to ask during assessment to evaluate the severity of the complaint and the urgency for treatment.

Table 11-7 Key Questions for Suspected CSF Shunt Malfunction

When was the CSF shunt placed?
Is the child acting the same as the last time there was a shunt problem (obstruction)?
Has the child had a fever?
Has the child complained of a headache, vomiting, or nausea?

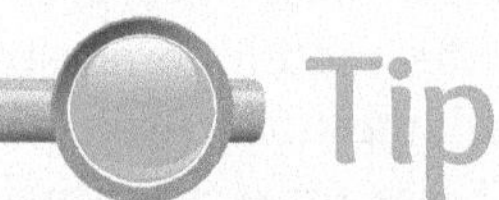

Many CSHCN, especially those with spina bifida, have a sensitivity or allergy to latex. Always use latex precautions with these patients. Reactions to latex can range from a localized skin reaction to anaphylaxis

Assessment of a Child with a Possible CSF Shunt Obstruction or Infection

Symptoms of a CSF shunt obstruction are the same as those of increased intracranial pressure and include headache, lethargy, sleepiness, irritability, nausea or vomiting, or trouble walking. Fever is usually a sign of a shunt infection or an intercurrent illness, but can occur with a shunt malfunction alone. Signs of a shunt obstruction are abnormal appearance, high-pitched cry, seizures, or altered mental status. A very worrisome finding is Cushing triad (bradycardia, elevated blood pressure, and irregular respirations), which indicates increased intracranial pressure caused by an obstructed shunt.

A child with a shunt infection may have a fever, headache, feeding difficulty, or altered behavior. Signs of a shunt infection include abnormal appearance, altered mental status, and shock.

Treatment

Make sure the child has a clear airway and effective breathing. Supply supplemental oxygen and transport the patient. Keep the head in midline position and elevate 30° to 45° whenever possible. If the child has bradycardia, irregular respirations, and elevated blood pressure (Cushing triad), there is increased intracranial pressure and herniation is imminent. Begin bag-mask ventilation and rapidly transport.

ALS

Hyperventilation for Suspected Increased Intracranial Pressure. Hyperventilation is a treatment for children with impending or frank herniation. However, the role of hyperventilation in treating out-of-hospital intracranial pressure elevation from hydrocephalus is not well understood. Hyperventilation, through carbon dioxide reduction and cerebral vasoconstriction, reduces brain

ALS

perfusion. However, overly aggressive ventilation may dangerously decrease perfusion and cause brain ischemia. If a child with a CSF shunt has signs of impending or frank herniation, treat with mild hyperventilation using capnography to keep $ETCO_2$ at 35 mmHg. This is the same treatment as outlined for traumatic brain injury in Chapter 7.

Ostomies

Some conditions, such as Crohn's disease, spinal cord injury, cancer, distal ureter or bladder defects, and necrotizing enterocolitis in an infant, interfere with regular elimination of urine and feces. Several types of ostomies are created to accomplish this bodily function. With a colostomy or ileostomy, an opening in the abdomen is formed when the small or large intestine is surgically brought out to the surface and sutured in place, creating a stoma. This procedure allows the digestive system to continue functioning while bypassing any inflamed or damaged bowel. An external pouch is placed over the stoma to collect digestive waste matter. The intestines below the colostomy site may not have been removed if there is a possibility of reconnecting the bowel at a later time. Colostomies can be temporary or permanent. With a **urostomy**, a stoma is surgically created to allow the elimination of urine.

Complications of Ostomies

Complications of ostomies include dehydration, infection, and pouch displacement. Because of an increased risk for dehydration, a child with a colostomy needs to be assessed carefully for clinical signs and symptoms of dehydration and shock, particularly if there is a history of diarrhea or decreased oral intake.

Signs of infection at the ostomy site include red, warm, tender skin spreading away from the stoma site. Ask the child or caregiver if the area is more tender than usual. If the child has signs of infection, transport the child for further evaluation.

Replacing a Pouch

Ask the caregiver to empty the pouch before transport, especially if the pouch is full. Before the pouch is emptied, document that amount of fluid in the pouch. Be sure the pouch is resealed after emptying to prevent leakage. In some instances, the pouch breaks or is torn off. If another pouch is not available, circle the stoma with moist gauze and then attach anything available that can serve as a substitute collection device. If no pouch is available, place several thicknesses of moist gauze over the stoma until a proper replacement is found. Another option is to secure a nonrebreather face mask over the stoma. The reservoir in the mask collects the excreted stool or urine.

Lastly, be respectful of the child's privacy. Keep the site, and pouch if in place, covered in public.

Internal Pacemakers and Defibrillators

Pacemakers are implanted medical devices that regulate the heart rate. Indications include bradycardia that does not maintain adequate perfusion, a previous cardiac arrest, and heart block especially after open heart surgery. They usually include a generator and leads. The generator houses the software and battery and supplies the electrical impulse. The leads are insulated wires that carry the electrical impulse to the heart and carry information about the heart's natural rhythm back to the pulse generator.

Complications of Internal Pacemakers

Several complications can occur for children with pacemakers. Some devices do not allow the child's heart rhythm to go above a certain rate. If that child is in shock or shock is impending, the body cannot compensate by increasing the heart rate. Begin treatment and transport immediately. Another complication is pacemaker failure. The child's heart rate drops and becomes too slow to maintain perfusion. Again, begin treatment and transport immediately. A third complication is pacemaker malfunction. The child may experience bradycardia if the pacemaker is not firing. In another instance, the leads may become dislodged and cause the child's diaphragm to contract instead of the heart muscle every time the pacemaker fires. The respiratory rate will equal the preset pacemaker rate. One unusual problem may be dislodgement of the leads after some type of chest trauma. Monitor the heart rate closely and transport.

Internal Cardiac Defibrillators

An automatic implantable cardioverter-defibrillator (AICD) or internal cardiac defibrillator (ICD) is an electronic device implanted under the skin. Its purpose is to monitor the heart rhythm and slow down or stop excessively fast heart rates that originate in the ventricles. Such rhythms include ventricular tachycardia and ventricular fibrillation.

The mechanical parts of an AICD include a generator and a lead. This generator is a tiny battery-operated electronic device located inside a case that monitors and records the heart rhythm. It sends out shocks to convert excessively fast heart rates when needed. The computer also records any shocks that it sends to the heart. A lead (or wire) is attached to the generator and is connected to the heart muscle to monitor the heart rhythm and carry shocks to the heart.

For any child with a pacemaker, ICD, or AICD, prehospital professionals should ask the caregivers the following questions:

- What type of heart problem does the child have?
- What rate is the child's underlying rhythm?

- What type of pacemaker, ICD, or AICD does the child have?
  - If a pacemaker, is the child dependent on the pacemaker? What are the settings?
  - If an ICD or AICD, what are the settings, at what heart rate does the ICD fire, and how many shocks has the child felt? In addition, has the child experienced any of the following:
    - More than three shocks in a row?
    - Continuation of unusual symptoms after experiencing a shock?
    - Sensations of dizziness, lightheadedness, palpitations, and so forth for a period of time yet has felt no shock?

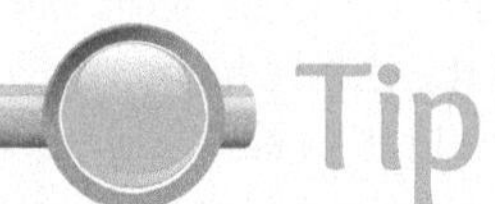

The internal pacemaker can easily be felt near the clavicle or in small children in the abdomen. Never place defibrillator paddles, "hands off" defibrillating-pacing patches, or automated external defibrillator (AED) patches directly over the internal pacemaker or defibrillator generator. The battery life for implanted pacemakers and defibrillators is 3–5 years.

Vagal Nerve Stimulator

The vagal nerve stimulator (VNS) was approved by the Federal Drug Administration (FDA) in 1997 for those patients with intractable epilepsy. Some children continue to have seizures despite conventional medication, surgical procedures, and diet. The VNS provides hope for better seizure control.

The VNS is an implantable device that looks like a pacemaker and is surgically placed by a neurosurgeon just under the skin in the left upper chest. It is programmed to provide baseline intermittent stimulation of the left vagus nerve, which leads directly to the brain. The patient or caretaker activates the device by placing over it a handheld magnet.

When responding to a call involving a CSHCN with an implanted VNS who is seizing, first assist the caregiver with activation of the VNS. Alternatively, contact medical control for guidance. Children with VNS devices should otherwise be treated as any other patient who is seizing with attention to airway, breathing, and circulation.

Dialysis Shunts

Chronic renal failure is a progressive and irreversible inadequate kidney function caused by permanent loss of nephrons. This disease develops over months or years and causes scarring in the kidneys, leading to diminished kidney function and the buildup of waste products and fluid in the blood. Renal dialysis is a technique for filtering toxic wastes from the blood, removing excess fluid, and restoring the normal balance of electrolytes. There are two types: peritoneal dialysis and hemodialysis.

In peritoneal dialysis, large amounts of specially formulated dialysis fluid are infused into and back out of the abdominal cavity. This fluid stays in the cavity for 1–2 hours, allowing equilibrium to occur. It is very effective yet carries a high risk of peritonitis. Many patients undergo peritoneal dialysis at home after the caregivers have received appropriate training. Prehospital professionals are not usually involved in this process.

In hemodialysis, the patient's blood circulates through a machine that functions much like a kidney and requires the use of some type of shunt or surgically created connection between a vein and an artery. External shunts may be located near the wrist, in the upper arm, or on the proximal anterior thigh. Some patients have an internal shunt also known as an arteriovenous (AV) fistula that is usually located in the forearm or upper arm (**Figure 11-13**).

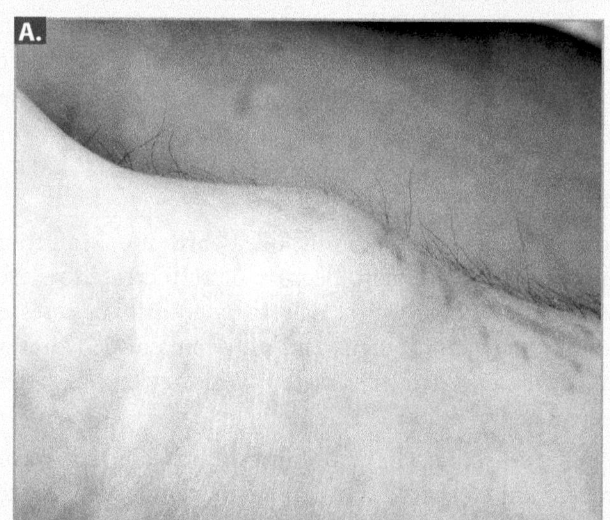

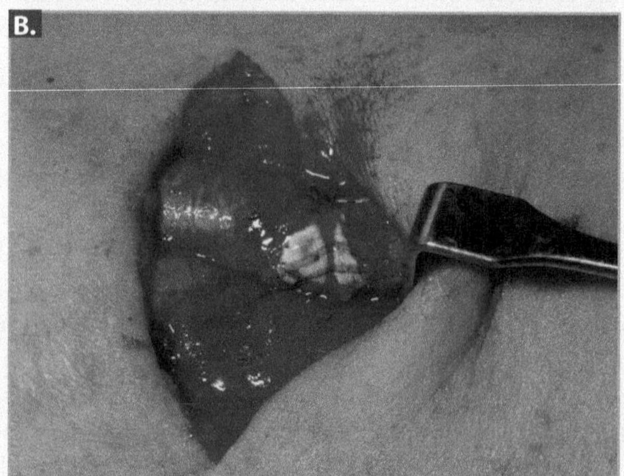

Figure 11-13 A. With an AV fistula, a bulge is created by arterial pressure. **B.** An AV graft creates a raised area that looks like a large vessel (operative photo).

When moving and transporting the patient, make sure the external shunt is protected and is not compromised by any straps. For all blood pressure measurements, use the arm without the device. If the patient has an internal shunt or AV fistula, do NOT attempt to access the fistula to draw blood or to infuse any fluids.

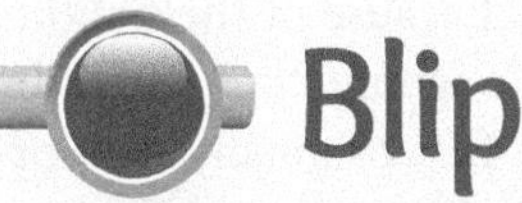

Never use an AV fistula for vascular access.

Summary of Children Assisted by Technology

Children assisted by technology may encounter many challenging problems with their equipment. The prehospital professional must be familiar with the basic purpose, design, and common complications of tracheostomy tubes, central venous catheters, feeding tubes, CSF shunts, and pacemakers and implantable defibrillators. Always ask the caregiver about the equipment, and transport all devices and infusions with the child to the ED. Ask whether the current problem has ever happened before, and how the situation was handled previously. Finally, remember that the child may be well-versed on the medical device that he or she uses. Consider asking the child your questions about the device; in doing so, you may gain his or her trust, which ultimately leads to better patient care.

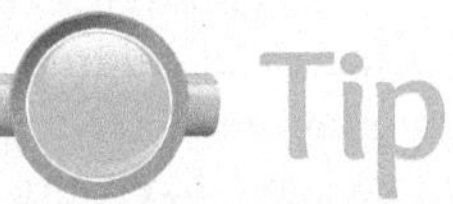

The best method of hyperventilation for out-of-hospital intracranial pressure elevation from hydrocephalus is guided by capnography. Aggressive ventilation may dangerously decrease perfusion and cause brain ischemia.

Behavioral Emergencies in Children

There has been an increase in the number of children suffering from behavioral and psychiatric conditions and a concomitant rise in the number of children presenting to EDs with these complaints. These children are a subset of CSHCN. There are many barriers to effective treatment, including few resources for inpatient and outpatient treatment of mental health problems, a lack of tools for screening in the ED setting, and a lack of education of health care providers. Many hospitals do not have psychiatrists or other mental health workers on staff to perform emergency evaluations. Psychiatric conditions are sometimes present in children with cognitive impairments and in children with normal intelligence. Sometimes the behavior of these children is "out of control" or violent. The child may be at school or at home at the time of the crisis.

Assessment and Transport of the Child with a Behavioral Emergency

First, consider provider safety. Attempt to establish a rapport with the child while assessing the likelihood for violence (**Figure 11-14**). If the child seems cooperative and gives permission to be touched for examination purposes, take a thorough history and perform a physical examination. Next, assess mental status. Is this child a risk to himself or others? Lastly, determine the need to transport the child. Consider restraints if the patient is a danger to himself or herself, or others. Always bring or ask the caregiver to follow the ambulance to the hospital.

Using Restraints for Assessment and Transport

Explain to the child's caregivers what you are doing and why you are restraining their child. Enlist their assistance. Talk to the child. Explain what you are doing and why, but do not negotiate. Do not attempt restraint placement alone. Often, securing the child in his or her car seat provides sufficient restraint, and may be preferable to the child, since he or she is already familiar with the seat. Before restraining a child, consider calling law enforcement officials. Do not allow the child to become positioned near an escape route. Should this happen, the child can escape, or worse attempt to injure the provider who has lost the ability to quickly escape. Apply restraint humanely, allowing the child as much dignity as possible. Document carefully the reasons for and the types of restraints in the medical record. Perform periodic assessments. Keep restraints as loose as possible to avoid injury.

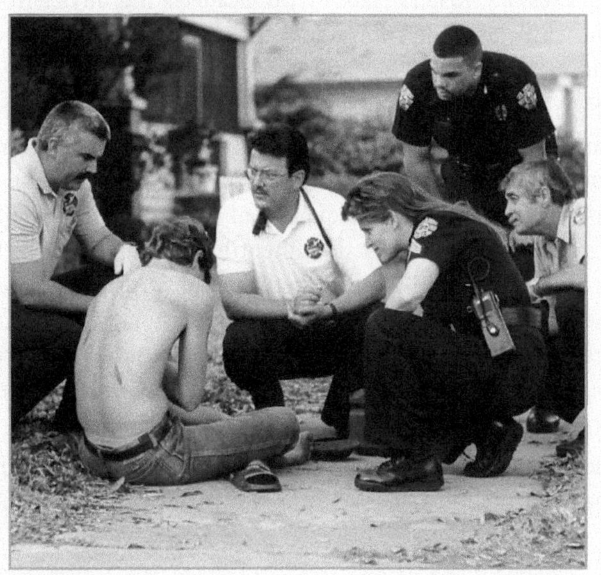

Figure 11-14 Establish a rapport with the child while assessing for the likelihood of violence.

ALS

The use of chemical restraint with medications such as midazolam has been used by some EMS agencies in adults. The use of chemical restraint in children may be considered if local protocols exist, with on-line medical direction.

There may be conflict between parental wishes and the needs of the child. If the child is in immediate danger of self-harm or is an immediate danger to others, notify law enforcement officials to help restrain if necessary and transport to the closest appropriate facility.

The Medical Home for CSHCN

Care coordination for CSHCN who often have involvement of multiple organ systems is quite complex. A specialist or general pediatrician's office can provide compassionate, comprehensive, continuous care in a culturally sensitive manner by being the child's family-centered medical home. Information is available at www.medicalhomeinfo.org.

CSHCN usually see multiple physicians, therapists, home care personnel, and other health care providers to manage their chronic conditions. To coordinate that care, these clinicians need to communicate with the medical home and one another in an effective manner. Traditionally, communication has occurred on paper with hospitals and offices faxing reports or sending copies to one another. This system is flawed in that some of these paper reports are lost, are misfiled, or do not arrive at the office or hospital in time for additional visits or procedures. For example, if the child sees the pediatric neurologist and is put on different medications to manage seizures, the primary care physician may not know about this change and prescribe another medication for an illness, which may cause a dangerous interaction that could be detrimental to the child. In addition to adverse drug reactions, the poor coordination of care may result in unnecessary hospitalizations, duplicate testing, advice from one clinician that contradicts that of another, and poor clinical outcomes.

The Institute of Medicine (IOM) identified ineffective care coordination as a cause of poor clinical outcomes and recommended electronic health records (EHRs) as one way to improve the quality of care for patients with chronic conditions. By documenting care and treatment in an EHR, the child's past medical and surgical histories, medications, allergies, contact information for multiple providers, schedule of preventive services, baseline neurologic status, and other information can be immediately available.

Electronic documentation can be beneficial, but sharing that information across systems of care presents yet another challenge. Some areas of the country have developed **health information exchanges (HIEs)** whereby electronic data are shared among hospitals, physician practices, and other entities where patients may be treated. The presence and use of these HIEs is sporadic at best, and many of them do not involve EMS systems.

In an emergency involving a CSHCN, obtaining accurate medical information is a priority because of the multitude of treatments, medications, and ongoing care. To address this, an electronic version of the EIF, originally developed by the AAP and ACEP, was offered through the Minnesota-based Midwest Emergency Medical Services for Children Information System (MEMSCIS).

Additional EMS Considerations for CSHCN

1. Many CSHCN, especially those with spina bifida, have a sensitivity or allergy to latex. Always use latex precautions with these patients. Reactions to latex can range from a localized skin reaction to anaphylaxis.
2. Speak quietly and calmly to the child, and explain what he or she can expect by using words appropriate for that child's developmental level. This approach decreases the child's anxiety and increases cooperation. Recognize that most CSHCN respond best with slower movements and firm, secure contact.
3. Children with musculoskeletal conditions, such as cerebral palsy or muscular dystrophy, need special care during preparation for transport. Children with cerebral palsy are often stiff and may have contractures. Do not force movements. Secure these children in their natural position, and pad any open areas. Children with paralysis or muscular dystrophy may not have regular sensation, so special care should be taken to ensure that their limbs are secured on the stretcher and do not hang off the edges.
4. Assess pain in CSHCN. If the child cannot communicate, then ask the caregiver if the child is in pain. Position the child for comfort. Use blankets under vulnerable areas of the body. If local protocols allow, administer medications for pain control after ensuring the caregivers did not give the child any pain medication before EMS arrival.
5. When leaving the home of a CSHCN:
    - Ask the parents or caregivers for the child's "go bag." This bag contains all of the supplies necessary (and that are not routinely stocked on ambulances) to manage the child's tracheostomy tube, feeding catheter, or central venous line.

Case Study 3

A distraught mother calls 9-1-1 because her infant son is having difficulty feeding and appears more blue than usual. She tells you that the child is a 2-month-old boy with Down syndrome and a heart defect. He has been home for a few weeks and is being allowed to grow before surgery to repair his heart. His mother confirms that he usually has a pulse oximetry reading in the 80s. She hands you a card with the child's medical history, medications, and hospital information, and states that he has been vomiting since the day before and has not kept down any of his medications.

You approach the child and note that he is cyanotic and poorly interactive. There are retractions and nasal flaring. The chest has crackles, and the pulse oximetry is 75%. His heart rate is 130 beats/min, respiratory rate is 70 breaths/min, and blood pressure is 86 mm Hg/palp.

1. What is the likely physiologic problem?
2. What are your primary interventions?

- Ask the parents for the child's daily medical information form, which contains pertinent medical information regarding the child's medical condition, baseline vital signs, allergies, doctors' names and numbers, medications, therapies, and necessary home support equipment. Ask how you can make the patient most comfortable.
- Ensure any compressed air or oxygen in the home is turned off before departure.

6. Request that the child's direct caregiver accompany the child to the hospital to continue assisting with the child's care. The caregiver not only becomes a valuable resource for repeated assessments and interventions, but also provides familiarity and reassurance to the child in the midst of an unfamiliar and potentially chaotic environment.
7. Recognize when the caregiver is overwhelmed with emotion or exhaustion. In these circumstances, it may be best to offer the caregiver a more passive role in the child's care while allowing him or her to continue to be with the child.

CASE STUDY ANSWERS

Case Study 1 — page 222

Assessment of the airway, breathing, and circulation suggests respiratory distress. Ask the child's caregiver about her baseline vital signs and activity level. Ask if there have been any changes and, if so, what is different.

Take the child off the ventilator and manually ventilate with a bag-mask device. Determine the ease of air entry through the tracheostomy tube and determine if aided respirations help the child's respiratory distress. Ask the caregiver when was the last tracheostomy tube change and the frequency of suctioning. Suction the tracheostomy to determine if this helps the child's breathing. Consider a tracheostomy tube change if there are copious secretions or there is difficulty with air entry during manual ventilations.

Consider an albuterol nebulizer treatment. Albuterol may help clear secretions and can open the child's airways to alleviate distress. In this case, the parent states that he has had to suction more frequently than usual and that he has already changed the tracheostomy tube that day. He states further that he thinks the child is getting sick and that her older sister has had a cold for the last few days. This history makes an exacerbation of the child's chronic lung disease more likely, and a mucous plug obstructing the tube less likely.

You decide to transport this child to her medical home hospital and continue the albuterol nebulizer treatment through her tracheostomy tube en route. You ask the caregiver to disconnect the feed through the gastrostomy tube to prepare for transport.

This patient has bronchopulmonary dysplasia (BPD), a chronic lung disease occurring in infants characterized by stiff lungs and chronic lung disease. BPD is a worldwide problem, affecting one of every three low-birth-weight (LBW) newborns, and ranking with cystic fibrosis and asthma as one of the most common chronic lung diseases in infants. BPD develops primarily in infants with a birth weight of less than 2 pounds or 1,000 grams who have respiratory distress syndrome (RDS), a lung disease common in premature babies. BPD occurs in 97% of all infants weighing less than 1,250 grams. Babies born before 32 weeks gestation may not have enough surfactant to keep these air sacs open. However, BPD development is not limited to RDS survivors; BPD may result from alveolar damage caused by lung disease, exposure to prolonged high oxygen concentrations, or mechanical ventilation after birth (caused by such conditions as neonatal pulmonary hypertension, pneumonia, or other infections or trauma to the lungs), all of which can cause harmful chemical reactions in the lungs.

A combination of fewer alveoli with a lack of surfactant can result in abnormally stiff lungs. This increases the work of breathing for affected infants, who can quickly tire out. As they progressively weaken, carbon dioxide builds up in the lungs and blood. Respiratory infections can also worsen the inflammatory response in the lungs, leading to more fluid in the lungs or bronchospasm. Wheezing results when tiny muscles in the bronchial tubes become narrower and spasm. Other emergencies directly related to BPD include pulmonary edema, aspiration of food or stomach contents into the lungs, and apnea. Signs and symptoms of BPD can vary in severity depending on the infant's lung maturity. They may include tachypnea, retractions, paradoxical respirations, abnormal posturing, and wheezing.

BPD causes the most difficulties during the first year of life. Most deaths from BPD also occur during this first year. Problems after the first year become increasingly uncommon. The most common long-term lung complication of BPD is asthma. Approximately one half of the children with BPD will have asthma. Other less common complications resulting from BPD include apnea during infancy, gastroesophageal reflux, pulmonary hypertension, high blood pressure, pulmonary edema, aspiration, subglottic stenosis, and tracheomalacia. Infants who have BPD are at risk for frequent hospitalizations because of their borderline respiratory reserve, hyperactive airway, and increased susceptibility to respiratory infection.

Case Study 2 — page 233

This boy is in no distress. The PAT is normal. His vital signs are stable. He is totally dependent on this central venous catheter for his nutrition and hydration. Ask the caregiver how long the catheter site has been bleeding. Check the catheter for dislodgement or breakage. Apply direct pressure to the site to stop the bleeding. Ask the caregiver to disconnect the catheter if it is still connected. Prepare the child for transport, preferably to his medical home hospital, so that the catheter can be repaired or replaced.

Another very common problem is dislodgement of a feeding catheter. This is especially true if the child is totally dependent on the gastrostomy tube (G-tube) for all nutrition and hydration. Also, the longer the tube is out, the more difficult it is to replace. Ask the family to bring the dislodged tube to the hospital, and if they have a replacement tube, bring that as well. Not all hospitals have the proper size tubes for children, so either call ahead to the local ED or transport the child to his home hospital.

Short gut syndrome results when a large section of the bowel has become necrotic and dies as a result of poor perfusion of the blood vessels. This phenomenon is more likely to occur in premature children, but can also occur in children who experience shock or hypoxemia to the bowel from infections, obstruction of the intestines, or trauma. These children often receive their nutrition through feeding catheters as this child did; however, if they have lost a significant amount of their bowel, they may need their nutrition (hyperalimentation and lipids) delivered through a central venous line. This boy no longer could receive all of his feeds through the gastrostomy tube and needed supplementation through his central venous catheter.

A young child who misses many hours of fluids may be tachycardic and have signs of dehydration, such as sticky mucous membranes and no tears, in the early stages of hypoperfusion. Interventions include oxygen supplementation, keeping the child warm, covering the stoma site with a dry gauze, and transporting the G-tube that fell out (along with any special adaptors) for sizing purposes. In addition, check fingerstick glucose level as it may be low.

ALS

ALS interventions include a 20 mL/kg crystalloid fluid by peripheral IV bolus in a child who seems dehydrated with a G-tube out or dislodged or a broken central venous line. If the glucose is low, provide IV dextrose or IM glucagon.

Case Study 3 — page 241

ALS

Assess airway, breathing, and circulation. You decide that this child needs assisted ventilations and begin to manually ventilate with a bag-mask device. As your partner is looking for an appropriate IV site, she notes that the child has pedal edema. You then consider that this child is in congestive heart failure and opt not to start this child on IV fluids without advice from medical control. Because blood pressure and perfusion are adequate, do not start a pressor drug. Transport immediately to the ED.

Down syndrome affects 1 in 800 births. This is lower than in the 1970s as a result of prenatal diagnosis and termination. Children with Down syndrome are at increased risk of medical complications. Some of the organ systems affected include cardiovascular, sensory, endocrine, orthopedic, dental, gastrointestinal, neurologic developmental, and hematologic systems. People with Down syndrome are developmentally delayed.

Cardiovascular defects are the leading cause of neonatal death caused by congenital abnormalities. When an infant is born with a severe cardiac anomaly, interventions are primarily directed toward home health care until definitive surgery can be performed or toward supportive treatment in the home of a child whose defect cannot be surgically repaired.

SUGGESTED READINGS

Textbooks

Adirim T, Smith E. *Special Children's Outreach and Prehospital Education (SCOPE)*. Burlington, MA: Jones and Bartlett Learning; 2006.

American Academy of Pediatrics and the American College of Emergency Physicians. *APLS: The Pediatric Emergency Medicine Resource*. 5th ed. Burlington, MA: Jones and Bartlett Learning; 2012.

Articles

American Academy of Pediatrics, Committee on Children with Disabilities. Care coordination: integrating health and related systems of care for children with special health care needs. *Pediatrics*. 2005;116:1238–1244.

National Task Force on Children with Special Health Care Needs. EMS for children: recommendations for coordinating care for children with special health care needs. *Ann Emerg Med*. 1997;30:274–280.

Spaite DW, Conroy C, Karriker KJ, et al. Improving emergency medical services for children with special health care needs: does training make a difference? *Am J Emerg Med*. 2001;19:474–478.

Spaite DW, Conroy C, Tibbitts M, et al. Use of emergency medical services by children with special health care needs. *Prehosp Emerg Care*. 2000;4:19–23.

Spaite DW, Karriker KJ, Seng M, et al. Training paramedics: emergency care for children with special health care needs. *Prehosp Emerg Care*. 2000;4:178–185.

CD-ROM

Center for Pediatric Emergency Medicine (CPEM). *Teaching resource for instructors in prehospital pediatrics (TRIPP), Version 2.0* [CD-ROM]. New York: Center for Pediatric Emergency Medicine; 1998.

References

Bhandari A, Bhandari V. Pitfalls, problems, and progress in bronchopulmonary dysplasia. *Pediatrics*. 2009;123:1562–1573. doi:10.1542/peds.2008-1962.

Burton LC, Anderson GF, Kues IW. Using electronic health records to help coordinate care. *Milbank Quarterly*. 2004;82:457–481. doi: 10.1111/j.0887-378X.2004.00318.x.

Institute of Medicine. Committee on Identifying Priority Areas for Quality Improvement. In: Adams K, Corrigan J, eds. *Priority Areas for National Action: Transforming Health Care Quality*. Washington, DC: National Academies Press; 2003:1–13.

McPherson M. A new definition of children with special health care needs. *Pediatrics*. 1998;102:137–139.

National Center for Medical Home Implementation. www.medicalhomeinfo.org. Accessed September 24, 2012.

National Down Syndrome Society. (2011). Down syndrome fact sheet. National Down Syndrome web site. http://www.ndss.org/Documents/NDSS%20Down%20Syndrome%20Fact%20Sheet%20English.ppt%20%5BCompatibility%20Mode%5D.pdf. Accessed September 12, 2012.

National Heart Lung and Blood Institute. (2011). Who is at risk for bronchopulmonary dysplasia. http://www.nhlbi.nih.gov/health/dci/Diseases/Bpd/Bpd_WhoIsAtRisk.html. Accessed March 26, 2011.

Wertz E. *Emergency Care for Children*. Albany, NY: Delmar; 2002.

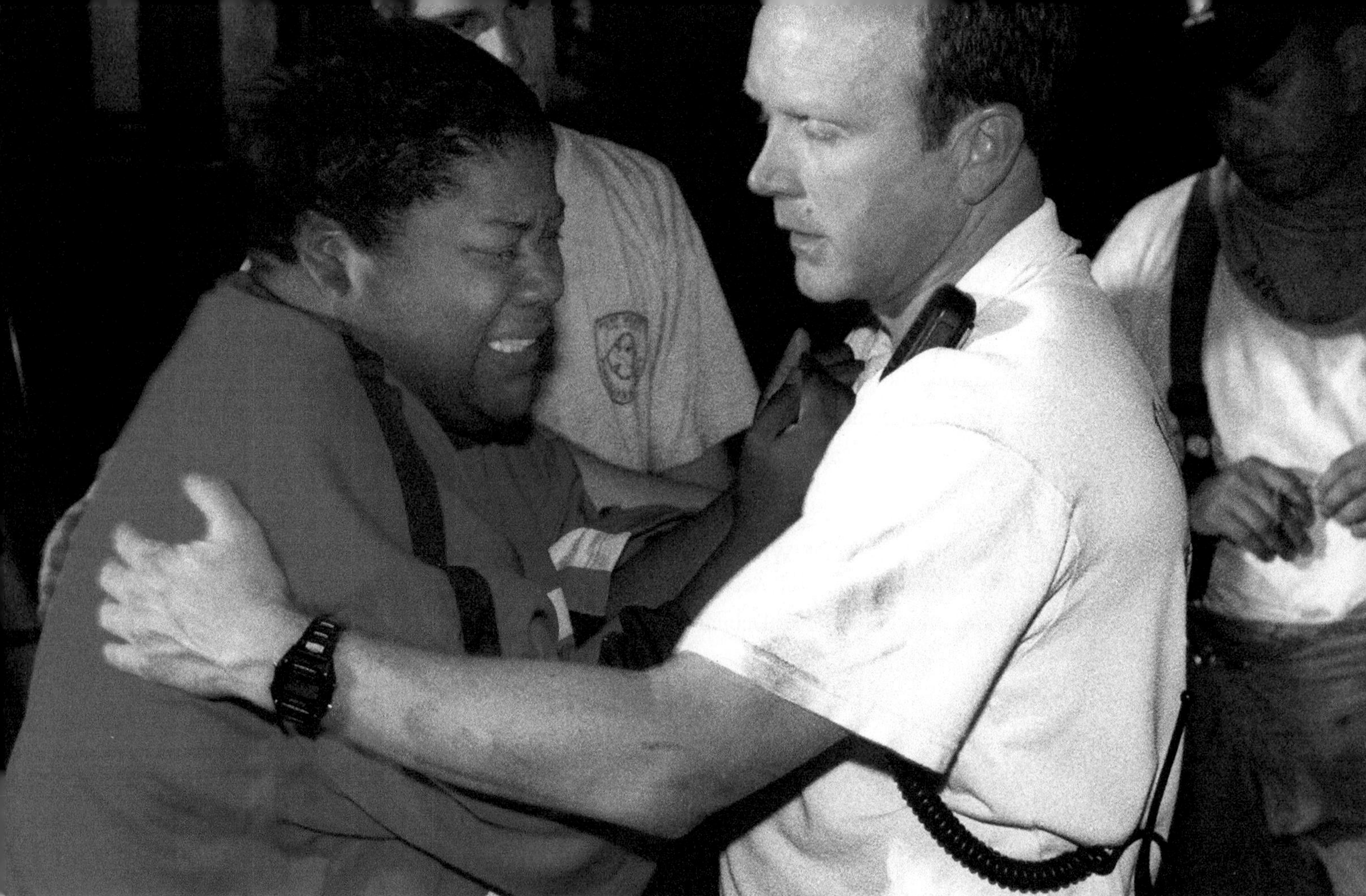

Learning Objectives

1. Describe the common clinical presentations and risk factors for sudden unexpected infant death (SUID).
2. Understand the differences between SUID and apparent life-threatening event (ALTE).
3. Discuss the actions of the prehospital professional in the setting of suspected SUID.
4. Define an ALTE and discuss assessment, management, and transport considerations.
5. Recognize responses of the family to the death of an infant or child.
6. Recognize emotional responses of prehospital professionals to the death of an infant or child.
7. List community resources for support after the unexpected death of an infant or child.

Sudden Unexpected Infant Death (SUID) and Death of a Child

Chapter 12

Introduction

Sudden unexpected infant death (SUID) and the death of a child are extremely difficult, emotional experiences for the prehospital professional. SUID is the leading cause of infant death between 1 month and 1 year of age and the fourth leading cause of death (followed by child maltreatment) in 2013.

The death of a child is an unparalleled family crisis and creates difficult emotional issues for the caregivers and the prehospital professional. The infant may be in the care of a parent, child care provider, or babysitter at the time of death and may not be at home. Absence of one or both parents may complicate field management and interactions at the scene.

Definition of SUID

SUID is the unexpected death of an infant less than one year of age that occurs suddenly and unexpectedly and whose cause of death is not immediately obvious before investigation. On the other hand, sudden infant death syndrome (SIDS) is defined as "the sudden and unexpected death of an infant under one year of age which remains unexplained after a thorough postmortem evaluation, including performance of a complete autopsy, examination of the death scene, and review of the clinical history." SUID is considered a broader term, as it encompasses SIDS, unknown cause of death, and accidental suffocation and strangulation in bed. Hence, SUID cannot be diagnosed at the scene or in the emergency department.

SUID Epidemiology

Sometimes a sudden, unexpected infant death is not caused by SUID, and the medical examiner identifies a specific illness or injury as the cause. This group includes deaths caused by child maltreatment, as discussed in Chapter 13. On the scene, the prehospital professional cannot determine the true cause of death of an infant. Treat every caregiver as a grieving parent. *Never*

Case Study 1

You are dispatched for an infant not breathing. On your arrival you find a 6-month-old boy in his mother's arms, with dark purplish bruising on his face and chest. He has pink frothy sputum around his mouth and nose, and he is cold, pulseless, and apneic. His arms and jaw are stiff. His mother is weeping, "I think he is dead."

1. **Is this a SUID death?**
2. **What can you do to assist the family with the death of their child?**

discuss child maltreatment as a possible cause of death while on scene. Be sure, however, to note details of the death scene and record observations in the patient-care report. To help identify deaths that may not be from natural causes, document any observations related to the scene size-up, physical assessment, or focused history that seem atypical or inconsistent with SUID. For example, dangerous or unclean home conditions, bruises or burn marks on the child's body, or changing or implausible stories are possible red flags for child maltreatment that require explicit documentation, as discussed in Chapter 13.

SUID is the leading cause of death in the post neonatal period (28 days-11 months). A breakdown of SUID cases in 2013 demonstrated that 45% were SIDS, 31% unknown, and 24% accidental suffocation/strangulation in bed.

Key information about mechanism for suffocation includes adults sharing a bed with the infant, soft bedding, and wedging and entrapment of the infant between two objects. Information provided by prehospital providers can assist in the later determination of the cause of death, so the scene survey is very important.

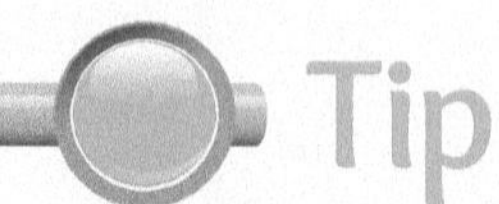

SIDS is the leading cause of infant death from age 1 month to 1 year.

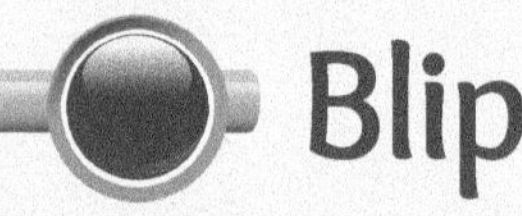

Never discuss child maltreatment as a possible cause of death on the scene.

Common Clinical Presentation of SUID

When evaluating an unresponsive infant, a thorough scene size-up is imperative. The scene may be potentially hostile because of the emotions present. Although emotional family members are rarely hostile toward prehospital providers, scene safety is a dynamic process, and the prehospital provider should constantly reevaluate the scene for hazards. A thorough scene evaluation can provide important clinical clues as to what may have caused the infant to become pulseless and apneic. Pay close attention to the environment. The provider should note any potential toxins that may have been within reach. Note any unusual conditions, such as high room temperature or odors. Look for street drugs, and if possible bring all medications to the ED. The provider should also pay attention to signs of abuse, as noted in Chapter 13.

The prehospital provider should note the time the infant was found, the position in which the infant was found, and the last time the infant was responsive. Pay close attention to the infant's position. Note if the infant is in a prone position. Evaluate how many pillows and plush toys are in the sleeping quarters. The provider should also note if the infant had a blanket over his or her head or if there was soft or loose bedding.

The infant will be unresponsive, pulseless, and apneic on arrival, and cardiopulmonary resuscitation (CPR) may be in progress. The provider should make it a point to evaluate central pulses. Pupils will be fixed and dilated. The ALS provider will also notice asystole on the electrocardiogram (ECG) monitor. This should be confirmed in at least two leads, and additional strips may be required to hand over to the coroner. Along with the signs listed previously, the provider may also note lividity or rigor mortis. Lividity is reddish blue mottling, caused by venous pooling, noted on the face and the dependent portion of the body. **Table 12-1** lists the signs of SUID. Some signs differ, depending on how long the infant has been dead. Some cases of SIDS do not show any of these signs.

Table 12-1 External Appearance of SUID Victims

Cold skin
Frothy or blood-tinged fluid in the mouth and nose
Lividity or dark, reddish blue mottling on the dependent side of the body
Normal hydration and nutrition
Rigor mortis
Vomitus (uncommon)

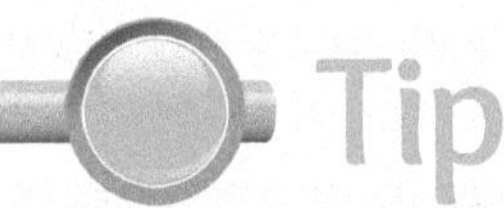

The typical SUID scenario is an apparently healthy baby, usually less than 1 year of age, who is found dead in his or her bed after having been seen alive a short time before.

Get a focused history at the scene if the child is not transported to the ED. *Refrain from asking judgmental or leading questions.* **Table 12-2** gives examples of key questions to ask. Always ask the baby's name at the beginning of the interview, and use his or her first name in all discussions with the caregiver.

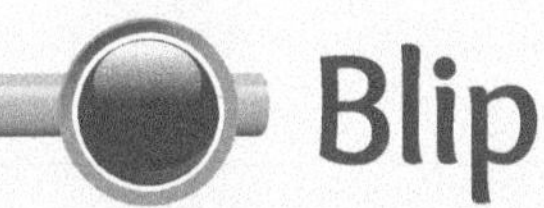

Refrain from asking judgmental or leading questions that suggest that the caregiver may be at fault for the infant's death.

A thorough history is important for identifying potential causes of the infant's death. The provider should pay close attention to the patient history, which may include recent infections, potential birth defects, or a variety of other complications. The infant's prenatal history and the maternal gestational history should be noted in detail.

Actions in Suspected SUID

The prehospital professional's first actions when SUID is suspected must always be to assess and treat the baby. Immediately begin resuscitation, using standard treatment protocols according to the current American Heart

Table 12-2 Key Questions in Focused History*

What happened?
Who found the infant and where?
What did the caregiver do?
Has the infant been moved?
What time was the infant last seen alive?
Had the infant been sick?
Was the infant receiving any medications?

*When asking these questions, use the infant's name rather than "the infant."

Association Guidelines and local protocols, unless the infant meets local emergency medical services (EMS) system criteria for death in the field. In many SUID cases, the baby has easily recognizable signs of death, and interventions or resuscitation are not indicated. If resuscitation is indicated, encourage the family to remain present during the resuscitative attempt, whenever possible.

After assessing the child's cardiopulmonary status, unless the patient meets local EMS system death in the field criteria, begin CPR if there is no detectable heart rate or other signs of life. If resuscitation is started and the child responds, transport as soon as medically appropriate, as discussed in Chapter 15.

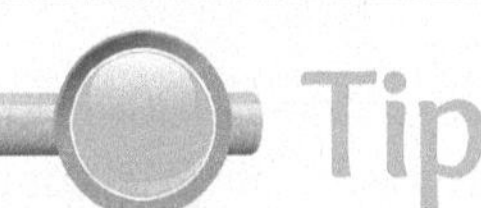

In all cases of cardiopulmonary arrest, immediately begin resuscitation using standard treatment protocol, unless the infant meets local EMS criteria for death in the field.

If resuscitation is considered to be futile on the prehospital professional's arrival at the scene or if the initial response to CPR is unsuccessful, it may be appropriate to leave the scene and allow the coroner or medical examiner to facilitate the death investigation. *The prehospital professional, however, should not leave the scene after a child has died until the appropriate authorities have arrived.* Notify medical oversight when there is uncertainty about treatment or transport. **Table 12-3** lists the pros and cons of transporting suspected SIDS infants. Because the prehospital professional cannot distinguish a child with SIDS from any other child in cardiopulmonary arrest, use standard principles of treatment and transport for children in cardiopulmonary arrest, as discussed in Chapter 5.

Table 12-3 Pros and Cons of Transporting Suspected SUID Infants

Pros	Cons
ALS capability in ED	Caregiver concern about infant's body
Facilitation of autopsy	Disruption of scene investigation by medical examiner
More medical personnel to manage infant and caregivers	High costs in dollars, personnel, and equipment
Physician involvement in management	Possible violation of family's culture
Religious services	Removal of family from familiar setting
Social services for grief counseling	Transport liabilities, especially ambulance crashes and adverse bystander reactions

ALS

Value of Transport After Failed ALS Treatment in Cardiopulmonary Arrest. The value of immediate or delayed hospital transport when a child does not respond to resuscitation is controversial. The chances of neurologic survival of a child in the ED, after failed ALS in the field, are almost zero, unless rare extenuating circumstances (e.g., profound hypothermia, barbiturate overdose) are present.

Sometimes, the child meets the EMS system's death in the field criteria or resuscitation is not successful, but grief counseling is not available at the scene. In this situation, consider transporting the baby to the hospital in a controlled transport mode (no lights or siren) with the caregiver, if possible. Transporting with lights and siren is the most dangerous transport that EMS providers perform and successful resuscitation on prompt transport for pulseless infants after failed ALS is extremely rare. The risks generally far outweigh the benefits of lights and siren transport. Allow the caregiver a chance to touch or hold the child before transport. This may be the last time the caregiver has to be with the child. This may not be possible if the scene is related to a crime but is an important step in the grieving process.

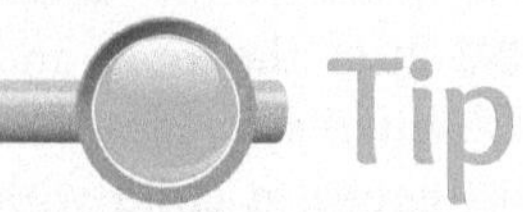

Encourage family presence during the attempted resuscitation.

The prehospital professional's emotional support of the caregivers is extremely important. When possible, have one person stay with the caregiver to provide information and support. Let family or caregivers stay with the child and do not separate them even during attempted resuscitation and transport. If family chooses to ride with the patient, ensure that they remain restrained with a seat belt according to manufacturer's recommendations and local protocols. *Be clear that the child is dead.* Do not use euphemisms, such as "your child has left us" or "she has gone to a better place." Avoid well-intentioned but inappropriate remarks, such as, "You can always have other children," "I know how you feel," or "You will get over this in time." **Table 12-4** suggests specific ways to communicate with caregivers when there is an unexpected death of a child.

It is vital that providers create a clear picture of the events that occurred through their documentation, which should be objective in nature. Any statements that are pertinent to the documentation should be captured with quotation marks. This patient-care report should be extremely detailed and include dispatch information, a scene size-up,

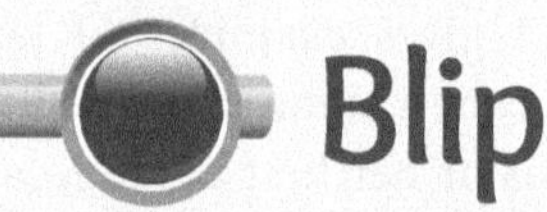

In discussion with the family, do not obscure the fact that the child is dead by using ambiguous language.

Table 12-4 Communicating About an Unexpected Death of a Child

Use the child's name.
Show **empathy** and express condolences.
Ask questions in a nonjudgmental manner. Never become hostile or angry.
Use a calm and directive voice.
Be clear with instructions and answers to questions.
Provide explanations to the caregivers about treatment and transport.
Repeat statements when necessary.
Reassure caregivers that there was nothing they could have done.
Allow the caregiver to accompany the baby if possible.

thorough head-to-toe assessment, interventions, response to interventions, transport decision and reasoning, and transfer of care. Also note any communication that occurs with the family, coroner, law enforcement, medical control, or any other entity involved. Failure to adequately document can cause a significant amount of stress on the provider and caregiver.

Summary of SUID

SUID is the most common cause of infant death. It is unpredictable and silent. The prehospital professional cannot "diagnose" SUID in the field, and the emergency physician cannot diagnose SUID in the ED. Determining the cause of death requires an autopsy. There are, however, common clinical signs and important risk factors that may be helpful in identifying probable SUID cases.

When faced with an infant in cardiopulmonary arrest, begin or continue CPR according to the local EMS system policies on death in the field. In some EMS systems, policy permits withholding or discontinuing resuscitation and focusing on the important tasks of talking to the family and helping them with their grief. **Figure 12-1** provides a typical sequence of events when there is a suspected SUID case. **Table 12-5** lists the responsibilities of the medical examiner and local health department in a case of suspected SUID.

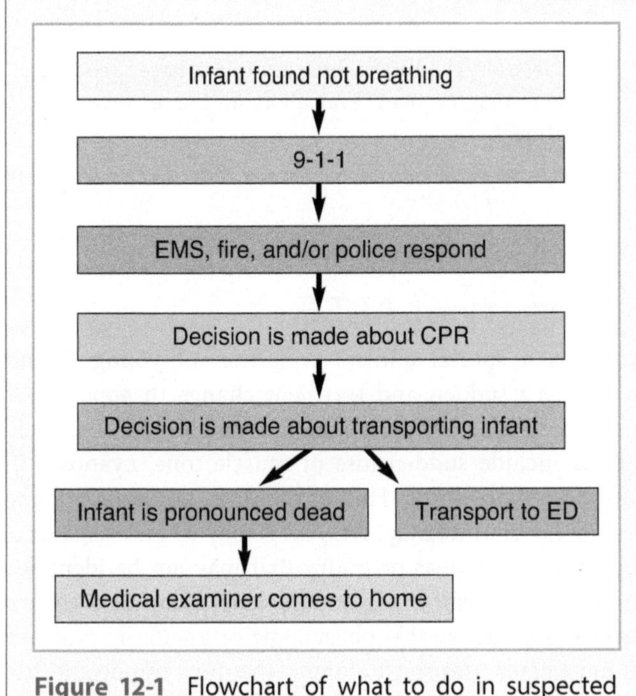
Infant found not breathing
9-1-1
EMS, fire, and/or police respond
Decision is made about CPR
Decision is made about transporting infant
Infant is pronounced dead
Transport to ED
Medical examiner comes to home

Figure 12-1 Flowchart of what to do in suspected SUID cases.

Table 12-5 Medical Examiner/Coroner and Local Health Department Responsibilities in Suspected SUID Cases

Medical Examiner/ Coroner Responsibilities	Local Health Department Responsibilities
Performs death scene investigation	Provides information and counseling
Performs autopsy	Provides referral information for peer support
Notifies local health department	Provides information to state program
Notifies state program	Performs periodic follow-up
Signs death certificate	Provides community education (with peer group)
Notifies parents of cause of death	

Definition of Apparent Life-Threatening Event

An apparent life-threatening event (ALTE) is an episode that is frightening to the observer and that is characterized by some combination of apnea (central or occasionally obstructive), color change (usually cyanotic or pallid but occasionally erythematous or plethoric), marked change in muscle tone (usually marked limpness), choking, or gagging. In some cases, the observer fears that the infant has died. Previously used terminology, such as "aborted crib death" or "near-miss SIDS," should be abandoned because it implies a possibly misleadingly close association between this type of spell and SUID.

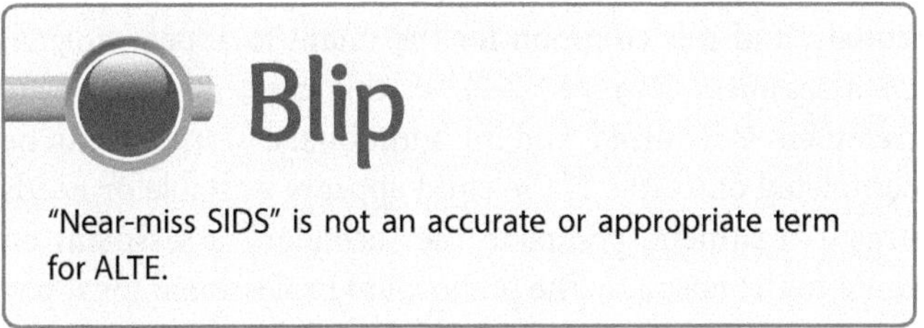
Blip

"Near-miss SIDS" is not an accurate or appropriate term for ALTE.

Common Clinical Presentation of ALTE

Similar to SUID, ALTE generally presents with a stressful scene. A thorough scene size-up should be used when evaluating scene safety, while ascertaining clinical clues that may have caused the event. Primary assessment should include evaluating the patient's airway for patency. The provider should evaluate the patient's breathing rate, depth, and quality. Breathing patterns may be slow, shallow, or have some other disruption in minute volume causing breathing to be inadequate. The circulation should be assessed by palpating pulses for rate, regularity, and quality; assessing capillary refills; and assessing skin color temperature and condition. Pulses may be bradycardic and weak, capillary refills may be greater than 4 seconds, and skin may show signs of hypoperfusion or hypoxia.

A thorough history should be assessed using the SAMPLE and OPQRST mnemonic. Onset should be noted so a timeline can be developed. The provider should note if anything makes the patient's symptoms better or worse. Pain is generally difficult to assess. SAMPLE history can be obtained from the patient's family. Identify the patient's signs and attempt to identify symptoms. If any allergies are known at this age, they should be noted. Any medications that the patient is taking should be evaluated for potential side effects and cross-referenced with any potential treatment plans. The patient's entire medical history is pertinent at this age. Identifying the patient's last oral intake and events leading up to it may help point toward a potential diagnosis.

Vital signs should be assessed on all ALTE patients. This should include pulse rate, respiratory rate, blood pressure, pulse oximetry, and possibly blood glucose analysis. A thorough, hands-on, head-to-toe assessment should be performed, noting any abnormalities. Auscultation of lungs and bowel should occur. Reassessments should be done every 5–15 minutes depending on severity and interventions.

Actions in Suspected ALTE

Clinical Interventions

Most ALTEs resolve before arrival of prehospital professionals, and it is common for the infant to appear normal on assessment (**Figure 12-2**). In this case, no immediate treatment is required, and the additional assessment can be completed on scene. If the child appears unstable or needs urgent treatment, complete the secondary assessment en route to the hospital. The prehospital professional must pay close attention to and protect the patient's airway as necessary. It is imperative that supplemental oxygen be placed on, or near if blow by is used, as early as possible if indicated. The advanced provider should be prepared to provide fluid resuscitation or cardiac medications as necessary and indicated. Always transport the baby, even if the complete assessment reveals no abnormalities. Serious illnesses in newly born and young infants are sometimes subtle and difficult to detect.

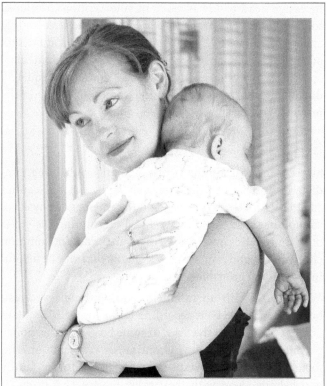

Figure 12-2 An ALTE is an episode in which an infant demonstrates a significant behavioral or physical change.

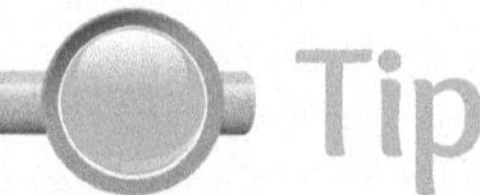

Tip

Consider every child with a reported ALTE to have a serious problem that requires evaluation in the emergency department.

Summary of ALTE

ALTE is a special clinical condition of young infants involving a sudden and transient change in appearance, respiratory effort, or perfusion. Examples of ALTE presentations include sudden loss of muscle tone, cyanosis, or cessation of breathing. Half of the time, no cause is found despite hospital workup. An ALTE may be an indicator of serious occult illness or injury that may not be identified in the field. Perform a standard assessment and treat if there is a demonstrable physiologic or anatomic problem. In most cases, transport alone is the most important field intervention.

Responses to an Infant Death

Caregiver's Response

The prehospital professional is often the first responder on the scene following the discovery of the dead infant. Responses of the caregiver to the sudden and unexpected death of an infant are not predictable and may vary from numb silence to rage. Common reactions include denial, anger, hysteria, withdrawal, intense guilt, or no visible response. The caregiver may or may not accept that the infant is dead and that resuscitation is not possible. The caregiver may cling to the hope that the prehospital professional can do something to save the infant, even though the child is obviously dead.

The death of a child is likely the most stressful and tragic moment in the life of a parent or caregiver. It is not uncommon for caregivers in this situation to express strong preferences or make "demands" of the prehospital professional. Remember, this is that individual's last chance to fulfill their role of protecting and caring for their infant. Respond to the caregiver gently and professionally. The caregiver may:

- Ask repeated questions
- Request that you not start care or that you stop resuscitation efforts
- Request to be alone with the infant
- Want to know the cause of death
- Physically interfere with care
- Insist on continuation of care or that resuscitation efforts begin

When the caregiver or family expresses their preferences or asks difficult questions, use a calm and professional approach. Keep explanations simple. Be honest and direct with family members. Follow EMS system protocol for death in the field and maintain an empathetic and nonjudgmental attitude. Allow room for the family to grieve. Be respectful of the family's religious beliefs, customs, or traditions.

If there is no indication to attempt to resuscitate the infant, while awaiting the medical examiner or coroner at the scene ask the family member or caregiver if someone can be called to give them support (**Figure 12-3**). This may involve calling friends, relatives, clergy, or public agencies to help care for other children at the home. If the scene is a child care setting, consider calling law enforcement to assist with other children and to contact the child's caregivers or the caregivers of other children present.

Prehospital Professional's Response

The prehospital professional has a difficult and sometimes agonizing role in the setting of unexpected infant or child death. After death is declared, comfort the parents. Never place blame on the parents or caregivers. Offering sensitive support to the family and gathering accurate information in a nonthreatening manner helps surviving family members. This is often challenging, because the prehospital professional may be struggling with overwhelming personal emotional responses related to the loss of a patient.

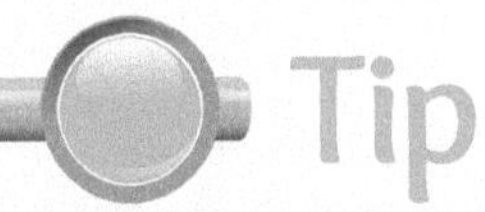

Tip

Responses of the caregiver to the sudden and unexpected death of an infant are not predictable and may vary from numb silence to rage.

Case Study 2

You are called to an apartment complex that is home to a large number of immigrant families. On arrival, there is a large, agitated group congregated at the doorway to the apartment, speaking in a language that you do not recognize. You enter the apartment to find a mother and father sitting on a couch, quietly weeping. They gesture toward a bassinet, where a stiff, cold 3-month-old infant with dependent lividity lies covered in a pile of blankets. Through a neighbor who speaks English, you explain that the baby is dead and ask if they would like to hold her. They decline, and seem offended by the proposal.

1. How should you react?
2. What steps do you take from this point?

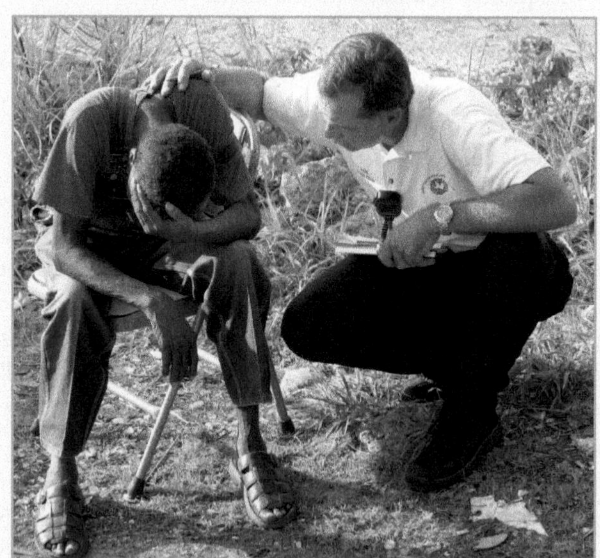

Figure 12-3 Caregivers can react to the death of a child in many ways, but all need support. Attempt to contact identified individuals who might give comfort.

Talking to the family or caregivers can be difficult. There are techniques that may improve the quality of these interactions:

- Use the child's name. This acknowledges the child as an individual rather than a "patient" and the unique, intensely personal nature of this child's death.
- Try to find a quiet area to talk to the caregivers. Often the scene can become noisy with activity. Finding an area where the caregiver can concentrate on your conversation helps to keep your message clear.
- Use concrete terms. The use of euphemisms to soften the news can make it harder for the caregiver to understand what has happened. "Your child has died" has a finite meaning, whereas "Your child is in a better place" has infinite possibilities (the hospital is a better place).
- It is okay to show emotion. Parents whose child has died often comment on how meaningful it was to them that a health care provider clearly cared. Expressing your emotions is appropriate in such tragic circumstances, so long as the focus remains on the family and child and you are able to fulfill your professional duties at the scene.

Sometimes there are cultural or language differences between the prehospital professional and the caregiver. There may be unfamiliar rituals and behaviors in how death is regarded or how grief is expressed. This presents another important challenge. *Respect cultural diversity. This is necessary to effectively communicate.* When cultural or language differences arise, attempt to find an interpreter to explain and translate.

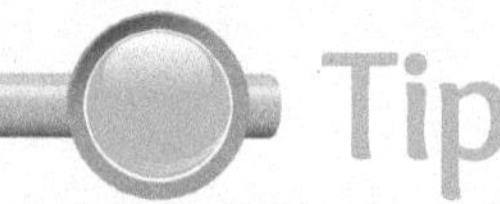

Ask the name of the child and use it in any discussions with the caregiver.

Responses of the prehospital professional to the sudden and unexpected death of an infant may include one or more of the following:

- Anger or blame
- Identification with the caregiver
- Withdrawal
- Avoidance of the caregiver
- Self-doubt (if resuscitation is attempted and the child does not recover)
- Sadness and depression

The prehospital professional may have unrealistic expectations of how the caregiver should behave and respond, or may believe that the caregiver was responsible for the baby's death. These feelings can become obstacles to communication, as outlined in **Table 12-6**.

Table 12-6 Responses of Prehospital Professionals That Hinder Communication With Caregivers After an Unexpected Death

Having stereotyped expectations of how the caregiver should respond to the event
Judging a caregiver who did not initiate CPR
Distrusting a caregiver who has recognized the infant is dead and does not want resuscitation
Misunderstanding the mourning and grief behaviors of persons of different cultures or religious beliefs

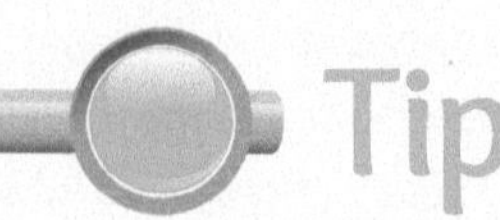

The unexpected death of an infant or child is one of the most stressful experiences for the prehospital professional.

Critical Incident Stress

Stress is an unavoidable part of the prehospital professional's job. The death of a child may be the most stressful situation in the prehospital professional's career (**Figure 12-4**). Acknowledging emotions is a key element in successfully coping with stress and maintaining a healthy mental attitude. **Table 12-7** lists the frequent signs and symptoms of stress.

There are many ways to decrease the impact of stress related to the death of an infant or child. Critical incident stress management (CISM) may be an important technique for helping cope with the emotional toll of SIDS and unexpected infant or child death. Other techniques to help decrease stress include the following:

- Talk to field supervisors and experienced prehospital professionals to share feelings.
- Maintain a well-balanced lifestyle outside of work. Exercise, plan leisure time, and limit overtime hours.
- Get adequate rest and eat a balanced diet.
- Avoid excessive alcohol or drugs.
- Write a personal journal.
- Obtain religious or peer counseling.
- Request professional psychologic assistance.

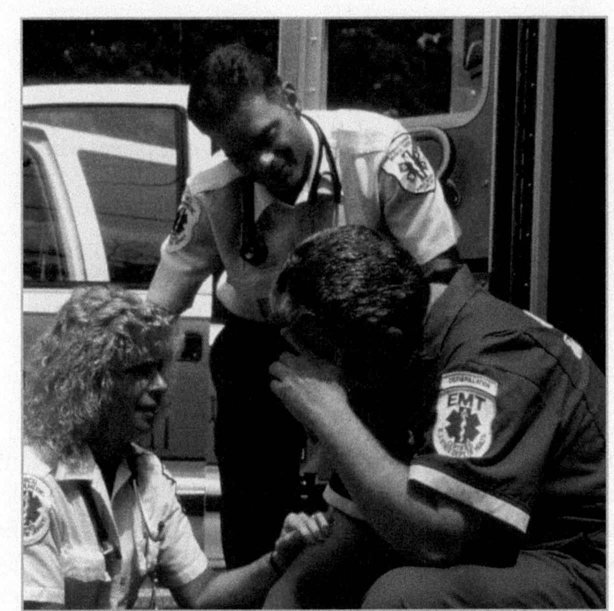

Figure 12-4 Stress is an unavoidable part of a prehospital professional's job. The death of a child can be agonizing.

Community Resources

Community resources available to caregivers and prehospital professionals to help them cope with the unexpected death of a child include the following:

- Local support groups
- Local public health departments
- First Candle (1-800-221-SIDS)
- American SIDS Institute
- Professional counseling
- Emergency Services Chaplain

Table 12-7 Signs and Symptoms of Critical Incident Stress

Anger and irritability
Changes in eating habits
Changes in sleeping patterns
Depression
Excessive alcohol consumption
Inability to concentrate
Mood changes and emotional instability
Physical illness
Recurring dreams or frightening images
Withdrawal

Case Study 3

You are dispatched to a coworker's home where a grandmother is weeping and largely incoherent. She leads you to a bedroom where a 3-month-old boy lies motionless in his crib, face down on a sheepskin. He is apneic and pulseless, has lividity on his chest and face, and is stiff. In between sobs, the grandmother tells you she put the baby to sleep 4 hours ago and found him this way when she checked on him 10 minutes ago. She asks you if he is dead.

1. What are your key medical actions?
2. How should you deal with the grandmother? The coworker?

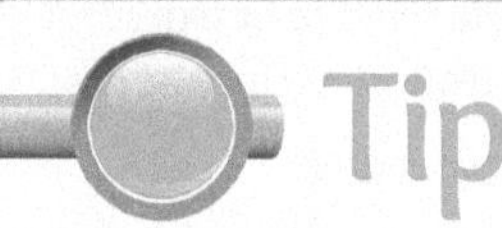

Critical incident stress management (CISM) may be an important technique for coping with the emotional toll of SIDS and unexpected infant or child death.

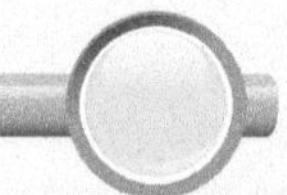

The value and appropriate timing of CISM is not known. Although the prehospital professional suffers predictable stress after the death of a child in his or her care, how and when such intervention should occur has not been studied.

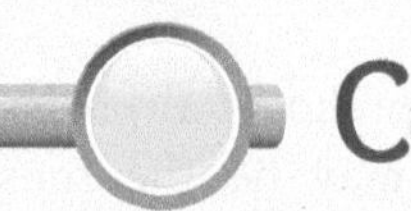

Risk reduction and risk counseling are important community prevention activities. Further research must help define the appropriate educational role of the prehospital professional at the scene of an injury or death.

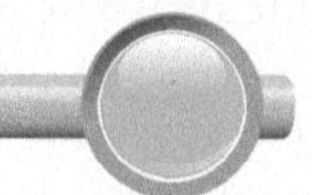

Prehospital professionals can play a key role in educating parents in the community on ways to decrease the risk of SIDS.

Risk Reduction Activities and Risk Counseling

In addition to community resource groups, prehospital professionals can also play a key role in educating parents in the community on ways to decrease the risk of SUID. This includes distribution of the American Academy of Pediatrics "Back to Sleep" brochures and active support of their recommendation to place babies on their backs to sleep. Although side-sleeping is several times safer than prone sleeping, the risk of SUID for the side-sleeping position is still double the risk of the supine position. Prehospital professionals can participate in community risk reduction by advocating for firm, flat mattresses in safety-approved cribs, and avoidance of soft or bulky blankets or comforters and overheating in the infant's sleeping area.

Recommendations for reducing the risk of SUID are:

- Place your baby to sleep on his or her back for every sleep.
- Place your baby to sleep on a firm sleep surface.
- Keep soft objects, loose bedding, or any objects that could increase the risk of entrapment, suffocation, or strangulation out of the crib. This includes pillows, blankets, and bumper pads.
- Place your baby to sleep in the same room where you sleep but not the same bed.
- Breastfeed as much and for as long as you can.
- Schedule and go to all well-child visits.
- Keep your baby away from smokers and places where people smoke.
- Do not let your baby get too hot.
- Offer a pacifier at naptime and bedtime.
- Do not use home cardiorespiratory monitors to help reduce the risk of SUID.
- Do not use products that claim to reduce the risk of SUID, such as wedges and positioners.

Support of antismoking campaigns is also important. Recent research shows that the risk of SUID doubles among babies exposed to cigarette smoke after birth, and triples for those exposed both during pregnancy and after birth. As for all infants, encouragement of breastfeeding is a useful action.

Prehospital professionals can also become involved in local or state child fatality review teams. These teams meet and discuss the community trends in infant and child deaths. They often review all sudden and unexpected deaths in children less than 2 years of age to improve the accuracy of SUID as a diagnosis versus other natural and nonnatural causes, especially child maltreatment.

CASE STUDY ANSWERS

Case Study 1 — page 248

The infant has many findings commonly associated with a SUID death. Sleeping prone (indicated by the lividity on the chest and face), the pink frothy sputum, and the absence of traumatic injuries are the initial clues to a SUID death. However, remember that SUID is a diagnosis of exclusion made by a medical examiner or coroner at autopsy and cannot be made in the field.

In this setting, provide a direct and calm explanation to the parent that the child is dead. Find out the child's name and use it. Do not ask questions in a way that suggests blame. Use controlled and supportive dialogue with the parent. If the child is not transported, try to get grief counseling for the parent, contact the medical examiner or coroner from the scene, and consider critical incident stress management for yourself and your partner. Gather family support resources.

Case Study 2 — page 253

Different cultures have different beliefs about death, afterlife, and the proper handling of a dead body. There may be rituals or taboos with which you are unfamiliar and different ways of coping with loss. Because there is no medical intervention that will help this child, your focus must be on providing support to the survivors. Obtaining a professional interpreter, where available, is an important part of the scene management and the death investigation. Through an English-speaking neighbor, you can inquire about family needs, who they might want you to contact, and any way that you might assist them at the scene. Remember that even with an interpreter present, concepts may be difficult to translate and the family may have a very different belief system than do you with regard to illness, health care, and cause of death. If you cannot communicate the rationale for your treatment or nontreatment to the family, transport.

Case Study 3 — page 255

In most EMS systems, this child would meet death in the field criteria and would not require any resuscitation attempt. If you are uncertain about whether resuscitation is indicated, begin CPR and call medical oversight to clarify treatment options.

The grandmother may need to be medically evaluated if she cannot be calmed down. Provide a calm and controlled environment. Do not place blame.

Try to minimize radio communications if your coworker may be listening. If the employee is at work, have a supervisor contact the coworker and provide safe transportation to the scene. Contact other family, friends, or clergy if the situation warrants. Watch for symptoms consistent with that of critical incident stress and initiate CISM if indicated.

SUGGESTED READINGS

References

American Academy of Pediatrics. SIDS and other sleep-related infant deaths: expansion of recommendations for a safe infant sleeping environment. http://pediatrics.aappublications.org/content/128/5/e1341.full. Accessed July 18, 2012.

American Academy of Pediatrics. AAP expands guidelines for infant sleep safety and SIDS risk reduction. http://www.aap.org/en-us/about-the-aap/aap-press-room/pages/AAP-Expands-Guidelines-for-Infant-Sleep-Safety-and-SIDS-Risk-Reduction.aspx. Accessed July 18, 2012.

Centers for Disease Control and Prevention. Sudden unexpected infant death and sudden infant death syndrome. Centers for Disease Control and Prevention web site. http://www.cdc.gov/sids/index.htm. Accessed November 17, 2015.

Mathews TJ, MacDorman MF, Thoma ME. Infant mortality statistics from the 2013 period linked birth/death data set. http://cdc.gov/nchs/linked.htm. Accessed November 18, 2015.

National Institutes of Health. Infantile apnea and home monitoring. NIH Consensus Statement Online 1986;6(6):1-10. National Institutes of Health web site. http://consensus.nih.gov/1986/1986InfantApneaMonitoring058html.htm. Accessed September 12, 2012.

Shapiro-Mendoza CK, Camperiengo L, Ludvigsen R, et al. Classification system for the sudden unexpected infant death case registry and its application. *Pediatrics.* 2014;134:e210-e219.

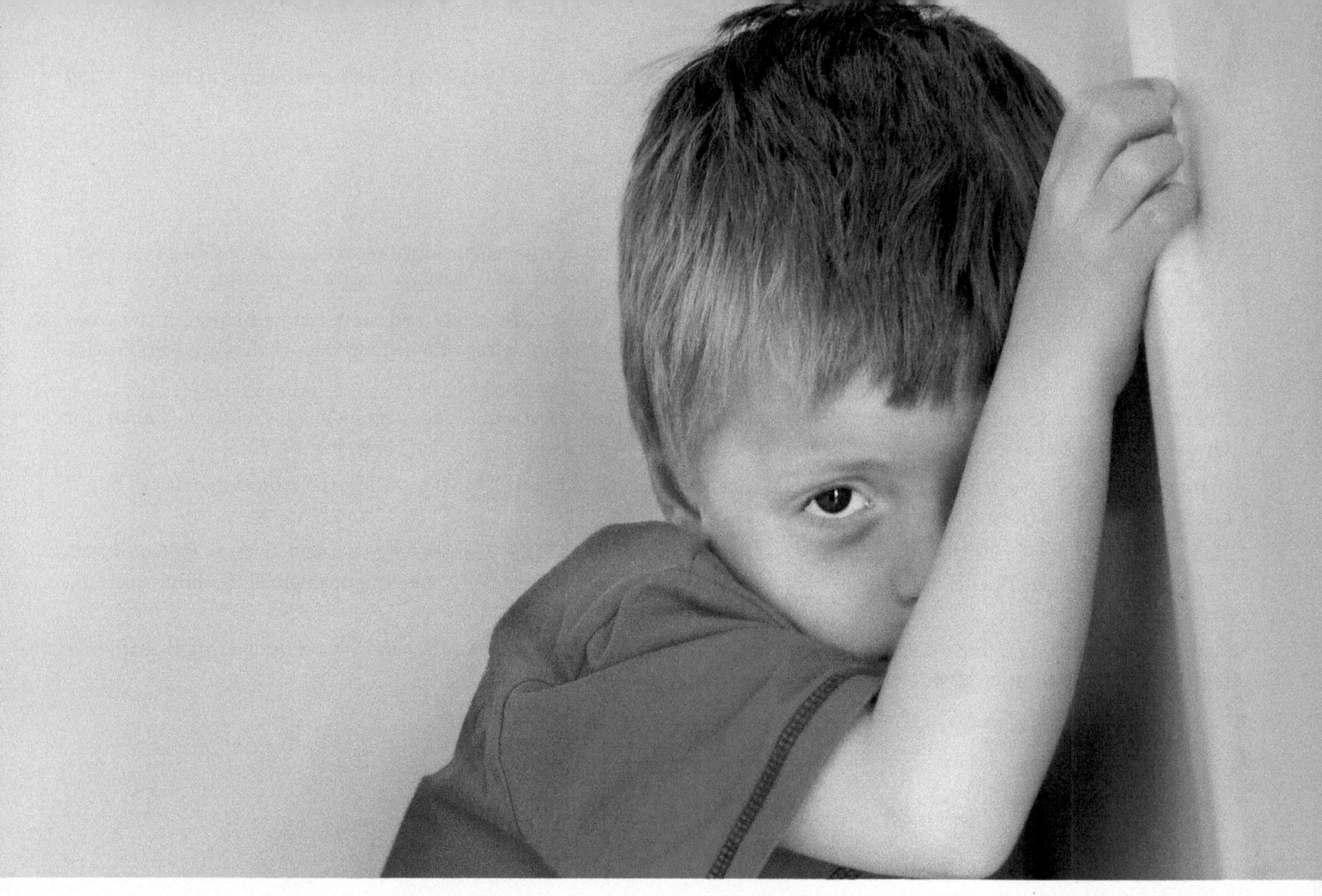

Learning Objectives

1. Discuss the known signs, causes, and complications of child maltreatment.
2. Define the terms physical abuse, emotional abuse, sexual abuse, and child neglect.
3. Explain the role of child protection services (CPS) in management of suspected child maltreatment.
4. Distinguish features in the scene size-up, in the history and physical assessment, and in the caregiver's behaviors that suggest child maltreatment.
5. Describe appropriate communication with caregivers of suspected victims of maltreatment.
6. Outline the prehospital professional's legal responsibility to document and report suspected child maltreatment.

Child Maltreatment

Chapter 13

Introduction

Prehospital professionals must know when to suspect child maltreatment. Although providing emergency medical care is always the top priority, prehospital professionals also provide valuable scene documentation and are often the first step in the reporting process of suspected cases of maltreatment. All of these actions are critical to protect vulnerable children and to break the cycle. When caring for a pediatric patient who has suffered obvious trauma, prehospital providers need to remain vigilant in looking for potential signs of abuse.

Unfortunately, child maltreatment is common. It is one of the leading causes of death in infants less than 12 months of age. Physical abuse and neglect are often detectable, but sexual abuse, emotional abuse, and child neglect may not be so obvious. Some children who die from maltreatment are known to local child protection services (CPS), the legal organizations established in every community to monitor, manage, and prevent child maltreatment. These deaths are sometimes preventable. Abused or neglected children have a high probability of being maltreated again. Early recognition is important to prevent future injury or death.

Background, Cost, and Definition

In 2013 there were 3.5 million referrals reported to CPS organizations in the United States through the National Child Abuse and Neglect Data System. Of those, 678,932 children were determined to have been abused or neglected. The highest prevalence is seen in infants from birth to 1 year (23.1 cases per 1,000). For each case of child maltreatment reported, it is estimated that there are one to two cases that go unrecognized. An estimated 1,520 children per year die of abuse or neglect, which is more than four children every day. Many survivors are negatively affected for the rest of their lives. After being physically and psychologically affected, survivors may themselves become abusive or neglectful to children, thus perpetuating the cycle of abuse. The number of children who suffer long-term effects from neglect is not as well documented, but is believed to be substantial. **Table 13-1** lists some of these long-term complications.

Younger children are at higher risk for fatal abuse and neglect than older children. About 74% of maltreated children who die are younger than 3 years of age, and 47% are younger than 1 year of age. Approximately half of these deaths occur in children who are known to CPS agencies as current or prior clients. It has been estimated that child maltreatment costs the United States $220 million every day or an estimated $80 billion for 2012.

Case Study 1

9-1-1 is called for an unresponsive infant. On arrival, you find a 10-month-old male infant who is unresponsive and has irregular respirations. The mother's boyfriend (mom is at work) tells you that he found the baby in this condition when he went to get him up from his nap. You note that it is 7 PM. The boyfriend is not holding the infant and when you pick the baby up from the crib, you also note that there is no muscle tone and the infant is flaccid. During your assessment and treatment, you note bruises on both upper arms. What are your initial patient management priorities?

1. What concerns you about the history reported by the boyfriend and the infant's injuries?
2. What do you suspect is the primary injury?

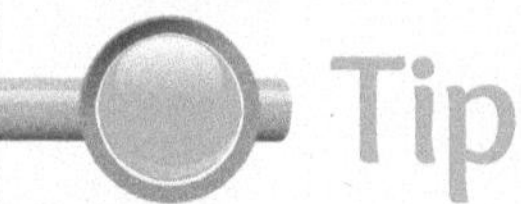

When adults with poor coping skills are faced with stressful situations, a cycle of child maltreatment may result.

Definition of Child Maltreatment

Child maltreatment is a general term that includes all types of abuse and neglect. Yearly, approximately 50% of substantiated maltreatment is classified as neglect, 25% is physical, and 12% is sexual abuse. The remaining types include emotional abuse, medical neglect, or combinations of the different types.

Physical Abuse

Physical abuse occurs when a person intentionally inflicts injury, or allows injury to be inflicted, to a child younger than 18 years of age or to a mentally disabled child younger than 21 years of age, which causes or results in risk of death, disfigurement, or distress.

Emotional Abuse

Emotional abuse occurs when there is an ongoing and consistent pattern of behavior that interferes with the normal psychologic and social development of a child. This includes unreasonable, excessive, or aggressive demands on the child that are not age-appropriate; setting tasks that are beyond the physical ability of the child; or the caregiver not providing the nurturing, guidance, and psychologic support critical for the growth and development of a healthy child. Verbal attacks, such as belittling, insults, rejection, and constant criticism, are a few patterns of emotional abuse.

Sexual Abuse

Sexual abuse occurs when an older child or adult engages in sexual activities with a dependent, developmentally immature child or adolescent for the older person's own sexual excitement or for the enjoyment of other persons (e.g., child pornography or prostitution).

In most cases of sexual abuse, the perpetrator is an adult who knows the child and is often living under the same roof. A common misconception is that child sexual abuse is perpetrated by strangers. According to the American Psychological Association, an estimated 60% of sexual abuse perpetrators are known by the child but are NOT a family member; 30% are family members, and only 10% are strangers.

Sexual abuse usually does not occur as a single incident. It does not always involve violence and physical force, and commonly leaves no visible sign. The perpetrator may use the power of adult–child authority or the parent–child bond instead of force or violence. The child may be manipulated into thinking that "it's OK" and a normal behavior or that the child is "special" for making the perpetrator feel good. The child may also be made to feel deeply ashamed and powerless or may even be kept silent by threats from the perpetrator. The insidious nature of this abuse makes it difficult to detect, unless the child discloses the information to a confidant or the prehospital professional.

Child Neglect

Child neglect occurs when a child's physical, mental, or emotional condition is harmed or endangered because the caregiver has failed to supply basic necessities or engages in child-rearing practices that are inadequate or dangerous. Child neglect may involve a caregiver's misuse of drugs or alcohol, or child abandonment. Neglect is the failure to act on behalf of a child and is an act of omission. Neglect may not have visible signs, and it usually occurs over a period of time rather than as a discrete episode.

Neglect may be physical or emotional. Physical neglect is a failure to meet the requirements basic to a child's physical development and safety, such as supervision, housing, clothing, medical attention, and nutrition. Some social service agencies subdivide this category into more specific acts of omission, such as medical neglect, lack of proper

Table 13-1 Potential Complications of Maltreatment

Low self-esteem and underachievement
Psychologic disorders or psychiatric symptoms
Abnormal growth and development
Permanent physical or neurologic damage
Poor school performance
Teen promiscuity and pregnancy
Social withdrawal
Eating disorders
Substance abuse
Negative learned behavior
Criminal behavior beginning in young adulthood
Vulnerability to further abuse
Suicidal tendencies
Increased survivor health care costs to family and society
Death

supervision, or educational neglect. **Emotional neglect** is failure to provide the support or affection necessary to a child's psychologic and social development.

Abuse Versus Neglect

The difference between abuse and neglect is that abuse represents an action against a child, whereas neglect represents a lack of action for the child. *Abuse is an act of commission; neglect is an act of omission.* In abuse, a physical or mental injury is inflicted on a child. In neglect, there is a failure to meet the basic needs of the child for adequate food, supervision, shelter, guidance, education, clothing, or medical care.

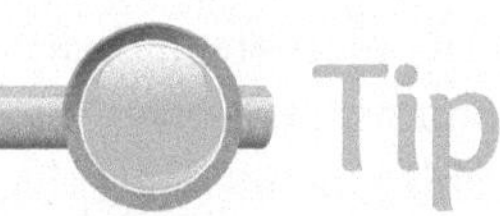
Tip

Abuse represents an action against a child (commission). Neglect represents a lack of action for the child (omission).

High-Risk Groups

Younger aged children are more vulnerable and at risk for maltreatment than older children who have more resources available to them and can better take care of themselves. The Centers for Disease Control and Prevention (CDC) reports that children younger than the age of 4 years are at greatest risk for severe injury or death from abuse (almost 80% who died from abuse in 2010 were younger than 4 years old). Child maltreatment involves risk factors and lapses in child protection at the individual, family, community, and societal levels. No geographic, ethnic, or economic setting is free of child maltreatment. The incidence rates for sexual abuse are similar for urban, suburban, and rural communities. Children from low-income or single-parent families, however, have more reported occurrences of neglect or physical maltreatment than children from higher-income families, and physically maltreated children are less likely to be identified in Caucasian, two-parent families. The 2013 data on child maltreatment show that 88% of the victims are represented by three races or ethnic groups (**Table 13-2**).

Table 13-2 Child Maltreatment Victims by Race or Ethnic Group

African-American	21.2%
Caucasian	44.0%
Hispanic	22.42%
TOTAL	87.6%

Source: U.S. Department of Health & Human Services. Children's Bureau. 2013. Available from http://www.acf.hhs.gov/sites/default/files/cb/cm2013.pdf. Accessed December 22, 2015.

The prehospital provider must consider maltreatment whenever circumstances suggest it, regardless of the family's socioeconomic status.

Other risk factors for child maltreatment, besides nonverbal toddlers and infants, include factors where additional stressors and insufficient resources are available to the parents or caregivers, such as children with special needs (mental and physical disabilities and developmental issues) and children with chronic medical conditions—all conditions in which there are increased responsibilities to care for the child and a financial impact that may also affect the level of stress in the home.

A perpetrator of child maltreatment can be any person who has care, custody, or control of the child. This can include the child's parents, relative, teacher, babysitter, or child care staff person, institution staff person, bus driver, playground attendant, coach, religious leader, caregiver, or boyfriend or girlfriend of the caregiver. Abusive head trauma (formerly known as shaken baby syndrome) may lead to seizures or apnea, but the person with the infant at the time emergency medical services (EMS) is called should not be assumed to be the perpetrator. *The caregiver with the child at the time of the 9-1-1 call or EMS arrival may not be the individual who injured the child.* This individual may be unaware of the abuse, or in denial, and unable to believe that the child has been harmed. He or she may also be a victim of abuse or afraid of the abuser. Maltreatment happens for many different reasons. Often the perpetrators genuinely care for the child, but lack the resources or the parenting skills to deal with frustration and cope with anger. Rarely does the prehospital professional have sufficient information to determine with certainty that maltreatment has occurred. Information gathered in the field can, however, be critical in the eventual confirmation of maltreatment. **Table 13-3** lists assessment factors that are suggestive of maltreatment. Particularly important is the documentation of the exact history given by the caregiver in cases of presumed injury. A changing story is one of the most common hallmarks of maltreatment. Recognizing and reporting suspected child maltreatment is one of the most important ways the prehospital professional can prevent childhood injury.

Table 13-3 Assessment Factors Associated With Maltreatment

Does the history change over time?
Was there a delay in seeking care, or was the closest treatment center bypassed?
Are there injuries of multiple ages?
Does the history fit the child's developmental ability?
Do the injuries fit the history?
Does the patient not seek comfort from the caregiver?
Does the caregiver inappropriately respond to the patient's needs?
What are the other sibling's involvements with the patient and caregiver?

Duties and Communication by the Prehospital Professional

The prehospital professional has an extremely important role at the scene. CPS and health professionals in the emergency department (ED) rely on the EMS scene assessment and documentation of suspected child maltreatment. **Table 13-4** lists the prehospital professional's duties in suspected maltreatment cases.

Table 13-4 Duties of the Prehospital Professional in Suspected Maltreatment

Recognition of suspicious circumstances at the scene
Physical assessment of the child
Assessment of the history given by the caregiver
Communication with the caregiver and family
Careful documentation
Notation of other children living at the scene
Reporting of maltreatment concerns to the proper authority

Mandatory Obligation to Report

In most states, licensed health care professionals, including prehospital professionals, have a legal obligation (mandate) to report suspected child maltreatment and other situations where a crime may have been committed or a vulnerable population is harmed. In other states, the duty of the prehospital professional is to ensure that a report is filed with the receiving hospital, law enforcement, or a designated state office. An agreement from the ED staff to report usually suffices. States with maltreatment laws may require health care providers to independently report suspected maltreatment to either law enforcement or CPS.

Although no law can forbid the filing of civil or criminal charges, most state laws protect the reporter of suspected child maltreatment from any decision or award in a lawsuit, if the report was made in good faith. *However, failure to report suspicion of child maltreatment may result in legal action against the mandated reporter.*

In small communities, especially when the prehospital professional knows the individuals involved, reporting suspected child maltreatment may have significant social implications. In many states, anonymous reports can be filed, and the identity of the person who reports maltreatment is protected. Remember that a report of suspected child maltreatment is not an attempt to harm or punish a family, but an attempt to help the child. All prehospital personnel should become familiar with the particular obligation to report laws in the state in which they practice.

Assessing the Caregiver's Behavior

Common characteristics among caregivers of maltreated children are drug use, poor self-concept, immaturity, lack of parenting knowledge, and lack of interpersonal skills. Although none of these factors in and of themselves mean that an individual has abused the child, be alert for these "red flag" behaviors, as noted in **Table 13-5**. Conversely, an "appropriate" caregiver who does not show any of these characteristics may still be maltreating a child. In some cases a caregiver may appear to be overreacting to the child's condition, such as in cases of Munchausen syndrome by proxy, in which a caregiver may intentionally inflict illness or injury on a child to obtain attention for herself or himself.

Never confront a caregiver with suspicions of maltreatment. Such an approach at the scene may delay care, endanger the child, and create a hostile and dangerous situation for

Table 13-5 "Red Flag" Caregiver Behaviors

Apathy
Bizarre or strange conduct
Little or no concern about the child
Overreaction to child misbehavior
Not forthcoming with events surrounding injury
Intoxication
Overreaction to child's condition

the prehospital professional. Instead, note the presence of alcohol or drugs in the prehospital report and document any statements from the caregiver that reflect apparent misinformation, inconsistency, or evasiveness. Watch interactions among the caregivers and document them if they seem noteworthy. Be careful, however, to keep the tone of the report objective and neutral. Report what you see and hear, but avoid making judgments or interpreting intent in the written documentation. Particularly note any comments made by the child about how he or she was hurt. However, be aware that young children may attribute injury to an abstract perpetrator, such as a monster or "bad man," rather than identifying the caregivers on whom they depend.

Documentation

There is no difference between basic and advanced level documentation of suspected child maltreatment. Be sure to document your findings of the scene assessment related to possible child maltreatment (e.g., whether there is child-appropriate food available, heat or air-conditioning, appropriate clothing, supervision, and any safety concerns). Make a note of the child's position and location when you first encountered him or her. It is also recommended to document who else is at the scene (e.g., caretakers) and their relationship to the child. When documenting the history and physical assessment, be thorough but objective. Interjecting feelings or interpreting the facts may make the documentation inadmissible in court. For example, write, "palms show a 1-cm circular burn" instead of "cigarette burn to hand." Use objective, clear, specific terminology. Place in quotation marks and note in the records any statements from caregivers (e.g., father states that "child climbed into hot bathtub").

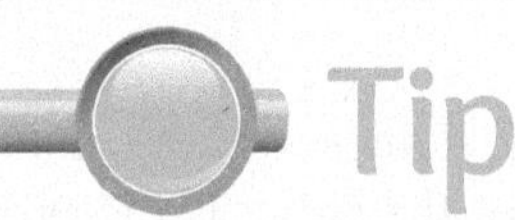

Tip

Document physical findings objectively. The facts speak for themselves in court.

Communicating With the Child and Caregivers

Communicate with the child in an age-appropriate manner. When assessing a stable child for whom there is concern of maltreatment, transport the child to the safe environment of the ED for full evaluation as soon as possible.

Communication with the caregiver in suspected maltreatment is a challenging task for the prehospital professional. Resist the impulse to "find out what really happened" or express anger at the caregiver. Do not make accusations or assume a judgmental tone. When confronted with suspicions of abuse, caregivers often respond defensively or angrily, whether or not they were the ones who inflicted the injuries.

Sometimes a caregiver may refuse to cooperate in further assessment, decline transport, or attempt to leave the scene with the child. If you believe the child to be in danger, immediately contact law enforcement for assistance. Never attempt to physically restrain a caregiver or to forcibly take possession of a child, because this may put everyone in danger. If the scene is chaotic but not dangerous, consider contacting medical control, who may be able to convince the caregiver to permit treatment and transport.

Patient Assessment

Scene Assessment

First, ensure that the scene is safe for the child and for the prehospital professionals. If you suspect maltreatment, make a mental note of any conditions at the scene, because you need to document the conditions in the patient care report (**Figure 13-1**). Record remarks or specific conversations with the caregiver and document specifics about the environment where injuries were reported to occur. For example, note the approximate height of furniture an infant

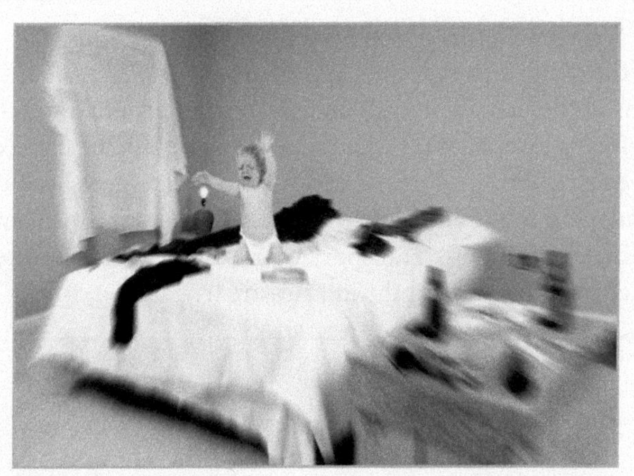

Figure 13-1 Document scene conditions that might support suspicion of maltreatment.

rolled off, the floor surface, or the location and condition of the sink or room where a child was burned.

Consider child maltreatment in every pediatric trauma call and every pediatric cardiac arrest situation in children less than 1 year of age. Suspicious circumstances in the environment, behavior of the child or caregiver, history, or physical examination may also raise concerns of abuse in responding to calls for unrelated complaints. Look for unsanitary or dangerous home conditions, such as guns, drug paraphernalia, or other unsafe care situations.

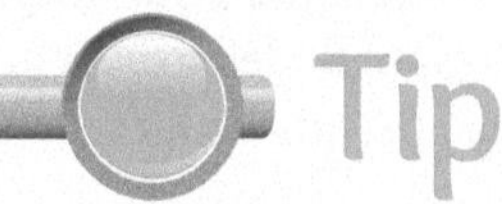

Consider child abuse in every injury case, as well as in illness cases with suspicious circumstances in the environment, behavior of the child or caregiver, history, or physical examination.

If the scene is safe, assess the child and provide appropriate medical care. If an infant with suspected maltreatment has an abnormal appearance (e.g., listlessness, inconsolability, weak cry) or altered mental status (abnormal response to verbal or painful stimuli), assess for a traumatic brain injury.

One cause of traumatic brain injury is abusive head trauma, formerly called shaken baby syndrome. Abusive head trauma involves diffuse intracranial hemorrhage, usually from violent shaking of the child with or without impact with another object. The signs, symptoms, and physical findings in abusive head trauma vary depending on the amount of trauma to the brain. These range from lethargy and irritability to seizures, coma, or death. Petechiae or hand grip patterns on the arms or chest (**Figure 13-2**) may also be found in abusive head trauma. The incidence of permanent neurologic damage from abusive head trauma is high. Seizures, learning disabilities, blindness, and other handicaps are common. The fatality rate in abusive head trauma is 20%–30%.

If the child with suspected maltreatment is physiologically unstable or has significant injuries, begin transport after the primary assessment. If the scene is unsafe for the child or prehospital professional, call for law enforcement back-up and move to the ambulance to complete the assessment and initiate treatment. Transport every child with suspected maltreatment, even if the injuries are trivial.

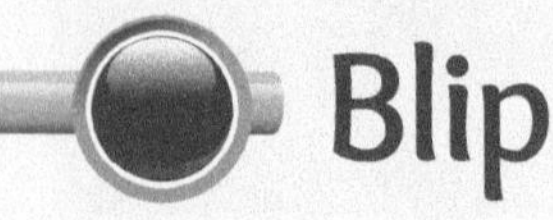

Never leave a suspected victim of child maltreatment. Transport every child, even if the injuries are trivial.

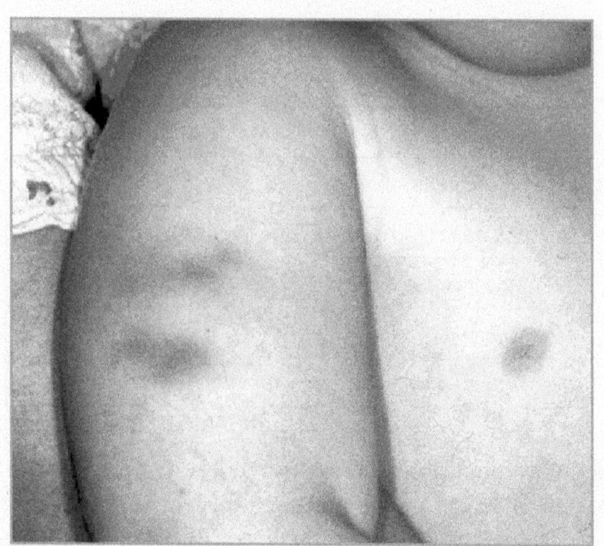

Figure 13-2 Human hand and fingertip marks can appear as oval bruises.

Additional Assessment

Stay on scene for additional assessment only if the child is stable and the scene is safe. Take a careful history, using the questions suggested in **Table 13-6**. *The history may be more important than the physical assessment.* Ask questions in a nonjudgmental way to maximize the quality of information and to avoid escalating the situation. Pay close attention to and document in detail the caregiver's description of the events leading to the call, noting inconsistencies or evasiveness. Consider the developmental capabilities of the child. Be concerned about inflicted trauma when the history does not account for the observed injuries (**Figure 13-3**), the caregiver's history changes over the course of the interview, or the mechanism of injury described is not plausible given the developmental level of the child. Note any unusual interactions between child and caregiver or other possible perpetrators. Although a child may seem wary or frightened of the perpetrator, at times a child may cling to or try to appease an abusive caregiver to avoid further abusive behavior.

If the injury is described as an "accident," determine the mechanism. For example, if the caregiver reports that the child fell, determine the distance, the stopping surface, and the initial reactions of the child (**Table 13-7**). The information obtained at the scene may be more accurate than that obtained by the ED staff, CPS agency, and law enforcement.

Physical Examination

The prehospital professional may note suspicious findings in the physical examination of the child. Up to 90% of physical maltreatment victims have some kind of skin injury. The physical examination may reveal the suspicious patterns and physical findings of child abuse. In cases of

Table 13-6 Focused History: Questions and Considerations in Evaluating Suspected Child Maltreatment

Question	Considerations
How did the injury occur?	• Is the caregiver's explanation plausible? • Do the physical conditions at the scene support the alleged mechanism of injury?
When did it happen?	• Was there a long delay before 9-1-1 was notified? • Does the injury appearance match the time frame?
Who witnessed the event?	• Do all of the caregivers' or witnesses' stories match? • Was there adequate supervision?
What is the child's medical history?	• Are there preexisting psychosocial, developmental, or chronic problems?
Does the child have a physician?	• When was the last visit? • Does the physician know the child?

Table 13-7 Distinguishing Fact From Common Fiction

History	Fact
"He fell off the couch, and then seized."	Fewer than 1 in 1,000 falls of 4 feet (1.2 m) or less result in serious injury.
"My 1-month-old rolled off the bed."	Most infants cannot roll over until 3–4 months of age.
"He must have bruised himself."	Bruises are rare in infants who are not yet pulling to a stand.
"I found him with his leg stuck in the crib slat."	Without an external force, either intentional or accidental, infants do not sustain fractures.

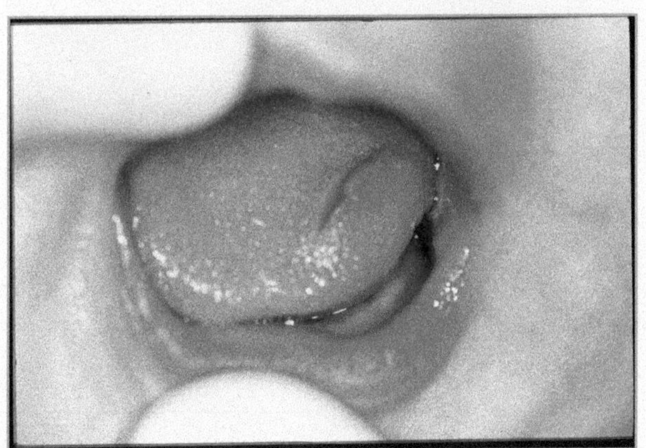

Figure 13-3 A caregiver's history of a child biting his or her tongue is not believable in an infant who has no teeth. This discrepant history suggests an inflicted injury.

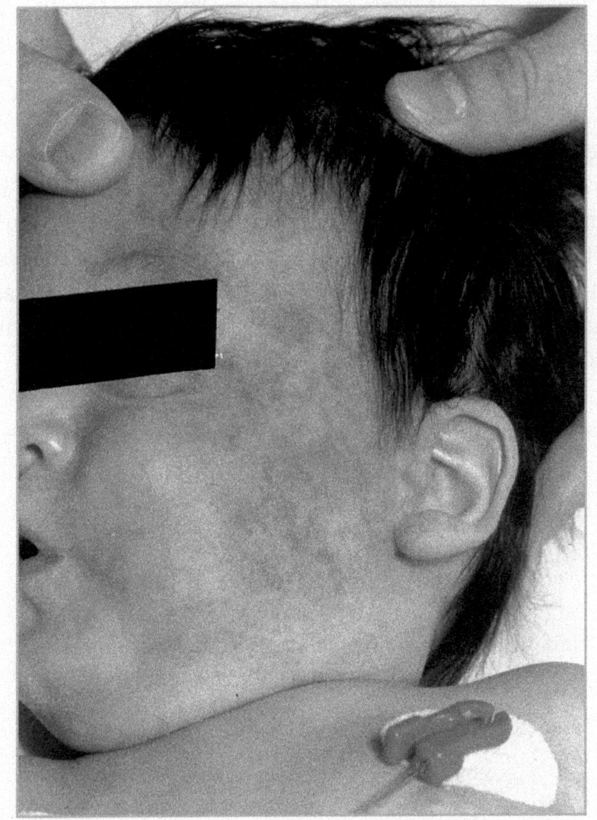

Figure 13-4 The face is a common target for physical abuse.

suspected sexual abuse, defer a genital examination to providers with specialized training.

Bruises

Physical findings that suggest inflicted injury include the following:

- Bruises located on soft tissues, such as neck, back, thighs, genitalia, or buttocks
- Bruises on or behind ears
- Bruises in a child less than 4 months of age
- Facial bruises from slapping (**Figure 13-4**)

In fact, the TEN-4 bruising rule has been developed in which any bruising of the **T**orso, **E**ars, **N**eck in any child 4 years or younger, or any bruising in an infant younger than 4 months are significant indicators of abuse.

Differentiating bruises resulting from maltreatment versus normal wear and tear depends on appearance, location, and developmental age of the child. Bruises over bony prominences, such as the elbow, forehead, or below the knees, are the common result of play injuries in children.

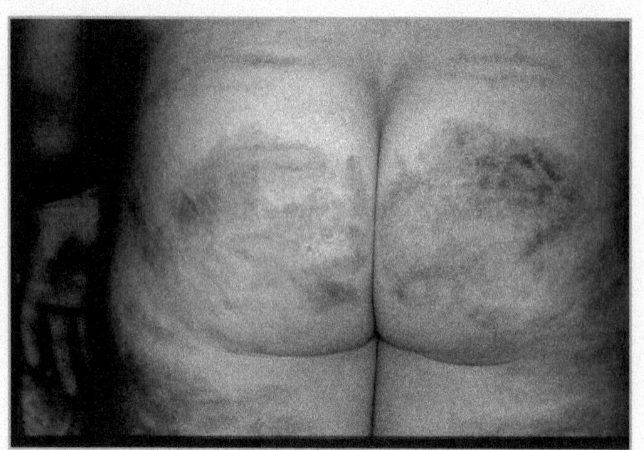

Figure 13-5 Bruises on the buttocks are usually inflicted injuries.

However, bruises over soft tissues, such as the thighs, buttocks, cheeks, ears, or on the back, are less common and should raise suspicions of inflicted injury (**Figure 13-5**).

ANY bruising in an infant who is not yet mobile may suggest inflicted injury. Most children are able to roll over by 4 months of age and able to pull to stand and cruise by 9 months of age. A child who is not yet cruising should not have unexplained bruises or fractures—*no cruising means no bruising.* As children become older and increasingly mobile, bruises and lacerations from normal activity become more common.

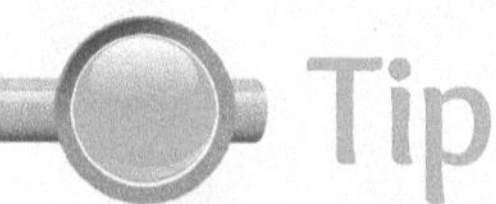

Tip

"Those who don't cruise rarely bruise." In a child who cannot yet pull up to stand and walk while holding onto furniture (cruise), bruising or injury is rare. Most infants do not start "cruising" until they are about 9 months of age.

Any bruise with an identifiable pattern is almost certain to have been inflicted. Common items include belts, cords, and hands. When an object hits the skin with high velocity, the edges leave an outline of petechiae. If a very thin object, such as a switch or a cord, hits the skin, parallel petechial lines form as an outline of the object.

It was previously thought that the time that a bruise was inflicted could be determined based on its appearance. This is now known to be inaccurate. Bruises resolve at differing rates based on their location and the mechanism of injury, and bruises of different colors can result from injuries sustained in one event. Still, document the location and colors of all bruises to provide a complete description of the injuries sustained.

Burns

Inflicted burns are usually from immersion in hot water (scalds) or from forced contact between the child and a hot object. Adult skin can develop a full-thickness burn from 2 seconds of exposure to 150°F water; children may burn even faster. Accidental scald burns typically have varying depths and irregular borders, with a "flow" pattern evident. They are rarely symmetric (i.e., both hands or both feet), and occur infrequently in the preambulatory child. In contrast, scalds from deliberately dipping a child in hot water are clearly demarcated, sparing flexural creases (e.g., the creases behind the knees or inside the elbows), because these areas are "protected" when the child reflexively tries to withdraw. "Donut burns" with sparing of the buttocks occur in children who have been dipped into hot water, but whose buttocks are pushed firmly down against the relatively cooler surface of the tub or sink (**Figure 13-6**). Children with inflicted burns may also have arm or leg bruises where they were restrained.

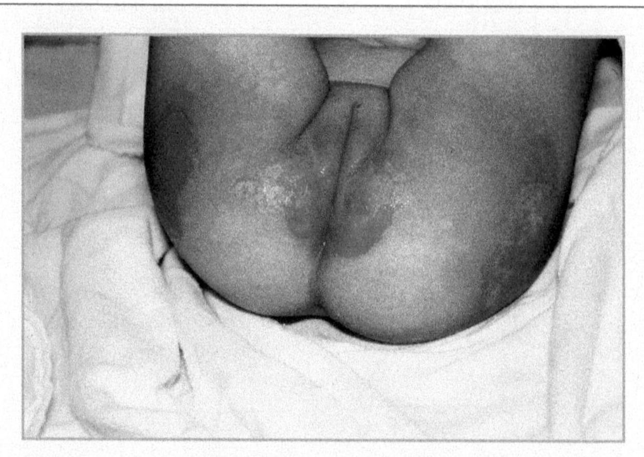

Figure 13-6 Donut burn.

Pattern burns that are an even thickness throughout or are repeated are red flags for maltreatment. Remember that any acute burn can be extremely painful. ALS providers should consider the administration of an analgesic as the local protocol allows.

Fractures

Fractures in children who are not yet ambulatory are also suspicious for maltreatment. Although an infant who is being carried and is unintentionally dropped may sustain a fracture, it is not plausible that an infant who is only crawling or cruising could develop sufficient energy on their own to fracture a bone. Infant fractures of abuse have typical patterns on hospital radiographs. A history of osteogenesis imperfecta or problems causing decreased bone calcification may increase fracture occurrence in some children. Include these conditions in the documentation of the child's history.

Deceptive Skin Signs Masquerading as Abuse

Sometimes, normal physical findings suggest an inflicted injury. For example, "Mongolian spots" are birthmarks frequently seen in children of color (e.g., African American, Asian, Latino) that can be easily mistaken for bruises (**Figure 13-7**). These birthmarks often take the form of large, flat patches of hyperpigmented skin, most commonly found on the low back or buttocks. Mongolian spots will blanch; bruises will not.

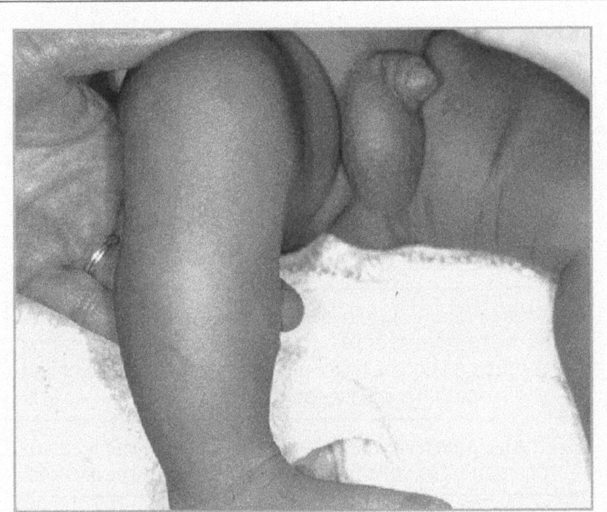

Figure 13-7 Mongolian spots appear on the buttocks, back, and extremities of many infants.

Certain disease states, such as leukemia, vasculitis, meningococcemia, or bleeding disorders (i.e., hemophilia), can rarely produce skin findings that appear to be bruises. Infectious processes, such as impetigo, can appear to be burns, but are much less painful. Insect bites in some children can cause redness and blistering. Distinguishing intentional injuries with certainty is sometimes impossible in the field.

Another benign skin finding that masquerades as abuse is the pattern of lesions produced by cultural rituals intended to treat illness. The most common of these patterns are associated with Asian practices called cupping (**Figure 13-8**) and coin rubbing (**Figure 13-9**). These superficial lesions have distinctive rounded edges. Caregivers of these children can explain the purpose for such practices—information that can help distinguish inflicted injuries that are intended to help from inflicted injuries that are intended to harm.

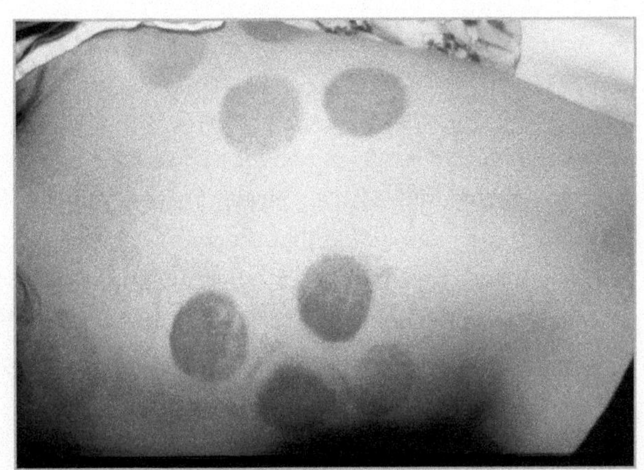

Figure 13-8 Cupping is the cultural practice of placing warm cups on the skin to pull out illness from the body. The red, flat, rounded skin lesions are often more intensely red at the borders.

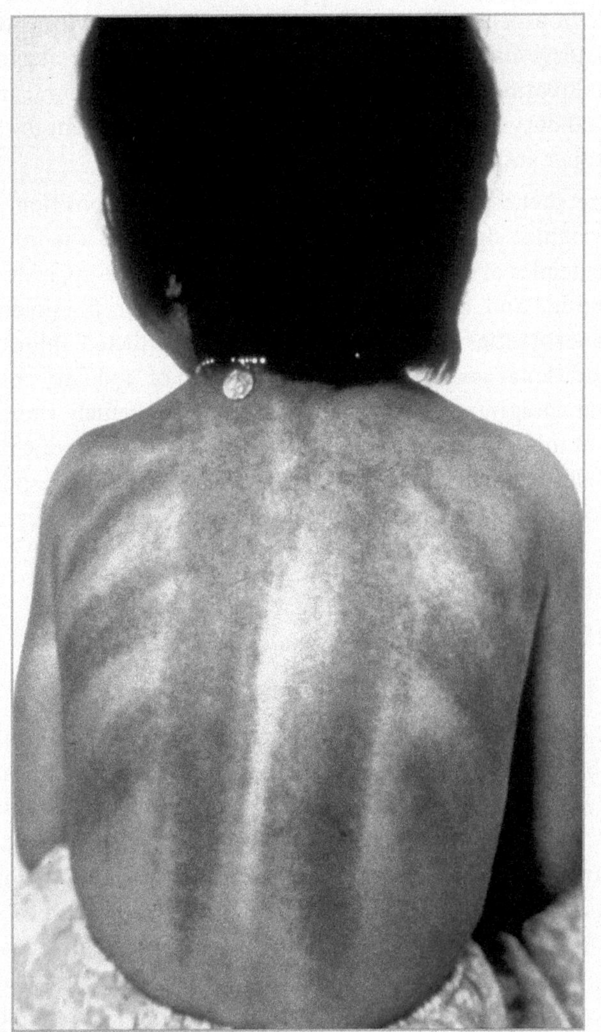

Figure 13-9 Rubbing hot coins, often on the back, produces rounded and oblong red, patchy, flat skin lesions.

Summary of Duties, Communication, and Assessment in Suspected Maltreatment

When child maltreatment is suspected, the prehospital professional faces a challenging and potentially explosive situation. Communication with the child may be difficult

Case Study 2

You respond to an apartment at 3 AM for a baby not breathing. On arrival, an apparently intoxicated female meets you at the door with an unresponsive 6-month-old female in cardiac arrest. Your partner begins treatment, and you are able to determine that the woman is the grandmother who is supposed to be watching her granddaughter while the baby's mother is working an overnight shift. The grandmother tells you that she and the infant must have fallen asleep on the couch, and she woke up "next" to the baby and that she found the baby this way. You also notice several beer cans in the room. There are at least three blankets and a pillow piled up on the couch.

1. **What are the red flags for maltreatment?**
2. **What are your medical and legal responsibilities?**

or limited, and interactions with the caregiver may be frustrating and sometimes hostile. A professional, nonjudgmental approach is necessary. Document conditions in the environment, the child's and caregiver's behaviors, the history, and relevant physical findings that may suggest maltreatment. The prehospital professional has a moral and legal duty to report suspected cases of maltreatment to the proper authorities.

The prehospital professional is in a unique position to recognize signs of possible child maltreatment. The initial principles of field care are the careful scene size-up, history taking, and careful physical assessment for physiologic abnormalities or anatomic patterns of inflicted injuries. Additional assessment and identification of "red flag" child and caregiver behaviors are sometimes extremely important to maltreatment investigations. The diagnosis of child maltreatment is rarely possible in the field. All cases require a complete investigation by the community CPS agency.

Legislation, Principles, and Protocols

Child Protective Services

The CPS agency is a legal community organization responsible for protection against child maltreatment. CPS has the legal authority to temporarily remove children at risk for injury or neglect from the home and to secure foster care placement. CPS is responsible for initial investigations of suspected maltreatment. They must make complicated and important decisions about the maltreatment accusations, at times remove children from the home and place them into foster care, and provide services for abusive and neglectful families. **Table 13-8** lists the initial actions of the CPS when a report is filed. CPS may work in concert with law enforcement to investigate the facts and determine who is responsible for maltreating the child. Ultimately, the judicial system determines if an accused individual is "guilty." Although emotions may run high when the prehospital professional suspects child maltreatment, it is neither appropriate nor safe to confront caregivers with these concerns at the scene.

The prehospital professional can provide scene information that helps CPS determine safe placement of the patient. When maltreatment is suspected, always note the presence of other children in the home. If a determination is made that an environment may be unsafe, contact law

Table 13-8 Initial CPS Actions

1. When a report of child abuse or neglect is received, either from a health care professional or a law enforcement agency, the protocols of the receiving agency determine the timing and scope of the initial response.
2. The facts are reviewed to determine if a home visit is appropriate and, if so, which members of the team will be involved.
3. The CPS caseworker assesses risk to the child, the family's ability to provide safety, and supportive resources available to the family.
4. After the investigation and assessment, a reported incident is determined to be founded, unfounded, or unable to be determined because of lack of information.

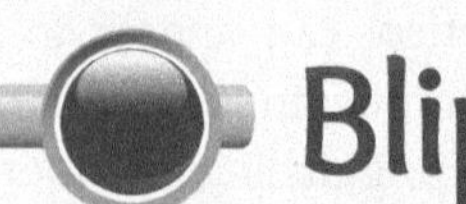

Judging or confronting caregivers or attempting to intervene in issues of dysfunctional parenting may interfere with patient care or a subsequent maltreatment investigation. The caregiver may in fact not know how the child was injured or by whom. Your interventions may put you at risk, and a confrontation does not help the child.

enforcement or CPS to evaluate the safety of any other children who are present, based on local EMS protocol. When a patient is transported to a hospital, communicate any concerns of maltreatment to hospital staff, which also have a mandatory obligation to report.

Another resource to know and be familiar with is the Child Abuse Prevention and Treatment Act (CAPTA). CAPTA is a federal law that provides funding, resources, grants, and guidance to states and organizations to protect children from child maltreatment. This law, among many other items, provides for a national clearinghouse to collect data (National Clearinghouse on Child Abuse and Neglect Information), establishes the Office on Abuse and Neglect, and coordinates activities and programs that serve this particular population. Other national resources of note include the Never Shake a Baby Campaign (National Center on Shaken Baby Syndrome; www.dontshake.org) and Healthy Families America (www.healthyfamiliesamerica.org; which provides education and support to expecting and new parents to help with the arrival of a newborn in the family).

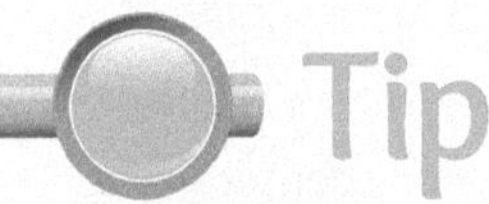

Note and report the presence of other children in situations suggestive of maltreatment.

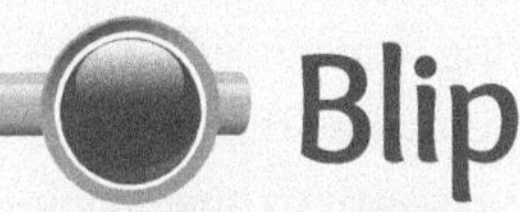

Never attempt to physically restrain a caregiver or to forcibly take possession of a child. Call law enforcement if the scene is unsafe.

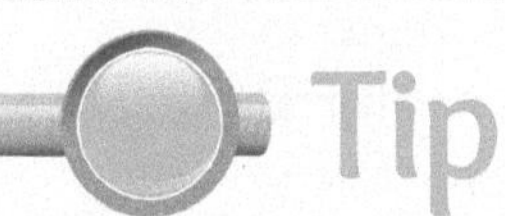

Even in the face of probable maltreatment, remain nonjudgmental with the caregiver and maintain control of the scene and transport.

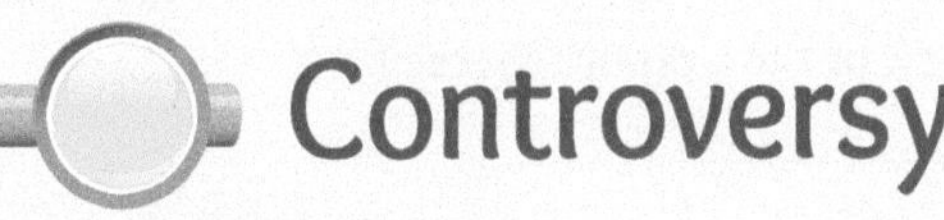

The on-scene role of law enforcement in suspected child maltreatment is controversial. In most cases, it is prudent to transport a child to the ED for physician and CPS evaluation. If the scene is not safe or caretakers are refusing transport, the prehospital professional must call law enforcement for protection and assistance.

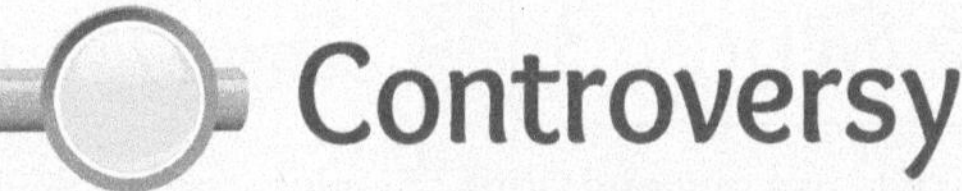

It is the duty of the prehospital professional to ensure that someone submits a CPS report when abuse is suspected. Depending on state law, this duty may be legal or it may be ethical. In some jurisdictions, a single report from hospital personnel is sufficient, whereas in others the prehospital professionals must file their own report.

Case Study 3

9-1-1 is called by a babysitter, because a child has been burned. On arrival at the scene, the EMS crew finds a teenage girl holding a sobbing 2-year-old boy. The teenager states that the child has been fussy and crying for the 2 hours in her care. On changing the child's diaper, the sitter noted what looked like burns on the buttocks, and on her mother's advice called 9-1-1.

The child is alert but upset and is not easily consolable by the babysitter. There are areas of denuded skin on the buttocks covered with diaper rash cream, with one unpopped blister near the sacrum. The centers of both buttocks, and the gluteal cleft, do not appear to be injured. Extremity examination shows no bruises or other abnormalities.

1. Is this injury caused from abuse?
2. What interventions are indicated?

CASE STUDY ANSWERS

Case Study 1 — page 262

Be alert for the signs of abusive head trauma in any infant or small child with a sudden onset of altered mental status and irregular respirations. Remember that grab bruises and marks may be found on the arms of children that are held and shaken, and their presence should be documented. Carefully document the scene, the comments of the caregiver, and the reported events leading to the injury.

Immediate transportation is critical. One common complication of inflicted head injury is respiratory failure or apnea as a result of elevated intracranial pressure and compression of the medulla (respiratory center in the brainstem). Be prepared to provide respiratory support. Ensure that the ED staff will make a report to the CPS agency, or file a report yourself.

Case Study 2 — page 270

This case may be the result of the grandmother accidently suffocating the infant. Co-sleeping, especially with a caregiver who is under the influence of alcohol or drugs, can have deadly consequences. Adults may roll over on top of infants and not realize it because of their intoxicated state. Infants do not have the strength to push back or to get the adult to notice that they are lying on them. Make a note of the scene and call law enforcement. Your attention needs to be focused on resuscitation efforts for the child.

Case Study 3 — page 271

This child has obvious signs of an inflicted scald injury. The lack of burn in the creases and the center of the buttocks (donut burn) may indicate the child was forcibly held in hot water. There is no way for the prehospital professional to know who inflicted the injury; nor is establishing responsibility part of his or her role.

Provide analgesia if possible. Large burns can lead to significant fluid losses, so ALS providers should start an intravenous (IV) line and begin fluid resuscitation. Document the scene size-up, the child's and caregiver's behaviors, and the history. Transport this child to an ED for burn care as well as an evaluation for inflicted injury. Treatment at a burn center may ultimately be necessary.

SUGGESTED READINGS

Textbooks

American Academy of Pediatrics and the American College of Emergency Physicians. *APLS: The Pediatric Emergency Medicine Resource*. 5th ed. Burlington, MA: Jones and Bartlett Learning; 2012.

Hazinski M, Zaritsky A, Nadkarni V, et al. *PALS Provider Manual*. Dallas: American Heart Association; 2011.

Reece R, Ludwig S. *Child Abuse: Medical Diagnosis and Management*. 2nd ed. Philadelphia: Lippincott, Williams & Wilkins; 2001.

Articles

Johnson CF. Child maltreatment 2002: recognition, reporting and risk. *Pediatr Int*. 2002;44:554–560.

Kairys S. Distinguishing sudden infant death syndrome from child abuse fatalities. American Academy of Pediatrics. Committee on Child Abuse and Neglect. *Pediatrics*. 2001;107(2):437–441.

Kempe CH. The battered child syndrome. *JAMA*. 1962;181:17–24.

Krug EG, Dahlberg LL, Mercy JA, et al. World report on violence and health. Geneva: World Health Organization; 2002.

Pierce MC, Kaczor K, Aldridge S, et al. Bruising characteristics discriminating physical abuse from accidental trauma. *Pediatrics*. 2010;125:67—74.

Web sites

American Psychological Association. Child sexual abuse: what parents should know. http://www.apa.org/pi/families/resources/child-sexual-abuse.aspx. Accessed September 28, 2012.

Krug EG, Dahlberg LL, Mercy JA, et al. World report on violence and health. Geneva, World Health Organization, 2002. Available in pdf format at: http://www.who.int/violence_injury_prevention/violence/world_report/en/FullWRVH.pdf. Accessed February 13, 2004.

U.S. Department of Health & Human Services, Childrens Bureau. 2013. *Child maltreatment*. Available from http://www.acf.hhs.gov/sites/default/files/cb/cm2013.pdf. Accessed December 22, 2015.

CD-ROMs

American Academy of Pediatrics. *Visual Diagnosis of Child Abuse* [CD-ROM]. Elk Grove Village, IL: American Academy of Pediatrics; 2001.

Lauridsen J, Levin A, Parrish R, et al. *Shaken Baby Syndrome: A Visual Overview*. Version 2.0. National Center on Shaken Baby Syndrome; 2003.

References

Child Welfare Information Gateway. 2012. Child maltreatment 2010: summary of key findings. http://www.childwelfare.gov/pubs/factsheets/canstats.cfm. Accessed September 11, 2012.

Gelles RJ, Perlman S. *Estimated Annual Cost of Child Abuse and Neglect*. Chicago, IL: Prevent Child Abuse America; 2012.

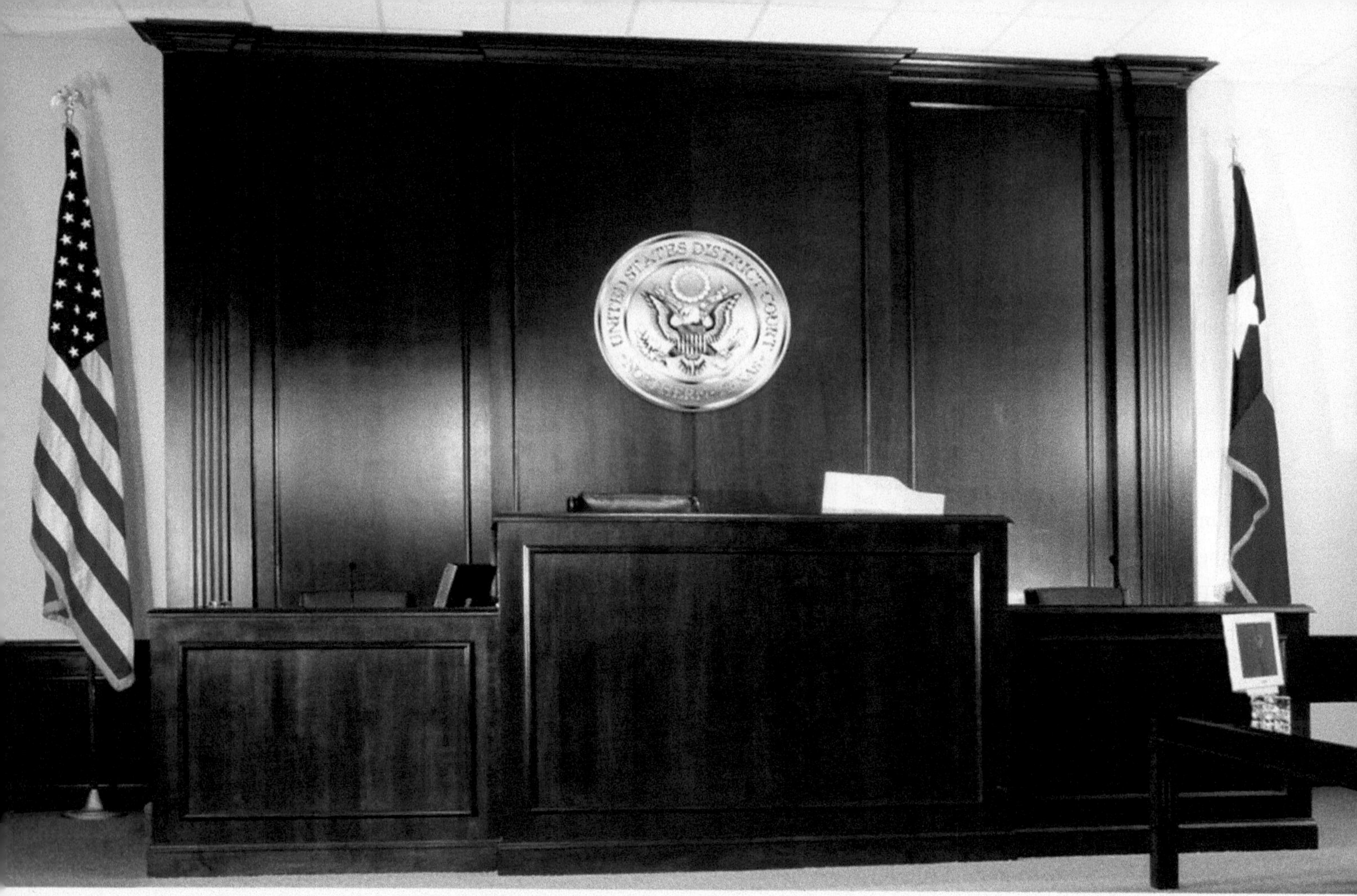

Learning Objectives

1. Identify out-of-hospital ethical and legal issues unique to pediatric emergency care.
2. Discuss the emergency exception rule, or the doctrine of implied consent, in the out-of-hospital treatment and transport of a minor.
3. Understand the different ethical and legal challenges in caring for older children and adolescents.
4. Outline the prehospital professional's responsibilities when a caregiver may refuse to grant consent to prehospital professionals to treat or transport a minor.
5. Review the legal and ethical considerations when faced with a child who has a "Do Not Resuscitate" status.

Medicolegal and Ethical Considerations

Chapter 14

Introduction

The prehospital professional frequently encounters ethical and legal issues while caring for children. These may include the inability to obtain the legal guardian's permission to treat a child, refusal of consent by parents or older children, challenges of confidentiality, issues related to telling the truth, and the identification of possible child maltreatment. This chapter discusses these issues and emphasizes the importance of protocols and policies for prehospital professionals to address common pediatric ethical and legal concerns.

Consent

The requirement to obtain **informed consent** from a patient or legal guardian before delivering medical care is a central feature of American health care law and ethics. A legally mature individual may not be touched, treated, or transported without his or her consent. **Minors** (children younger than 18 years of age), however, present a special problem because they do not have the legal authority to give or refuse consent. Therefore, in most states, a parent or legal guardian must give permission before a minor can be medically treated or transported (**Figure 14-1**).

State law designates certain minors as "emancipated" and grants these **emancipated minors** the right to make decisions, including health care decisions. Children who are legally emancipated may give consent for medical treatment and transport. They may also refuse medical care or transport. Although emancipated minor laws vary from state to state, most states recognize minors to be emancipated if they are married, are pregnant, have a child, are economically self-supporting and not living at home, or are on active-duty status in the armed services.

In situations where a minor who is not emancipated yet has a medical condition that represents a threat to life or health and a legal guardian is not readily available to provide consent, prehospital professionals can assess the child, provide necessary medical treatment, and transport the child. The legal basis for taking action in an emergency when consent is not available is known as the **emergency exception rule**.

The emergency exception rule is also known as the doctrine of **implied consent**. For minors, this doctrine means that the prehospital professional can presume consent and proceed with appropriate treatment and transport if all of the following four conditions are met:

1. The child is suffering from an emergent condition that places his or her life or health in danger.
2. The child's legal guardian is unavailable or unable to provide consent for treatment or transport.
3. Treatment or transport cannot be safely delayed until consent can be obtained.
4. The prehospital professional administers only treatment for emergency conditions that pose an immediate threat to the child.

Case Study 1

You are called to an apartment where you find a 3-year-old girl in mild respiratory distress. She is interactive and consolable, but has bilateral wheezes and a pulse oximeter reading of 94%. She is home alone with a 16-year-old babysitter who tells you that the child's parents will not return for several hours and did not leave information about their destination or contact information.

1. **Can the babysitter give you legally valid consent to treat the child?**
2. **Can you legally provide care and transport this child?**

The emergency exception rule is based on the principle that if the legal guardian knew the severity of the emergency, he or she would consent to medical treatment of the child. Any time a minor is treated without consent, the burden of proof falls on the prehospital professional to justify that the emergency actions were necessary. The prehospital professional must fully and clearly document on the prehospital record the nature of the medical emergency, attempts to contact the legal guardian, and the reasons the minor required immediate treatment or transport.

If possible, contact on-line medical control for assistance when consent is unclear or unavailable. If the guardian is unavailable or cannot be notified, provide information about the destination emergency department (ED) to the most responsible person on scene (in writing whenever possible), with instructions to pass the information on to the minor's legal guardian. As a general rule, when the prehospital professional's authority to act is in doubt, always do what is in the best interest of the minor.

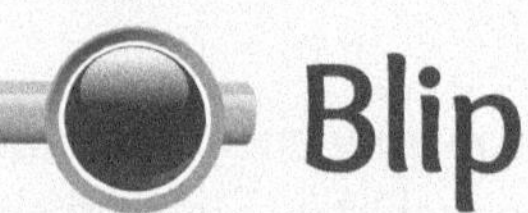

Blip

When a legal guardian is not readily available to provide consent for a minor, the prehospital professional must provide only treatment and transport for emergency conditions that pose an immediate threat to the child.

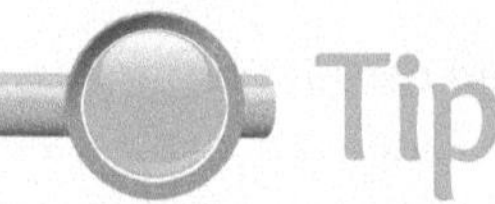

Tip

When the prehospital professional's authority to act is in doubt, always do what is in the best interest of the minor.

Refusal of Care or Transport

Guardian Refusal

A special situation occurs when the prehospital professional is faced with a legal guardian who refuses to give permission for medical treatment or transport of a child with an acute illness or injury. As long as a child's legal guardian is alert, oriented, and mentally competent, he or she has the right to refuse medical care for the child. However, the guardian must act in the best interest of the child.

When a guardian refuses to allow provision of care or transport of a child whose life or health might be threatened, an important legal and ethical issue arises. In such circumstances, attempt to contact medical control for guidance. The medical control physician may speak directly to the legal guardian to convince the guardian to allow treatment and transport. If medical control agrees that the child's condition requires immediate treatment to prevent serious harm, yet the legal guardian continues to refuse consent for care, it may be necessary to notify law enforcement and enlist their assistance in placing the child in temporary protective custody. Likewise, when a legal guardian seems to be intoxicated or otherwise impaired, involvement of law enforcement officers may be necessary to place a minor in temporary protective custody. Local emergency medical services (EMS) pediatric policies should guide the prehospital professional's procedure in such situations.

Although temporary protective custody may allow the prehospital professional to transport a minor to a medical facility for purposes of medical evaluation, it does not give the prehospital professional the right to treat a minor for medical conditions that are not serious or life-threatening. *A prehospital professional can provide medical treatment without consent only when the child has a medical condition that poses a risk of death or serious harm, when immediate specific treatment is necessary to prevent that harm, and when only those specific treatments are provided.* Discuss these situations with medical control before initiating treatment, whenever possible. Sometimes an intermediate solution is possible. Document everything fully and clearly about the medical condition of the child, the need for emergency care, and the basis for overriding the wishes of the legal guardian.

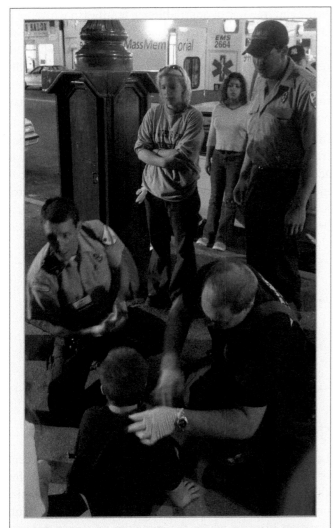

Figure 14-1 In most states, a parent or legal guardian must give permission before a minor can be transported.

Every case of unclear consent or refusal requires careful scene management, notification of medical control if available, and full and accurate documentation in the prehospital record.

Never confront the caregiver with accusations, moral judgments, or threats when difficult circumstances develop at the scene. This approach only aggravates the situation and does not help the child. Try to establish whether the caregiver refuses all care and transport or only certain aspects of care. For example, some caregivers may prefer that prehospital professionals not initiate therapy, but permit the child to be transported to the hospital. If the child can be safely transported without initiating care, respect the caregiver's wishes concerning care. It may be appropriate for the caregiver of a child with a terminal illness or significant disabilities to restrict certain kinds of care for the child. Discuss these difficult situations with medical control.

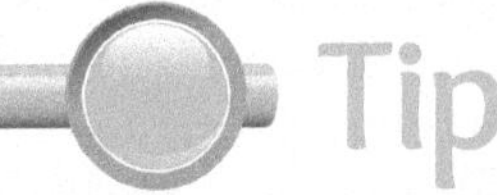

Get police assistance when a guardian who is impaired or intoxicated refuses care or transport of an ill or injured child.

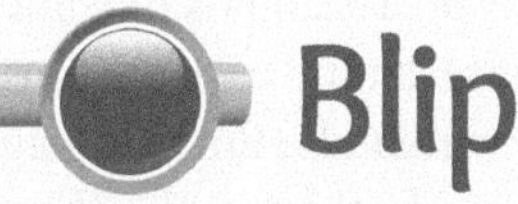

Never confront the caregiver with accusations, moral judgments, or threats.

Child Refusal

There are two situations in which a minor has the legal authority to refuse care and make decisions regarding his or her health care. The first situation is when the child is an emancipated minor, as previously discussed. A second situation in which a minor might have legal status to make decisions arises when a court has declared an individual a mature minor. This is different than an emancipated minor. In most states, mature minors are older than 14 years of age and have been formally declared adults by the court. **Table 14-1** lists the legal circumstances in which pediatric patients can provide or refuse consent for medical care and transport in most states. *Since these laws vary, the prehospital professional should be familiar with the specifics of emancipated and mature minor laws in the state in which care is being provided.*

Table 14-1 Characteristics of Emancipated or Mature Minors

Emancipated Minor
Married
Pregnant
Has a child
Active-duty status in the armed services
15 years or older, economically self-supporting, and living apart from parents
Mature Minor
14 years or older and declared a mature minor by the state Superior Court
AND patient is not on a psychiatric hold
AND patient demonstrates competency to refuse

If a child is not an emancipated or a mature minor, then he or she has no legal capacity either to give consent or to refuse medical care. Regardless of whether a child has the legal authority to provide or withhold consent, it is always prudent to try to get the child's agreement or "assent" to treat and transport. This approach respects the personal dignity and self-determination of the child-patient and minimizes confrontation. A willingness to provide the child with some control and some choices may allow for a compromise that helps prehospital professionals to achieve a safe transfer. Reserve force or restraint to transport a child only for those situations in which all efforts to negotiate respectfully with the child have failed and the child is at risk of serious harm if he or she is not transported.

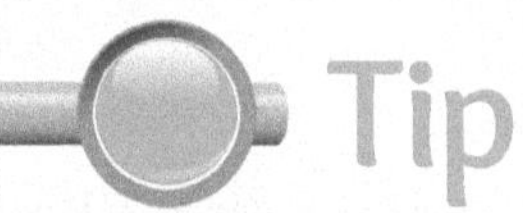

Tip

A minor child cannot legally refuse care or transport when care is required.

Caregivers Who Disagree

One rare but confusing situation arises when the prehospital professional is confronted by caregivers who disagree about whether to consent to treatment and transport of a sick or injured child. In these cases, establish whether one or both caregivers are legal decision-makers for the child. If both caregivers have legal authority, the prehospital professional may need to negotiate a plan that both find acceptable. Focus on the child's needs and the common desire to assist the child, while deflecting attention from the disagreement. Medical control may need to be involved to assist the prehospital professional in determining the proper course of action and to determine the need for law enforcement.

Custody Issues and Nontraditional Families

Parents who are legally divorced may disagree about the child's care or access to the child's medical records. One parent may accuse the other of harming the child or being a poor influence. There may be differing viewpoints between the biologic parent and the step-parent. In another case, the biologic mother at the scene may refuse to allow the step-mother, also at the scene, to participate in the child's care, give permission for any treatment, or have any access to knowledge about the child's condition. Perhaps one parent is the legal guardian and the other parent's rights have been terminated. Another parent may refuse transport because he or she does not want to be billed, because that responsibility rests with the parent who is not available.

Many children live in nontraditional families in which they are cared for by grandparents, older siblings, two same-sex parents, or foster parents. It may not be clear who has the responsibility of consenting for the minor child. In addition, these caregivers may be the only adults involved with the child on a regular basis despite the fact that they may not be legally accountable for that child.

In these situations, determining legal guardianship for treatment and transport may be difficult. If the child is acutely ill or injured, there is not time to look at legal documents, if they are even available. Contact medical control for advice, and involve law enforcement if the situation becomes violent or may cause harm to the child.

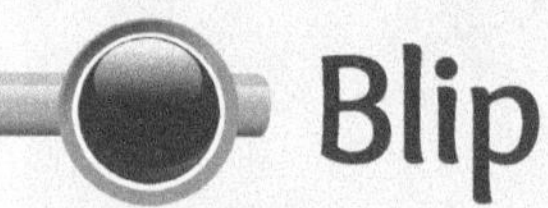

Blip

Many children live in nontraditional families, and it may be unclear who has responsibility for consenting for the minor child.

Summary of Consent

Laws strictly protect the right of adult patients to accept or reject medical care. Interpreting these consent laws for children in a prehospital setting, however, can pose special problems. The prehospital professional faces a difficult situation in cases where the caregiver refuses to consent or where consent to provide care and transport for a child cannot be readily obtained. Every case requires careful scene management, notification of medical control if available, and accurate documentation in the prehospital record. EMS systems should provide clear policies, procedures, and protocols based on state law to guide the prehospital professional or medical control. Local EMS policy on consent should clearly define the following:

- Who can refuse ambulance transport according to state law
- The process for field evaluation, consultation, and documentation
- The method for enlisting police and medical control when the patient or guardian is dangerous and refuses transport, or when a child has a life-threatening problem and the guardian is refusing transport

Confidentiality

Medical information is private. Carelessly or inadvertently revealing identifiable information is an ethical and legal risk that prehospital professionals face, because they frequently care for individuals in a public environment.

It is essential to remain aware of the potentially sensitive nature of identifiable information and to take every possible precaution to protect confidentiality. Conduct all sensitive discussions, when possible, in a setting where bystanders cannot overhear. Avoid using last names, if at all possible, at the scene. Do not share private information with concerned bystanders (other than those legally responsible for the patient).

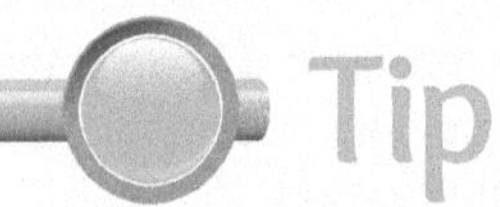

Prehospital professionals must be aware of the potentially sensitive nature of protected health information and take every possible precaution to protect confidentiality.

Respect for Cultural or Religious Differences

Cultural differences and religious beliefs may present exceptionally difficult situations. Although the care of the patient is always of primary concern, the prehospital professional must attempt to respect requests from the family or patient regarding preferences that may originate from their religious or cultural beliefs, especially when these do not interfere significantly with the provision of treatment to the child. The prehospital professional must always remain nonjudgmental about requests that stem from cultural or religious beliefs, acknowledge the importance of these requests to the family, and attempt to accommodate them when possible. When the prehospital professional cannot accommodate requests that are based on cultural or religious beliefs because they would put a child at risk of serious harm, the reasons the requests cannot be accommodated must be respectfully explained. Medical control and police may need to be involved if parents refuse to consent to necessary care and the child is at risk of harm.

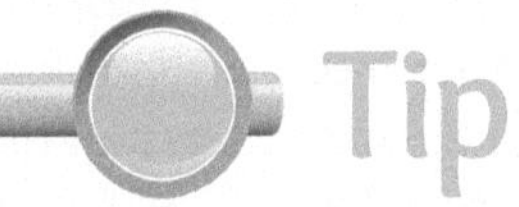

The prehospital professional must always remain nonjudgmental about cultural or religious beliefs, acknowledge their importance to the family, and attempt to accommodate them whenever possible.

Language barriers may also present a challenge as the prehospital professional attempts to communicate with a child's caregiver. The prehospital professional should be familiar with what resources are available locally to provide translation in a timely manner. Miscommunications can have a significant impact on a child's care, especially if the prehospital professional is unable to obtain information about a child's underlying medical conditions, allergies, current medications, or other factors relevant to field care. If professional translation services are available, use these rather than family members or bystanders. If translation services are not available, a family member or neighbor may be asked to assist with translation, with the understanding that the information transferred may be inaccurate or incomplete, especially with regard to medical terminology.

Patient Rights and Advocacy

For children, patient rights may be dependent on the wishes of the child's parents or legal guardians. However, emancipated minors have the ability to make decisions about their medical care and treatment even though these decisions may not be accepted by other members of the family or the general public. The EMS system, the medical director, and the community's standard of care can compete with the wishes of the patients. These competing interests can create an ethical conflict that needs to be resolved.

The decision to accept medical treatment may be a difficult one. Give the parents, guardians, or the emancipated minor time to consider what is most appropriate. In some

Case Study 2

You are called to care for a homeless 15-year-old boy whose friends called because he was not feeling well and was not acting normally. You find the young man lying on the sidewalk, complaining of a severe headache. When you attempt to assess him, he starts cussing, pushes you away aggressively, and demands to be left alone. He screams that he has rights and that he does not have to talk to you. He will not even answer questions that would allow you to assess his level of consciousness and orientation.

1. What rights does the teenager have to refuse care and transport?
2. What methods of persuasion can you use?

instances, this emergency may be the first time the patient has had to face the reality of his or her medical condition. When in doubt, try to do what is in the best interest of the patient and rely on medical control for advice.

End of Life Issues

The caregivers of some children who are terminally ill, usually in consultation with their primary physician, may decide on limitations to treatments and interventions. These decisions usually arise from the child's underlying condition and the desire to avoid futile or burdensome interventions if the child develops a life-threatening condition. Prehospital professionals, in responding to a call about a sick child, may be confronted with a Do Not Resuscitate (DNR) order. A DNR order must be signed by a physician to be valid (**Figure 14-2**). These orders inform health care providers that cardiopulmonary resuscitation (CPR) or additional resuscitation, such as defibrillation or advanced airway control, should not be initiated in the event of a cardiopulmonary arrest. Some local EMS regions do not recognize DNR orders for children. *Prehospital professionals must know the limits of the DNR law governing their area of coverage and develop protocols for dealing with them.*

Regardless of the nature of the local DNR law or prehospital policy, a legal guardian may always revoke a DNR order written on behalf of a child. When faced with a valid DNR order written for a child and a legal guardian requesting that the child be resuscitated, always follow the legal guardian's wishes. Even in the face of a valid DNR order, clarify with the legal guardian what kinds of interventions he or she does and does not consider acceptable. For example, oxygen delivery and transport may be acceptable and expected for some children with DNR orders.

Resuscitation

Sometimes resuscitation attempts are ineffective for children in cardiopulmonary arrest, and occasionally such attempts are unnecessary, as discussed in Chapter 5, *Resuscitation*. Resuscitation policy should define circumstances when cardiopulmonary resuscitation must be initiated, when it may be withheld, and when it may be stopped. Personnel in rural and wilderness situations must also consider the time it takes for a patient to reach definitive care at the hospital. For pediatric patients, the policy should take a medically conservative approach, but allow appropriate withholding of resuscitation to focus on grief management and family interactions.

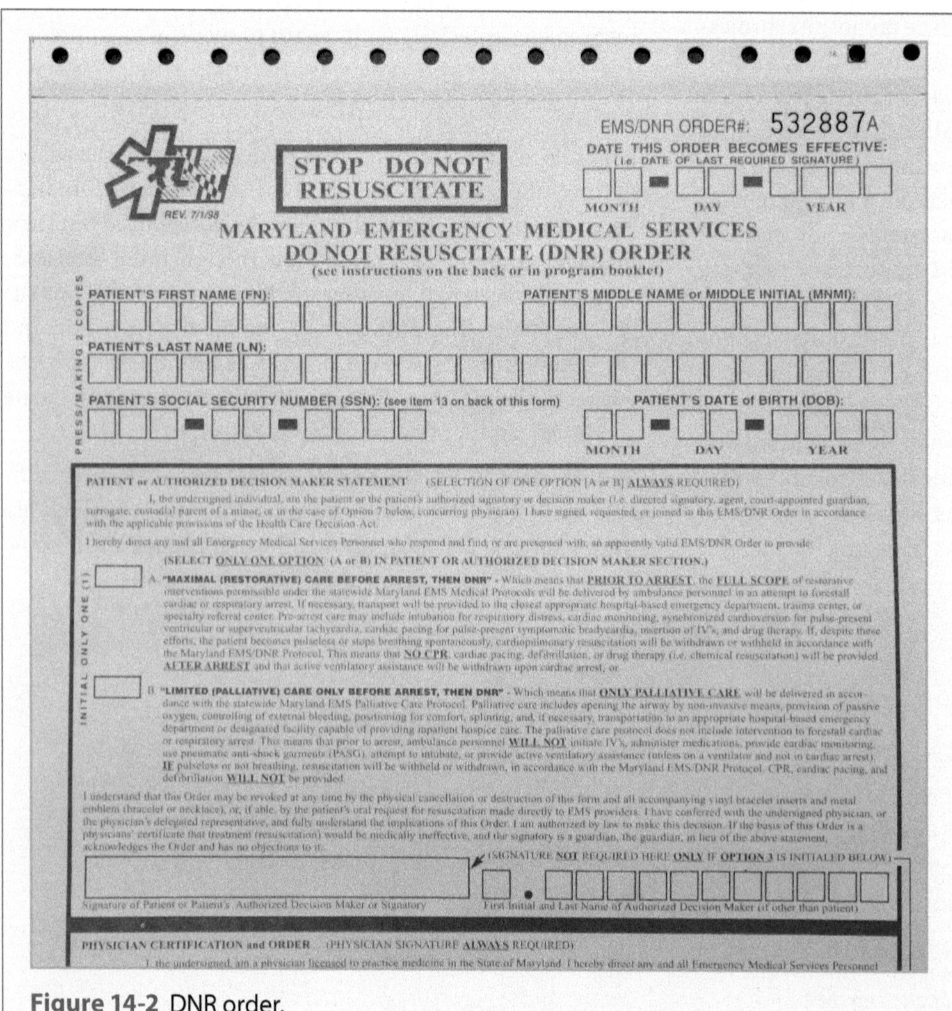

EMS/DNR ORDER#: 532887A

DATE THIS ORDER BECOMES EFFECTIVE: (i.e. DATE OF LAST REQUIRED SIGNATURE)

MONTH DAY YEAR

STOP DO NOT RESUSCITATE

REV. 7/1/98

MARYLAND EMERGENCY MEDICAL SERVICES

DO NOT RESUSCITATE (DNR) ORDER

(see instructions on the back or in program booklet)

PRESS/MAKING 2 COPIES

PATIENT'S FIRST NAME (FN):

PATIENT'S MIDDLE NAME or MIDDLE INITIAL (MNMI):

PATIENT'S LAST NAME (LN):

PATIENT'S SOCIAL SECURITY NUMBER (SSN): (see item 13 on back of this form)

PATIENT'S DATE of BIRTH (DOB):

MONTH DAY YEAR

PATIENT or AUTHORIZED DECISION MAKER STATEMENT (SELECTION OF ONE OPTION [A or B] ALWAYS REQUIRED)

I, the undersigned individual, am the patient or the patient's authorized signatory or decision maker (i.e. directed signatory, agent, court-appointed guardian, surrogate, custodial parent of a minor, or in the case of Option 7 below, concurring physician). I have signed, requested, or joined in this EMS/DNR Order in accordance with the applicable provisions of the Health Care Decision Act.

I hereby direct any and all Emergency Medical Services Personnel who respond and find, or are presented with, an apparently valid EMS/DNR Order to provide:

(SELECT ONLY ONE OPTION (A or B) IN PATIENT OR AUTHORIZED DECISION MAKER SECTION.)

INITIAL ONLY ONE (1)

A. **"MAXIMAL (RESTORATIVE) CARE BEFORE ARREST, THEN DNR"** - Which means that **PRIOR TO ARREST**, the **FULL SCOPE** of restorative interventions permissible under the statewide Maryland EMS Medical Protocols will be delivered by ambulance personnel in an attempt to forestall cardiac or respiratory arrest. If necessary, transport will be provided to the closest appropriate hospital-based emergency department, trauma center, or specialty referral center. Pre-arrest care may include intubation for respiratory distress, cardiac monitoring, synchronized cardioversion for pulse-present ventricular or superventricular tachycardia, cardiac pacing for pulse-present symptomatic bradycardia, insertion of IV's, and drug therapy. If, despite these efforts, the patient becomes pulseless or stops breathing spontaneously, cardiopulmonary resuscitation will be withdrawn or withheld in accordance with the Maryland EMS/DNR Protocol. This means that **NO CPR**, cardiac pacing, defibrillation, or drug therapy (i.e. chemical resuscitation) will be provided **AFTER ARREST** and that active ventilatory assistance will be withdrawn upon cardiac arrest; or

B. **"LIMITED (PALLIATIVE) CARE ONLY BEFORE ARREST, THEN DNR"** - Which means that **ONLY PALLIATIVE CARE** will be delivered in accordance with the statewide Maryland EMS Palliative Care Protocol. Palliative care includes opening the airway by non-invasive means, provision of passive oxygen, controlling of external bleeding, positioning for comfort, splinting, and, if necessary, transportation to an appropriate hospital-based emergency department or designated facility capable of providing inpatient hospice care. The palliative care protocol does not include intervention to forestall cardiac or respiratory arrest. This means that prior to arrest, ambulance personnel **WILL NOT** initiate IV's, administer medications, provide cardiac monitoring, use pneumatic anti-shock garments (PASG), attempt to intubate, or provide active ventilatory assistance (unless on a ventilator and not in cardiac arrest). **IF** pulseless or not breathing, resuscitation will be withheld or withdrawn, in accordance with the Maryland EMS/DNR Protocol. CPR, cardiac pacing, and defibrillation **WILL NOT** be provided.

I understand that this Order may be revoked at any time by the physical cancellation or destruction of this form and all accompanying vinyl bracelet inserts and metal emblem (bracelet or necklace), or, if able, by the patient's oral request for resuscitation made directly to EMS providers. I have conferred with the undersigned physician, or the physician's delegated representative, and fully understand the implications of this Order. I am authorized by law to make this decision. If the basis of this Order is a physicians' certificate that treatment (resuscitation) would be medically ineffective, and the signatory is a guardian, the guardian, in lieu of the above statement, acknowledges the Order and has no objections to it.

(SIGNATURE NOT REQUIRED HERE ONLY IF OPTION 3 IS INITIALED BELOW)

Signature of Patient or Patient's Authorized Decision Maker or Signatory

First Initial and Last Name of Authorized Decision Maker (if other than patient)

PHYSICIAN CERTIFICATION and ORDER (PHYSICIAN SIGNATURE ALWAYS REQUIRED)

I, the undersigned, am a physician licensed to practice medicine in the State of Maryland. I hereby direct any and all Emergency Medical Services Personnel

Figure 14-2 DNR order.

Local resuscitation policy may allow prehospital professionals to withhold or stop resuscitation when a child is clearly dead, as defined by specific criteria (e.g., rigor mortis or injuries incompatible with life). This situation may be emotionally difficult for the prehospital provider, and all crew members must be in agreement with the decision to stop or to forego a resuscitation attempt. Likewise, it may be difficult emotionally for family members if prehospital professionals do not attempt resuscitation. *In cases where family members of the child are clearly distressed by the decision to forego resuscitation, consider providing resuscitative efforts as a gesture to the family that every effort has been made to save their child.* In such cases, the child can be treated with basic life support (BLS) measures only and transported to the ED, where physicians can formally pronounce the child dead and terminate resuscitation.

EMS systems should have, as part of educational and training requirements for field personnel, a formal training program regarding SUID (see Chapter 12). Local EMS policies should clearly establish the responsibility of the prehospital professional at death scenes regarding care of the body, notification of the coroner or medical examiner, and interaction with caregivers.

Organ Donation

A major issue in medical ethics involves the potential for patients with mortal injuries to donate organs. Donor organs are badly needed within the medical system, and many patients wait years or die while waiting for a match (**Table 14-2**).

Table 14-2 Organ Donation Statistics

• As of May 2015, nearly 124,000 people were waiting for an organ transplant to survive. Of this number, 2,146 were pediatric patients.
• Another person needing a transplant is added to the waiting list every 10 minutes.
• Each day, approximately 21 people die waiting for a transplant.
• In 2014, there were 29,532 organ transplants performed, which is only a 3% increase over 28,663 in 2010.
• Approximately 90% of Americans are supportive of organ donation, yet only 30% know what to do to become an organ and tissue donor.

Source: Donate Life America. Organ donation. http://donatelife.net/understanding-donation/organ-donation/. Accessed June 30, 2015.

Whether or not a child should be kept alive for the sole purpose of organ donation is an issue that prehospital professionals should discuss with medical control and the local hospital system. The parameters for viable organs should be clearly spelled out within the individual EMS system. Understanding state laws regarding organ donation helps the prehospital professional decide how to proceed.

Another helpful resource is the local organ transplant programs within the EMS service area. They may offer workshops or agree to come to the service to provide continuing education to increase awareness of the vital role of prehospital professionals.

Telling the Truth in Difficult Situations

Prehospital professionals should deal as honestly as possible with children and their caregivers. It is not unusual for caregivers to ask about the condition of a child or request information about a child's "chances of survival." In such situations, refrain from speculating, but respond instead with honest reassurance. For example, the statements "We'll take the best possible care of your child," or "He is in good hands; everything is being done to help him," provide an honest and reassuring response without speculating about uncertain outcomes.

The prehospital professional may also face situations in which multiple patients have sustained injuries and the parent or child requests information about others involved in the incident. It may be appropriate to deflect such questions, especially when the other party has suffered severe injuries or has died. The best tact may be to offer an honest statement of reassurance, such as "I need to focus on taking the best care of you right now. My partners are doing their best to take care of the others." Although there is an ethical obligation to be honest, it may be appropriate to delay

Case Study 3

You respond to the scene of a motor vehicle crash where you find a 10-year-old child with facial bruising; a tense, tender abdomen; and an obviously deformed left thigh. The child is seat belted in the rear passenger seat of the car, which has been struck on the driver's door by a truck. The child seems scared and begins to cry as you begin your assessment. The adult woman who had been driving the car has obvious head injuries and lacks a pulse. Another team begins work on the adult while you tend to the child. As you stabilize the child for transport, she asks you if her mother is okay.

1. **Would it be appropriate to tell the child her mother is okay to enable a safe and efficient transport?**
2. **How should you respond to this child's question?**

sharing particularly distressing information until a patient has been transported safely and other sources of emotional support are available.

Physician On Scene

Out-of-hospital care is under the authority of EMS medical control. Unless specifically authorized by medical control or the medical director of the EMS agency, prehospital professionals cannot carry out orders from other physicians, even the patient's private physician. This policy is sometimes controversial. *Medical control may either allow the on-scene physician to assist prehospital professionals or transfer total authority to the on-scene physician.* If the on-scene physician takes responsibility for treatment, he or she must be available to accompany the child to the ED.

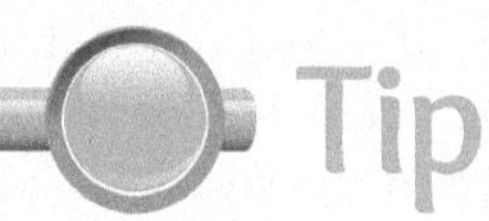

Tip

If the on-scene physician takes authority for care, he or she must be available to accompany the child to the ED.

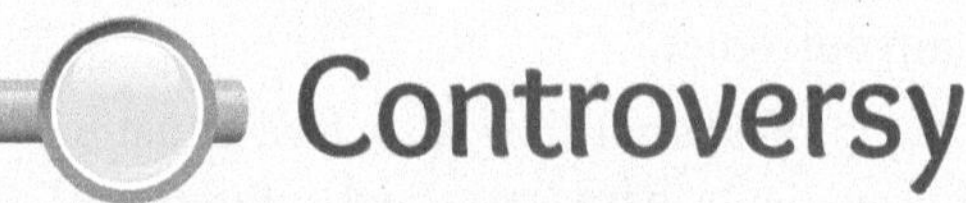

Controversy

The role of the child's private physician in on-scene care is controversial. The prehospital provider must abide by local EMS system policy, but the precise limitations to an on-scene physician providing assistance are sometimes unclear. Always act in the best interests of the child when the policy is confusing.

Hospital Destination

The hospital destination policy for children must define the following components:

1. Field triage criteria (which patients with what conditions go where)
2. Designated receiving hospitals
3. Specialized pediatric centers

The appropriate ED for a sick or injured child may differ from the ED appropriate for an adult with a similar condition. Some EMS systems may identify specialized pediatric centers (e.g., general trauma centers with pediatric capability, pediatric critical care centers, or pediatric trauma centers) as primary receiving facilities for certain pediatric patients. In some cases, a child may meet multiple conflicting triage criteria (e.g., should a severely burned child be transported to a regional children's hospital or a nonpediatric hospital with a regional burn center). The destination policy must either provide guidance on where such patients should be transported or specify that medical control makes all complex triage decisions. The prehospital professional must transport the child to the ED preferred by the legal guardian unless hospital destination policy requires an alternative facility. If disagreement persists, try to explain your reasoning for choosing the destination. If not successful, call medical control and have them speak to the guardian.

Pediatric Policies and Procedures

EMS systems should provide clear guidelines for common problems related to ethical and legal issues involving children. In addition, when available, on-line medical control provides the prehospital professional with the ability to obtain real-time consultation regarding particularly difficult situations, such as the inability to obtain consent, refusal of consent by a child or guardian, presence of a physician on scene, resuscitation decisions, and suspected child maltreatment or sexual assault.

Protocols, Policies, and Procedures

Operations are the administrative backbone of the EMS system. The goal of operations is to manage day-to-day field care with standards established by the EMS system. An important part of operations is the policies, procedures, and protocols that define the medical responsibility and legal authority of the prehospital professionals and medical director within the EMS system. These written directives assist the prehospital professional in knowing what to do in complicated out-of-hospital situations. These written directives, along with education and training, also help set performance standards.

Because the needs of children differ from those of adults, pediatric-specific protocols, policies, and procedures are necessary tools for a comprehensive EMS system. Protocols define explicit field treatments or the order and type of medical interventions for specific illness and injury conditions. They give the appropriate pharmacologic options, including drug doses, routes of delivery, and methods of administration. Most EMS systems have out-of-hospital pediatric advanced life support (ALS), medical emergency, and trauma treatment protocols. Appropriate treatment protocols for out-of-hospital BLS personnel and for first responders are also important. **Table 14-3** lists some common EMS pediatric treatment protocols.

Policies and procedures reflect the medicolegal expectations of the community for out-of-hospital care, quality management, and system accountability. These forms of regulation consist of clear, written directives to guide

Table 14-3 Examples of Pediatric Treatment Protocols

Examples of Pediatric Treatment Protocols
Airway obstruction
Allergic reaction and anaphylaxis
Altered mental status
Bradycardia
Burns
Cardiopulmonary arrest
Hypoperfusion or shock
Neonatal resuscitation
Respiratory distress
Seizures
Tachycardia
Toxic exposures
Trauma

prehospital professionals. They are intended to help with decision-making in difficult or legally sensitive pediatric field situations, such as those discussed previously in this chapter. Policies usually explain how the prehospital professional should handle certain situations, rather than medical treatment. Procedures describe the sequence of actions for the prehospital professional in applying medical protocols or medicolegal policies. The field policies with the most frequent application to pediatric care include:

- Consent for care or transport
- Refusal to consent for care or transport
- Death in the field
- Triage guidelines
- Hospital destination
- Child maltreatment

State statutes and the state EMS authority usually set basic requirements for local EMS systems; provide guidelines for quality management, accountability, and enforcement; and establish EMT scope of practice. Local policies, procedures, and protocols may be very different from one EMS system to the next. Mutual aid agreements between bordering geographic areas are especially useful because resources, equipment, and personnel for specialized care of children are not evenly distributed. Indeed, specialized trauma care and critical care centers for children are usually only available at major hospitals in large urban areas. In some states, no specialized centers at all exist for children.

Child Maltreatment and Sexual Assault

Education of prehospital professionals in identifying possible maltreatment is an essential component of initial education and continuing medical education in pediatrics (see Chapter 13). A policy and procedure for reporting suspected cases of maltreatment and for appropriate patient transport to an ED are important components of every EMS system. The prehospital professional must ensure that victims of maltreatment or sexual assault are initially evaluated in a careful, compassionate, and respectful way. Transport these patients to an ED staffed by clinicians experienced in working with child victims of maltreatment and sexual assault and equipped with the appropriate ancillary and follow-up services. Never confront the caregiver or others with accusations, moral judgments, threats, or suspicions. Although these situations are emotionally difficult, the immediate goal must always be to provide necessary treatment and ensure the safe transport of the child.

Medical Control for Pediatrics

Medical control, medical direction, or medical oversight are the mechanisms by which physicians, nurses, and EMS officials supervise field practice. Medical control includes direct and indirect methods.

On-line (Direct) Medical Control

On-line or direct medical control refers to any communication between the prehospital professional and medical control by telephone or radio. This form of control is required by some local EMS systems for many or all cases involving children younger than 18 years of age (**Figure 14-3**) because decisions about pediatric ALS treatment (e.g., intravenous lines [IVs], drug routes, and doses), triage, scene control, and transport are often difficult. **Table 14-4** lists some examples of problems in pediatric field practice that often require on-line physician input or direct medical control.

Off-line (Indirect) Medical Control

Off-line or indirect medical control involves prospective and retrospective guidance. Prospective indirect control consists of planning for expected educational and operational requirements within the prehospital professional's scope of practice. Retrospective indirect control involves review of individual and overall system performance against expectations or standards of care to provide accountability. **Table 14-5** lists common examples of how indirect control creates and monitors different types of policies, procedures, and protocols for children.

Table 14-4 Possible Pediatric Issues Needing Direct Medical Control

Pediatric Issue	Possible Scenario
Type of field treatment	IV or rectal diazepam for status epilepticus
Hospital destination	Appropriate ED for infant trauma patient
Specialized scene control	Hazardous materials exposure in school
Transport	Requirement for ED care after minor poisoning

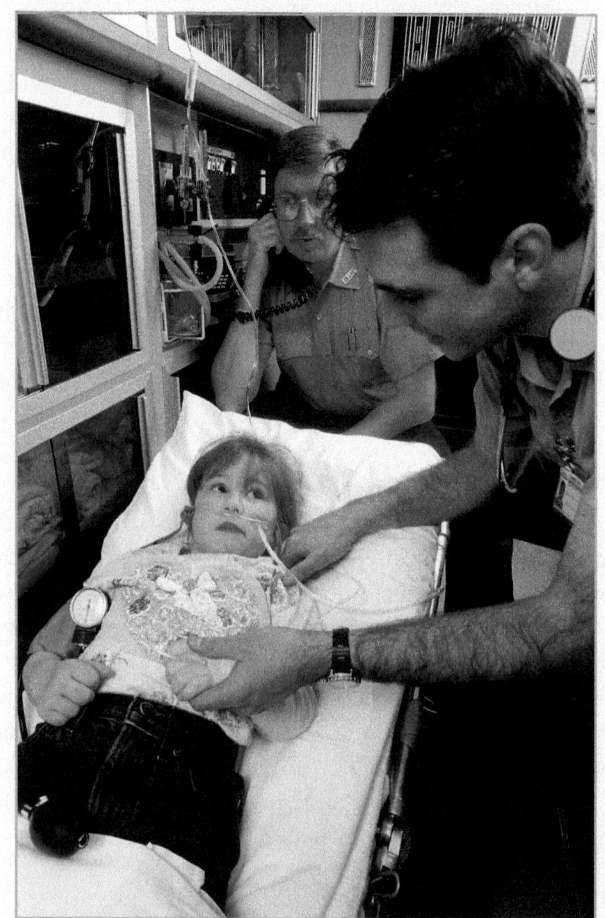

Figure 14-3 Direct medical control can be extremely helpful when the prehospital professional confronts medical and legal problems with children.

Table 14-5 Indirect Medical Control

Examples of Prospective Control
Pediatric BLS and ALS ambulance equipment and drugs
Pediatric out-of-hospital treatment protocols
Skills training
Airway foreign body removal
Endotracheal intubation
IO needle insertion
Rectal diazepam
Pediatric-specific policies
Hospital destination
Triage
Transport
Refusal of care
Suspected SIDS
Maltreatment
Examples of Retrospective Control
Review of compliance with treatment, triage, and transport policies
Review of success, failure, and complications of pediatric procedures and patient outcomes
Epidemiologic data on types of pediatric illness and injury
Review of ED or hospital capabilities for the care of children

Summary of Rationale for Protocols, Policies, and Procedures

Pediatric-specific guidelines (as defined in protocols, policies, and procedures) help set standards of care for children. Medical control is especially important in the delivery of out-of-hospital services to families and children because of the unusual circumstances that often arise medically and legally.

CASE STUDY ANSWERS

Case Study 1 — page 276

Although a babysitter (even an adult babysitter) cannot provide valid consent to treat, the emergency exception rule allows you to treat and transport this child who is in respiratory distress. She suffers from an emergent condition that places her at risk, her legal guardian is unavailable, and it would be unsafe to delay treatment. If the babysitter has a telephone number for the parents, call them, apprise them of the situation, and ask permission to provide necessary treatment and transport. If there is no way to reach the parents, you should provide treatment for the child's wheezing and respiratory distress with oxygen and a bronchodilator and transport her to an appropriate facility. Finally, make sure this 16-year-old babysitter is safe, and leave a note with her to give to the child's caregivers that explains what happened and where you have transported the child.

Case Study 2 — page 279

Unless you can persuade the child to allow you to deliver care, this will be a difficult situation. As a homeless adolescent, most states would consider this child to be a ward of the state, not an emancipated minor. However, despite the fact that he cannot legally refuse treatment and transport, every effort must be made to show respect, involve him in decisions, and avoid the use of force. If he persists in his refusal to be evaluated, contact medical control. If his "combativeness" seems to be the result of a medical condition that impairs judgment (i.e., meningitis, a head injury, intoxication), call law enforcement to provide assistance in restraining the adolescent sufficiently to allow a safe assessment and transport.

As a practical matter, respect the boy's dignity but be firm that transport to an ED is necessary. Try to establish rapport and do not be judgmental. If a friend or counselor is available, try to get assistance in persuading the teenager to agree to care and transport.

Case Study 3 — page 281

Carefully consider your answer to this child's concerned question. On the one hand, avoid being dishonest. Since you do not know whether her mother will survive, you should not assure the child that her mother will be okay. On the other hand, it would be appropriate to withhold your concerns and suspicions about the mother's condition until the child has been transported safely, more is known about the mother's condition, and there are resources (e.g., a social worker) available to assist the child in receiving what may be terrible news. One honest answer might be, "I know you are worried about your mother. My partners are taking good care of her. I need to take good care of you, and I'm going to take you to the hospital. Once we get there, we'll try to find out more about your mother."

SUGGESTED READINGS

Textbooks

American Academy of Orthopaedic Surgeons. *Nancy Caroline's Emergency Care in the Streets.* 7th ed. Burlington: Jones & Bartlett Learning; 2012.

Wertz Evans EM. Children and youth with special health care needs. In: Thomas D, Bernardo L, eds. *Core Curriculum for Pediatric Emergency Nursing.* 2nd ed. Chicago: Emergency Nurses Association; 2009.

Articles

Larkin G. Essential ethics for EMS: cardinal virtues and core principles. *Emerg Med Clin North Am.* 2002;20:887–911.

Schears R, Marco C, Iserson K. "Do not attempt resuscitation" in the out-of-hospital setting. *Ann Emerg Med.* 2004;44:68–69.

References

American Medical Association. What you need to know about the new HIPAA Breach Notification Rule. http://www.ama-assn.org/ama1/pub/upload/mm/399/hipaa-breach-notification-rule.pdf. Accessed September 12, 2012.

Center for Democracy and Technology. Stronger protections for, and encouraging the use of, de-identified (and "anonymized") health data. http://www.cdt.org/policy/stronger-protections-and-encouraging-use-de-identified-and-anonymized-health-data.asp. Accessed May 22, 2010.

Centers for Medicare and Medicaid Services. HIPAA—General information, 2010. http://www.cms.gov/HIPAAGenInfo/01_Overview.asp. Accessed September 12, 2012.

Donate Life America. Organ donation. http://donatelife.net/understanding-donation/organ-donation/. Accessed June 30, 2015.

Donate Life America. Statistics. http://donatelife.net/understanding-donation/statistics/. Accessed June 30, 2015.

McWay DC. *Today's Health Information Management: An Integrated Approach.* Clifton Park, NY: Delmar Cengage Learning; 2008.

Privileged Communication. *Encyclopedia Britannica.* http://www.britannica.com/EBchecked/topic/477379/privileged-communication. Accessed April 1, 2011.

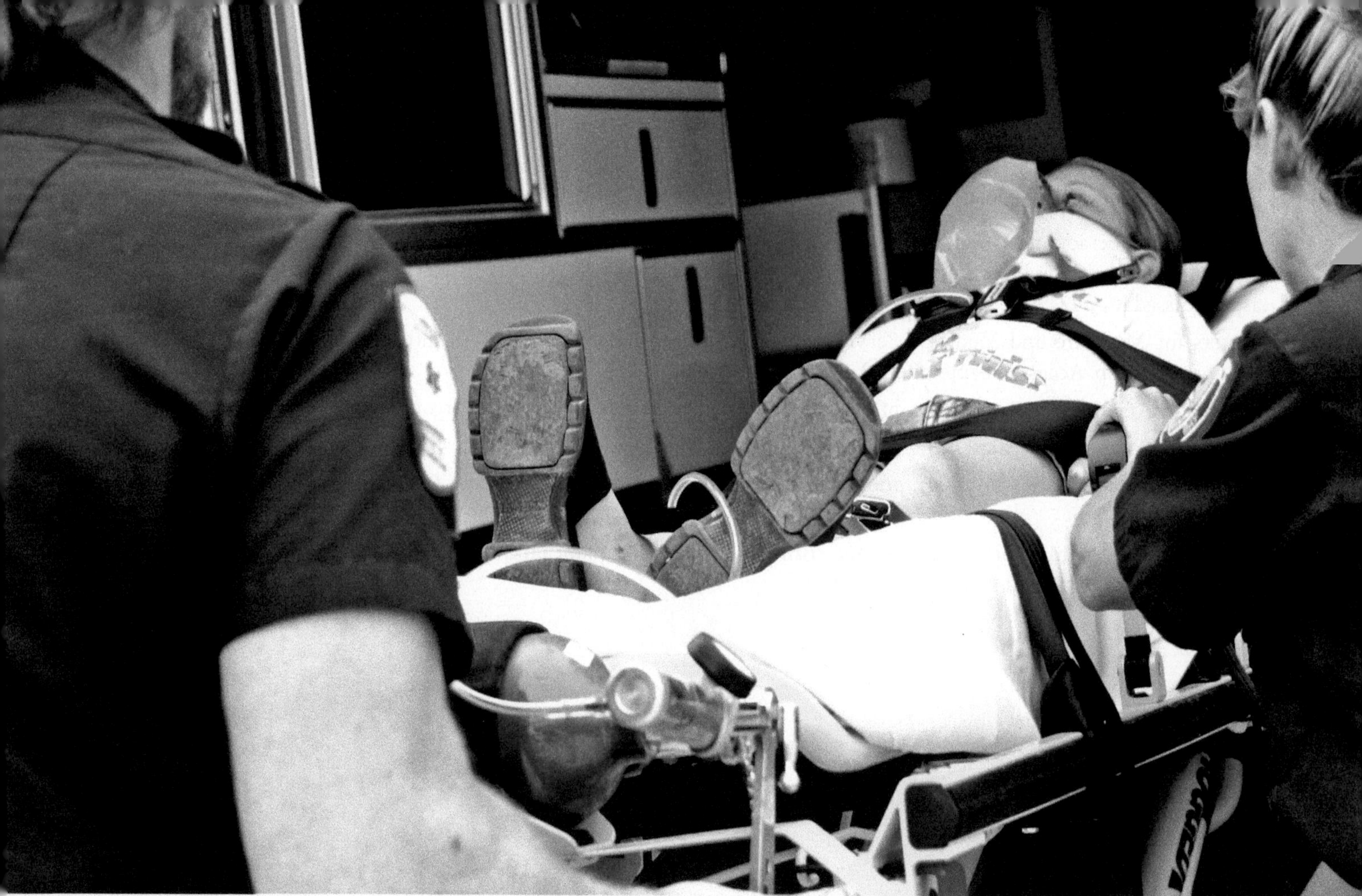

Learning Objectives

1. Discuss transport considerations for pediatric encounters in an ambulance.
2. List the considerations used to determine the mode of transport for children in an ambulance.
3. Identify issues related to choice of destination when making pediatric transport decisions.
4. Discuss advantages and disadvantages of transporting caregivers in the ambulance.
5. Identify and discuss current guidelines for child restraint systems in ambulances.
6. Outline issues involved in transporting multiple children.

Transportation Considerations

Chapter 15

Pediatric Transport

At some point in their career, every prehospital professional is faced with the decision of when and how to transport a child. Whether the child is a patient, or accompanying an adult, the transport decision involves many facets. Consideration of all circumstances current and potential should go into making the decision. The prehospital professional must know the local emergency medical services (EMS) protocols for safe transport of children, the local motor vehicle laws addressing child occupants in vehicles, the local resources and equipment that may be available, and the EMS regulations that govern the treatment of children en route. Most importantly, the prehospital professional must also meet the sometimes urgent and changing medical needs of the patient while considering the operational issues involved in transport.

The decision process about whether a child should be transported in the ambulance if they are accompanying an adult patient should be handled through policies and protocols, with forethought and resource guidelines before an on-scene decision. If that is not available in the system, it is important to understand that ambulances were not designed to transport pediatric occupants and ambulance design challenges even the most experienced personnel with safe options for nonpatient pediatric occupants.

When the child is the patient and transport is necessary, the position in which the patient is secured usually depends on the stability of the child, and whether or not interventions are needed en route. Rapid transport depends on multiple factors. In a basic life support system, early transport is appropriate if the scene is unsafe for the child, caregiver, or prehospital professional, or if the child has any of the following:

- A serious mechanism of injury
- A history compatible with serious illness
- A physiologic abnormality noted during the primary assessment
- A potentially serious anatomic abnormality
- Significant pain

In an advanced life support (ALS) system with more extensive treatment options in the field, the transport decision is often complicated. Major factors to consider include:

- Type of clinical problem (injury versus illness)
- Expected benefits of ALS treatment in the field
- Local EMS system treatment and transport policies
- The ALS provider's comfort level

Case Study 1

You arrive on scene to find a 25-year-old single mother who has fractured her leg while playing in the backyard with her children. She is holding her infant daughter, who she states is uninjured. Her lower leg is obviously fractured, and she requires transport. Her two children, aged 10 months and 3 years, are scared but cooperative. The patient agrees to be transported, but not without her children. No other family members or neighbors are available at this time.

1. **Is it appropriate to transport the children with the mother?**
2. **What issues are involved when transporting children who are not patients?**

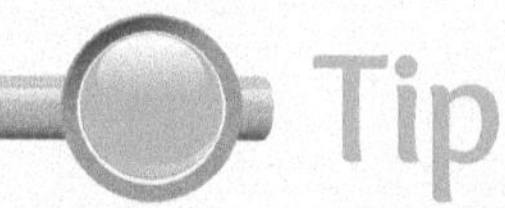

All EMS systems do not have clear policies that define pediatric transport practices. National guidelines about safe transport of children in ambulances have recently been released.

Another consideration is choice of destination; not all areas have pediatric centers and rely on local hospitals for stabilization. This should be addressed within local EMS protocols. Many states have pediatric hospital designation agreements and other pediatric-specific programs accomplished through the Emergency Medical Services for Children (EMSC) program.

How to Begin Transport

Is the Child the Patient?

Why a child is being transported is the first factor in determining how to transport. Is the child the patient or is the child with a caregiver who needs ambulance transport? *Children who are not patients and only need transport because they must accompany the patient are best transported in a vehicle other than an ambulance.* There are few safe options available to secure a child properly, and there may be risk of injury while transporting any patient in an ambulance. Ambulances are not designed for transporting children who are not patients.

Many communities have coalitions for pediatrics that may be able to act as resources to transport children who are not patients in alternate vehicles. Reviewing the public safety disaster plans and school resources in the local area is a good place to start when looking to developing partnerships. Agreements can be set up ahead of time to have alternate transport options when these situations arise. Working together, the prehospital professional may be able to provide a system that affords a variety of child restraints and safe vehicles. Providers should explain that the need for safe transport of additional family members may require separating the family temporarily.

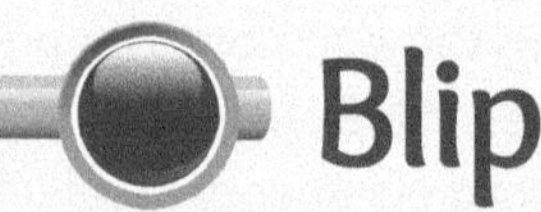

Avoid transporting a child who is not a patient in an ambulance.

When a Sick Child Is the Patient

If the child requires airway, breathing, or circulatory support more than simple oxygen delivery or nebulized bronchodilators, or if the child requires ALS monitoring or treatment, secure him or her to the stretcher in a supine or semi-Fowler's position. This is a position that best and most safely allows the prehospital professional to perform ongoing assessment and treatment en route.

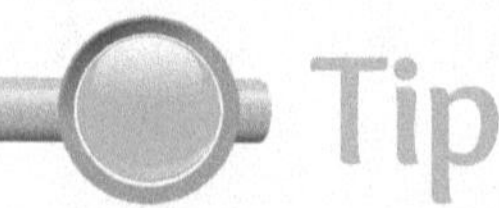

Except in the case of mild illness or injury, transport a sick child secured on a stretcher in a supine or semi-Fowler's position. This provides the safest and most effective position for ongoing assessment, monitoring, and treatment.

When the Child Is the Patient but Not Sick

Often the primary assessment reveals that the child has only minimal or mild illness or is not seriously injured but requires transport to a medical facility. There are numerous options on how to transport that protect the child's safety, permit appropriate monitoring, and provide comfort. Many children who are strapped supine to a

Case Study 2

You arrive on the scene of a 3-year-old girl who has altered mental status. She is limp in her mother's arms and does not respond to your arrival in the room. She is pale but does not seem to have increased work of breathing or noisy respirations. The patient has been sick for 24 hours with nausea and vomiting and could not be awakened from her afternoon nap. The child responds to painful stimuli and is wearing a dry diaper. Vital signs show heart rate of 150 beats/min, respiratory rate of 36 breaths/min, and blood pressure of 70 mm Hg/palp. She weighs 33 lb (15 kg).

1. Should this child be transported in a car seat?
2. Should the mother be transported with the child?
3. Discuss the possible transport modes and destination for this patient.

stretcher become distressed from the effects of restraint, stranger anxiety, fear, and pain. When possible, attempt to transport children who are only mildly ill or injured in an upright position, to minimize the emotional distress and discomfort from an uncomfortable stretcher. Integrated child restraints for the EMS provider seat and pediatric transport devices that attach to stretchers are becoming more readily available and can provide more options for safe transport.

Avoid transporting a child who is not a patient in an ambulance. Determine another safe means to care for the child or arrange transport by another vehicle. When a child is the patient, consider carefully how to position him or her to maximize effectiveness of interventions, to allow appropriate monitoring, and to preserve comfort. If the child has any immediate or anticipated requirements for interventions other than oxygen delivery or simple wound care, secure the child to a stretcher in a supine position. If the child only requires monitoring, attempt to transport the child in an upright position that allows observation, enhances safety, and promotes comfort. Do not secure the child in the parent's arms.

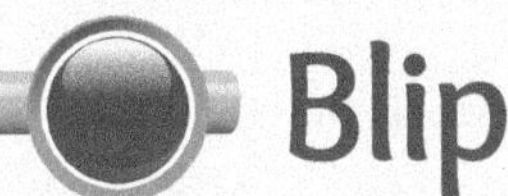

Blip

It is never acceptable to secure the child in the parent's arms.

Taking Caregivers in the Ambulance

Taking parents or caregivers in an ambulance is usually regulated by local EMS protocols. Often the caregiver can decrease the anxiety of the child during the transport, especially age groups who are more likely to experience emotional distress when transported without familiar caregivers. Dealing with emotional distress of children is an important principle in prehospital pediatric care and represents a key ingredient in quality care. The effect of the presence of family or a caregiver on the effectiveness and comfort level of the prehospital professional is not known, but in other settings has been associated with higher satisfaction in pediatric care delivery (**Figure 15-1**).

Some prehospital professionals may feel less comfortable when a caregiver is present in an ambulance during a resuscitation or when an advanced procedure, such as endotracheal intubation, is being performed. One way for the prehospital professional to help address his or her own comfort level is to get involved with child advocacy and increase pediatric training and exposure.

If local EMS policy allows caregiver transport with the child, it should specify where the child and caregiver should be positioned during the transport. One common place for a caregiver during transport is in the front seat of the

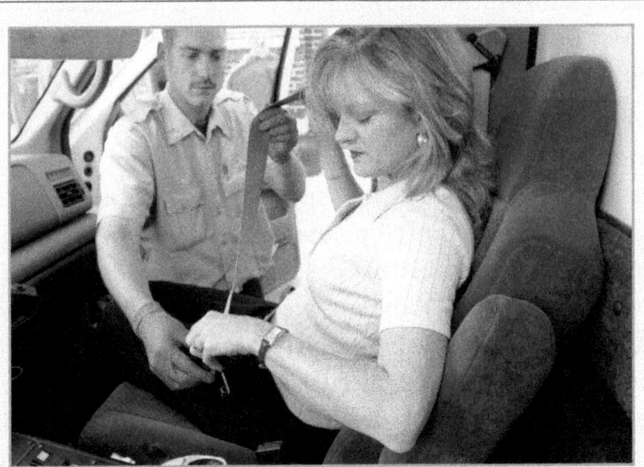

Figure 15-1 Allowing a parent to accompany a child may reduce the child's anxiety, but make sure all occupants are safe.

ambulance. As with any passenger, make sure the caregiver fastens his or her seat belt correctly and remains seated. Another possible place to seat a caregiver is in the rear of the ambulance when it is appropriately configured with secure seating options for both crew and the caregiver. This allows a child to visualize the caregiver and may provide some emotional consolation. Ensure that all occupants and equipment are secured; unsecured items and occupants have been shown to pose a great threat to the patient's safety in the event of vehicular events (**Figure 15-2**).

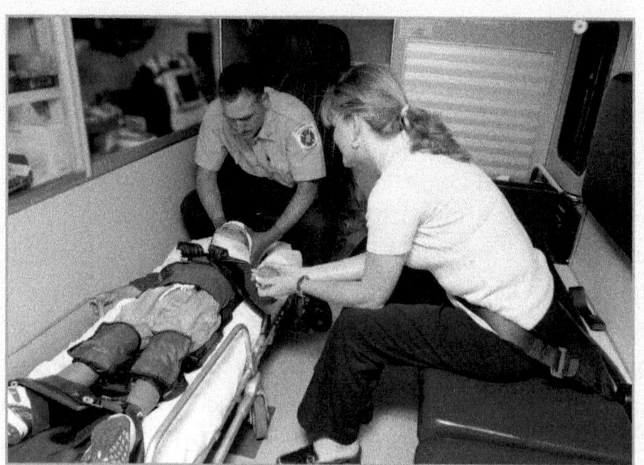

Figure 15-2 If caregivers are allowed to ride in the ambulance with the child, make sure all equipment and personnel are securely fastened.

Child Restraint Systems in Ambulances

Dangers Facing Children During Transport

There are several factors that can decrease the possibility of additional injury to a child during ambulance transport. These factors include how the child is secured, the configuration of the ambulance, and whether the crew and the equipment are secured.

The first step in deciding how to transport a child is to determine what assessment, monitoring, and treatment are necessary during transport. *If the patient is stable and weighs less than 40 pounds and no interventions are anticipated, then transport the infant or child using a child restraint system (CRS) that meets the injury criteria of the Federal Motor Vehicle Safety Standard No. 213.* This consists of a car seat secured with appropriate restraining devices in the ambulance. If an ambulance-specific child restraint device is available for children over 40 pounds (approximately 18 kg), the provider should use it to secure the patient for transport. Otherwise, secure children over 40 pounds to the ambulance stretcher in a seated position using the existing straps altered to meet the size requirements of the child. Some circumstances make this standard approach impossible, such as transporting a child on a backboard. If the child requires a backboard, or if no other safe position is possible, transport the child in the supine position. Secure the child to the backboard. Secure the backboard to the cot with three horizontal restraints across the torso (at the chest, waist, and knees) and a vertical restraint over each shoulder. When possible, tether the foot end of the backboard to the cot to prevent forward movement during rapid decelerations.

If EMS policy allows a CRS in the ambulance, decide where to position the device in the ambulance. Car seats are designed to restrain a child during a front end or rear end collision. They provide only moderate lateral stability. This means that these seats cannot be secured sideways to a bench seat. This limits the choices about where to position the CRS in the rear of an ambulance to the cot or the EMS provider's seat at the head of the stretcher.

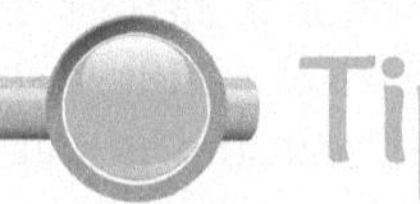

Convertible child restraint devices are acceptable seats for use on the cot or rear-facing or forward-facing EMS provider seat.

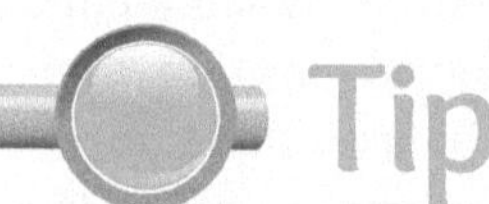

If EMS policy allows, transport stable children weighing less than 40 pounds with a CRS when possible. This consists of a car safety seat properly secured in the ambulance.

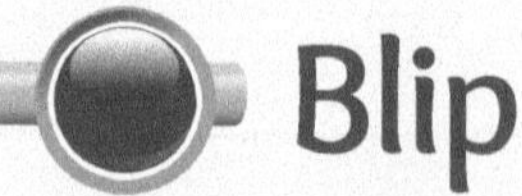

Never secure car seats to a bench seat in the ambulance. There is no way to safely secure a car seat to a bench seat.

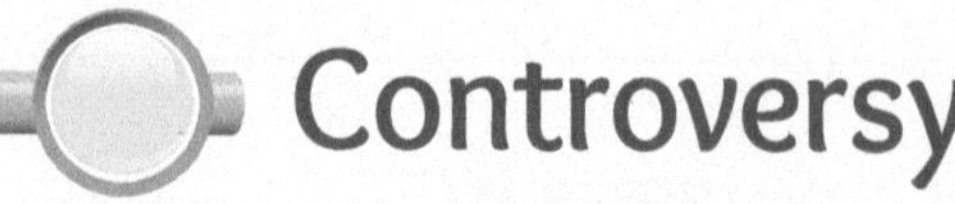

"Rear-facing only" or "infant only" child restraint seats cannot be secured properly to the ambulance cot or rear-facing EMS provider seat because they have only one belt pathway to secure the device and are not engineered to be restrained on a rear-facing seat.

Choosing a CRS

While there are many car safety seats and child restraint systems available for the ambulance, there are no federal regulations and very limited testing of these devices. Car safety seats designed for passenger vehicles are tested to meet Federal Motor Safety Standard 213 (FMVSS 213), and convertible car safety seats carrying weights to 40 pounds and a car bed using two belt paths have been tested and meet the injury criteria of FMVSS 213 (Ref Bull, MJ, 2001). There are a few integrated seats and restraints that are permanently mounted on the rear-facing captain's chair (**Figure 15-3**), and some restraint systems designed to be secured on a rear-facing stretcher. These options have variable recommendations for use, and some have been tested to ensure they meet the injury criteria of FMVSS 213, as no standards have been developed that are ambulance-specific. *Convertible car safety seats are for children of different ages and weighing up to 40 pounds. They are usually recognized by having two belt paths for both forward and rear facing.* Some recently manufactured seats have raised the limit to 80 pounds, but none have been tested for use on an ambulance stretcher by children over 40 pounds. In addition to securing the child in the car safety seat, the seat must be attached to the ambulance stretcher using two belt paths to prevent rearward and forward motion. Only convertible car safety seats have two belt paths and are the only seats that can safely be secured to a stretcher. The back of the stretcher is elevated to an upright position, and the seat is secured to the stretcher with belts through both the forward-facing and rear-facing belt paths (**Figure 15-4**).

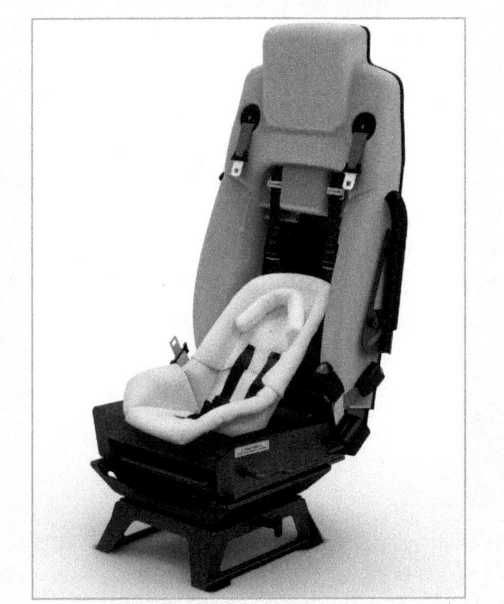

Figure 15-3 An integrated child restraint system.

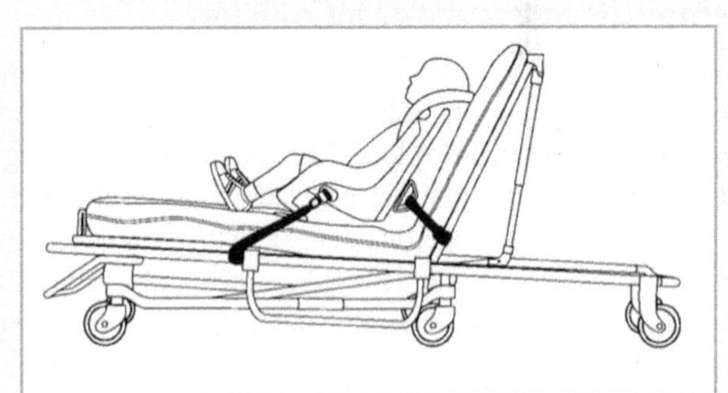

Figure 15-4 Convertible child safety seat for children 5–40 pounds.

Source: National Highway Traffic Safety Administration. Working Group Best-Practice Recommendations for the Safe Transportation of Children in Emergency Ground Ambulances, DOT HS #811 677, Appendix D.

Used with permission, Automotive Safety Program, Riley Hospital for Children.

Rear-facing only seats are usually limited to those infants weighing less than 30–35 pounds and are designed only to be used in a rear-facing position. They cannot be secured to the stretcher safely, as they have only one belt path. However, there is one infant car bed that can be secured to the stretcher in a side-facing orientation (**Figure 15-5**).

If a booster seat is used, it should only be used on forward-facing captain's chairs with lap/shoulder belts available. *Other specialty restraints include vest and harness devices that may be available to specialty crews with additional training in how to install and secure a patient for transport.*

Case Study 3

You are called to the scene of a vehicle crash involving two automobiles that collided at moderate speed in a downtown intersection. There are three patients. One is the restrained driver of the vehicle that struck another vehicle broadside. The other patients are the restrained driver of the second vehicle and an 11-month-old boy, who was fully restrained in a rear-facing convertible car seat on the opposite side of the point of collision. The two drivers have minor wounds and no significant physiologic abnormalities. Assessment of the child reveals a crying infant with no signs of injury.

1. Should the child be transported?
2. Should the child be transported in his own car seat or an ambulance car seat?

Detailed instruction for selection and installation of ambulance restraints is available from EMS providers who have taken the EMS training course on child transportation in ambulances.

A CRS should be cleaned and maintained. Pads that are removable and surfaces that can be wiped down are preferable. Check with the manufacturer to see what cleaning materials are acceptable for the seat. If there is a dedicated ambulance CRS, check with the EMS policy and the manufacturer to make sure there have been no safety recalls.

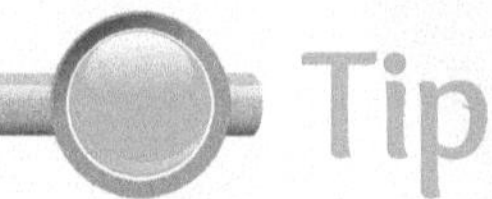

Tip

Practice installing child seats to the stretcher as part of training, or bring in a certified child passenger safety technician with training in ambulance transport to help familiarize the service with the installation process.

Using Car Seats After a Collision

If the ambulance does not have a CRS and a stable child requires transport, an important dilemma arises when the child's own car seat is available. If local EMS policy permits using a personal car seat, be sure that it is fully intact. If the device shows any signs of damage, do not use it in the ambulance. The National Highway Traffic Safety Administration (NHTSA) recommends that child restraints should be replaced after a moderate or severe crash to ensure a continued high level of crash protection for child passengers; however, reuse of a child safety seat that has been involved in a minor crash is recommended if the crash meets certain criteria (**Table 15-1**).

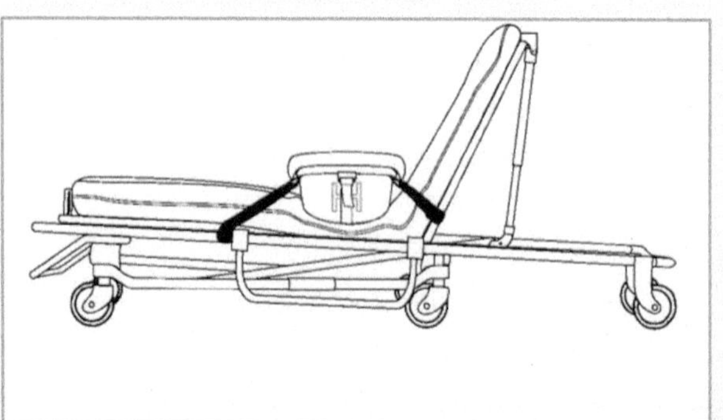

Figure 15-5 Car bed for children 5–20 pounds.

Source: National Highway Traffic Safety Administration. Working Group Best-Practice Recommendations for the Safe Transportation of Children in Emergency Ground Ambulances, DOT HS #811 677, Appendix D.

Used with permission, Automotive Safety Program, Riley Hospital for Children.

Securing a Car Seat to the Stretcher

Transport children weighing less than 40 pounds in a rear-facing convertible car seat unless medical attention is indicated. This is easily accomplished using the ambulance stretcher. Use a convertible car seat that meets the national standard and place it flush with the raised back of the cot. Secure the car seat tightly to the cot using straps through both the forward-facing and the rear-facing belt paths of the seat (**Figure 15-6**). Adjust the car seat harness to be at or below the shoulders of the child, connect the harness and pull it snug. Then place the harness clip at the level of the child's armpit (**Figure 15-7**).

Table 15-1 Recommendations for the Use of a CRS After a Crash

It is safe to reuse a child safety seat that has been involved in a minor crash if:
• The vehicle was able to be driven away from the crash site.
• The vehicle door nearest the safety seat was undamaged.
• There were no injuries to any of the vehicle occupants.
• The airbags if present did not deploy.
• There is no visible damage to the safety seat.

Source: http://www.nhtsa.gov/people/injury/childps/childrestraints/reuse/restraintreuse.htm

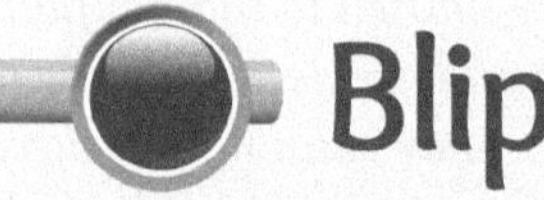

Blip

If a child's personal car seat shows any signs of damage, or does not meet NHTSA criteria, do not use in the ambulance.

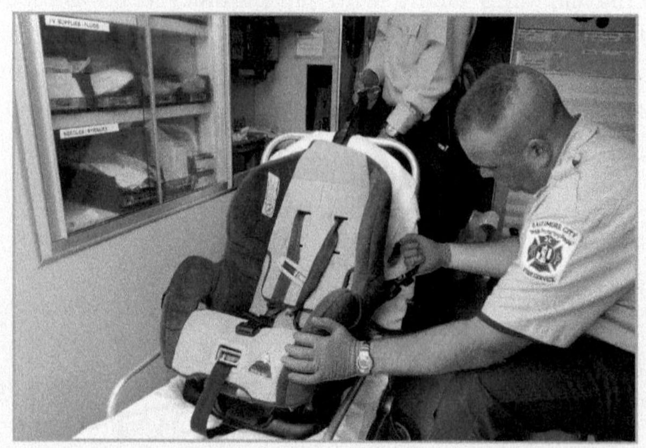

Figure 15-6 Place the car seat on the stretcher and use one belt through the rear-facing belt path and one through the forward-facing belt path of the car safety seat.

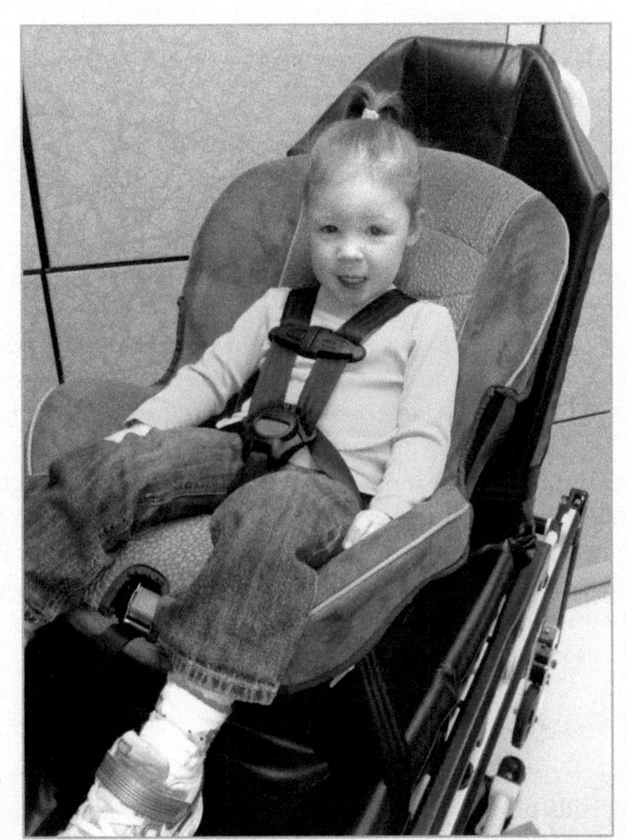

Figure 15-7 Child properly positioned in convertible car seat with harness snug and chest clip at level of the armpits.

Securing Older Children to the Stretcher

Children weighing more than 40 pounds are too large for a car safety seat on a stretcher, but they are NOT yet large enough to fit into adult-sized restraint systems. When ambulance-specific child restraint systems that fit larger children are available, children should be transported in an appropriate device secured to the cot. If a CRS is unavailable, the child needs to be secured to the stretcher. The position of the stretcher straps needs to be adjusted for the size of the patient.

During an ambulance crash, children can slide up the stretcher. The use of shoulder straps can help minimize this effect, but there are some difficulties with these straps because they do not fit tightly on a child's shoulders or prevent the child from moving upward during a crash. Ideally the straps should be secured similarly to those used in a car seat, adjusted at or below the shoulders. The straps should enter through the padding and be secured to the frame of the stretcher at the height of the shoulders. Unfortunately, this is not possible with most of today's stretchers. There are a few ambulance-specific restraint systems now available that make securing a child to the stretcher safer. These devices must be first secured to the stretcher, and then adjusted to fit the patient (**Figure 15-8** and **Figure 15-9**). The use of the pediatric restraint devices made for stretcher application helps to more properly secure most pediatric patients.

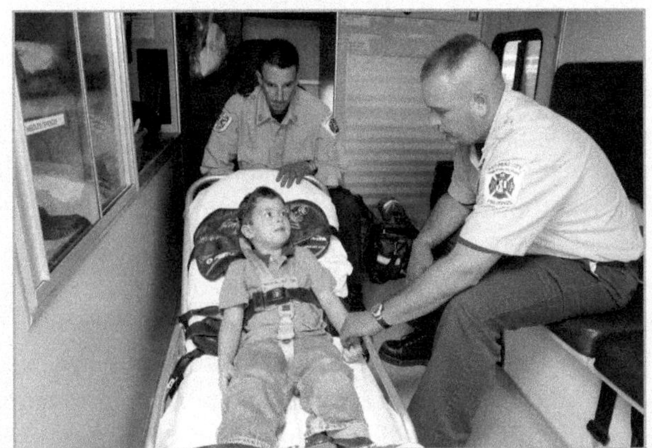

Figure 15-8 Ambulance-specific child restraint accommodating children 10–40 pounds.

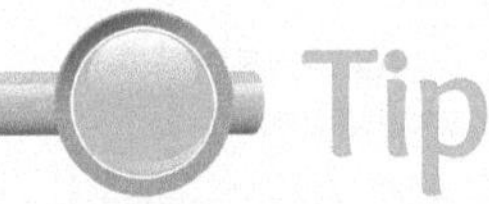

It is extremely important to secure all occupants and equipment during transport. Just applying the brakes hard can cause harm to the patient by unrestrained objects.

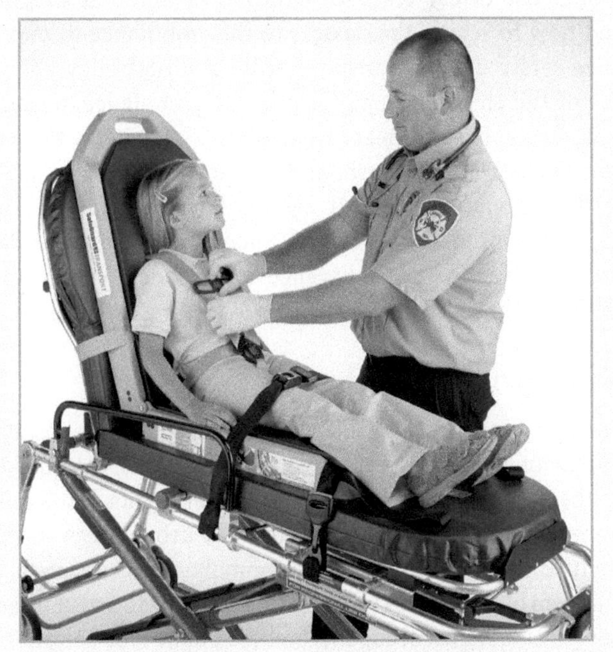

Figure 15-9 Ambulance-specific child restraint accommodating children 22–100 pounds.

Other Dangers in Transporting Children

Placing the child in an appropriate transporting device is the first means of creating a safe mode of transport. It is important to recognize that crew members and flying debris can create a significant hazard to the patient during a collision. When transporting a child, secure or store all loose equipment before leaving the scene. Monitors, portable oxygen containers, equipment bags, and all other loose pieces can create missile-like objects that have been shown to be potentially dangerous to crew members and patients. Keep crew members secured in a seat-belted position throughout the transport. Crash testing of ambulances has shown that unrestrained passengers in the patient compartment present a risk to the patient during a collision by being launched and landing on the patient.

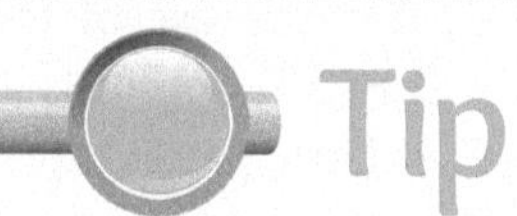
Tip

Crash tests of ambulances have shown that unrestrained passengers in the patient compartment present a risk to the patient during a collision by being launched and landing on the patient. All occupants should be restrained.

Summary of CRSs

Whenever possible, use a size-appropriate CRS to transport a stable child in an upright position. This is the preferred position for transport. There are important guidelines for proper use of car seats for children of different weights and how to secure the devices to the ambulance to maximize safety during transport. If local EMS policy allows use of the child's own car seat in the ambulance, be sure it is not damaged, meets all the NHTSA criteria for use of a car seat after a crash, and that it is properly secured to the ambulance. Also, if EMS policy allows and he or she can be properly restrained, encourage the presence of the caregiver in the ambulance to provide comfort and solace to the child, and to improve ongoing assessment.

Transport Mode

Emotions can run high in pediatric calls, and prehospital professionals may feel a strong desire to transport quickly to the emergency department. However, lights and sirens transport, especially through crowded urban areas in the daytime, is fraught with risk to ambulance occupants and innocent bystanders. A way to minimize the dangers of transport to ambulance occupants and the public is to determine the best mode of transport before moving. Transport mode should be based on the type of call, the presenting illness or injury, and the degree of physiologic instability of the patient. The child with the highest priority for rapid transport is the critically injured child who needs blood products and/or operative interventions. This child always requires a time-sensitive response and a lights, and sirens transport is often indicated. Children with severe illness or physiologic abnormality are also important candidates for lights and sirens mode.

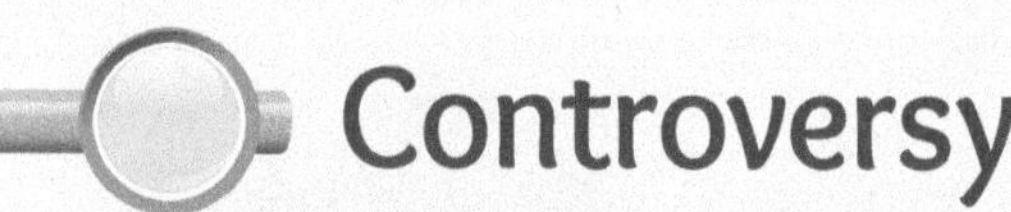
Controversy

Lights and sirens transport poses significant risks to the ambulance occupants and innocent bystanders. Hence, the benefits of shorter transport time must be carefully weighed against the dangers.

Transport Destination

The decision of where to transport the pediatric patient depends on the physiologic condition of the patient, the cause of the illness or injury, and the stability of the patient, coupled with local EMS policy, weather, and resources. It is important to be aware of all the factors that affect the decision based on the situation. Air transport may be appropriate for some patients, but add in the extra facet of potential separation from the caregiver because not all air transport can accommodate caregivers. For further guidance on making transport destination decisions, consult local protocols.

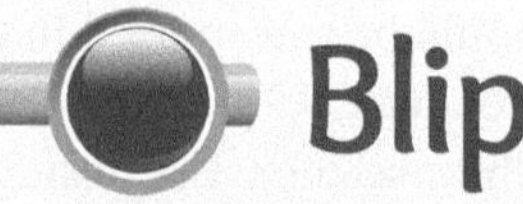
Blip

Rotary wing transport for pediatric patients can be a very useful and lifesaving tool. It can also add to the stress of the patient and caregiver if both cannot travel aboard the aircraft. It is important to weigh all factors when considering method of transport based on condition and needs of the patient.

Multiple Patients

If there are multiple pediatric patients, extra transportation units may be required to transport the children safely. There are limited locations to properly secure a car seat or to be able to adjust the adult straps to fit the child in the patient compartment of the ambulance.

Summary of Transport Mode and Multiple Patients

Children are often the source of great provider stress. Transport mode is best determined before beginning transport. Although lights and sirens are the fastest method, this mode is more dangerous and is best reserved for unstable trauma cases and physiologically unstable illness cases. When there is more than one child at the scene, activate additional units to avoid logistical problems with safely securing multiple child restraints in the ambulance.

CASE STUDY ANSWERS

Case Study 1 — page 290

This case demonstrates an important dilemma. Although family-centered care is highly desirable, this must take place without placing the patient, family member, accompanying child, or provider at increased risk. Whenever possible, arrange alternative safe care and/or transportation for the child so that attention of the medical providers can be centered on the patient. This includes care by or transportation with a competent adult, ensuring that appropriate child restraints are available and in use. Additional potential options for transporting the child could include a supervisor's, auxiliary, or child service's transportation vehicle. Transporting the child in the front seat of the ambulance or in the rear seat of a police car or other emergency vehicle is dangerous. A vehicle where the CRS is to be used in the front seat must have an airbag deactivation switch.

Parent and child separation, however, may cause undue distress to the mildly injured parent. In that case, if the system allows the transport of the child in the ambulance, follow proper procedures to secure the child in the appropriate restraint system and in the correct position. This method of transportation must include enough participants to meet the child's and the patient's needs, and ensure that observation or immediate needs of either one does not detract from those of the other. This is an option that is often unavailable because of space or personnel resource limitations.

Case Study 2 — page 291

This is a case where the patient needs appropriate positioning, airway and vascular access, monitoring, and perhaps intervention during the transport process. "Stabilization" in a car seat affords none of those requirements and therefore should not be used. This is a child who should be restrained in a standard fashion on the ambulance stretcher, with attention to airway positioning, vascular access, and appropriate observation. Here, accompaniment of the parent can often be advantageous to parent and child. Although the medical team can attend to the physiologic needs of the child, they cannot meet their emotional needs. Be sensitive to the parent's need to offer support to his or her child and the mother's ability to keep the child calm. The parent may also be able to provide additional history and assist in reassessments. The parent cannot be allowed to carry the child during transport, either on his or her lap while seated or with the parent and child secured together to a stretcher.

Local protocol often dictates where and how this patient should be transported, and whether a parent can accompany his or her child and specific requirements for this process. These protocols should include preferred parental seating location and safety instructions for the parent before transport. Parents must be instructed that the primary role of the providers is to care for the sick child, and that precious attention cannot be diverted from that task. Having the parent sit in the front is one way to include him or her in the environment, while allowing some separation for the providers.

Providers may express concern that parents will critique their techniques or skills during the transport or that the providers will be nervous when confronted with this environment. Parents, however, generally report very positively about the experience and comment mostly on the caring nature of the providers, not their technical capabilities.

Case Study 3 — page 293

Assessment of infants after a collision is very difficult in the best of environments. The significant mechanism of this incident necessitates assessment during the transport process and medical evaluation of the infant at the appropriate emergency department. The question then is how to best transport the child. If a careful inspection of the child yields no physiologic or anatomic abnormality requiring further stabilization or intervention, and the child is accessible to completely assess and reassess as needed when secured in the car seat, this method is appropriate. If a detailed inspection of the child's convertible car safety seat does not yield evidence of fracture or abnormality, it is an appropriate seat for the child's weight, is not damaged and meets NHTSA criteria, and EMS policy allows, then use this seat and secure in the usual rear-facing position in the emergency vehicle, unless the ambulance has its own CRS or local EMS policy forbids this practice. If there is any question as to the appropriateness or the structural integrity of the child's car seat, then use another more appropriate car seat. Remember that a rear-facing only or infant car seat cannot be safely secured to the ambulance cot and may only be secured to a forward facing attendant seat.

SUGGESTED READINGS

Textbook

Bledsoe BE, Porter RS, Cherry RA. *Essentials of Paramedic Care.* 2nd ed. Upper Saddle River, NJ: Prentice Hall; 2011.

Articles

Becker LR. Relative risk of injury and death in ambulances and other emergency vehicles. *Accid Anal Prev.* 2003;35(6):941–948.

Bledsoe BE. Emergency EMS Mythology, Part 4. Lights and sirens save a significant amount of travel time and save lives. *Emerg Med Serv.* 2003;32(6):72–73.

Bull MJ, Weber K, Talty J, Manary M. Crash protection for children in ambulances. *Annu Proc Assoc Adv Automot Med.* 2001;45:353–367.

Kahn CA. Characteristics of fatal ambulance crashes in the United States: an 11 year retrospective analysis. *Prehosp Emerg Care.* 2001;5(3):261–269.

Warren J. Guidelines for the inter- and intrahospital transport of critically ill patients. *Crit Care Med.* 2004;32(1):256–262.

References

Automotive Safety Program. Improving Occupant Protection for Non-Critical Pediatric Patients in Ambulances: A Training Curriculum for EMS Personnel. Child passenger safety: about child safety seats. http://www.preventinjury.org. Accessed January 9, 2013.

Health Resources and Services Administration and National Highway Traffic Safety Administration. The Do's and Don'ts of Transporting Children in an Ambulance. Washington, DC: 2009. http://www.childrensnational.org/files/PDF/EMSC/PubRes/Dos_and_Donts_of_Transporting_Children_by_Ambulance.pdf. Accessed October 5, 2012.

National Highway Traffic Safety Administration. Working Group Best-Practice Recommendations for the Safe Transportation of Children in Emergency Ground Ambulances, DOT HS # 811 677, September 2012. http://www.nhtsa.gov/staticfiles/nti/pdf/811677.pdf. Accessed October 5, 2012.

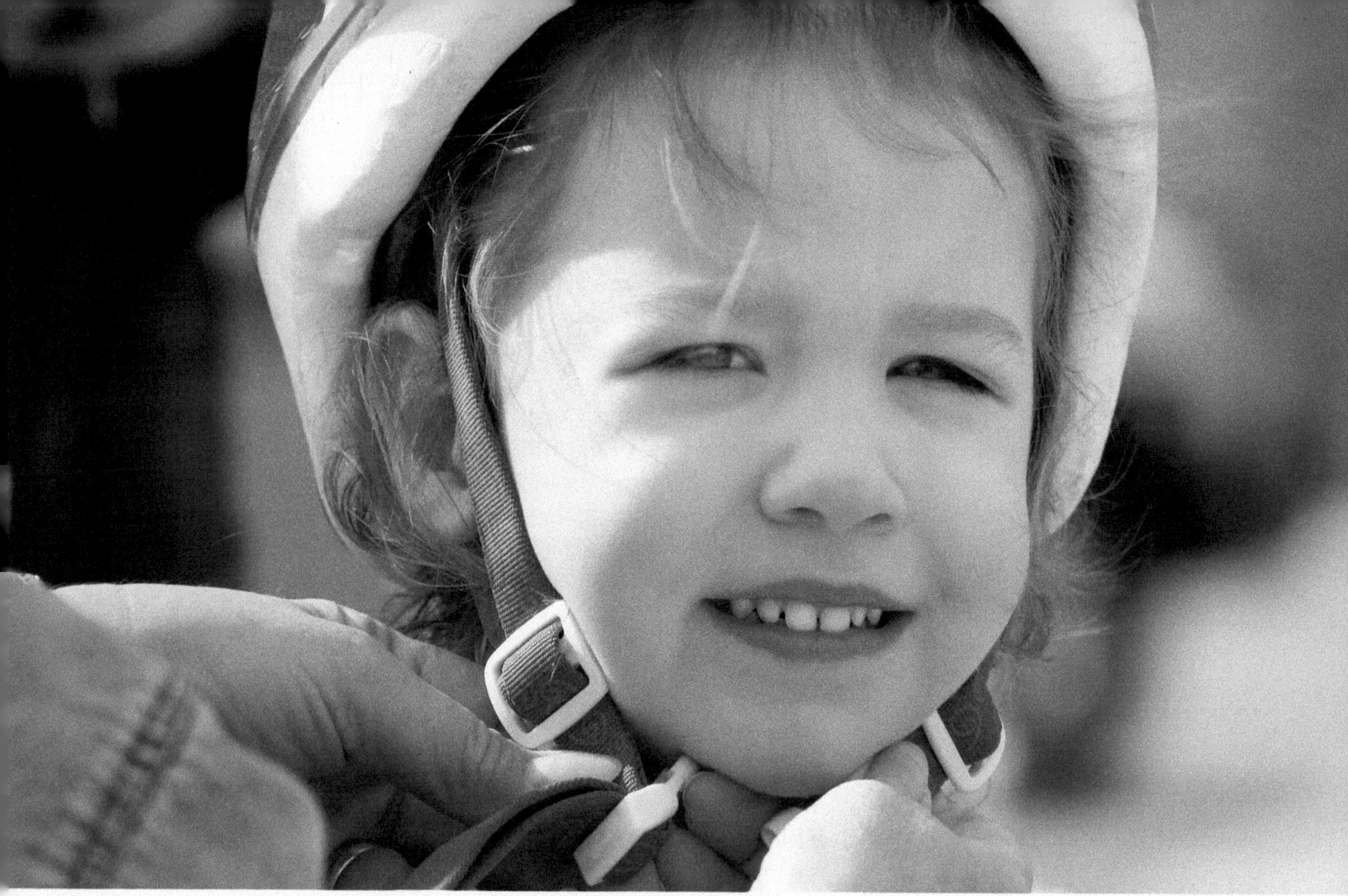

Learning Objectives

1. Describe Emergency Medical Services for Children (EMSC) and the EMS-EMSC continuum.
2. Discuss how EMS can interface with public health and the EMS role in injury and illness prevention and promotion.
3. Identify primary and secondary prevention strategies involved in injury prevention.
4. Outline the three components and the three phases of an injury event.
5. Discuss EMSC partnerships with other injury prevention agencies and programs.
6. Define the role of the child's "medical home" and identify its importance in the EMS-EMSC care continuum.
7. Identify unique quality and safety issues for children in out-of-hospital care.
8. Discuss the importance of data collection and information management in EMSC.

Making a Difference

Chapter 16

Introduction

Emergency care for children involves the work of many health care professionals, inside and outside of the community's hospitals. To provide safe and effective emergency care, these professionals must work together as a team to develop and implement comprehensive clinical services and oversight mechanisms designed specifically for children suffering acute illness and injury. Professionals must also recognize the limitations of an emergency care system largely oriented toward treatment after an illness or injury occurs, and embrace the essential role of prevention. Of all community activities that can improve children's overall health and well-being, prevention of acute injury and illness is by far the most cost-effective. Making a difference means practicing prevention as part of day-to-day work duties and stepping into a role as a community leader and health advocate. Making a difference entails professionals getting involved in injury and illness prevention in innovative ways. This includes understanding and supporting the prevention and safety programs conducted through Emergency Medical Services for Children (EMSC) and prevention programs within local EMS systems. EMS has the opportunity to make a substantial difference in a community through advocacy and involvement. Prehospital providers can act as the link between programs and intended recipients, bringing resources and education to those who are in need. Although one provider can make an incredible difference, together an EMS system can create a stable infrastructure for its community through advocacy.

Emergency Medical Services for Children

Children are a unique group of EMS patients. They have special needs and problems that are different from those of adults. They require equipment, tools, and medications designed for smaller bodies with different anatomy and physiology. Children also have different emotional and developmental needs that require a modified approach to assessment and treatment. Although children younger than 18 years of age account for only 10% to 20% of out-of-hospital transports; evaluating, treating, triaging, and transporting this group can create significant stress and multiple challenges for prehospital professionals.

EMSC is a federal program initiated more than 25 years ago to ensure high-quality care of children within the EMS system. With federal grant funds and sustained EMSC program support, EMS communities across the country have developed pediatric-specific policies, procedures, and protocols to assist prehospital professionals in pediatric care at the local level. These pediatric considerations may be outlined in a state or local EMSC plan or in pediatric components within

Case Study 1

You have been called to the scene of a motor vehicle crash between a compact car and a minivan. A 2-year-old girl, who was not properly restrained at the time of the crash, was thrown from the minivan and lies approximately 15 feet from the vehicle. She is unconscious and has no abnormal airway sounds, retractions, or nasal flaring. Respiratory rate is 8 breaths/min, heart rate is 50 beats/min, and blood pressure is 40 mm Hg by palpation. You transport the child to the nearest emergency department (ED), but the child dies shortly after arrival.

1. **How could this have been prevented?**
2. **What could you do to help others avoid this type of tragedy?**

a general EMS plan. For example, most EMS systems now have pediatric triage, treatment, and transport policies. Most systems have pediatric-specific equipment and supplies, and allow special pediatric procedures, such as intraosseous infusions and rectal diazepam administration. In addition, most EMS systems also have specialized operational policies that address unique pediatric legal considerations, such as a pediatric refusal policy that recognizes the legal issues surrounding consent and provision of care to unaccompanied minors.

The umbrella of EMSC is broad and includes out-of-hospital and in-hospital care within general hospitals and specialized pediatric hospitals. Because there are relatively few specialized pediatric centers (pediatric critical care centers and pediatric trauma centers), most children receive emergency care in general hospitals. Hence, universal standards for pediatric emergency care in all EDs within an EMS system (urban and rural, general and specialized) are an important part of EMSC development.

The EMS-EMSC continuum (**Figure 16-1**) is the planned and organized interface between the clinical services of the EMS system itself, other out-of-hospital emergency care resources, the community's primary child health services, and the in-hospital system. The five major phases in the overall continuum include (1) prevention, (2) primary care and the child's "medical home," (3) out-of-hospital care, (4) hospital care, and (5) rehabilitation. These phases represent a cycle of care for a single event that should bring the child back to prevention and the child's medical home. The prehospital professional has the responsibility to support children's emergency care throughout all phases of the continuum. An active partnership with public health programs, collaboration with the community, and continued advocacy through prevention and training empower EMS to make a difference.

Summary of EMSC

EMSC began as a federal grant program to improve out-of-hospital pediatric services, within the community EMS system. Over two decades, the prolific work in the field has forged a broad concept of EMSC as a continuum of multiple clinical services in the community that are coordinated and child-specific. The essential phases of the EMS-EMSC continuum include prevention, the medical home, out-of-hospital care, in-hospital care, and rehabilitation.

Public Health Interface

EMS systems have been evolving as an important part of the public health interface. Prehospital professionals can directly affect disease prevention through vaccination and education, and through continued screening and care aimed at limiting disease progression. Prehospital-care reports act as disease surveillance in helping to identify disease and symptom patterns identifying outbreaks earlier than otherwise available through current means. Proper documentation and participation in screenings, health fairs, clinics, and education forums give prehospital professionals an opportunity to better prepare their community. In the event of a disaster, act of terrorism, or other major response, it is important to be familiar with your partners in public health.

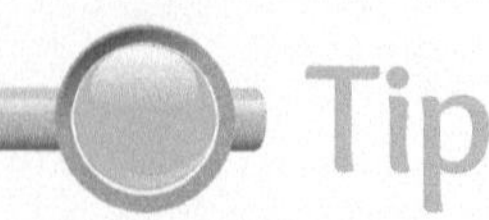

Tip

The umbrella of EMSC is broad and includes general hospitals and specialized pediatric hospitals.

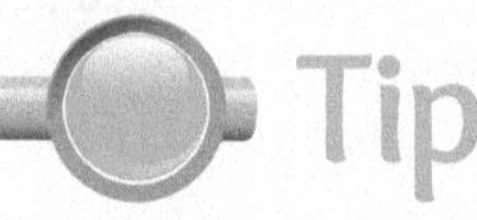

Tip

Standards for pediatric emergency care in the emergency department are an important part of EMSC development.

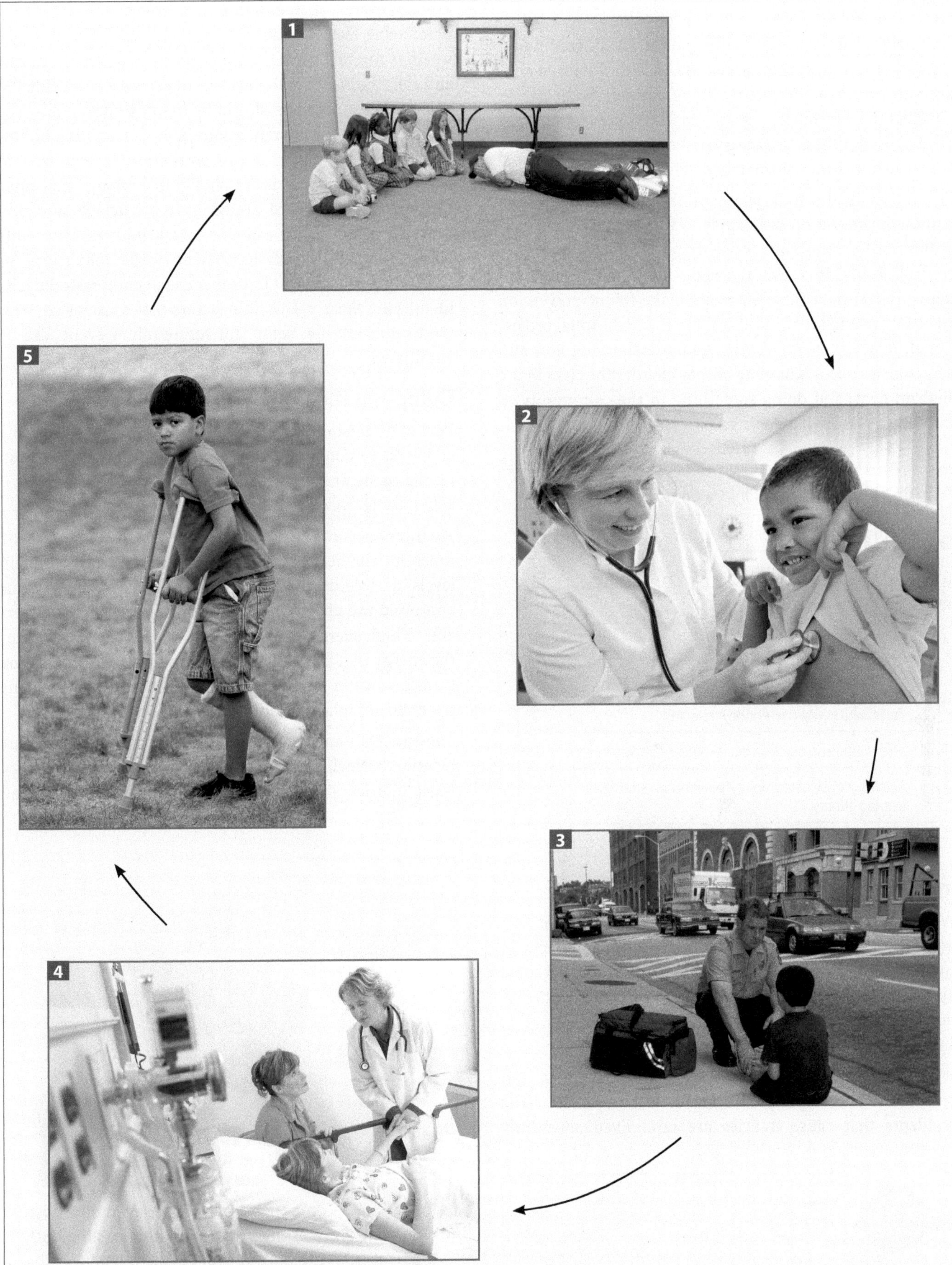

Figure 16-1 EMS-EMSC continuum: **1.** prevention, **2.** primary care and the medical home, **3.** out-of-hospital care, **4.** hospital care, and **5.** rehabilitation.

Injury and Illness Prevention

An integral part of public health and the EMSC continuum is injury and illness prevention. Many ill and injured children die each year, despite receiving optimal medical care. To affect these numbers, injury and illness prevention must be increased. Illness and injury prevention is more effective at saving lives than optimal medical care.

Prevention is the first phase of the EMSC continuum. Although prevention does apply to illness and injury, out-of-hospital services have concentrated primarily on injury control. **Table 16-1** lists the eight identified elements of injury prevention; these elements make injury prevention an objective and scientific effort. For the prehospital professional, injury prevention involves understanding how and why injuries occur, knowing how to identify the risks in the environment, and doing something in the community to stop injuries from happening.

Table 16-1 Elements of Injury Control

1. Recognize injury as a disease process.
2. Maintain a reliable database.
3. Identify problem injuries and high-risk groups.
4. Identify the factors in injury causation.
5. Practice appropriate injury **assessment**.
6. Formulate injury-prevention strategies.
7. Select efficient, practical injury-prevention strategies.
8. Reevaluate selected injury-prevention strategies for the desired effects.

Injuries Are Not Accidents

When injury patterns are carefully studied, it is clear that injuries, like illnesses, vary with the seasons, can occur in epidemics, and often have local trends and demographic distributions. Injuries are largely predictable, whether they are unintentional (e.g., drowning) or intentional (e.g., handgun assaults) and are potentially preventable.

Webster's Dictionary defines the word accident as, "an unforeseen and unplanned event or circumstance." True accidents that cause injuries are rare. Even apparently random events, such as lightning strikes or tornados, have predictable features and can be anticipated. For example, weather forecasting can predict potentially deadly storms and alert the public to their path. "Injuries are not accidents" has become a common slogan by injury professionals. The slogan reflects the current scientific understanding of how injuries really happen. Injury prevention experts refer to automobile accidents as "crashes" rather than "accidents," because crashes almost always have predictable and preventable features. For example, crash injuries commonly occur because of persons driving while intoxicated or speeding, or because of improper use of child restraints. By identifying these predictable factors that cause or contribute to injuries, the "setup" for future injury events can be eliminated.

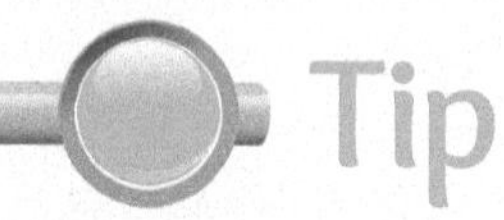

Tip

Injuries are not accidents. They are usually predictable and preventable.

Components of an Injury Event

Part of understanding how injuries occur involves looking at the three components of an injury event: (1) the host, (2) the agent, and (3) the environment (**Figure 16-2**).

The **host** is the person who is the recipient of the injury. An injury occurs when potentially destructive energy is too much for the host to tolerate. Human hosts have different levels of tolerance. Children, because of their unique **anatomic** and **physiologic** features, are particularly vulnerable to high energy transfers. Their smaller body size means the energy that is transferred to the body during a collision transfers over a larger percentage of body surface, placing the child at higher risk for multiple trauma.

The **agent** is a form of energy. The major agents of injury are kinetic, thermal, chemical, electrical, and radiation energy. Most injuries are associated with these types of energy.

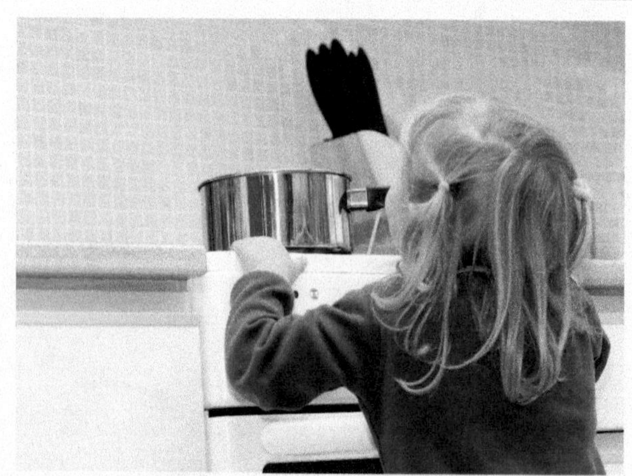

Figure 16-2 Components of an injury event: the host, the agent, and the environment. The child is the host, the heat from the boiling water is the agent, and the dangerously placed handle is the environment for a burn injury.

Kinetic energy is the most common injury agent in circumstances that involve prehospital professionals. For example, falls, automobile-passenger injuries, pedestrian versus automobile, and bicyclist versus automobile events all involve a human as the host and kinetic energy as the agent. Burns, in contrast, involve thermal, chemical, or electrical energy.

The **environment** is the setting where the agent meets the host. The environment causes or influences the injury event. Some examples are an unfenced swimming pool, a poorly maintained road, or an open upper-story window without a protective barrier. Any of these factors may provide the environment for an injury event to occur that might involve a young child as a host and kinetic energy as the agent.

Looking at injury events, the prehospital professional should consider what components of an injury can be modified to prevent future occurrences (**Figure 16-3**). Modifying the host's behavior to prevent drowning or head injury, for example, may involve education in swimming skills or driving techniques. Modifying the agent may include providing bicycle helmets (**Figure 16-4**) or installing soft stopping surfaces in playgrounds to reduce the effect of kinetic energy on vulnerable brain tissue. Modifying the environment may include fencing of swimming pools or setting up window bars.

Phases of Injury

Just as there are three components in every injury event, there are also three separate phases of every injury that need to be considered when devising control strategies: (1) the pre-event period, (2) the event itself, and (3) the postevent period (**Figure 16-5**).

Pre-event factors are conditions in the host, the agent, or the environment that make an injury more or less likely to occur. For example, riding a bicycle with a helmet is a pre-event factor that might significantly decrease the probability of injury. Event factors are conditions that increase or decrease the effect of the agent on the host. An event factor that decreases the risk of injury in a vehicle crash is seat belt use in the automobile at the time of the crash. Postevent factors are conditions that increase or decrease the effect of the agent on the host after the injury event. An example of a postevent factor that affects the outcome in a severely head-injured child is on-scene airway management by the prehospital professional.

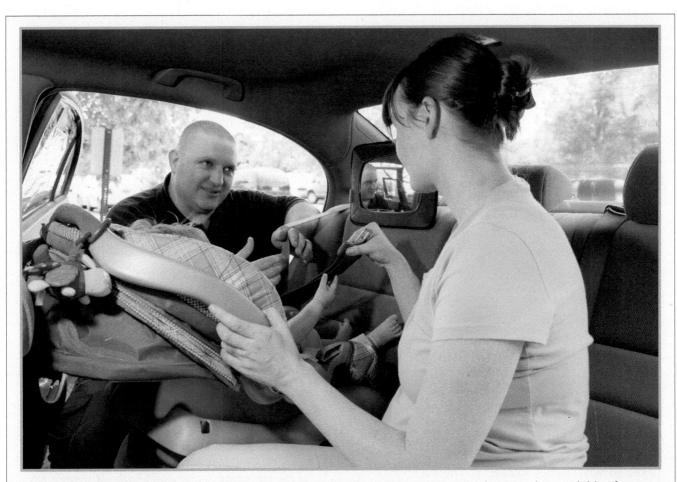

Figure 16-3 EMS professionals can become involved directly in injury prevention by attending a child safety seat technician training program and then by providing a child safety seat checkpoint program.

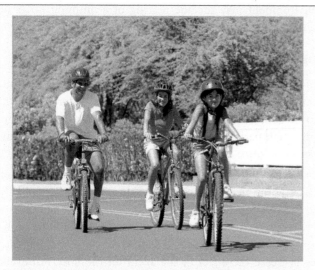

Figure 16-4 When worn correctly, bicycle helmets significantly reduce the complications and incidence of death from closed-head injuries. Prehospital professionals have an important community role in teaching simple injury-control strategies.

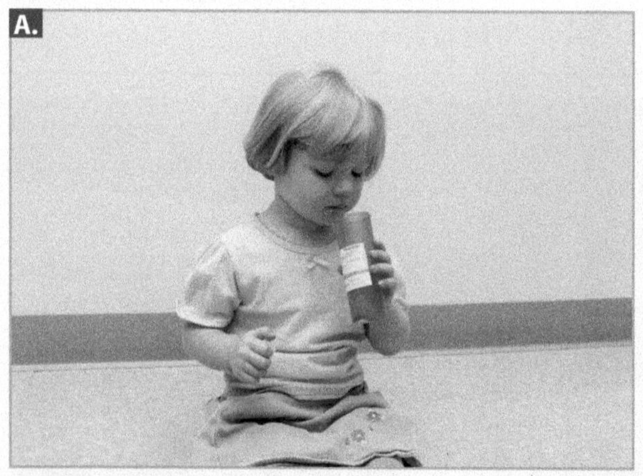

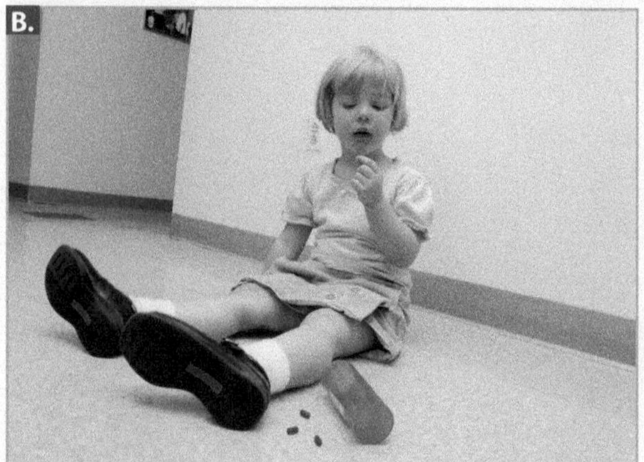

Figure 16-5 The first two phases of an injury. **A.** The pre-event period. An unlocked medicine cabinet invites an adventurous toddler. **B.** The event itself. A toddler will put anything into her mouth, including dangerous medications.

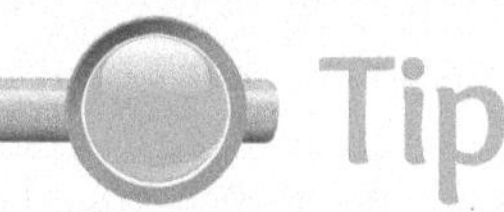

Prevention is an essential feature of all EMS systems and represents an opportunity for prehospital professionals to profoundly affect the health and well-being of their own children and every child in their community.

Traditionally, out-of-hospital care has focused almost exclusively on the postevent period, or medical care and transport after the injury has occurred. Prehospital professionals must now recognize their potential to influence the pre-event and event phases of injury by acting as community educators and advocates. Data collected from patient-care reports help identify patterns and incidences that can steer prevention programs. **Table 16-2** provides examples of injury control strategies aimed at modifiable factors in different phases of injury. The prehospital professional has an important role in all of these prevention strategies. Prevention is enhanced through partnerships accentuated through EMSC.

Table 16-2 Modifiable Factors in Different Phases of an Injury

Phase	Examples of Modifiable Factors
Pre-event	Maintaining child restraint seats Installing proper fencing around pools Ensuring that smoke detectors work in homes Wearing bicycle helmets
Event	Properly using child restraint seats Deployment of front and side air bags
Postevent	Performing pediatric airway management skills Proper cervical spine stabilization Choice of an appropriate transport destination for an injured child

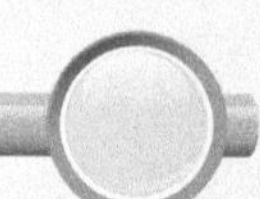

Controversy

Until recently, prehospital professionals were not taught injury or illness prevention. Although adding prevention to the prehospital professional's scope of practice has exciting potential, the role of EMS in injury prevention has not yet been fully explored.

Case Study 2

You are dispatched to a local elementary school for a 7-year-old girl with a history of cerebral palsy and seizures. On arrival the nurse states the patient has been seizing for 15 minutes and she has just administered phenytoin (Dilantin) through the patient's G-tube. The patient is no longer seizing and has respirations of 20 breaths/min, a heart rate of 130 beats/min, a blood pressure of 94/60 mm Hg, and a blood glucose of 88 mg/dL. The child's father arrives and states the patient is acting like normal after a seizure. He requests transport to the children's hospital 45 minutes away and states he will take her if you cannot go that far, refusing ambulance transport to the local ED. The child is now awake, alert, and medically stable.

1. What are your options in the care and transport of this child?
2. How can you assist the parents with safe transportation for this child?

Summary of Prevention and Injury Control

Injury and illness prevention are key features of EMSC, and the first phase of the EMS-EMSC continuum. Injuries are not "accidents" and are almost always predictable. Prehospital professionals have a unique role in community injury control. They are at the scene and able to assess accurately the principle components in an injury or illness event. This includes assessing the child or host, the energy type or agent of injury, and the environment, and understanding the pre-event, event, and postevent phases of injury. National and state EMSC resources allow for collaboration with other programs to provide additional resources.

The Medical Home

The second vital link in the EMS-EMSC continuum is the child's primary care provider, or medical home. The American Academy of Pediatrics (AAP) defines a medical home as the child's primary source of medical care. Creating an effective medical home requires that infants, children, and teenagers have accessible, continuous, comprehensive, family-centered, coordinated, compassionate, and culturally effective services in a geographically close location. The child and family need to know the primary care provider and develop a partnership of mutual responsibility and trust. This is especially important for children with special needs (see Chapter 11) who often require specialized medical care. Trained pediatricians and family physicians create the medical home. They should not only manage and facilitate ongoing pediatric primary care, but also have a linkage to the EMS system in case a child requires emergency services beyond what is offered by the office or clinic. In some offices, there are written protocols and procedures that define how to identify an emergency requiring EMS services, when to summon 9-1-1, and what care should be immediately provided in a medical emergency. The providers in the medical home should have an accurate understanding of the pediatric capabilities of the prehospital professional and EMS system, know the closest hospital for pediatric care, and know the local EMS system's policies and procedures regarding triage, transport, and treatment of children.

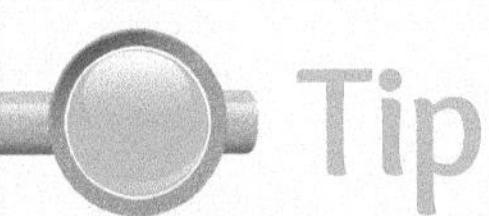

Communication and teamwork are essential features in the linkages between all components of the EMS-EMSC continuum.

The Prehospital Professional and the Medical Home

Traditionally, prehospital professionals have had little contact with primary care physicians who provide the medical home, although both are part of the community settings in the EMSC continuum. There are many opportunities for collaboration between the physicians and providers in the child's medical home and the prehospital professionals in the EMS system. Under some conditions, with the permission of a parent or guardian, the primary provider can offer valuable history and information to the prehospital professional. This may be especially important in evaluating and treating children with special health care needs. This information may be communicated in the form of a written care plan or by a telephone consultation on scene. This does not require the prehospital professional to delay care or transport of a critically ill or injured child, but can take place as part of an EMS system optional procedure for history gathering in stable patients. Sometimes the primary physician can deliver emergency care on scene with the prehospital professionals, and accompany the child

Emergency Information Form for Children With Special Needs

American College of Emergency Physicians® American Academy of Pediatrics

Date form completed By Whom | Revised | Initials | Revised | Initials

Last name:

Name:	Birth date: Nickname:
Home Address:	Home/Work Phone:
Parent/Guardian:	Emergency Contact Names & Relationship:
Signature/Consent*:	
Primary Language:	Phone Number(s):

Physicians:	
Primary care physician:	Emergency Phone:
	Fax:
Current Specialty physician: Specialty:	Emergency Phone:
	Fax:
Current Specialty physician: Specialty:	Emergency Phone:
	Fax:
Anticipated Primary ED:	Pharmacy:
Anticipated Tertiary Care Center:	

Diagnoses/Past Procedures/Physical Exam:	
1.	Baseline physical findings:
2.	
3.	Baseline vital signs:
4.	
Synopsis:	Baseline neurological status:

*Consent for release of this form to health care providers

Last name:

Diagnoses/Past Procedures/Physical Exam continued:	
Medications:	Significant baseline ancillary findings (lab, x-ray, ECG):
1.	
2.	
3.	
4.	Prostheses/Appliances/Advanced Technology Devices:
5.	
6.	

Management Data:

Allergies: Medications/Foods to be avoided	and why:
1.	
2.	
3.	

Procedures to be avoided	and why:
1.	
2.	
3.	

Immunizations

Dates						Dates					
DPT						Hep B					
OPV						Varicella					
MMR						TB status					
HIB						Other					

Antibiotic prophylaxis: Indication: Medication and dose:

Common Presenting Problems/Findings With Specific Suggested Managements

Problem	Suggested Diagnostic Studies	Treatment Considerations

Comments on child, family, or other specific medical issues:

Physician/Provider Signature: Print Name:

Figure 16-6 Emergency information form.

to the ED. *Effectively treating a child with the assistance of prehospital professionals requires that the primary physician understand the local scope of practice, drugs, equipment, and supplies available for children within the local EMS system.* The prehospital professionals should have a "physician on scene" policy that defines the relative roles and responsibilities of the parties in such circumstances.

Communication from the medical home is especially important when assisting children with special needs and should include the emergency information form, as described in Chapter 11 (**Figure 16-6**). This form can provide invaluable information to the prehospital provider when called on to care for a patient. Communicating with the family before the emergency can also allow for familiarity with the child's "regular" status, thereby allowing for a higher comfort level during an emergency response for all involved. Communication and teamwork are essential features in the linkages between all components of the EMSC continuum.

Summary of the Medical Home

The medical home is the child's primary medical provider, usually a pediatrician or family physician, sometimes in concert with other medical practitioners. The medical home is the source of key information and decision making for the child. When appropriate, use the expertise of the primary provider in information gathering and in decision making about emergency care. Always ask caregivers of a child with special needs if they have an emergency information form. Primary care physicians should be aware of the pediatric capabilities and scope of practice of the prehospital professionals and local hospitals and about the services of the other components of the EMSC continuum.

Quality and Safety in EMSC

Quality assurance (QA) and quality improvement (QI) have long been recognized as methods of ensuring efficiency, decreasing waste, and increasing customer satisfaction in industrial settings. Over the last few decades, the concept of continuous QI has been adopted by the health care industry. The ingredients of health care quality now defined in health institutions include: *patient-centered care, efficiency, effectiveness, timeliness, equity,* and *safety.* All of these domains are relevant to pediatric out-of-hospital care:

- *Patient-centered care* is "respectful of and responsive to individual patient preferences, needs, and values."
- *Efficiency* avoids waste, including waste of equipment, supplies, ideas, and energy.

- *Effectiveness* entails treatment grounded in the best scientific evidence that links clinical practice to improved patient outcome. To date, there has been limited research on the effectiveness of prehospital interventions for children. A commitment to participating in clinical research studies is an important element of an EMS program.
- *Timeliness* has always been a primary goal of EMS systems, where treatment and transport delays have long been linked to adverse outcomes for cardiac and trauma patients.
- *Equity* implies providing the same level of care to all patients and families, regardless of socioeconomic status, race or ethnic background, disability, or language barriers.

Safety is a paramount concern for every health care professional, and certainly for the prehospital professional, who faces unique risks in the out-of-hospital setting. Medical error and safety in the prehospital environment are issues now receiving increasing attention. Error rates—in terms of medication dosing and administration, performance of critical procedures, and misdiagnosis—are higher in children than in adults. This discrepancy is probably related to the limited number of pediatric calls and limited opportunities to reinforce pediatric knowledge and skills in the field. EMS efforts to improve pediatric patient safety might include competency-based pediatric training modules, use of length-based tapes or medical software to assist in equipment sizing and medication dosing, the development and dissemination of guidelines of care for common or critical pediatric emergencies, and routinely run reviews to identify factors that contribute to adverse outcomes related to field care. The emerging availability of computer-based decision support systems that prehospital professionals can access by mobile computers or personal digital assistants (**Figure 16-7**) may help to reduce pediatric errors.

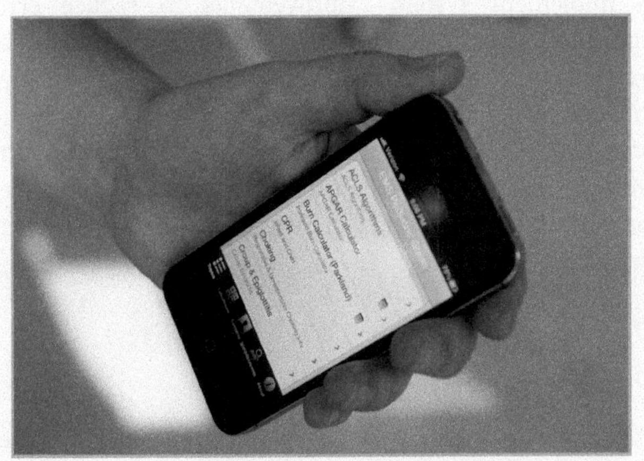

Figure 16-7 Pediatric medical decision support software systems will soon be available for prehospital professionals on vehicle computers and PDAs.

EMSC has been instrumental in the development of regional prehospital pediatric protocols for offline medical control, pediatric hospital destination agreements, and pediatric care policies. These resources better prepare the prehospital professional for pediatric calls.

Data and Information Management

To improve systems of care, providers must have substantive knowledge of how the system currently works. This requires collection and analysis of data on system performance at baseline and after a process or procedure has been introduced or modified. Change for the sake of change does not necessarily represent improvement. Therefore, before any QI initiative is undertaken, the following three questions should be answered:

1. What are we trying to accomplish?
2. What changes can we make that will result in improvement?
3. How will we know that a change is an improvement?

A Prehospital QI Case Study

Consider the following hypothetical scenario: An ED physician contacts the manager of your EMS agency with concerns about two children who were transported over the past month after scene endotracheal intubations following apparent febrile seizures. Both had been treated in the field with intravenous (IV) diazepam, suffered brief respiratory depression, received endotracheal intubations, and were extubated shortly after arrival in the ED. A query of your agency's electronic database reveals a total of 10 children over the past year with a diagnosis of seizure who were intubated in the field after treatment with IV diazepam. Knowing that most febrile seizures are brief and self-limited, you are concerned that the potential complications of intubation likely outweigh the benefits of diazepam therapy. You bring this to the QI committee for review. They ask the following questions:

Question #1: What are we trying to accomplish?

Answer #1: We want to decrease the incidence of children experiencing respiratory depression and intubation caused by benzodiazepine treatment for seizures.

Question #2: What changes can we make that will result in improvement?

Answer #2: Possible changes might include education of advanced life support (ALS) personnel on indications for benzodiazepine administration in children with seizures, adding computer-based decision-support software or length-based resuscitation tapes to each drug box to promote accurate dosing of benzodiazepines, switching from IV to rectal diazepam administration for prolonged seizures, and teaching the technique of nasal airway placement and bag-mask ventilation.

Case Study 3

You are called to a recreational complex for a 12-year-old male student who was hit in the chest with a baseball and collapsed. Before your arrival, his coach and teammates started CPR and attached an automated external defibrillator (AED), and the patient was subsequently defibrillated. As you arrive on scene, you are told what happened and what care was rendered up to your arrival. As you continue resuscitation efforts, you calculate medications and equipment size with a length-based tool. The patient regains a pulse and recovers, and you transport him to the ED.

1. **How did the community prepare for this event? How did EMS?**
2. **What resources are available in a community?**

Question #3: How will we know if a change is an improvement?

Answer #3: Our intubation rate for children with seizures will drop, without an associated increase of children with low oxygen saturation on arrival to the ED.

Together with your medical control physician, you develop a new protocol for assessing and managing seizures in children, provide in-service training with your ALS personnel, and develop a data sheet to be filled out after every seizure call. After 6 months, you find that your intubation rate for children with febrile seizures has been cut by 75%.

This data-driven approach is based on examining the status quo and looking for opportunities to improve prehospital practice.

Importance of Data Collection and Information Management in EMSC

Injury prevention begins with an understanding of the community's injury problems. Data, when correctly collected, integrated, and interpreted, become useful information. A properly maintained injury database can be analyzed to identify patterns of preventable injury in a community, which then can be used to generate financial and political support for focused prevention programs. These data also allow an evaluation of the effectiveness of targeted programs in reducing the frequency and severity of injuries.

Elements of an injury database that would be useful in EMS system management include the type, severity, and frequency of fatal and nonfatal injuries; persons at risk; geographic location; time of day and year; and contributing factors, such as alcohol, weather, and lack of (or improper use of) protective devices. Analysis of these data can help set the agenda for program planning and evaluation. For example, the data indicate that a community is experiencing a high rate of injury among unrestrained young children in car crashes. An injury prevention effort must then examine why the injured children are not restrained. The problem may be an issue of education or accessibility. Perhaps the problem is a community cultural belief that a baby is always safest in a mother's arms. Understanding the basis of the problem is critical in determining the best intervention strategy.

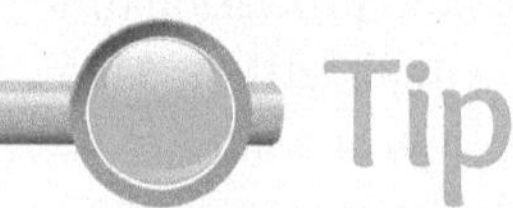

Data, when correctly collected, integrated, and interpreted, become useful information.

Summary of Quality, Safety, Data Collection, and Information Management

QI is now a key feature of EMSC. There are many opportunities to evaluate clinical practice with children and to implement system improvements to reduce error. Appropriate data collection is a key to improvement. There are many types of EMS data that pertain to children. Simply collecting data is not enough. For data to be useful, they need to be accurately collected and then reviewed with a problem orientation. When data are effectively managed, the essential information can be used for focused education and program development.

Prevention: The Prehospital Professional's Role

Prehospital professionals have a responsibility to affect their communities through illness and injury prevention. *They can have a greater impact on health by reducing illness and injury through prevention than they can through*

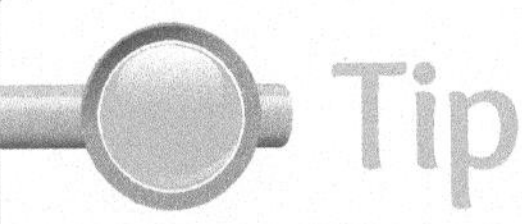

Prehospital professionals can have a greater impact in reducing the incidence and impact of illness and injury through prevention than through treatment.

treatment alone. However, to be effective in this new role, prehospital professionals need education and training. Recognizing how injuries can be avoided is the first step in developing prevention activities in the community.

Before the Call

Prevention can be started before the call through preparedness. Working with your community on such programs as Community Emergency Response Team (CERT), the emergency information form, CPR and first aid training, babysitting classes, and car seat safety checks helps to strengthen the infrastructure needed to handle emergencies. Educational programs and skills training also serve to hone your response to pediatric calls. The better prepared your community is to recognize and respond to an event, the more likely prevention programs and response will be successful.

Role On Scene

Prevention actions of the prehospital professional begin during the "scene size-up" and include ensuring scene safety and performing an environmental assessment. Ensuring scene safety involves prevention of injury and illness to the prehospital professional and to other medical and law enforcement personnel. This includes identification of possible communicable diseases in the child that can be transmitted to unwary scene personnel unless proper body substance precautions are observed. Ensuring scene safety also may prevent an injury to the child or to the caregiver.

Performing an environmental assessment adds a crucial piece to the overall picture at the scene. ED providers cannot do an environmental assessment. Observation and documentation of the physical and interpersonal environment by the prehospital professional may provide the basis for important prevention actions. Such actions may include providing information directly to the caregiver on safety hazards in the home.

Another type of environmental assessment involves observing and noting any evidence of possible maltreatment by the caregiver and then communicating these concerns to the ED physician. This preventive action may be lifesaving to the child, as explained in Chapter 13.

Role in Safe Transport

Another important aspect of childhood injury prevention for the prehospital professional is safe vehicular transport. *Most serious and fatal vehicular injuries occur to occupants who are improperly restrained.* This pertains to ambulance transport and automobile transport. The key step for safety of the prehospital professional AND the patient is the simplest: wear a seat belt, secure all equipment, and secure the pediatric patient in a proper restraint device for the entire transport.

For a child who requires spinal stabilization, use a stabilization device secured to the ambulance stretcher to package the child safely, as described in Chapter 15. If the child is critically ill, treat and transport the child secured in a supine or semi-Fowler's position on a stretcher. This position allows rapid management and monitoring of the child's airway, breathing, and circulation. For a child with mild-to-moderate illness or injury not requiring spinal stabilization or a supine position, transport in an upright position on the stretcher or, use an age-appropriate and locally approved approach to restraint, as described in Chapter 15, if available. For some children with respiratory problems, an upright position of comfort is important, as explained in Chapter 3. The child with cardiopulmonary or neurologic disabilities may require a specialized child seat to breathe effectively, as described in Chapter 11.

In addition to passengers, unsecured items and equipment move like unsecured people in the back of an ambulance. If the transport requires additional equipment for special patient care, such as a drug box or medication pump, then secure the items before transport. There is always the potential for an ambulance crash, or even just a hard stop, and preparation and prevention avert damage and injury.

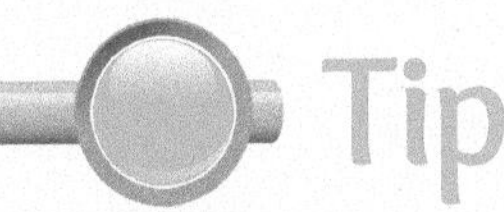

Wear your seat belt and secure all portable items in the ambulance.

Role in the Community

Detailed and accurate observations at the scene may serve to start or support community-wide strategies for injury and illness control. For example, in Europe and Australia, prehospital professionals played a key role in recognizing the relationship between sleep position and sudden unexpected infant death (SUID). Scene observations were part of the scientific studies that confirmed the increased risk of SUID in babies who slept prone and assisted in the campaign that has decreased SUID mortality. Chapter 12 discusses SUID in more detail.

Prehospital professionals can help in the understanding of community injury and illness patterns by documenting the mechanism and scene circumstances of an acute event in the prehospital record and by assisting in other local data-collection efforts. **Table 16-3** lists some specific community injury prevention activities that prehospital professionals might consider in their expanded roles as community advocates, public educators, and teachers.

Table 16-3 Examples of Common Injuries and Possible Prevention Strategies

Injury	Prevention
Vehicle trauma	Infant and child restraint seats
	Seat belts and air bags
	Pedestrian safety programs
	Motorcycle helmets
Cycling	Bicycle helmets
	Bicycle paths separate from vehicle traffic
Recreation	Appropriate safety padding and apparel
	Cyclist/skateboard/skater safety programs
	Soft, energy-absorbent playground surfaces
Drowning	Four-sided locked pool enclosures
	Pool alarms
	Immediate adult supervision
	Caretaker CPR training
	Swimming lessons
	Pool/beach safety instruction
	Personal flotation device
Poisoning and household items	Proper storage of chemicals and medications
	Child safety packaging
Burns	Proper maintenance and monitoring of electrical appliances and cords
	Fire/smoke detectors
	Proper placement of cookware on stove top
Other	Discouragement of infant walker use
	Gated stairways
	Babysitter first aid training
	Child care worker first aid training

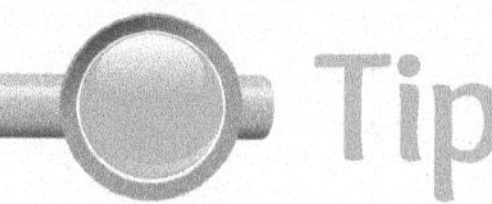

Scene observations were part of the scientific studies that confirmed the increased risk of SIDS in babies who slept prone.

Summary of Roles in Prevention

The prehospital professional has many opportunities to teach and practice prevention on the job and as a community member (**Figure 16-8**). Recognition of scene safety issues, documentation of suspicious home circumstances, and recording of injury mechanisms are fundamental information for EMS systems. Error reduction through careful equipment sizing and drug dosing prevents adverse outcomes as a result of medical care delivered in the field. Fulfilling the dual agendas of ensuring the child passenger's safety in the event of an ambulance crash and permitting ongoing monitoring and treatment continues to represent a challenge for EMS professionals. Last, there are many opportunities as a community member to advocate for injury control and illness prevention as a member of the EMSC continuum.

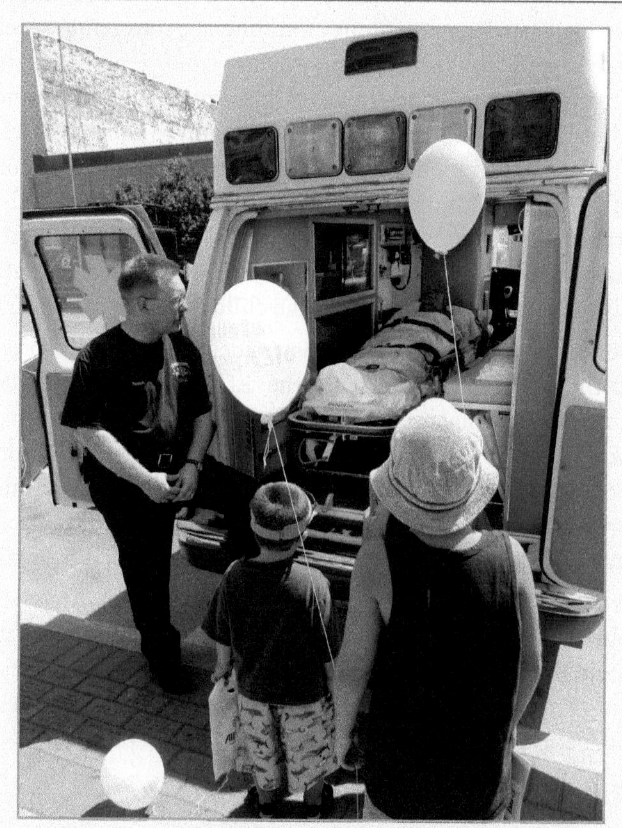

Figure 16-8 Prehospital professionals have the opportunity to teach prevention.

Call to Action: Advocacy for EMSC

Advocates can support EMSC on and off the ambulance. There are numerous roles for the prehospital professional in the clinical and operational aspects of EMSC, and there are endless problems to undertake in every community. National and state EMSC programs offer many excellent models and templates for system improvement and often provide funding to support new programs for children. New pediatric-specific software is available to support bedside clinical care of children. In addition, many funding agencies, public and private, have resources to support children's services and enhancements in pediatric emergency care in the community. Advocacy for EMSC includes looking creatively for sources of support outside traditional EMS to help or strengthen pediatric services.

Possible roles to advance children's issues within EMS may involve participation on EMSC committees and advocating on a day-to-day basis for training, equipment, policies, procedures, and protocols that pertain exclusively to children. Other roles may include serving as a volunteer educator at school, developing school first aid services, becoming a CPR trainer, or joining community programs on injury control and children's health issues. National associations, such as the American Academy of Pediatrics, American College of Emergency Physicians, and the Emergency Nurses Association, and local fire departments and prehospital organizations sponsor programs for pediatric illness and injury prevention, but these visionary programs require advocacy and participation for success.

Partnerships created within your community can help empower tomorrow's generation through education today. A child who understands he or she is not helpless in times of emergency becomes a powerful ally on the scene, while allowing for less psychological trauma. Civil organizations have been successful with affecting lives through preparedness, and EMS has an opportunity to further those efforts exponentially. Through training and education, we can make a difference.

There is unprecedented potential for exciting improvements in saving lives, decreasing pain and suffering, preventing injury and illness, and facilitating the complex interface of out-of-hospital pediatric care with community and in-hospital services through participation with public health. Preserving the health and safety of children demands constant advocacy and vigilance from all prehospital professionals to sustain quality pediatric services in EMS systems now and to continue the evolution of EMSC tomorrow.

CASE STUDY ANSWERS

Case Study 1 — page 302

Factors that may have helped prevent or modify the injuries include car safety education in schools and communities, especially use of seat belts and child restraint seats; reduced vehicle speed; and better traffic signs for drivers.

For the prehospital professional, the key prevention steps in this case are to do the scene size-up, document the important scene conditions, provide appropriate on-scene care, and rapidly transport the child to the appropriate facility. Documenting the mechanism and informing hospital professionals of the preventable aspects of the injury (unrestrained child) have many benefits. It is highly unlikely that any type of medical care would have changed this child's outcome. Hence, although the prehospital professional's interventions after an injury event are few and futile in such cases, there are many useful preventive interventions before the event.

Careful documentation of the circumstances of injury also contributes to vital data collection and helps define patterns of injury within the community. The prehospital professional can become a community advocate for injury prevention, helping to educate parents and policy makers about known risks and identifying and promoting solutions to the important public health problems of childhood injury.

Case Study 2 — page 307

This child's primary care physician plays an active role in managing her chronic illness and is likely best qualified to make care decisions. Given the child's medically stable status after treatment, contact with medical control to discuss transport destination is reasonable. Effective out-of-hospital care is a phase of the EMS-EMSC continuum and requires not only appropriate equipment and education of prehospital personnel, but also teamwork, knowledge of community resources, and expert communication. Transport of this child to her "medical home" if allowed by local EMS policies may have advantages that must be weighed against potential risks of further physiologic compromise. When local protocols do not allow transport beyond local facilities, alternative safe transport should be sought. If the patient has an emergency information form, it also can act as a resource to the patient's regular status and response, and provide information before the parent's arrival.

Case Study 3 — page 310

The rapid response, scene efficiency, and lifesaving skills provided by the community before EMS arrival serve the patient and the bystanders. Through education, training, equipment procurement, and emergency preparedness, the potential for a community to handle an emergency with the best outcomes is allowed. The ability to respond and react appropriately ensures the continuum of care is served. CPR training, AED placement, community response teams, pediatric training, and tools create a community empowered to make a difference. Access to a computer-based decision support software program or length-based tool can assist the prehospital professional in choosing the appropriately sized equipment and the correct dosages of medications. Having pediatric equipment well organized and accessible facilitates the search for the correct equipment size and safeguards the care of the child. Using computer software tools or length-based tapes may elevate critical thinking, reduce cognitive load, and allow the prehospital professional to focus on assessment, prioritization, medical interventions, and transport.

Training and education allow the community to take an important role in the patient's care and subsequent outcome. Prehospital professionals have the ability to help prepare and empower their communities through EMSC resources and community collaboration.

SUGGESTED READINGS

Textbooks

Aehlert B. *Paramedic Practice Today: Above and Beyond.* St. Louis: Elsevier-Mosby-JEMS; 2010.

Barss P, Smith G, Baker S, Mohan D. *Injury Prevention: An International Perspective.* New York: Oxford University Press; 1998.

Seidel J, Knapp J. *Childhood Emergencies in the Office, Hospital, and Community: Organizing Systems of Care.* 2nd ed. Chicago: American Academy of Pediatrics Committee on Pediatric Emergency Medicine; 2000.

Articles

American Academy of Pediatrics. Medical Home Initiatives for Children with Special Needs Project Advisory Committee: the medical home. *Pediatrics.* 2002;110(1):184–186.

Gausche M. Out-of-hospital care of pediatric patients. *Pediatr Clin North Am.* 1999;46(6):1305–1327.

Horowitz L. Mental health aspects of emergency medical services for children: summary of a consensus conference. *J Pediatr Psychol.* 2001;26(8):491–502.

Sia C. The medical home: closing the circle of care. In: Seidel JS, Henderson DP, eds. *Emergency Medical Services for Children: A Report to the Nation.* Washington, DC: National Center for Education in Maternal and Child Health; 1991.

Resources

EMSC National Resource Center. http://www.childrensnational.org/emsc. Accessed December 4, 2012.

Procedure 1: Field Reporting

Introduction

Gathering and organizing pertinent information about children to report to other prehospital professionals, medical oversight, and the receiving emergency department (ED) requires pediatric terms. Clear, concise communication helps ensure an orderly flow of out-of-hospital tasks: describing children and their clinical problems accurately to medical oversight personnel; informing the receiving ED personnel about incoming patients; and making an effective transfer of information about the patient's assessment and care. Each emergency medical service (EMS) region has unique requirements for field reporting to medical oversight and to the receiving ED. The patient criteria requiring field reporting are variable in different EMS systems. Sometimes the reporting is not by radio, but rather by telephone or another form of real-time communication. Many local EMS agencies have reporting or communications protocols that specifically address on-line medical oversight and ED notification requirements for children.

In addition to the spoken presentation format for field reporting, pediatric-specific documentation is also essential for later review and analysis. Each EMS agency has its own reporting form on which the prehospital professional must record clinical facts, as well as the necessary information for billing and for detailed incident or system analysis.

Indication

Use good field reporting procedure in any radio, telephone, facsimile (fax), personal, or other communication with medical oversight, the receiving ED, or other prehospital providers regarding on-scene or inbound pediatric emergency patients. Good reporting technique is also indicated for chart documentation.

Contraindication

The only relative contraindication to appropriate field reporting is the child with a physiologic abnormality requiring constant hands-on care. This situation may make it difficult for the prehospital professional to communicate fully with a receiving ED or medical oversight while on the way to the ED. In most cases, a coworker, such as a partner, can assist with notifying the ED that a distressed child is on the way, although complete reporting of patient assessment, treatment, and response to treatment may not be possible. There are no contraindications to accurate reporting through chart documentation.

Equipment

Equipment requirements vary depending on the EMS system. Equipment may include telecommunications equipment, computerized real-time data transmission, or video. The patient care record is essential, as are other assessment worksheets in some EMS systems.

Rationale

A logical and descriptive format for presentation of key information about ill or injured children is essential for everyday field practice. It promotes the cost-efficient use of communications equipment and personnel time. Proper field reporting also integrates efforts from all emergency care professionals (prehospital professionals, nurses, and doctors) and helps ensure that vital data are transmitted completely and concisely. Pediatric-specific reporting techniques complement appropriate age-related modifications in assessment, treatment, triage, and transport.

Preparation

1. The prehospital professional should prepare for and practice field reporting about children.
2. It is helpful to have a field reporting format that is agreed on by the EMS agency, medical oversight, and the ambulance providers. The desired format can be printed on small

pads as a checklist. This may help in the flow and understanding of patient information during situations when the prehospital professional has multiple tasks and when the environment or equipment makes communicating difficult.

3. Such notes may be useful not only during transport, but also when transferring care at the ED.

Possible Complications

Using incorrect, deceptive, or unclear terminology, or failing to distinguish the pediatric report from the more frequent adult-oriented report, may confuse medical oversight and delay preparation by the receiving ED.

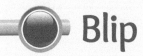

Blip

Do not give long field reports when there is a distressed child in the ambulance.

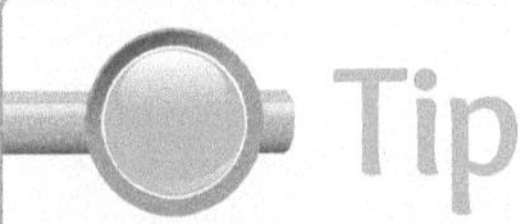

Tip

Report the patient's assessment using the PAT.

Procedure 1-1

Field Reporting

1. State the child's age, gender, and estimated body weight. Using the patient's name is generally not pertinent to treatment, triage, or transport, so do not use names in the field report. Emergency medical channels are easily monitored, and omitting the patient's name protects his or her identity and medical confidentiality.

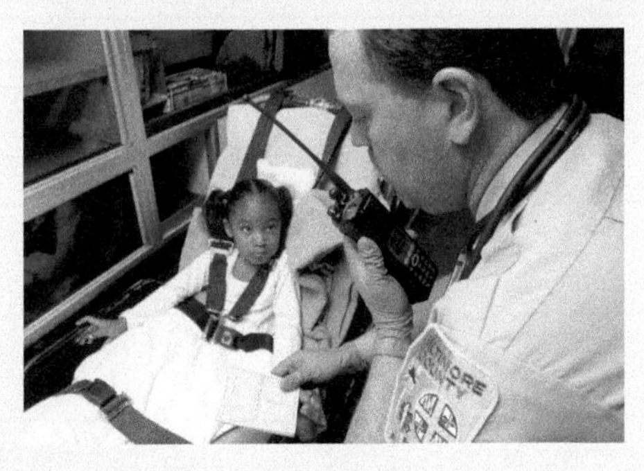

2. Give the child's chief complaint.
3. Provide in one sentence the mechanism of injury or history of illness, and state pertinent past medical history (usually none or brief).
4. Summarize the assessment and establish the level of severity and urgency for treatment using the Pediatric Assessment Triangle (PAT). Address all three elements of the PAT, using appropriate descriptive words and terms, as listed in **Table P1-1**.

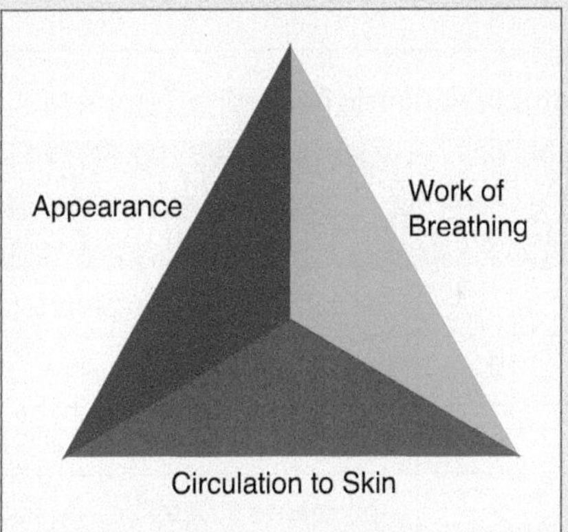

5. Report any abnormalities in the ABCDEs. Avoid focusing on vital signs.
6. State treatment and response, using the PAT.
7. Estimate time of arrival and state the proposed receiving ED.
8. Request agreement from medical oversight with interventions and request additional orders as per local EMS protocol.
9. Repeat medical oversight orders to confirm understanding. **Table P1-2** is a sample pediatric reporting template.

Table P1-1 Examples of Pediatric-Specific Terminology for PAT

Appearance (use TICLS mnemonic to recall individual features)	Work of Breathing	Circulation to Skin
Tone Active, vigorous, good muscle tone Limp, listless, motionless, will not sit or walk	Apneic	Pink, good color
Interactiveness Alert, interactive, attentive, playful Restless, agitated, screaming	Abnormal positioning (sniffing position, tripoding)	Mottled, dusky
Consolability Consolable or distractible by caregiver, comfortable Cannot be consoled	Abnormal airway sounds (snoring, stridor, wheezing, grunting)	Pale
Look/Gaze Fixes gaze, maintains good eye contact Will not engage or make eye contact	Retractions (supraclavicular, intercostal, subxiphoid)	Cyanotic
Speech/Cry Strong cry, normal speech Weak cry, cannot speak	Nasal flaring	

Table P1-2 Sample Pediatric Reporting Template

We are [on scene] or [en route to (name of ED)] with a [state age in days, weeks, months, or years as appropriate] [state boy or girl] patient weighing [state approximate body weight in kilograms].	
CC	The patient's chief complaint is [state chief complaint in one or two words].
HPI	State brief history of present illness/injury.
PMH	State brief, pertinent, medical history (note: usually there is none).
PAT	Appearance: Describe the patient's appearance using descriptive terms.* Work of breathing: Describe the work of breathing using descriptive terms. Circulation to skin: Describe the circulation to skin using descriptive terms.
Initial ABCDEs assessment	Summarize key findings from the ABCDEs.
TX	Report the treatment and the patient's response. Use these elements as the basis for ongoing assessment: the PAT, the ABCDEs, repeating vital signs, and reassessing of positive anatomic findings in distressed children who have received the focused and detailed exams.
ETA	Our ETA to [state receiving ED] is ______ minutes. Do you have any advice or questions? [Request additional orders as per local protocol at this point.]

*See Table P1-1 for examples of pediatric-specific descriptive terminology.

Procedure 2: Length-Based Equipment Sizing and Drug Dosing

Introduction

Selecting the appropriately sized piece of equipment or drug dose is often challenging during pediatric resuscitations. Errors are common, and may be dangerous or life-threatening. Several types of devices are useful for determining the correct equipment sizes and drug doses. The pediatric length-based resuscitation tape is a simple and effective tool to measure body lengths and to determine approximate weights. Knowledge of the child's body length and approximate weight is the basis to calculate appropriate equipment sizes and drug doses.

Computerized methodologies that use length and weight for instantaneous equipment sizing and drug dosing may include pediatric-specific software on a computer or hand-held personal digital assistant (PDA). Software has the advantage of including essential resuscitation information, such as algorithms, drug doses, and equipment sizes for a wide range of clinical problems. Computerized calculation of drug or fluid doses facilitates precise equipment sizing and drug dosing.

Indication

Children requiring equipment, medication, or fluids, weighing from 3–36 kg body weight

Equipment

Pediatric resuscitation tape

Pediatric decision support software on a computer or PDA

Rationale

Treatment of infants and children in the out-of-hospital setting is difficult because children of different ages require different sizes of equipment, doses of medications, and volumes of fluids. Mistakes are common when selecting appropriate equipment and medications in critical pediatric emergencies without the benefit of an accurate weight. Pediatric resuscitation equipment for such calculations uses weight or length as a valid marker of size-specific equipment and medication needs. These devices are portable, easy to use, and applicable to all out-of-hospital equipment and medications.

Computerized Calculations

Indication

Children requiring equipment, medication, or fluids

Contraindications

None

Equipment

Length-based resuscitation tape

Computerized software specific to pediatric resuscitation

Possible Complications

None

Preparation

Length-Based Resuscitation Tape

1. Place the patient in a supine position.
2. Extend the patient's legs.

Computerized Technology

1. Knowledge of the particular software application for the PDA or computer.
2. After entering the patient's data (weight, length, and age), the device provides equipment information, and drug and fluid calculations specific to the clinical problem.

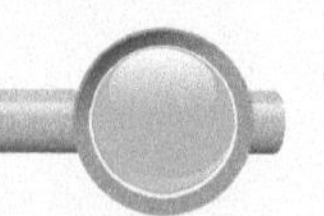

Store the length-based resuscitation tape in a place that is easily accessible, such as the pediatric equipment kit.

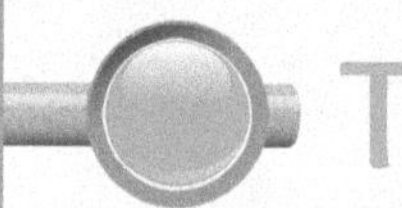

Practice using the computerized applications prior to resuscitation events to allow easy use during resuscitation.

Procedure 2-1

Length-Based Resuscitation Tape

1. Measure child's length—from head to heel—with the tape (with the red portion at the head). Note and say weight in kilograms that corresponds to the child's measured length at the heel. If the child is longer than the tape, use adult equipment and medication doses. From the tape, identify appropriate equipment sizes. From the tape, identify appropriate medication doses.

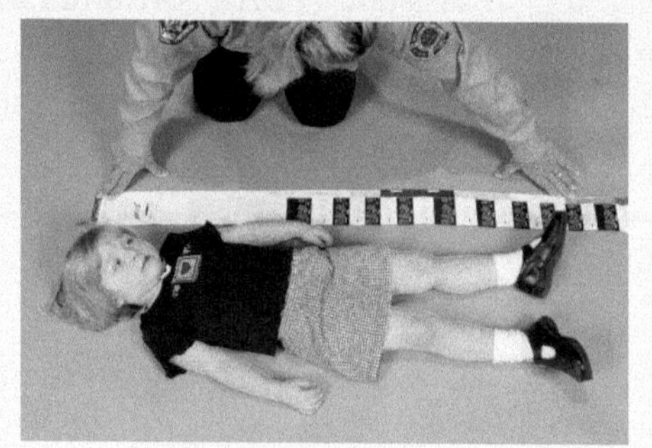

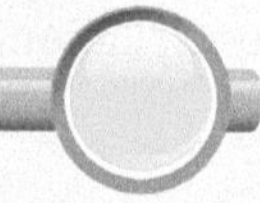

There are several different brands of length-based pediatric resuscitation tapes; these have not been compared for speed, accuracy, or safety.

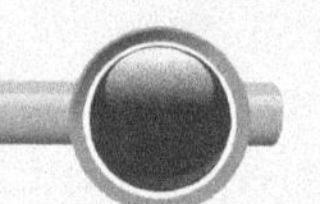

Measuring to the child's toes (instead of heel) adds a number of kilograms to the estimated weight and may result in equipment sizes that are too large or excessive drug doses.

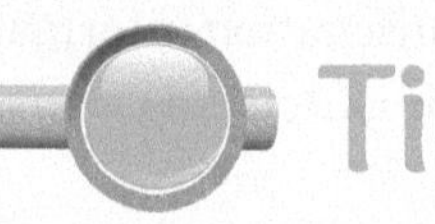

"Red to the head" provides proper alignment of the length-based Broselow tape.

Procedure 2-2

Pediatric Resuscitation Software

1. Enter the child's length into the software program, then select the clinical condition or type of resuscitation. The software calculates the equipment size and drug dose for the child's size.

Procedure 3: Oxygen Delivery

Introduction

Hypoxia in the infant or child causes cardiopulmonary distress and may lead to organ failure. Careful assessment of the child's cardiopulmonary status includes standard physical assessment techniques and pulse oximetry. A normal room air pulse oximetry reading is 95% or greater. A pulse oximetry value of less than 95% on room air is an indication for supplemental oxygen. A value less than 90% with the child on 100% oxygen is usually also an indication for ventilatory support. Acute hypoxia is usually easy to treat. Rapid intervention may slow or reverse cardiopulmonary distress or failure and avoid the need for ventilatory support. Although respiratory disease is usually the cause of hypoxia in children, other conditions, such as hypovolemic shock, severe poisonings, or seizures, may also result in hypoxia.

There are different procedures for giving oxygen to children that vary the amount of actual oxygen supplementation. Use an oxygen delivery technique that matches the child's clinical condition, age, and need for oxygen. For example, give oxygen by nasal cannula or simple mask to the child in no or mild distress who has an open airway. Give oxygen by a nonrebreathing mask or bag-mask device to the child with moderate to severe respiratory distress. Rarely, a critical child requires endotracheal intubation for positive pressure ventilation and oxygen administration. When supplemental oxygen does not improve the child's condition, consider other possibilities, such as a cardiac disorder (e.g., cyanotic congenital heart disease); a circulatory disorder (e.g., hypovolemic shock); or, rarely, a toxicologic disorder (e.g., methemoglobinemia).

Be creative in delivering oxygen to young children. Under some circumstances, giving blow-by oxygen may avoid agitating the child and increasing his or her distress. In the newly born be careful about oxygen delivery, because it is unnecessary if the newborn has a normal pulse oximetry and supplemental oxygen may be harmful to the immature brain.

Indications

- Respiratory distress
- Pulse oximetry less than 95% on room air
- Respiratory failure
- Partial upper airway obstruction
- Partial lower airway obstruction
- Worsening of chronic lung disease
- Status epilepticus
- Overdose
- Shock from any cause
- Multiple trauma
- Any condition possibly causing decreased oxygen delivery to tissues
- Smoke inhalation
- Carbon monoxide poisoning

Contraindications

There are few absolute contraindications to oxygen delivery to a child who may be hypoxic. There are, however, rare relative contraindications to certain oxygen delivery techniques that do not match the child's clinical condition. For example, shunted cyanotic cardiac patients whose saturation goals are 75%–85% should not receive oxygen to increase saturation greater than 85%. Oxygen has proper doses and routes of administration for maximum benefit, minimum toxicity, optimal feasibility, and reasonable cost.

Rationale

A child's immature anatomy and physiology make respiratory distress and failure common pediatric emergencies. When apnea or hypoventilation occurs, hypoxia develops quickly. Therefore, give oxygen to any child with clinical signs of cardiopulmonary distress or failure, or with a history suggesting possible abnormalities in gas exchange. *Children seldom have a condition where excess oxygen turns off their respiratory drive, so it is better to overtreat with oxygen than to undertreat.*

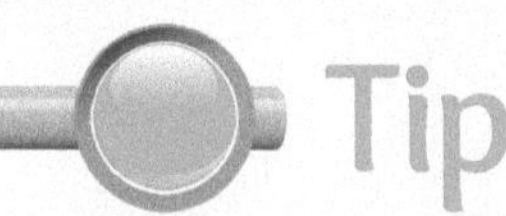

The appropriate oxygen delivery technique is based on the child's condition, age, and need for oxygen.

Preparation

1. Connect the pressure regulator and flow meter to the oxygen source. Turn on the tank.
2. Match the correct oxygen delivery device with the patient assessment (child's condition, age, and need for oxygen; **Table P3-1**).

Equipment

Infant and pediatric nasal cannula

Pediatric mask sizes

Pediatric nonrebreathing mask

Oxygen connecting tubing

Oxygen source

Possible Complications

Injury, if the pressurized tank is punctured or a valve breaks off

Potential for fire, because oxygen supports combustion

Respiratory arrest if high concentrations of oxygen are given to the child with chronic lung disease (rare)

Agitation and worsening of hypoxia, if delivery technique is overly aggressive

Hypothermia in an infant younger than 6 months of age with an endotracheal tube in place, who receives cool, unhumidified oxygen for more than 30 minutes

In newly borns with normal pulse, brain injury may occur because of unnecessary supplemental oxygen

Table P3-1 Oxygen Delivery Technique and Patient Assessment

Device	Flow Rate	Concentration Delivered	Considerations
Nasal cannula	1–6 L/min	Up to 44%	• Low-flow system • Least restrictive • Slowly start flow of oxygen after cannula is secured to avoid frightening child • May help to tape cannula to child's cheeks • Use in infants who are obligatory nose breathers or if there is difficulty in obtaining a correctly sized mask
Simple mask	6–10 L/min	35–60%	• Low-flow system • Infant, pediatric, and adult sized masks are available • Use minimum flow rate to flush the mask
Nonrebreathing	12–15 L/min	60–90%	• High-flow system mask • Consists of face mask and reservoir bag with a valve on the exhalation mask port to prevent drawing in room air during inhalation and a valve between the reservoir bag and mask to prevent exhalation of air into the reservoir bag • Use in spontaneously breathing patients who require highest concentration of oxygen available (children with respiratory distress and shock) • Make sure the flow rate keeps the reservoir bag inflated • With a snug fit, delivers highest oxygen concentration available by mask • Pediatric and adult masks are available • Partial rebreather masks are indicated in neonates and infants who cannot overcome valve resistance
Blow-by	6–10 L/min	Depends on flow rate and proximity to face	• Indicated for infant or young child requiring oxygen who will not tolerate mask on the face • Start oxygen flow through simple mask, corrugated tubing, or oxygen tubing threaded through the bottom of a cup • Hold the delivery device as close to the child's nose and mouth as tolerated

Source: Emergency Nurses Association. Respiratory distress and failure. *Emergency Nursing Pediatric Course, Provider Manual.* Park Ridge, IL; 1999.

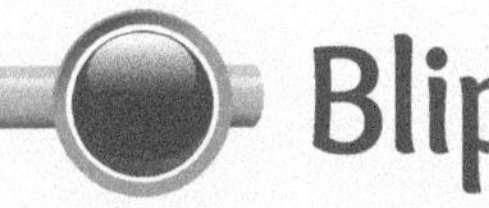

Do not give oxygen to a newly born who is not hypoxic. It may cause injury in immature patients.

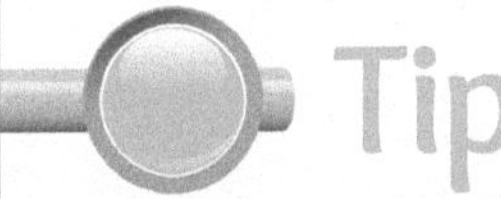

Add humidification to nasal cannula flow greater than 5 L/min to avoid nasal irritation and bleeding.

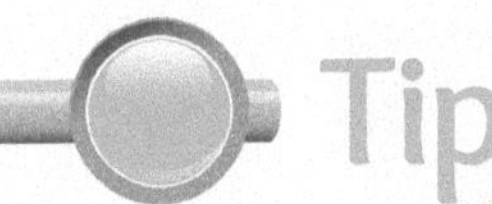

An oxygen mask may frighten a child.

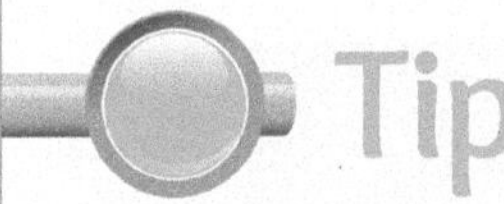

For nasal cannula: percent oxygen delivered is affected by respiratory rate, tidal volume, and extent of mouth breathing. An infant may receive higher FiO_2 concentration than older patients (e.g., 30%–35% with 1 L/min oxygen, 26%–32% with 0.5 L/min oxygen).

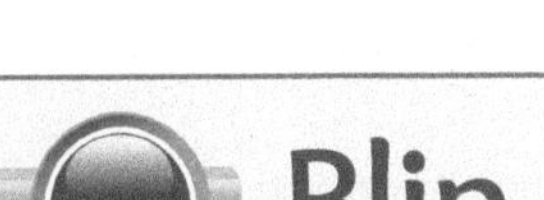

Do not force the child to lie down because it may increase the child's anxiety and agitation.

Procedure 3-1

Oxygen Delivery

1. Explain to the child and family why oxygen is needed and how the device works. Use developmentally appropriate language. **Table P3-2** suggests methods to ease anxiety in the child who does not want to cooperate with oxygen delivery. For blow-by oxygen using a paper cup, punch a hole in the bottom of the cup and insert the tubing through the hole. Placing stickers on the cup or drawing smiley faces may decrease the child's anxiety.

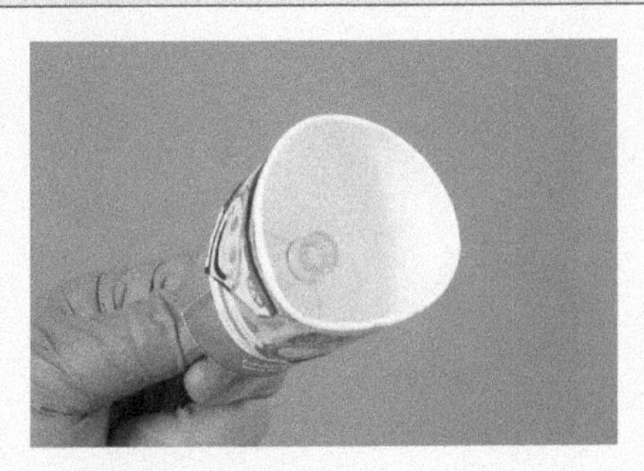

2. Allow the child to remain in a position of comfort, which may be sitting on the caregiver's lap. In the ambulance, the child must be safely restrained.

3a. To apply a mask, select the correct size. The mask should extend from the bridge of the nose to the cleft of the chin. Avoid placing pressure on the eyes.

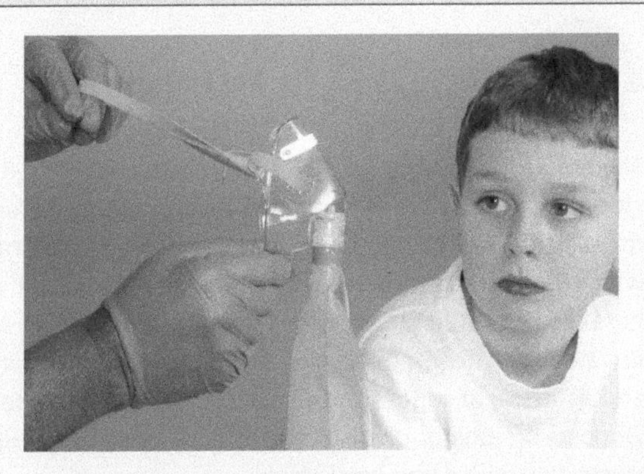

(continues)

Procedure 3-1 *(continued)*

3b Place the mask over the child's head, starting from the nose downward. Squeeze the nose clip and adjust the head strap.

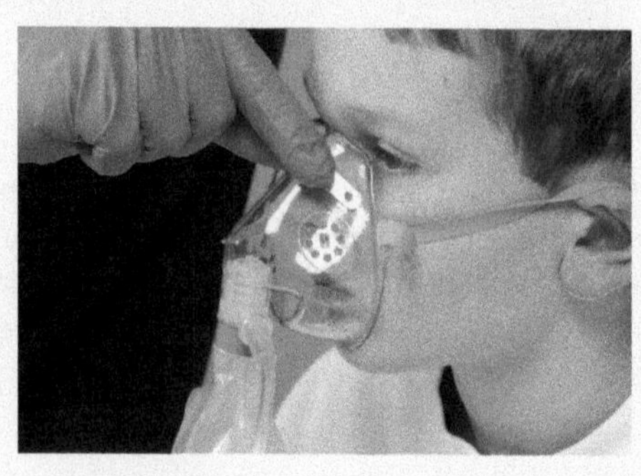

4 To apply a nasal cannula, curve the plastic prongs back into the nostrils. Loop the tubing around the ears.

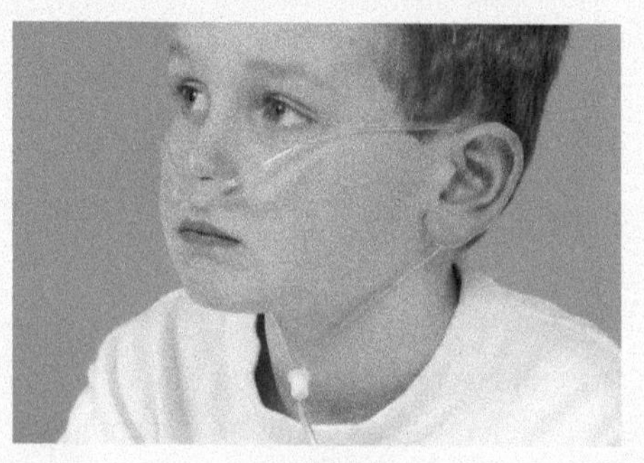

5 For blow-by oxygen, instruct the caregiver to hold the tubing or paper cup close to the child's face to maximize oxygen delivery.

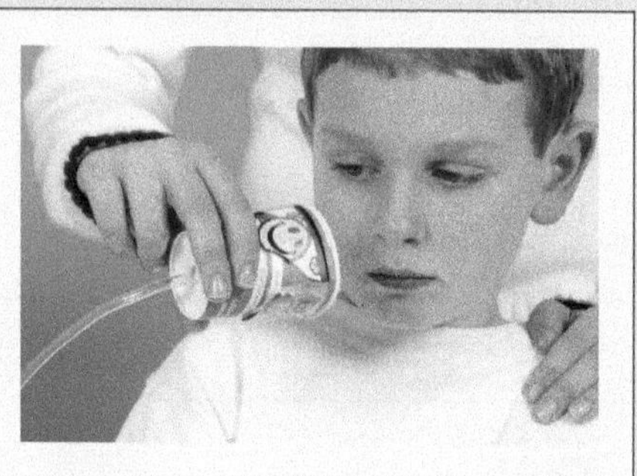

Table P3-2 Methods to Gain Child's Cooperation for Oxygen Delivery

Allow the child to hold the mask before placing it on his or her face.
Allow the child to feel the flow of oxygen before placing the mask on his or her face.
Describe the mask in appealing terms, such as a space mask or Santa Claus beard.
If the child struggles, consider using the blow-by technique to avoid agitation and increasing the oxygen demands. Placing stickers or drawing smiley faces on the cup may decrease the child's anxiety.

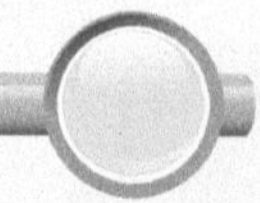

Controversy

The amount of oxygen to give routinely to children with chronic lung disease is unknown and probably differs for each individual. Administration of oxygen to patients with chronic lung disease who retain carbon dioxide at baseline can result in hypoventilation, but rarely does so in actual practice in pediatrics. If the child has a history and assessment suggesting acute hypoxia and increased work of breathing, give oxygen but be ready to assist ventilation with a bag-mask device.

Procedure 4: Suctioning

Introduction

Children of all ages are prone to airway obstruction from secretions, vomitus, pus, blood, edema, and foreign bodies. In newly borns, airway obstruction from amniotic fluid, meconium, and blood is a common and potentially critical problem that is usually treatable with suction alone. In infancy and childhood, conditions, such as closed head injury or status epilepticus, may cause the loss of airway protective reflexes, and put the child at risk for loss of airway patency from aspiration or airway obstruction. Children needing endotracheal intubation often have diseases or trauma associated with fluid in the endotracheal tube, airways, or air sacs; this fluid must be removed to ensure adequate oxygenation and ventilation. Children with tracheostomy tubes may get fluids or foreign bodies in the tubes, which must be evacuated.

Indications

All newly borns

Infants or children with fluids or foreign bodies in the nasopharynx or oropharynx

Intubated patients with fluids or secretions in the endotracheal tubes

Patients with tracheostomy tubes with fluids or mucus in the tubes

Contraindications

Children with severe airway obstruction and suspected airway foreign body, prior to seeing the airway with laryngoscopy

Minimize suctioning in intubated children with increased intracranial pressure and herniation

Equipment

Bulb syringes, one- and two-piece types

Endotracheal tube suction catheters, sizes 8 to 14 French

Feeding tubes, size 5 or 7 for small infants

Large-bore rigid suction catheter

Rationale

Suctioning is a basic technique to maintain an open airway. Children have tiny airways that are easily obstructed. The type of suction device and suctioning procedure to use depends on the child's age and clinical problem (**Table P4-1**). Bulb syringes remove thin secretions from newly borns or infants, but do not permit deep suctioning. When suctioning newborns, avoid suctioning vigorously or deeply. Deep suctioning can cause vagal stimulation, bradycardia, and laryngospasm in the newborn, particularly in the first hours during initial transition to extrauterine life. Brief, gentle suctioning with a bulb syringe (mouth, then nose) is usually adequate to remove secretions. Suction catheters remove thin secretions from the mouth, nose, or throat, and are useful in all age groups. Suction catheters are also necessary for endotracheal tube suctioning. Large-bore rigid suction catheters are useful in infants and children (not newly borns) to remove thick secretions, vomitus, pus, blood, or particulate matter from the mouth.

Table P4-1 Suction Technique Based on Age and Type of Obstructing Material

Newly borns	Bulb syringe or suction catheter
Infants and children with thin secretions	Bulb syringe or suction catheter
Newly borns, infants, and children with endotracheal tube	Suction catheter
Infants and children with thick secretions or particulate matter	Large-bore suction catheter

Preparation

1. Select an appropriate suction device based on clinical condition or type of obstruction and age. If there is no functioning negative pressure or suction source (vacuum outlet, battery-powered or electric portable suction, or hand-powered portable suction), use a bulb syringe for thin secretions.

2. Make sure the suction device is operational.
3. Determine correct catheter size with the pediatric length-based resuscitation tape. The suction catheter should be smaller than the nostril.
4. Open catheter package.
5. Connect suction tubing or rigid suction catheter to connecting tubing and suction source.
6. Set suction force (maximum, 120 mm Hg), being careful to avoid injuring sensitive tissues.
7. Maintain sterile technique.

Possible Complications

Injury to the mouth, nose, airway, or lung
Gagging, vomiting
Aspiration of stomach contents
Hypoxia from prolonged suctioning
Pushing foreign body into trachea with suction device
Increased intracranial pressure

Procedure 4-1

Oropharyngeal/Nasopharyngeal Suctioning with Bulb Syringe

1. Squeeze the bulb away from the infant to remove air. Suction the mouth, then the nose.

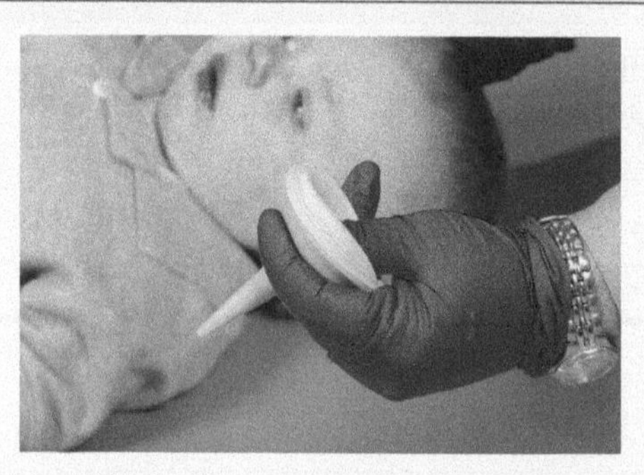

2. Open the mouth and insert the syringe tip at the side of the mouth, and then advance the syringe to remove thin secretions. Avoid inserting the syringe tip into the deeper soft tissues at the back of the mouth. Do not use a two-piece bulb syringe in the mouth because it may come apart.

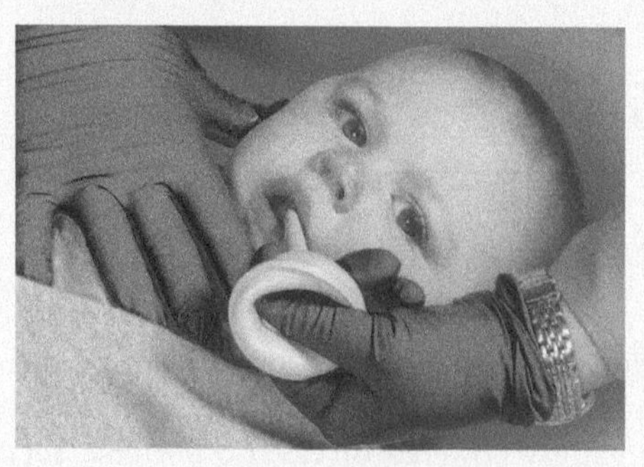

3. Lift the nostril slightly and suction the nose. Insert the syringe tip straight back into the nostril or at a right angle to the face.

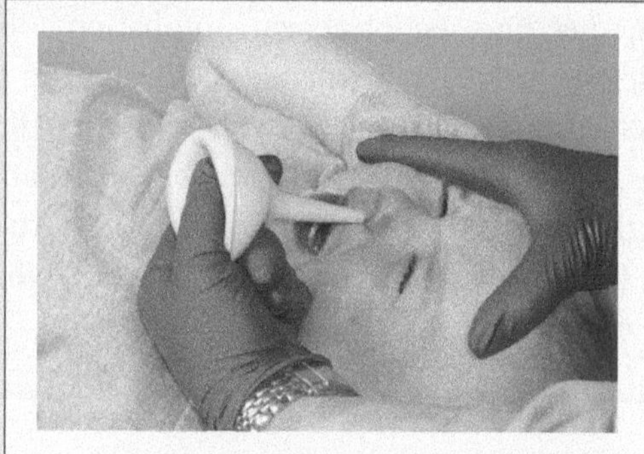

Procedure 4-2

Oropharyngeal/Nasopharyngeal Suctioning with Suction Catheter

1. Suction the mouth, then the nose. Open the mouth and advance until the tip touches secretions.

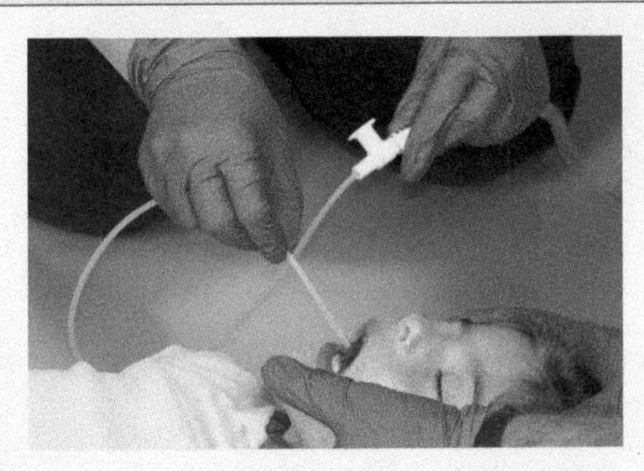

2. Block the side port and begin suctioning. Do not do deep suctioning beyond what is in direct vision. Remove catheter with twisting motion.

3. Insert the catheter into the nostril.

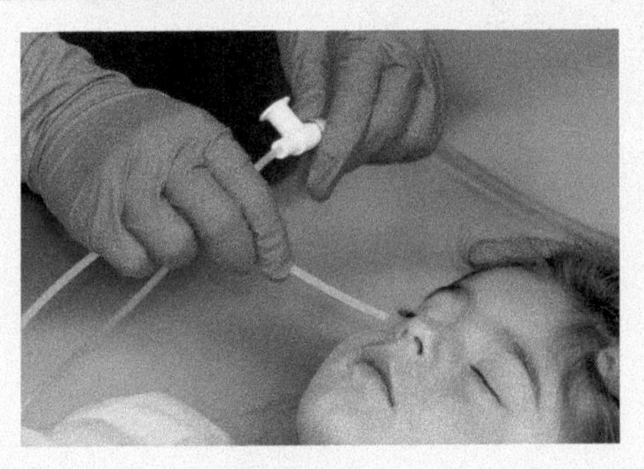

4. Block the side port to begin suctioning when the tip touches secretions. Remove the catheter with a twisting motion. Never suction longer than 5 seconds.

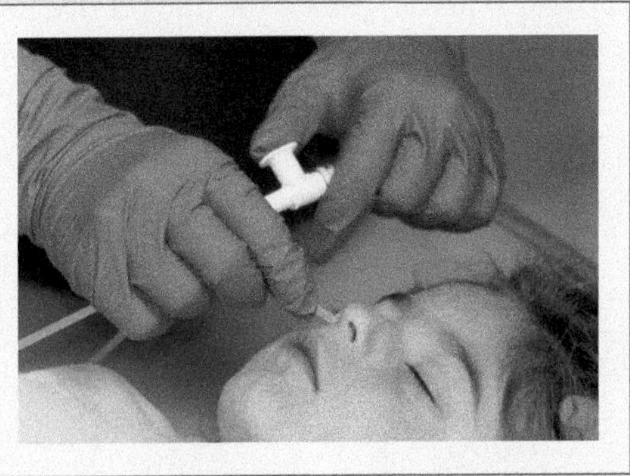

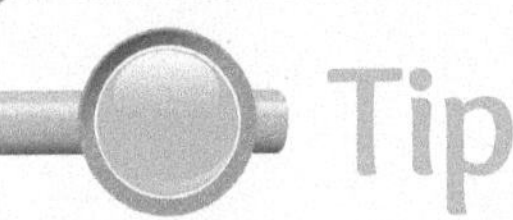

In suspected foreign body aspiration, look at the airway prior to suctioning.

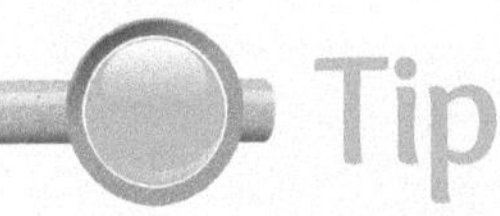

Suction for less than 5 seconds, but use enough time to remove secretions.

Procedure 4-3

Tracheal Tube Suctioning with Suction Catheter

1. Ask partner to preoxygenate the patient five to six times with a bag-mask device using 100% oxygen.

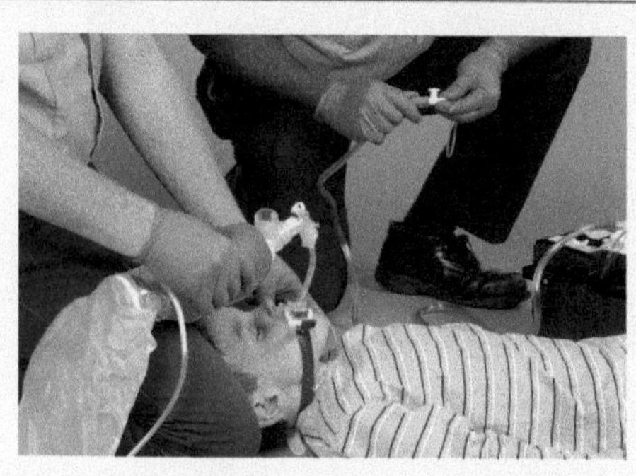

2. With thumb off the side port, insert suction catheter through endotracheal tube and down the trachea until resistance is met.

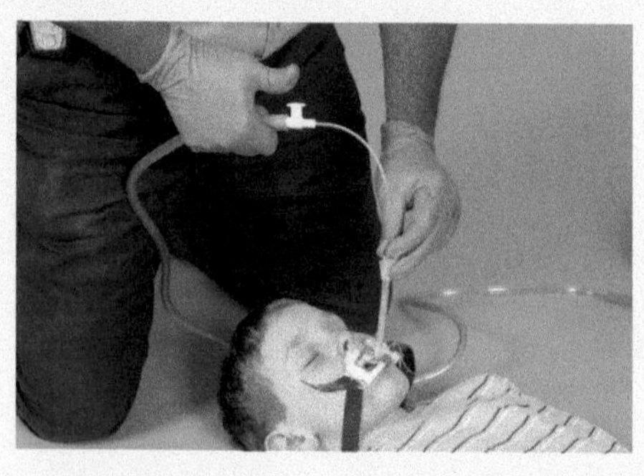

3. Apply suction off and on by placing thumb over the side port while withdrawing and twisting catheter (maximum, 5 seconds).

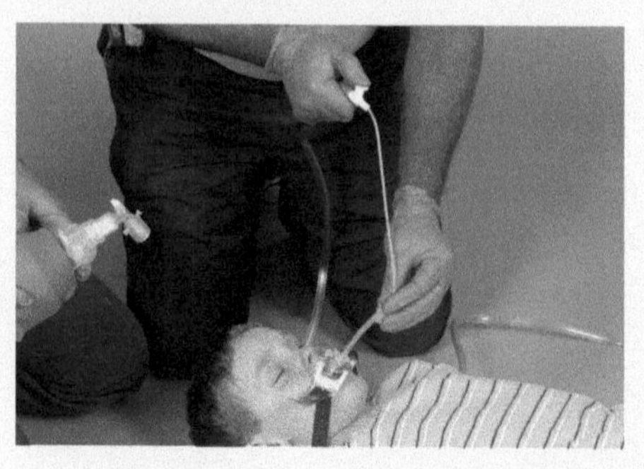

4. Irrigate catheter with normal saline.

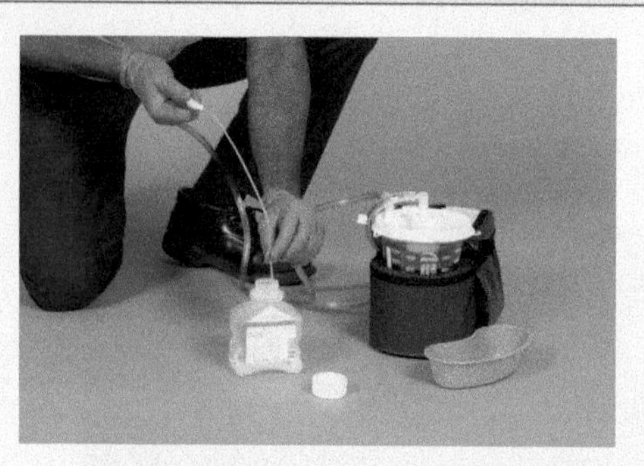

5. Ask partner to oxygenate five to six times. Repeat, as necessary.

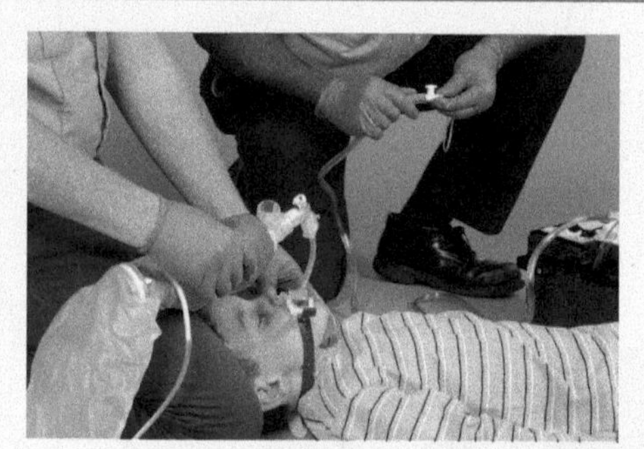

Procedure 4-4

Oropharyngeal Suctioning with Large-Bore Rigid Suction Catheter

1. Open the mouth and advance catheter until it touches secretions.

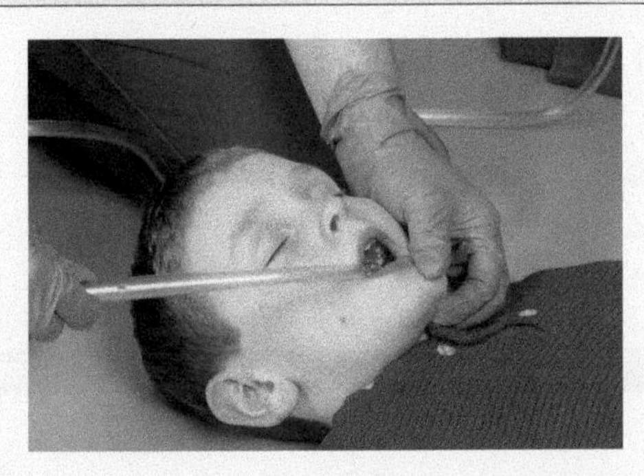

2. Close the side port or turn on suction to begin suctioning. Remove the catheter with a twisting motion. Do not suction more than 5 seconds.

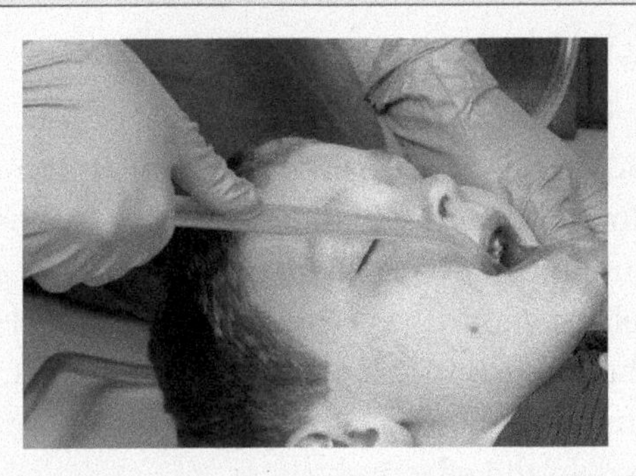

Reference

American Academy of Pediatrics, American Heart Association. *Textbook of Neonatal Resuscitation*. 6th ed. Elk Grove, IL: AAP; 2011.

Procedure 5: Airway Adjuncts

Introduction

An oropharyngeal (OP) or nasopharyngeal (NP) airway adjunct is often helpful to maintain an open airway for optimal ventilation. Sizing is important, because improperly sized OP or NP airways may cause further obstruction. The prehospital professional must know when to use an OP or NP airway adjunct, how to determine the proper size, and how to insert the adjunct safely and effectively.

Indications

Respiratory insufficiency

NP or OP airway obstruction

Seizures, including postictal state (NP airway)

Contraindications

OP airway

- Intact gag reflex
- Ingestion of a caustic or petroleum product

NP airway

- Complete nasal obstruction
- Possible basilar skull fracture
- Major nasofacial trauma

Equipment

NP airways

OP airways

Rationale

Opening the airway of a small infant or child by positioning alone, with the head-tilt/chin-lift maneuvers or jaw thrust, may not keep the tongue from obstructing the airway. Adequate ventilation often requires placement of airway adjuncts. They are easy to insert and may markedly improve airway patency. Adjuncts may immediately improve the efficacy of the child's spontaneous ventilation. In addition, they may allow more effective bag-mask ventilation, reduce gastric inflation, and avert the need for endotracheal intubation.

Preparation

1. Position patient's airway:

   Medical patient

   - Perform the head-tilt/chin-lift maneuver to open the airway. Avoid hyperextension of the neck because it may cause airway obstruction.
   - Use a towel under the shoulders of an infant or small child to get neutral airway position.

   Trauma patient

   - Use the modified jaw thrust maneuver with in-line spinal stabilization to open the airway.

2. Select the properly sized adjunct:

   OP airway

   - Use resuscitation tape or refer to resuscitation software (see Procedure 2) OR
   - Measure the device on the patient:
     - Place OP airway next to face with the flange at the level of the central incisors, and the bite block segment parallel to the hard palate.
     - The tip of the appropriate-sized OP airway should reach the angle of the jaw.

   NP airway

   - Use resuscitation tape or refer to resuscitation software (see Procedure 2) OR
   - Measure the device on the patient:
     - The outside diameter of the NP airway should be less than the diameter of the nostril.
     - Place the NP airway next to the face and measure from the tip of the nose to the tragus of the ear.
     - Adjust movable flange (if present) up or down to get appropriate length.

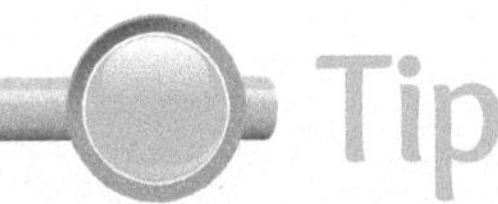

An NP airway is useful in maintaining an open airway during an active seizure.

Procedure 5-1

OP Airway Insertion

1. Depress tongue with a tongue blade (if available). Then insert oral airway with the tip down to avoid injury to the palate until the flange rests against lips.

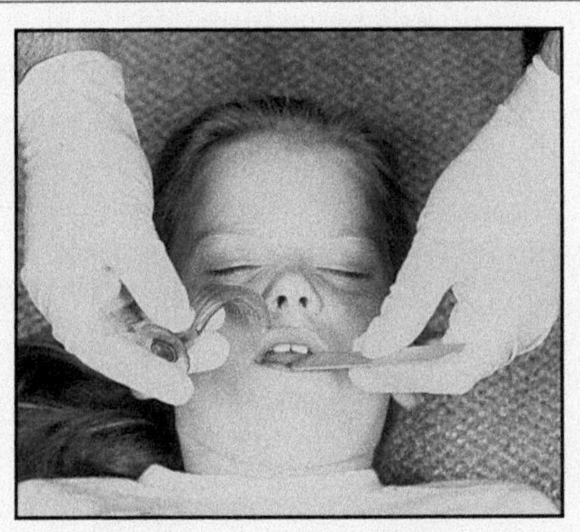

2. If a tongue blade is not available, insert the airway sideways, with the tip to the side. Then rotate down over the base of the tongue.

3. Insert OP airway until the flange is resting against the lips.

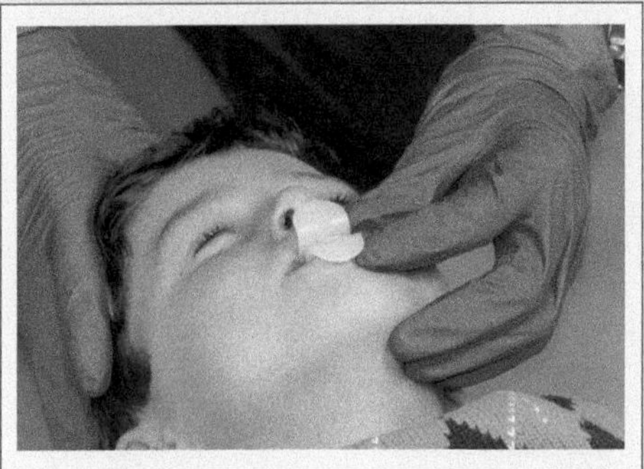

Procedure 5-2

NP Airway Insertion

1. Lubricate NP airway.

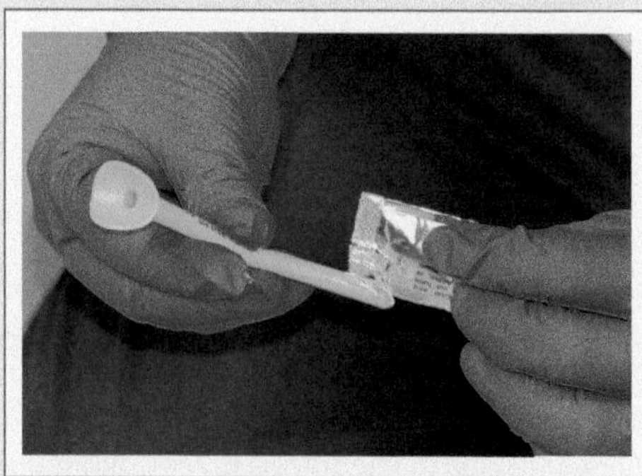

2. Insert with bevel toward septum (center of nose).

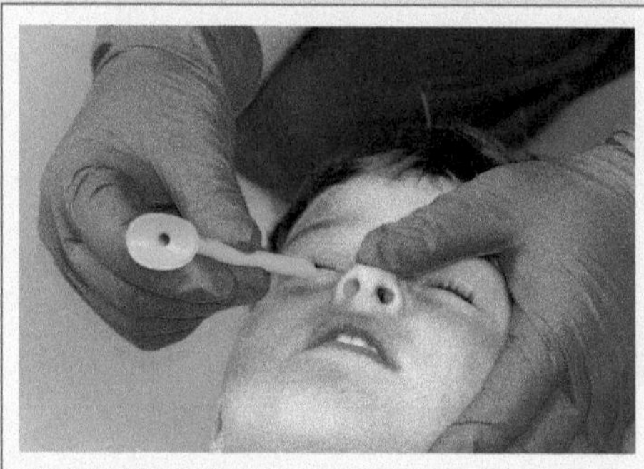

3. Advance tip along floor of nasal cavity.

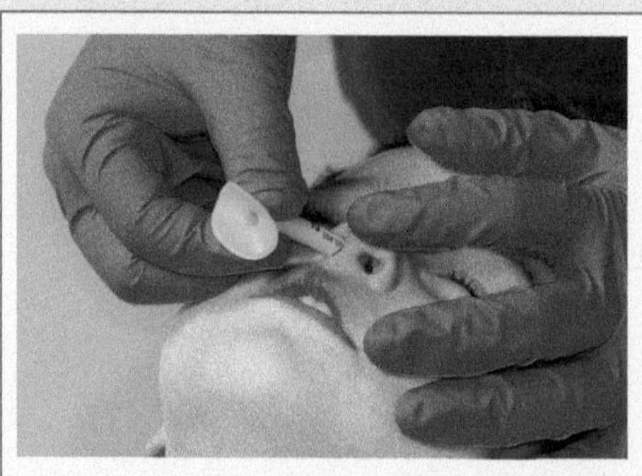

4. If using the right nostril, advance until flange is seated against outside of nostril. The tip should be in the nasopharynx.

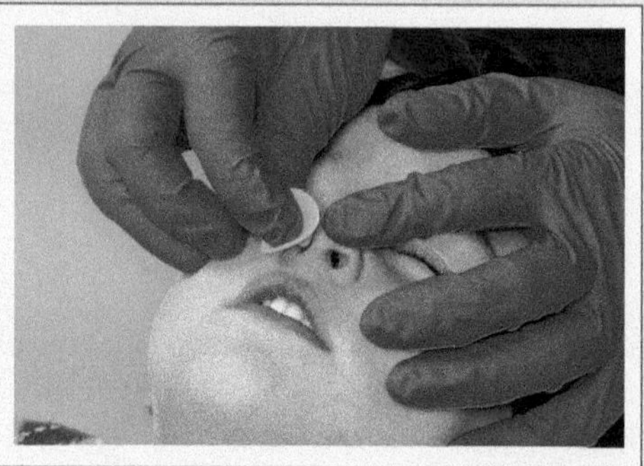

5. If using the left nostril, begin inserting the airway with the curvature upward until resistance is felt (about 2 cm), and then rotate the device 180 degrees and advance until flange is against outside of nostril.

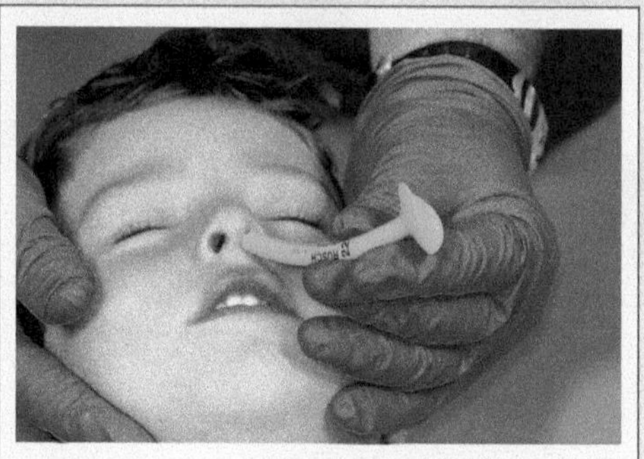

Possible Complications

OP Airway

If OP airway is too small, the tongue may get pushed back into the pharynx, obstructing the airway

If OP airway is too large, it may obstruct the larynx

Pharyngeal bleeding

Laryngospasm

Vomiting

NP Airway

Adenoidal tissue laceration

Pharyngeal bleeding

Obstruction of tube with fluids or soft tissues, causing airway obstruction

If an NP airway is too long, vagal stimulation or esophageal entry with gastric distention may occur

Laryngospasm

Vomiting

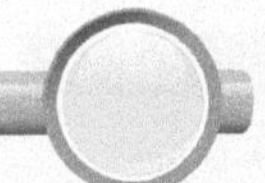

Controversy

The use of airway adjuncts in facial trauma is controversial. If the child has an open fracture of the craniofacial bones, the device could penetrate into the brain and cause further brain injury or hemorrhage. The devices must be used cautiously or not at all in the setting of suspected facial bone injury.

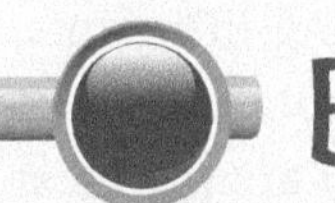

Blip

Do not insert an OP airway that is too small, or it will push the tongue back and obstruct the airway.

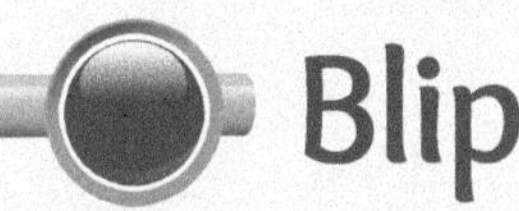

Blip

Never attempt to insert an OP airway in a conscious child.

Procedure 6: Foreign Body Obstruction

Introduction

Indications
Severe airway obstruction
Severe partial airway obstruction and respiratory failure

Contraindication
Partial airway obstruction with maintenance of the airway

Equipment
Laryngoscope and straight blades (Miller sizes 1 and 2)
Pediatric Magill forceps
Bag-mask devices (infant and pediatric)

Foreign body obstruction of the airway is an uncommon cause of hypoxic brain injury and death in toddlers and preschool children, who place objects in their mouths as part of the exploratory behavior normal for patients in these age groups. Liquids are the most common cause of choking in infants, whereas balloons, small objects, and food (e.g., hot dogs, round candies, nuts, and grapes) are the most common causes of foreign body airway obstruction (FBAO) in children. The infant or child with a completely obstructed airway poses the ultimate medical challenge because a moment's delay can result in permanent disability or be fatal. When treating a patient with foreign body obstruction, it is important to begin with basic maneuvers to clear the airway, but sometimes more advanced techniques are necessary.

Rationale

In the setting of severe airway obstruction, prehospital professionals can make the difference between life and death. Immediate removal of an airway foreign body can often be achieved using basic life support (BLS) procedures, yet every year many children suffer grave injury and death because of failure to use basic clearance maneuvers. Sometimes, the foreign body is deeper in the airway or embedded in tissue, so that basic maneuvers are unsuccessful. In such cases, using Magill forceps and direct laryngoscopy may be the best option for removal.

Preparation

1. Attempt BLS maneuvers first (see Procedure 6-1).
2. Move to advanced life support (ALS) maneuvers if BLS maneuvers fail.
3. Attach appropriately sized straight blade to laryngoscope handle.
4. Ensure light is working on laryngoscope blade.

Possible Complications

Hypoxia

Foreign body is pushed farther into airway

Laryngeal and tracheal injury

Teeth and mouth injury

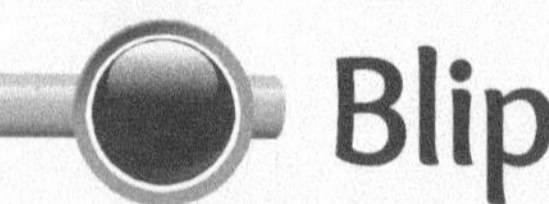

Do not perform blind finger sweeps, which may push the foreign body further into the airway.

Procedure 6-1

BLS Maneuvers

1. If FBAO is mild, do not interfere. Allow the victim to clear the airway by coughing while you observe for signs of severe FBAO.
2. If the FBAO is severe (i.e., the victim is unable to make a sound), you must act to relieve the obstruction.
3. For a child, perform subdiaphragmatic abdominal thrusts (Heimlich maneuver) until the object is expelled or the victim becomes unresponsive.

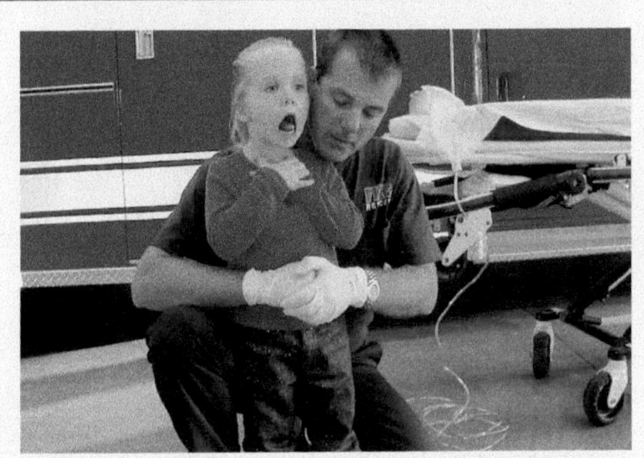

4. For an infant, deliver repeated cycles of five back blows (slaps) followed by five chest compressions until the object is expelled or the victim becomes unresponsive. Abdominal thrusts are not recommended for infants because they may damage the infant's relatively large and unprotected liver.

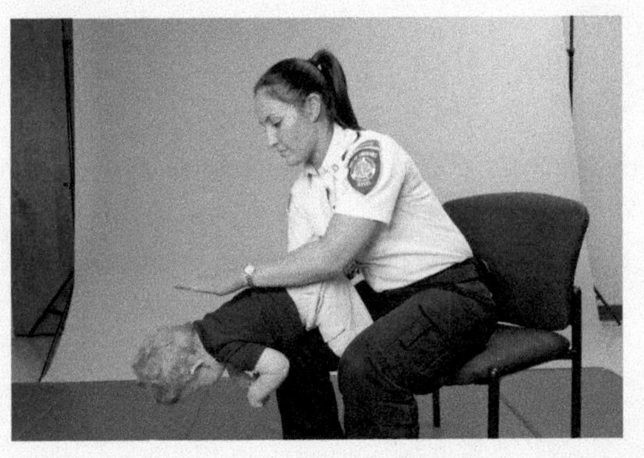

5. If the victim becomes unresponsive, start CPR with chest compressions (do not perform a pulse check).

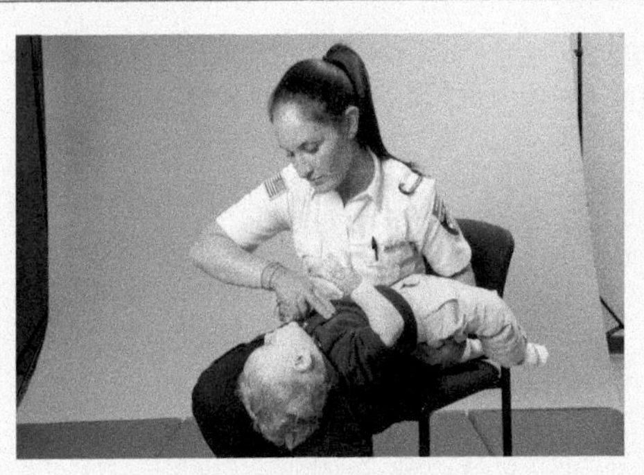

6. After 30 chest compressions, open the airway. If you see a foreign body, remove it but do not perform blind finger sweeps, because they may push the obstructed object farther into the pharynx and may damage the oropharynx. Attempt to give two breaths and continue with cycles of chest compressions and ventilations until the object is expelled.

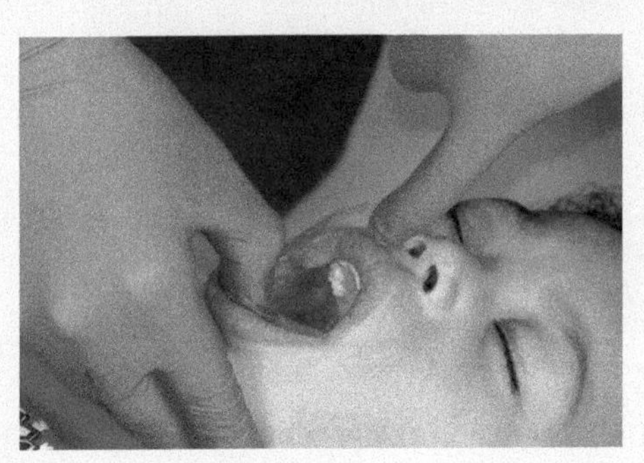

Procedure 6-2

Laryngoscopy and Magill Forceps

1. Grasp laryngoscope handle in the left hand. Use trigger-finger technique.

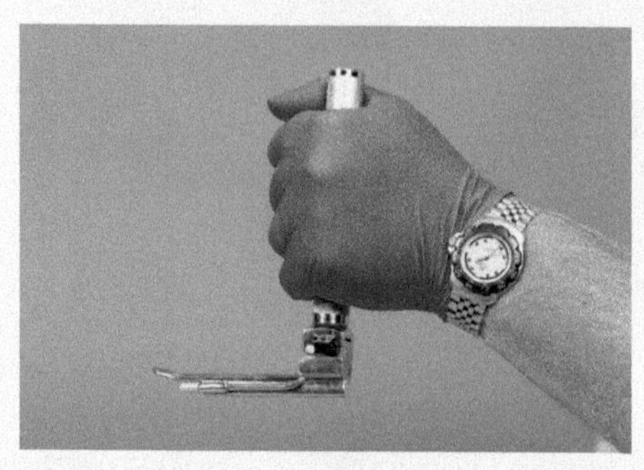

2. Open mouth by using thumb pressure on chin. Insert pediatric straight laryngoscope blade into mouth.

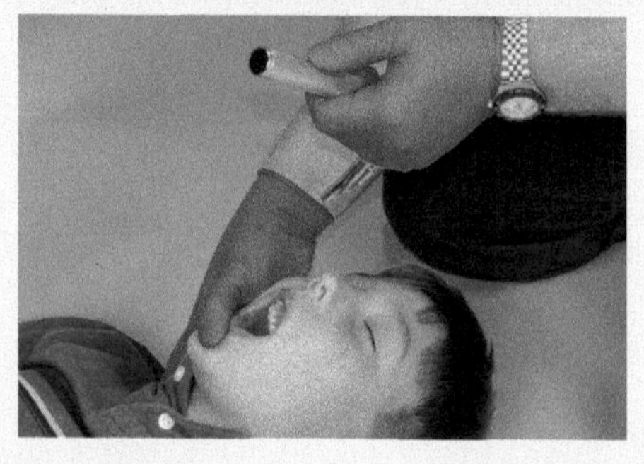

3. Lift tongue with blade. Exert gentle traction upward along the axis of the laryngoscope handle at a 45-degree angle. Do not use teeth or gums for leverage. Advance blade. Watch the tip until foreign body is visible. Do not go past vocal cords. Use suction to improve visibility and maintain airway.

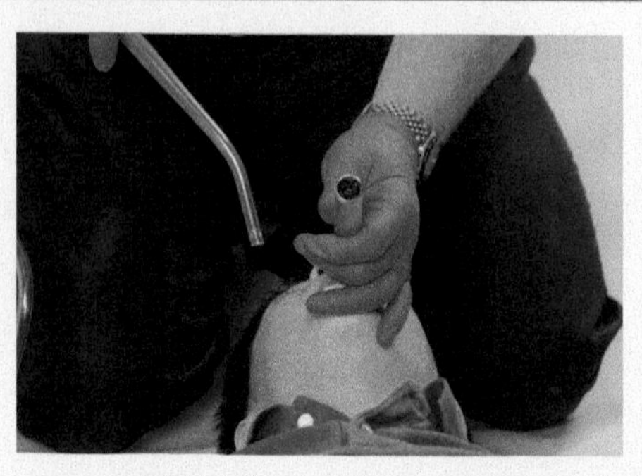

4. Grasp closed Magill forceps in right hand, palm down. Insert Magill forceps into mouth, tips closed. Open forceps and move tips around foreign body. Grasp foreign body and remove while looking directly at it. Look at the airway and make sure it is clear of foreign bodies or debris. Remove laryngoscope blade. After removal of foreign body, reassess respiratory status. Use suction if needed. Attempt to ventilate if the child does not breathe spontaneously. Return to BLS maneuvers if no foreign body is seen by direct laryngoscopy.

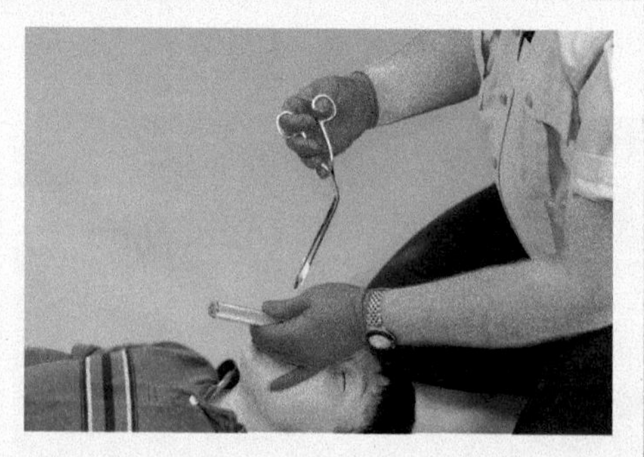

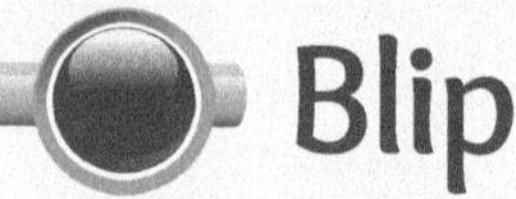

Blip

Suctioning may push the foreign body farther into the airway, so look at the airway before suctioning.

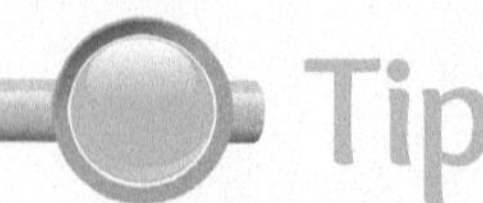

Tip

Repeat BLS procedures if no foreign body is seen by direct laryngoscopy.

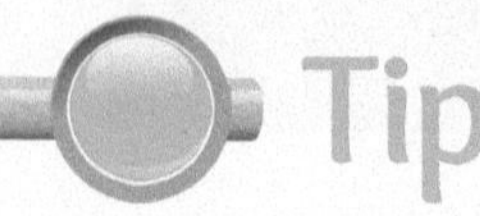

Tip

Attempt BLS maneuvers before using Magill forceps.

Reference

Berg MD, Schexnayder SM, Chameides L, et al. Part 13: Pediatric basic life support: 2010 American Heart Association Guidelines for Cardiopulmonary Resuscitation and Emergency Cardiovascular Care. *Circulation*. 2010; 122(suppl 3): S862–S875.

Procedure 7: Bronchodilator Therapy

Introduction

Wheezing from bronchospasm is one of the most common out-of-hospital pediatric problems. Children who are wheezing are usually in acute respiratory distress and are often anxious, agitated, and uncooperative. The prehospital professional must use a developmentally appropriate approach with the child and the caregiver when giving general noninvasive respiratory care and using a bronchodilator with or without anticholinergic medication. The caregiver can help by holding, soothing, and supporting a scared child. One way to give aerosolized bronchodilators is with an oxygen-powered nebulizer. Another way is the metered dose inhaler (MDI; in children via a spacer), although this inhalation technique has not been studied in the out-of-hospital setting. If the child is uncooperative or unable to use inhaled bronchodilator therapy, or intramuscular (IM) drug delivery is another possibility.

Indication

Wheezing

Contraindication

Known sensitivity to bronchodilator drugs

Equipment

Inhalation therapy (nebulizer)

- An oxygen-powered nebulizer that aerosolizes the liquid bronchodilator to small particle size that can reach the bronchioles
- Oxygen source
- Mask or mouthpiece with liquid reservoir
- *Bronchodilator*
  - **Albuterol** solution (1.25 mg/3 mL, and 2.5 mg/3 mL, prediluted solutions for nebulization and 5 mg/mL solution for nebulization [dilution required]).
- *Anticholinergic*
  - **Ipratropium** solution 0.02% (500 mcg/2.5 mL)

Inhalation therapy (MDI)

- MDI, mask, and spacer
- *Bronchodilator*
  - Albuterol MDI (90 mcg/puff)
- *Anticholinergic*
  - Ipratropium (MDI) (17 mcg/puff)

IM therapy

- Tuberculin (TB) or 3-mL syringe
- 22- to 27-gauge needle
- *Bronchodilator*
  - **Epinephrine** 1 mg/mL concentration

Rationale

For asthma, early bronchodilator therapy, on the scene and on the way to the emergency department (ED), helps immediately open airways, relieve respiratory distress, and improve oxygen delivery. Early bronchodilator therapy may reduce the need for more aggressive hospital therapy, shorten ED and hospital times, and decrease chances of complications or death. The addition of anticholinergic medication may also be beneficial. *Continuous inhalation treatment with a nebulized beta agonist is the best initial approach with severe wheezing and respiratory distress.*

Preparation

Inhalation Therapy

1. Have the caregiver hold the child on his or her lap. An older child can sit alone.
2. Have the child in an upright position of comfort.
3. Explain what is happening. Most children need only inhalation bronchodilator therapy by oxygen-powered nebulizer or with an MDI and spacer.

Intramuscular Therapy

1. Position the child on the caregiver's lap or straddling the caregiver's leg.
2. Expose the thigh or deltoid area for injection (see Procedure 14, Intramuscular Injections).

Possible Complications of Albuterol and/or Ipratropium

Anxiety	Nausea
Chest pain	Nasal stuffiness
Cough	Palpitations
Dizziness	Restlessness
Dry mouth	Tachycardia
Dysrhythmias	Tremors
Headache	Vomiting
Hypertension	

Procedure 7-1

Inhalation Therapy

1. If the child can cooperate, deliver nebulized bronchodilator, with or without anticholinergic medication, through a mouthpiece or mask. The caregiver can hold the mask to the child's face, if necessary.

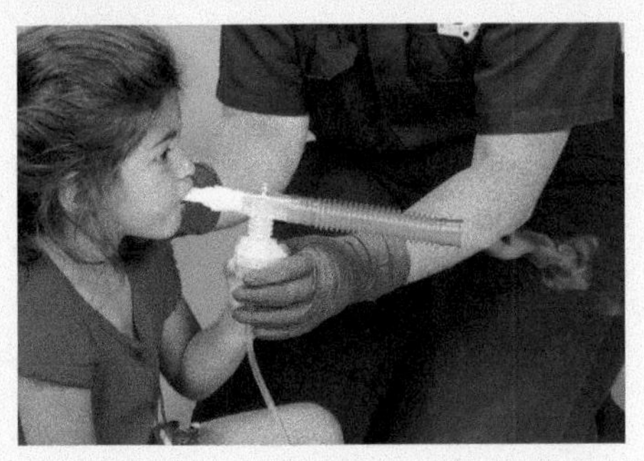

2. If an MDI is used, attach spacer and mask when the child is too young or unable to trigger aerosol effectively.

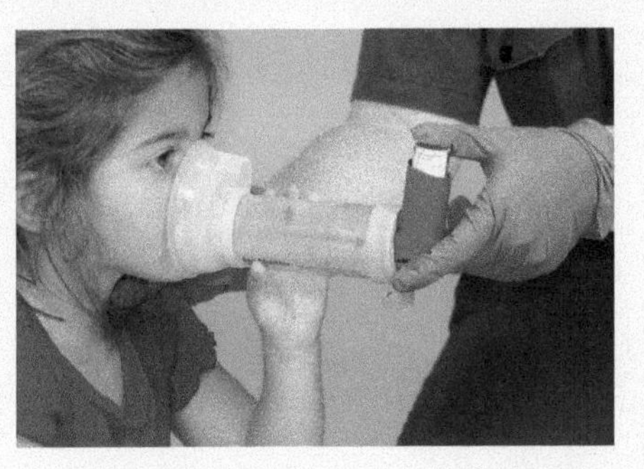

3. Monitor respiratory rate, heart rate, and pulse oximetry during therapy.

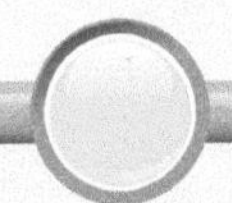

Controversy

The role of the MDI in out-of-hospital bronchodilator therapy is not known. Although ED studies have shown that the MDI is as effective as inhaled drugs for most children, it has not been studied in the out-of-hospital setting. MDI with mask and spacer, however, can probably deliver an adequate bronchodilator dose to most children.

Procedure 7-2

Intramuscular Therapy

1. If the child is in significant respiratory distress or if the child cannot cooperate with inhalation therapy, give epinephrine by IM injection. Use one of two anatomic locations: lateral aspect of deltoid in upper arms (older child) or anterolateral thigh.
2. Inject the medication into the IM area.

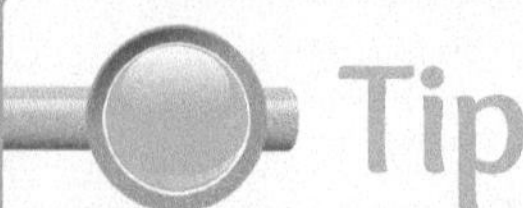

Avoid injectable drugs in cooperative, wheezing patients. The procedure is painful and is no more effective than inhaled bronchodilators.

Procedure 8: Bag-Mask Ventilation

Introduction

Bag-mask ventilation is a highly effective way to deliver assisted ventilation to a child in respiratory failure. Oxygen at 60%–95% concentration can be given safely by choosing a well-fitted mask, connecting the oxygen reservoir to a supplemental oxygen source at 15 L/min, disabling the pop-off valve, and ventilating at an age-appropriate rate.

Indication

Apnea or respiratory arrest

Respiratory failure

Cyanosis despite supplemental oxygen*

Consider when oxygen saturation (SaO_2) less than 90% despite administration of 100% oxygen by nonrebreathing mask

Equipment

Transparent masks with soft rim, sizes neonate through adult

Self-inflating resuscitator (bag), at least 450 mL volume

*N.B. children with uncorrected cyanotic heart disease may have low oxygen saturations at baseline.

Rationale

Assisted ventilation is a way to oxygenate and ventilate a child who is unable to breathe adequately on his or her own. Although the technique does not provide the definitive airway control that endotracheal intubation does, in many cases bag-mask ventilation will be the best technique for assisting ventilation during resuscitation and transport. Effective bag-mask ventilation is one of the prehospital professional's most useful skills in pediatric out-of-hospital care.

Preparation

1. Measure the mask on the patient. The mask should extend from the bridge of the nose to the cleft of the chin, avoiding compression of the eyes. The right sized mask will have a small volume to minimize dead space and to prevent rebreathing of expired carbon dioxide. Transparency allows the rescuer to observe the child for cyanosis of the lips and for emesis.
2. Select an appropriate resuscitator bag. Although a small child can be safely and effectively ventilated using a big bag, a small bag will not work for a large child. Pediatric tidal volume is approximately 8 mL/kg. The bag should have a volume of 450–750 mL. An adult bag is acceptable for larger children or adolescents.
3. If a pop-off valve is present, it may need to be disabled to permit higher inspiratory pressures and achieve chest rise.
4. Connect one end of oxygen tubing to the resuscitator bag and the other end to the flow meter, set to 15 L/min.

Possible Complications

Hypoxia

Barotrauma

Gastric distention

Emesis and aspiration

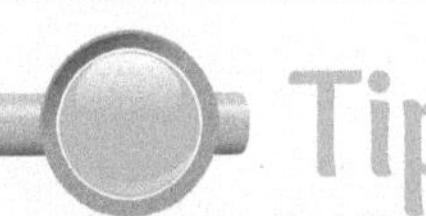

Tip

In children with pending respiratory failure due to an obstructive process (i.e., status asthmaticus), listening for the end of expiration may minimize risk of barotrauma.

Procedure 8-1

Bag-Mask Ventilation

1. Open airway. *Medical patient*: Use head-tilt/chin-lift maneuver. *Trauma patient*: Use jaw thrust with in-line manual stabilization.

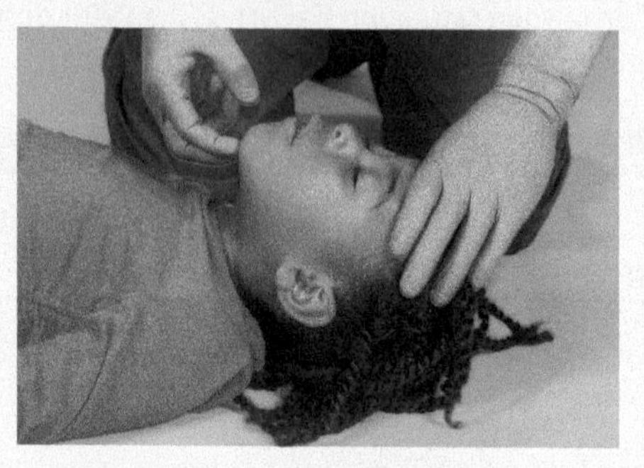

2. Ensure neutral positioning (sniffing position). Because infants and toddlers have large heads, place a small roll under the shoulders to achieve the sniffing position. Avoid hyperextension of the neck because this may cause airway obstruction or spinal injury.

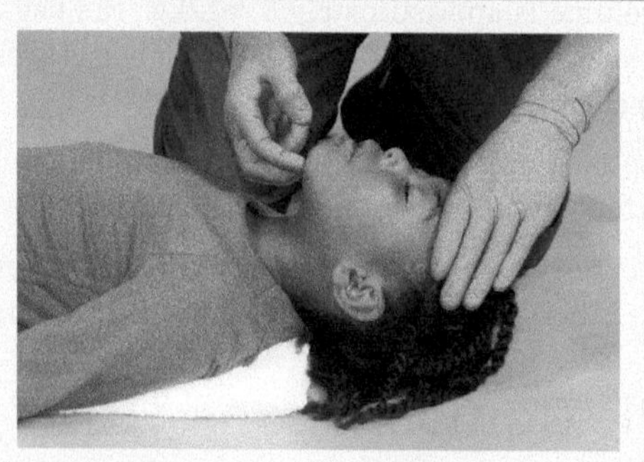

3. Insert appropriate airway adjunct if airway patency cannot be maintained with the head-tilt/chin-lift or jaw thrust maneuvers (see Procedure 5, Airway Adjuncts). Use an oropharyngeal (OP) airway if the patient does not have a gag reflex, or use a nasopharyngeal (NP) airway if the patient has an active gag reflex.

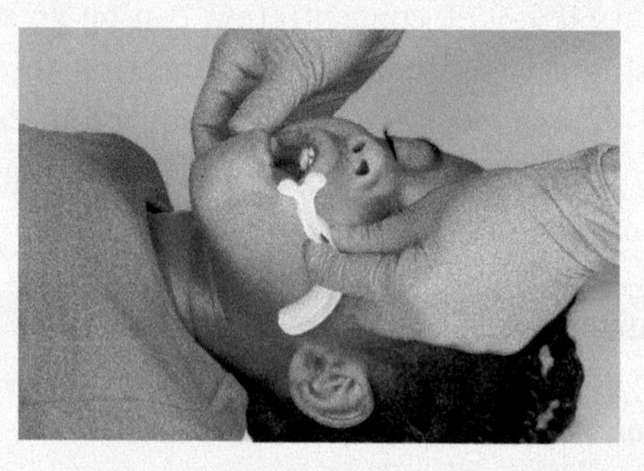

4. Begin ventilation.

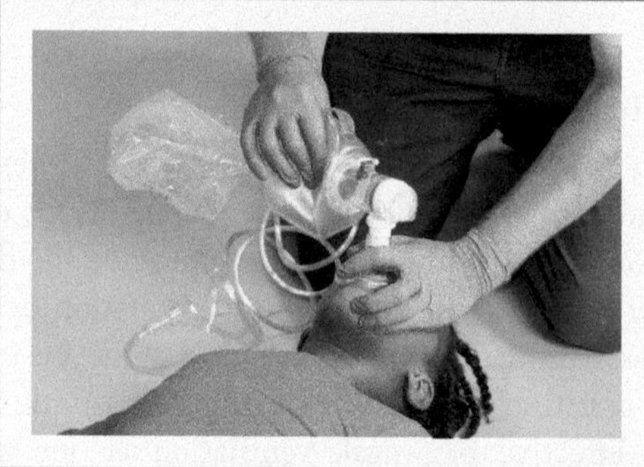

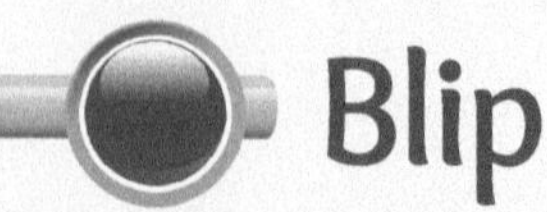

Avoid hyperextension of the neck, which may cause airway obstruction or spinal injury.

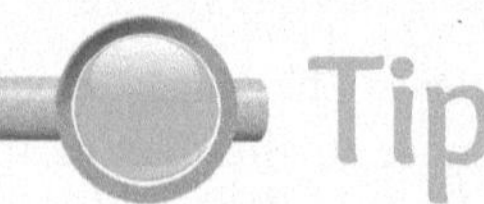

In children with pending respiratory failure due to an obstructive process (i.e., status asthmaticus), listening for the end of expiration may minimize risk of barotrauma.

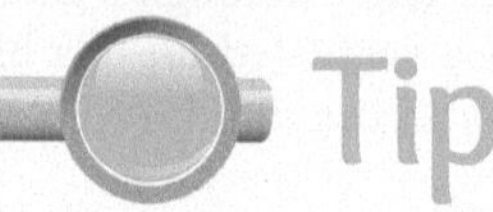

Use an OP or NP airway with the bag-mask device if airway patency cannot be maintained with the head-tilt/chin-lift or jaw thrust maneuvers.

Procedure 8-2

Bag-Mask Ventilation Using One-Rescuer Technique

1. Apply the mask to the face and get an airtight seal by placing the thumb and index finger on the mask, and place the third, fourth, and fifth fingers on the bony portion of the jaw (mandible). This is called the E-C clamp technique.

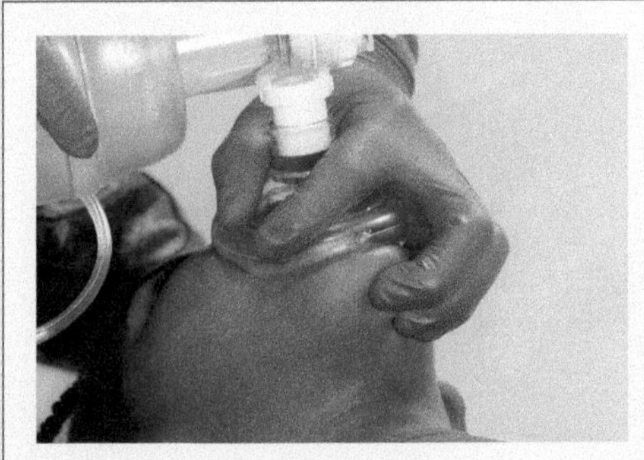

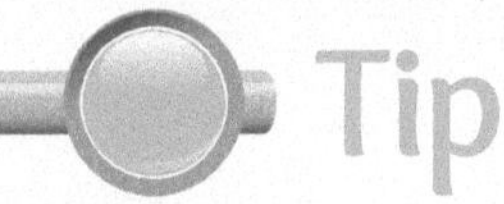

Pull the jaw into the mask, instead of pushing the mask into the face.

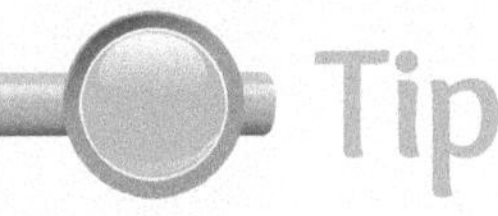

Seeing the chest rise is the best indicator of adequate tidal volume.

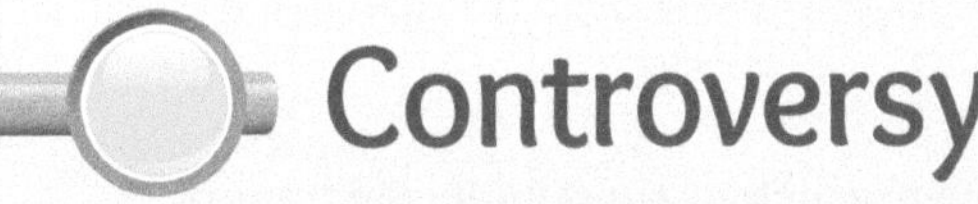

Few studies have assessed the relative value of BMV versus endotracheal intubation in the out-of-hospital setting. Gausche Hill et al demonstrated no significant benefit from endotracheal intubation compared to BMV in children.

2. Pull the child's jaw into the mask, instead of pushing the mask into the face, to establish a seal. Failure to provide a tight seal may result in delivery of lower oxygen concentrations or an inadequate volume of air. Avoid placing pressure on soft tissues under the chin because this may compress the airway. Squeeze the bag with the dominant hand, watching for chest rise. Squeeze the bag only until the chest rise is visible, then release. Say, "Squeeze, release, release" during ventilation to achieve the correct inspiratory volume and to allow for expiration.
Child and infant: 12–20 squeezes/minute.
Adult: 12–16 squeezes/minute.
3. Assess effectiveness of ventilation. Look for adequate bilateral rise and fall of chest. Auscultate for lung sounds at the midaxillary line bilaterally. Monitor oxygen saturation.

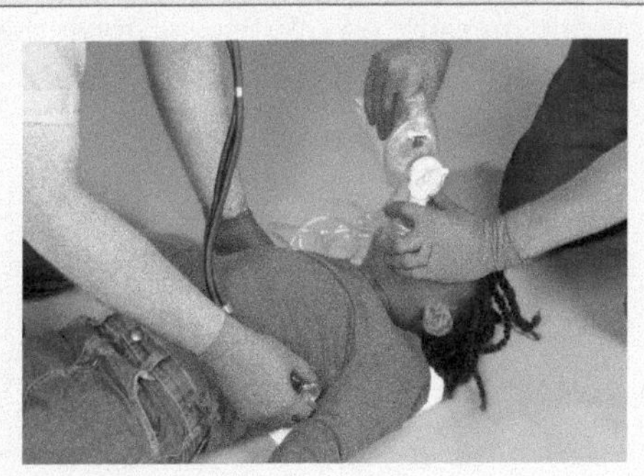

Procedure 8-3

Bag-Mask Ventilation Using Two-Rescuer Technique

The two-rescuer technique is preferable in trauma patients or if the one-rescuer technique does not create an effective seal.

1. Rescuer applies the mask to the face and maintains a seal. *Medical patient*: Hold the mask to the face with the thumb and index fingers of both hands; use the other fingers to perform a chin lift (bilateral E-C clamp technique). *Trauma patient*: Perform a jaw thrust maneuver, lifting the jaw into the mask with both hands, while maintaining in-line manual stabilization.

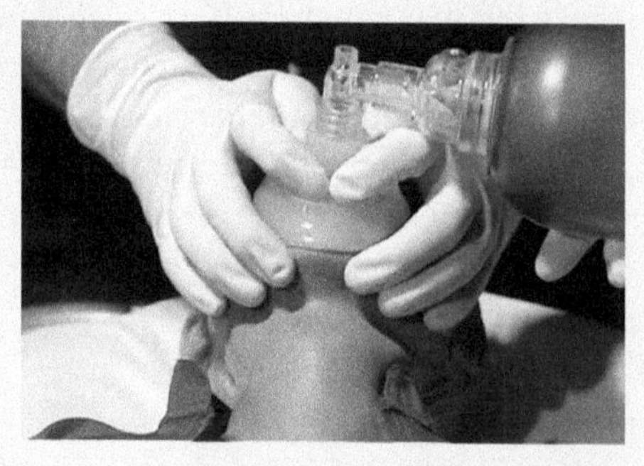

2. Pull the child's jaw into the mask, instead of pushing the mask into the face, to establish a seal. Avoid placing pressure on soft tissues under the chin because this may compress the airway.

3. Second rescuer ventilates. Avoid gastric distention. Watch the abdomen for signs of enlargement during ventilation. If this happens, reposition the airway and observe the chest rise carefully, squeezing the bag only until the chest starts to rise. If bag-mask ventilation is to be considered during transport, consider placement of an orogastric or nasogastric tube for gastric decompression.

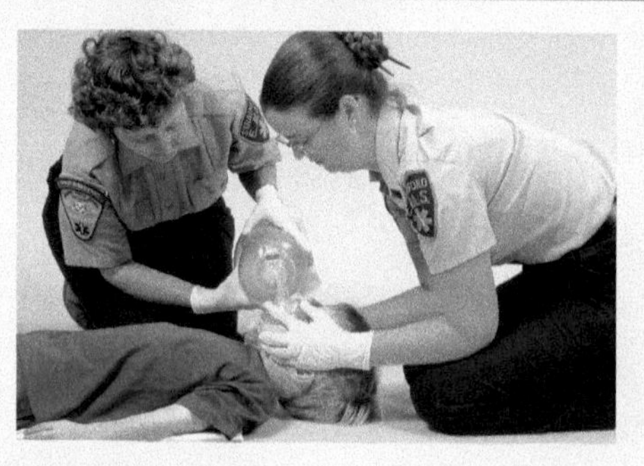

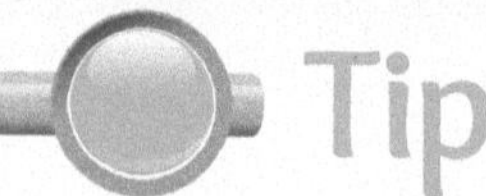

Tip

The two-rescuer technique is preferable in a trauma patient or if the one-rescuer technique does not get a good seal.

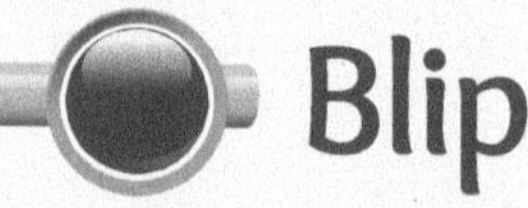

Blip

A bag less than 450 mL will not generate enough inspiratory pressure to ventilate a large child.

Procedure 9: Pulse Oximetry

Introduction

Pulse oximetry, which measures oxygenation and pulse rate, can be a useful adjunct in the management of the ill or injured child. Use of the pulse oximeter does not replace clinical assessment of the child. Monitoring changes in pulse oximetry readings may help the prehospital professional to determine the patient's response to interventions and guide additional interventions.

However, there are caveats. If the child is in shock, inadequate circulating red blood cells may have such low flow states that the pulse oximeter probe will be unable to sense flow, resulting in an inability to obtain a reading or waveform. Where there is suspected carbon monoxide (CO) poisoning, do not rely on pulse oximetry. The probe detects gaseous saturation of the hemoglobin molecule and does not discriminate between oxygen and CO. A child with CO poisoning may have a pulse oximetry reading of 100% and be hypoxic.

Indications

Hypoxia

Need for oxygen therapy

Respiratory distress

Major trauma or other clinical conditions with the potential for hypoxia

Equipment

Pulse oximeter probes in sizes for newborns, infants, and children

Monitoring cable and pulse oximetry monitoring device

Preparation

1. Prepare the child for application of the pulse oximeter probe. This may be explained as being similar to putting on a band-aid.

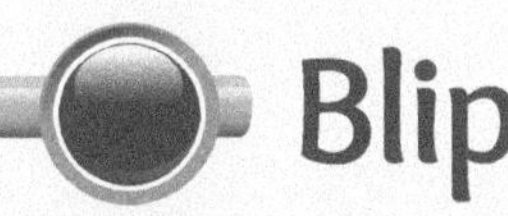

Blip

Do not rely on pulse oximetry in carbon monoxide poisoning.

Possible Complications

Using incorrect probe placement

Poor perfusion with poor tracing or waveform

Inability to obtain a SpO_2 reading

Causes of Inability to Obtain a Reading or Waveform

- Using incorrect probe placement
- Poor perfusion with poor tracing or waveform

Procedure 9-1

Pulse Oximetry

1. **Obtain equipment in the appropriate size. Place probe on a fingertip, toe, earlobe, or wrist as indicated on the manufacturer's instructions.**

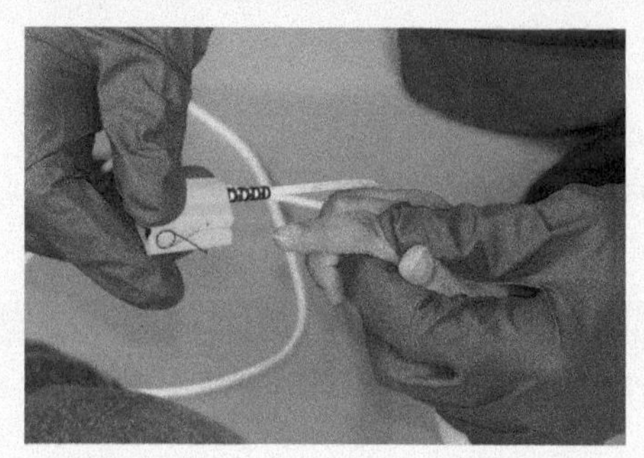

2. **Connect the probe to the monitoring cable. Some portable monitoring devices have a reusable probe that has a spring-loaded clip for use only on a fingertip or toe. Note oxygen saturation (SpO_2) and document. If the monitoring device being used shows a waveform, observe for correlation with heart rate.**

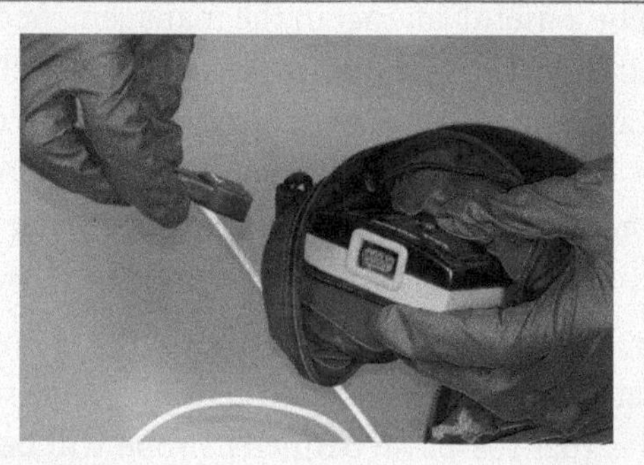

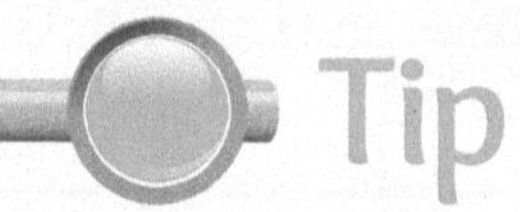

Tip

Use pulse oximetry in the primary assessment of every acutely ill or injured child.

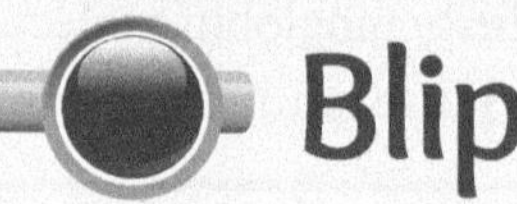

Blip

Even when the pulse oximetry is normal, if there is increased work of breathing or significantly increased respiratory rate, the child may need additional therapy.

Procedure 10: Orogastric and Nasogastric Tube Insertion

Introduction

Gastric tube insertion has many purposes, but in the out-of-hospital setting, gastric tube insertion has only one indication: decompression of the stomach during assisted ventilation. The tube may be placed into the stomach through the nose (nasogastric [NG] insertion) or through the mouth (orogastric [OG] insertion).

Indication

Abdominal distention associated with assisted ventilation

Contraindications

NG and OG insertion

Unconscious child with poor or no gag reflex and unsecured airway: In this case, do endotracheal intubation first to decrease risk of vomiting and aspiration

Caustic ingestions: In a child who has ingested a caustic substance, there is a risk of esophageal damage with passage of the tube.

NG insertion

Perform OG insertion to avoid intracranial passage of the NG tube when the child has any of the following findings: Severe head or facial trauma, especially with midfacial injuries, nasal bleeding, or clear nasal secretions.

Infants with nostrils too small to accommodate the tube: OG insertion is preferred for infants younger than 6 months of age.

Equipment

Gastric tube (a double-lumen sump tube is the best device for removing stomach contents)

30- to 60-mL syringe with funnel-tipped adaptor for manual removal of stomach contents through tube

Mechanical suction

Adhesive tape

Nonpetroleum lubricant

Rationale

During assisted ventilation, it is common to inflate the stomach as well as the lungs with air. Gastric inflation with air slows downward movement of the diaphragm and decreases tidal volume, making ventilation more difficult and necessitating higher inspiratory pressures. In addition, inflation of the stomach with air increases the risk that the patient will vomit and aspirate. Gastric tube insertion with a NG or OG tube decompresses the stomach and makes assisted ventilation easier.

Preparation

1. Select the proper size tube. Sizing techniques are outlined in **Table P10-1**.
2. Measure the tube on the patient. The length of the tube should be the same as the distance from the lips or tip of the nose (depending on if the route OG or NG is used) to the left ear PLUS the distance from the left ear to the left upper quadrant of the abdomen, just below the costal margin (**Figure P10-1**).
3. Mark this length on the tube with a piece of tape. When the tip of the tube is in the stomach, the tape should be at the lips or nostrils.
4. Place the patient in a supine position.
5. Assess the gag reflex. If the patient is unconscious and has a poor or no gag reflex, perform endotracheal intubation before gastric tube insertion.
6. In a trauma patient:
   - Maintain in-line stabilization of the cervical spine if a neck injury is possible.
   - Choose the orotracheal route if the patient has severe head or facial trauma or has serious midfacial injuries.
7. Lubricate the end of the tube.

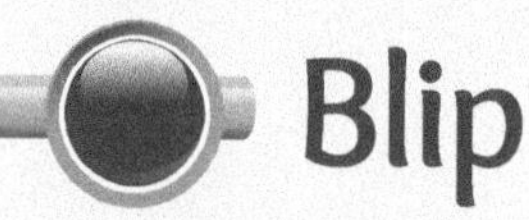

Do not perform orogastric tube insertion on a conscious patient because he or she is at risk for aspiration.

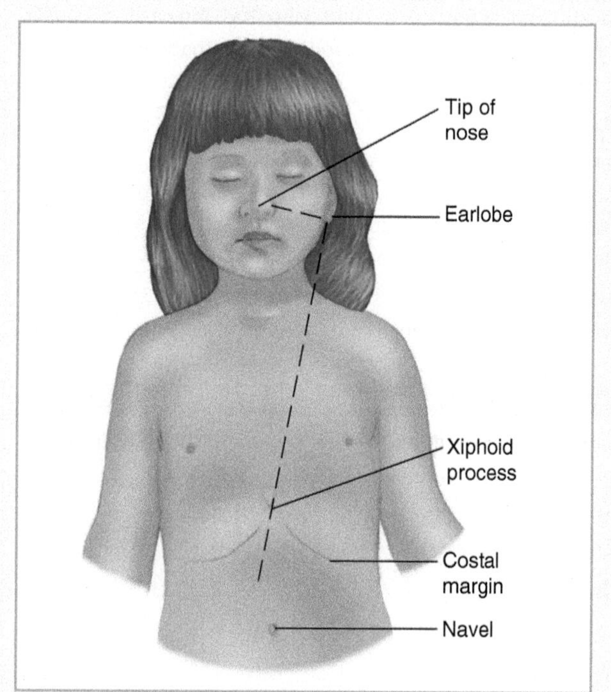

Figure P10-1 Technique for measuring the distance to insert an NG or OG tube.

Table P10-1 Methods for Determining NG/OG Tube Size

1. Refer to a length-based resuscitation tape or resuscitation software (see Procedure 2).
2. Select a tube size that is the same as the size of the patient's nostril, through which it should pass with minimal resistance.
3. Use a tube size twice the endotracheal (ET) tube size (a child who needs a 5.0-mm ET tube needs a 10 French NG or OG tube).

Possible Complications

Placement of the tube into the trachea with hypoxia

Vomiting and aspiration of stomach contents

Airway bleeding or obstruction

Passage of tube into brain

Controversy

The value of NG and OG insertion is unproven. Although these procedures are routine in emergency departments, no studies have tested the benefit of easier ventilation against the potential complications of hypoxia from endotracheal intubation or aspiration of stomach contents.

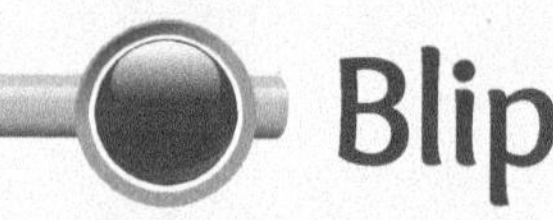

Never use force to pass an NG tube.

Procedure 10-1

NG Insertion

1. Pass the tube gently through the nostril, directing the tube straight back. Do not angle the tube superiorly.
2. If the tube does not pass easily, try the opposite nostril, or a smaller tube. Never force the tube. If NG passage is unsuccessful, use the OG approach.

Procedure 10-2

OG Insertion

1. Insert the tube over the tongue, using a tongue blade if necessary to help insertion.
2. Advance the tube into the hypopharynx, then insert rapidly into the stomach. If coughing, choking, or change in voice occurs, immediately remove the tube. It may be in the trachea.

Procedure 10-3

Check Placement of NG or OG Tube

1. Check tube placement by aspirating stomach contents. An additional method of checking tube placement is to use a syringe with appropriate adaptor to quickly instill 10–20 mL of air through the tube while auscultating over the left upper quadrant. If there is a rush of air over the stomach region, the placement is correct. If correct placement cannot be verified, remove the tube.

2. Secure the tube to the bridge of the nose or to the cheek, using adhesive tape. Aspirate air from stomach, using a 30- to 60-mL catheter-tipped syringe, or connect to mechanical suction at low, continuous, or intermittent setting.

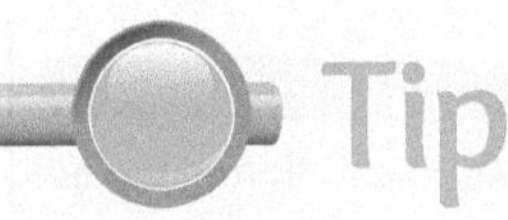

Tip

Perform OG insertion in infants younger than 6 months of age.

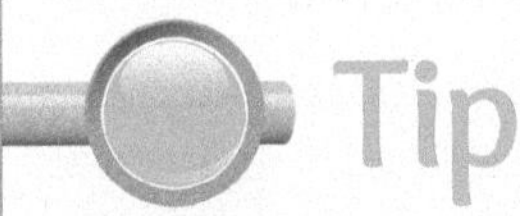

Tip

Talking or crying during the procedure is a good indication that the gastric tube is not in the trachea.

Procedure 11: Endotracheal Intubation

Introduction

Endotracheal intubation is the definitive advanced airway maneuver that is often a life-saving procedure for some critical patients. However, this procedure has important modifications and pitfalls in children. There are several anatomic considerations that make the pediatric airway different from the adult airway:

- The child's vocal cords are more anterior and superior.
- The tongue is proportionally larger.
- The mandible and oral cavity are smaller.
- The diameter and length of the trachea are less.
- The soft tissues are more fragile.
- The narrowest area of the airway for children 5 years of age and younger is the cricoid cartilage

Performing the procedure quickly and safely in the field can be tricky. Inappropriate or unsuccessful intubation attempts may result in hypoxia or injury to the child's airway.

Indications

Respiratory or cardiopulmonary arrest

Respiratory failure

Inability to maintain patent airway

Loss of protective airway reflex

Need for controlled ventilation as in traumatic brain injury

Need for endotracheal administration of resuscitative medications

Severe shock (to decrease myocardial oxygen demand)

Contraindications

Permanent tracheostomy (relative)

Good response to bag-mask ventilation and short transport time (relative)

Anatomic abnormalities that would probably prevent successful intubation (large tongue hematoma, massive facial injuries) (relative)

Equipment

Uncuffed ETTs in pediatric sizes (2.0–5.0), in addition to cuffed tubes (2.5–7.0)

Pediatric laryngoscope with fresh batteries

Pediatric laryngoscope blades, curved (sizes 2–4) and straight (sizes 0–4)

Laryngoscope bulb

Large-bore rigid suction catheter

Suction catheters, sizes 5–12 French

Pediatric stylets

Water-soluble lubricant

Oropharyngeal airways

Pediatric bag-mask device, at least 450 mL volume

Pediatric face masks

Adhesive tape

Commercial ETT securing devices

Skin adhesive

Pulse oximeter

Oxygen source

Device for confirmation of ETT placement (e.g., capnography, end-tidal CO_2 device)

Rapid Sequence Intubation (RSI)/ Drug-Assisted Intubation (DAI)

Rapid sequence intubation (now known as drug assisted intubation) is a technique for relaxing a child's muscles and central nervous system in preparation for intubation. The medications available can be divided into neuromuscular blockers (succinylcholine, rocuronium) and analgesic/sedative/anxiolytics (midazolam, diazepam, fentanyl, ketamine). See **Table P11-1**. Local protocols define the medications used. It is important to realize that each drug or combination of drugs have important benefits and risks. The use of atropine as a premedication to prevent bradycardia can be used in infants. The induced muscular paralysis allows the prehospital professional to insert an ETT with no resistance, and hence, improve success and decrease complications. However, it is not appropriate to induce paralysis without the addition of a medication (awake intubation) that provides some degree of sedation and even unconsciousness. One must also realize that the induction of muscular paralysis renders the patient apneic. *Therefore, if RSI/DAI fails, bag-mask ventilation is essential for the child to survive. Medication doses vary with the changing weight of the child. Medication doses are important causes of error.*

Table P11-1

Drug	Type	Dose
Succinylcholine	Paralytic/ neuromuscular blockade	1–2 mg/kg IV/IO/IM
Rocuronium	Paralytic/ neuromuscular blockade	1 mg/kg IV/IO
Lorazepam	Anxiolysis/ sedative	0.1 mg/kg IV/IO/IM or 0.2 mg/kg IN
Diazepam	Anxiolysis/ sedative	0.1 mg/kg IV/IO
Fentanyl	Analgesia	1 mcg/kg IV/IO or 1–2 mcg/kg IN
Ketamine	Analgesic/ anesthetic	1–2 mg/kg IV/IO or 3–5 mg/kg IM
Atropine (infants)	Anticholinergic	0.02 mg/kg IV/IO 0.1 mg min

Indication

Failed ETI

Severe head trauma requiring hyperventilation

Contraindication

Abnormal airway anatomy

Upper airway obstruction

Laryngeal fracture

Equipment

ETI equipment

RSI medications

Procedure 11-1

RSI/DAI Steps

1. Prepare equipment and medications.
2. Preoxygenate.
3. Premedicate with atropine (as needed).
4. Administer sedation/analgesia/anxiolysis.
5. Administer a neuromuscular blockade.
6. Intubate (can apply cricoid pressure as needed for visualization).
7. Confirm ETT placement (chest rise, breath sounds, end tidal CO_2).
8. Tape ETT in place (or use commercial device if available).

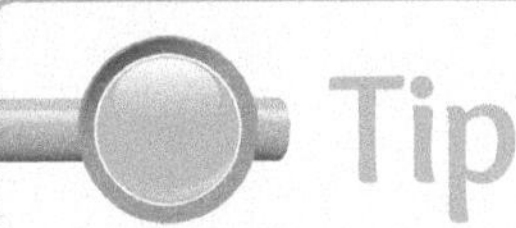

Tip

The induced muscular paralysis from RSI allows the prehospital professional to insert an ETT with no resistance, and hence improves success and decreases complications from forced insertion attempts.

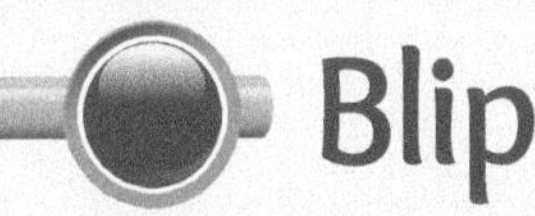

Blip

If RSI fails, bag-mask ventilation is essential for the child to survive.

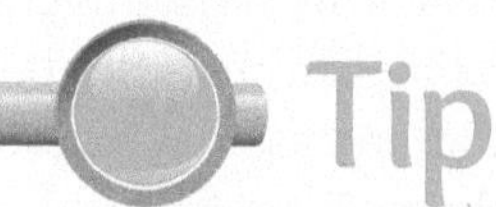

Tip

Preferred resuscitation medication delivery is by intraosseous (IO) or intravenous route (IV), and only LEAN (lidocaine, epinephrine, atropine, and naloxone) medications can be given through the endotracheal tube route (and doses must be increased two to three times for lidocaine, atropine, and naloxone, and increased 10 times for epinephrine).

Rationale

Successful endotracheal tube (ETT) placement allows optimal oxygenation and ventilation, provides a tube for medication delivery, and decreases the risk of aspiration and loss of airway control. A properly placed and secured ETT is a good tool for managing critical patients, but the procedure can take a long time, and there are frequent and serious complications.

Preparation

1. Make sure oxygen delivery equipment is connected to an oxygen source.
2. Select an appropriately sized ETT (**Tables P11-2** and **P11-3**) for oral endotracheal intubation.
3. For a properly selected uncuffed ETT:
   - Allow a minimal air leak. The absence of an air leak may indicate excessive pressure at the cricoid cartilage.
   - Tracheal perfusion pressure is between 35 and 40 cm H_2O, such that the cuff pressure should be less than 25 cm H_2O.
4. For a properly selected cuffed ETT: Check cuff for leaks, maintaining aseptic technique, as follows:
   - Inflate cuff with appropriate volume of air
   - Remove syringe
   - Feel cuff for integrity
   - Deflate cuff before insertion
5. Attach blade to laryngoscope handle, and make sure the bulb is secure and works.
6. Test the large-bore rigid suction catheter.
7. Insert stylet into the ETT, stopping the stylet at least 1 cm from the end of the ETT.
8. Bend the ETT into a gentle upward curve. In some cases, bend the tube into the shape of a hockey stick.
9. Lubricate tube with a water-soluble lubricant (optional).
10. Prepare device for confirmation of ETT placement.
11. To predict correct ETT tube position at gum line, either:
    - Check resuscitation tape, or refer to computer software
    - Calculate ETT position with formula: gum line position (in cm) = ~3 × tube size
12. Have partner prepare for:
    - Ongoing patient assessment
    - Providing time counts for ventilation rates
    - Watching monitors (heart rate, pulse oximetry)
    - Handling suction devices
    - Handling ETT
    - Applying gentle cricoid pressure
    - Stabilizing neck, if child has possible spinal trauma
13. Position patient (avoid hyperextension or hyperflexion of neck).
    - Medical patient: Place the child in the "sniffing" position.
    - If spinal trauma is a possibility, place the child in neutral position with in-line manual stabilization.

Procedure 11-2

Insert Endotracheal Tube

1. Oxygenate and ventilate patient five to six times with bag-mask device and 100% oxygen, at a rate of one ventilation every 3 seconds. Say "squeeze, release, release" to reinforce proper rate.

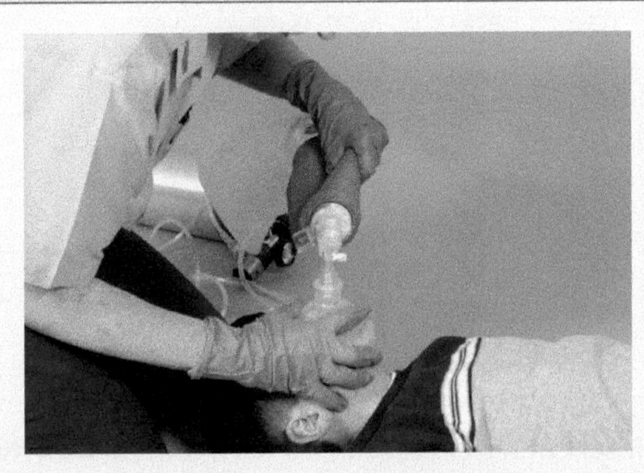

2. Grasp laryngoscope in left hand. Stop ventilating and begin timing, giving 20- to 30-second counts.

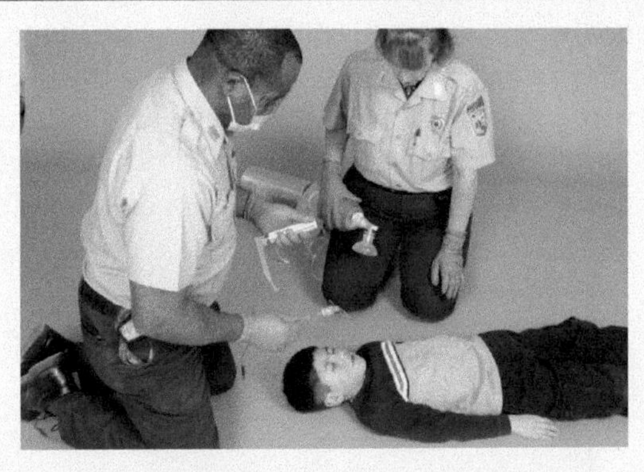

3. Open mouth by applying thumb pressure on chin; check mouth for foreign bodies or loose teeth; remove oropharyngeal airway if present.

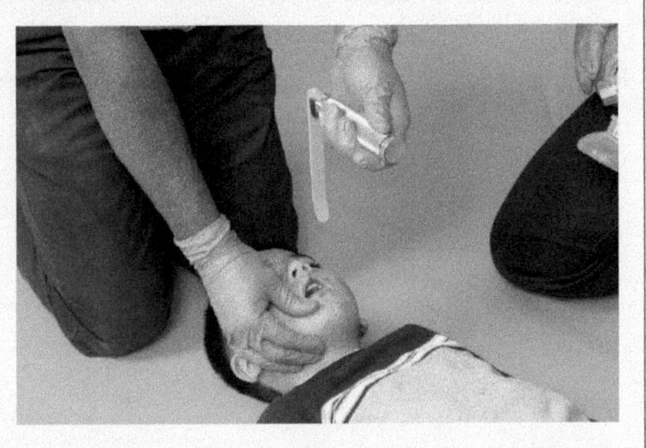

4. Hold laryngoscope in trigger finger position.

5. Insert pediatric straight laryngoscope blade into mouth.

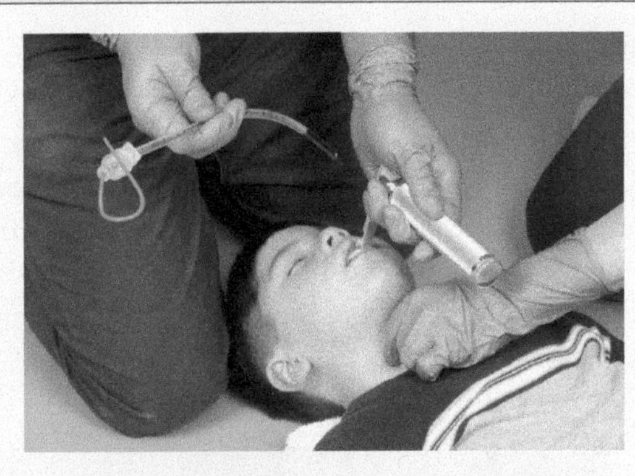

6. Lift tongue with blade.

7. Exert gentle traction upward along the axis of laryngoscope handle at a 45-degree angle. Do not use teeth or gums to gain leverage.

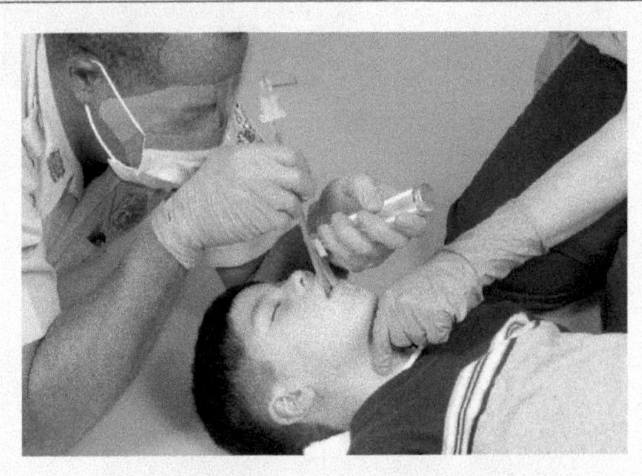

(continues)

Procedure 11-2 *(continued)*

8 Advance blade straight along tongue. Continue looking at blade tip, until tip is just beyond epiglottis. Do not take your eyes off of the vocal cords once visualized. Your partner should be handing the ETT to you while you are maintaining visualization.

9 Have partner apply gentle cricoid pressure if there is difficulty seeing the vocal cords. If there is difficulty seeing the vocal cords, you have four options: (1) advance or retract laryngoscope blade; (2) modify amount of cricoid pressure (Sellick maneuver); (3) remove vomitus, blood, other fluids, or particulate matter with rigid, large-bore suction device; or (4) repositioning of the head or degree of extension.

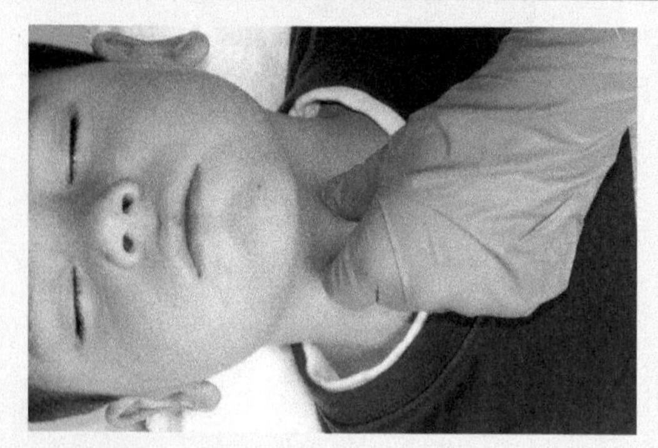

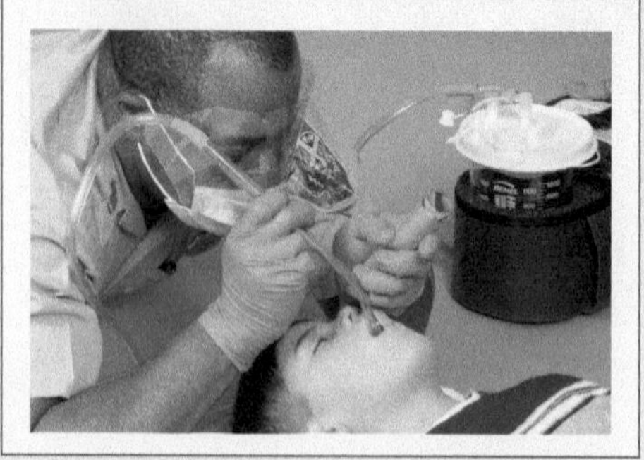

10 If gastric reflux appears near, increase cricoid pressure or stop laryngoscopy attempt.

11 Continue to look at vocal cords and suction.

12 Remove large solid matter with pediatric Magill forceps.

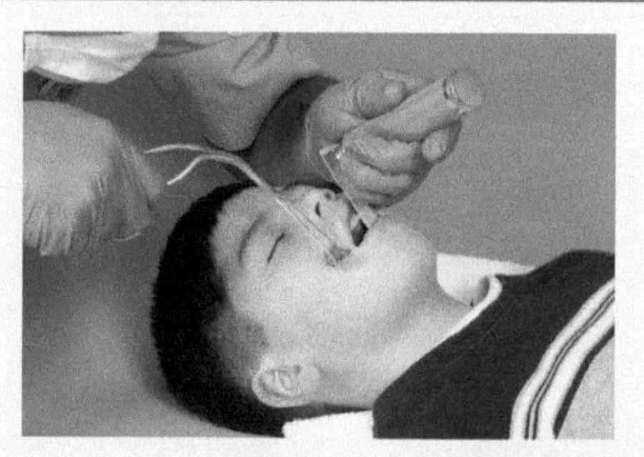

13 Insert ETT. Hold tube in dart-like fashion with right hand and insert tip of tube from right corner of mouth down between vocal cords. Do not insert tube in channel of laryngoscope blade because this blocks the view of the vocal cords. Watch the ETT go through the vocal cords. Advance tube until vocal cord marker on ETT is situated beyond the vocal cords with an uncuffed tube. Advance a cuffed tube until the balloon passes through the vocal cords. Look for centimeter marking on ETT in relation to the gum line.

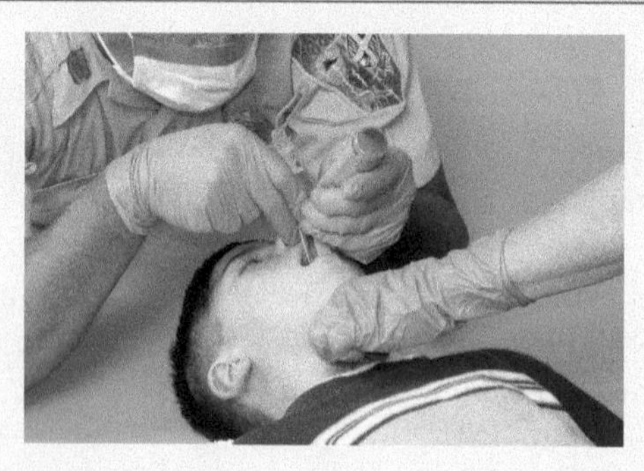

14 Remove laryngoscope blade, holding ETT in place.

(continues)

Procedure 11-2 *(continued)*

15 Remove stylet from ETT.

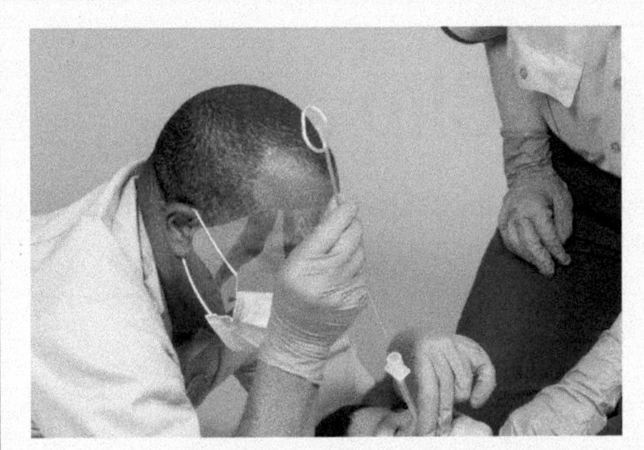

16 If using an ETT with a cuffed end, inflate cuff with pilot balloon. Maintain tube position by holding ETT against upper lip. If large amount of fluid is evident in ETT, use a suction catheter to clear the airway. Have partner maintain ETT position and ventilate patient with bag-mask device.

17 Confirm ETT correct placement using an end-tidal CO_2 device or quantitative capnography as explained in Procedure 12.

18 Assess correct position in trachea. Do general patient evaluation (appearance, heart rate, pulse oximetry). Look for bilateral chest rise. Make sure there are no bubbling, gurgling sounds in epigastric area indicating air-water interface (check for two breaths). Auscultate for bilateral lung sounds at the midaxillary line, third intercostal space (check for two breaths on right and then two breaths on left). Use device to confirm endotracheal positioning. If breath sounds are heard only on one side (usually the right), pull back ETT slightly until breath sounds are heard on both sides.

19 Record tube position on permanent record. Use centimeter mark at teeth or gum line or mark on ETT with indelible pen.

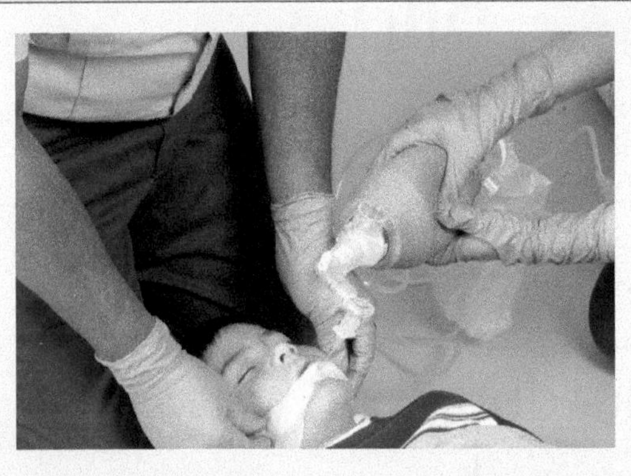

20 Secure tube with tape or commercially available ETT securing device. Reassess proper location of tube and make sure the patient is stable.

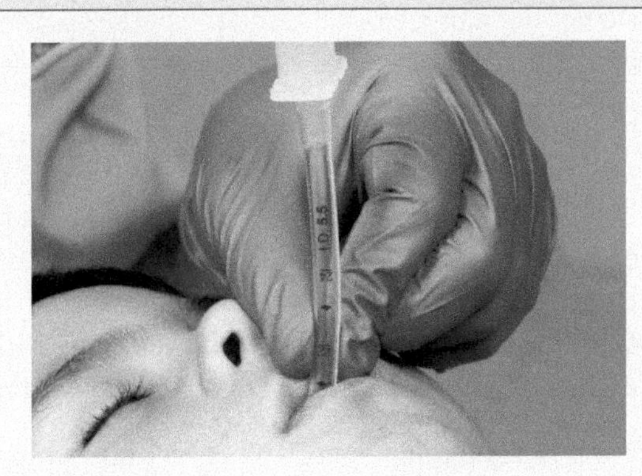

(continues)

Indications for Tube Removal

Immediate Tube Removal

- No chest rise with ventilation.
- Presence of epigastric gurgling sounds.
- Failure to confirm endotracheal placement with detection device.

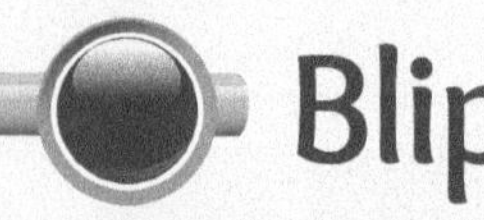

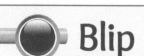

Beware of inadequate spinal stabilization during intubation attempts in trauma patients.

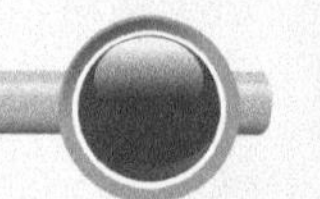

Never assume the ETT is in the trachea unless you see the tube passing through the vocal cords.

Procedure 11-3

Secure Endotracheal Tube

1. Insert correctly sized oral airway (see Procedure 5, Airway Adjuncts) and make sure ETT is not compressed. Do not use a bite block in pediatric patients. Carefully hold the ETT in place while the second rescuer secures.
2. If a commercial device is available, it can be used; otherwise, in medical patients, one method of securing the ETT is by wrapping the tape around the back of the patient's neck. In trauma patients, cut two pieces of tape into a Y: secure one end around the tube and the other on the face. Do the same with the other piece of tape from the other side of the face.
3. Bring tape up to opposite side of face and wrap around the tube twice, crimping end of tape so it can be easily removed.

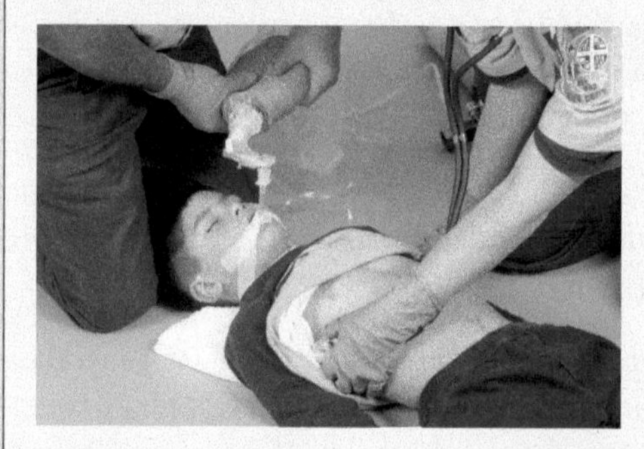

Procedure 11-4

Reconfirm Endotracheal Tube Placement

1. Recheck to make sure there is no bubbling, gurgling noise in epigastric area (air-water interface) for two breaths.
2. Reassess breath sounds bilaterally at the midaxillary line, third intercostal space (two breaths on right and then two breaths on left). Take extra care handling an ETT in a pediatric patient because it can be easily dislodged. Reassess after patient is in ambulance (and after change of position or change in patient status). Report and record findings.

Possible Complications

Aspiration of stomach contents

Dislodgment of ETT from trachea

Esophageal intubation

Hypoxia

Increased intracranial pressure

Laryngeal, tracheal, pharyngeal, or esophageal injury

Teeth and mouth injury

Vocal cord injury

Procedure 11-5

Extubation

1. Postresuscitation extubation is rarely indicated in the field. All three situations must be present: (1) spontaneous breathing with adequate rate and tidal volume; (2) conscious patient; and (3) coughing and gagging causing inability to maintain oxygenation and ventilation. Ensure rigid large-bore suction device is functioning.
2. Suction oropharynx.
3. Turn patient on left side.
4. Deflate cuff completely (if cuff is inflated).
5. Remove ETT quickly at end-inspiratory phase, while suctioning.

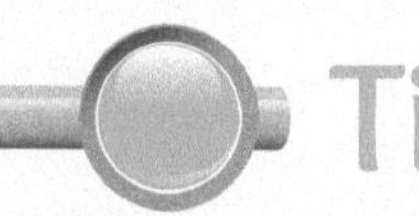

Tip

Make sure proper equipment is available and functioning before intubation attempt.

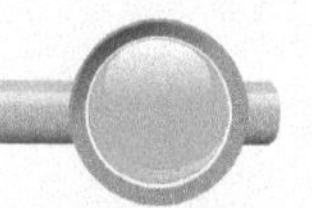

Tip

Chest rise is the best indication of correct endotracheal placement of the ETT. Qualitative end-tidal CO_2/capnography is also useful.

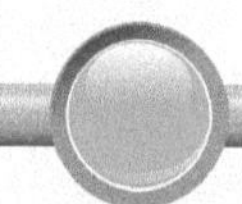

Tip

Always reassess tube location after patient movement or when there is a change in patient status.

Table P11-2 Suggested Uncuffed Endotracheal Tube and Suction Catheter Sizes

Age	ETT Size (mm)	Suction Catheter Size (French)
Premature newborn	2.0–2.5	5
Newborn	3.0–3.5	6–8
6 months	3.5	8
12–18 months	4.0	8
3 years	4.5	8
5 years	5.0	10
6 years	5.5	10
8 years	6.0	10
12 years	6.5	12
16 years	7.0–8.0	14

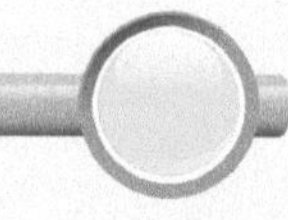

Controversy

The value of performing endotracheal intubation in children in the out-of-hospital setting is controversial. More studies are necessary to define which groups of children benefit from this procedure, especially in light of the well-known risks of hypoxia, esophageal intubation, tube dislodgment, airway injury, and transport delay.

Table P11-3 Selecting Endotracheal Tube Size

Uncuffed	Cuffed
Remembering numbers Newborns and infants Preterm infants: 2.0- or 2.5-mm tube Term newborns or small infants: 3.0- or 3.5-mm tube Infants 6–12 months: 3.5-mm tube Infants 12–18 months: 4.0-mm tube Children >1 year: OR Use the resuscitation tape or resuscitation software (see **Procedure 2**). OR The diameter of the tracheal tube is approximately the same size as the child's fingernail on the fifth finger. $\text{Size} = \frac{\text{(age in years)}}{4} + 4$ (formula for child older than 2 years of age)	For a child younger than 2 years old $\frac{\text{(age in years)}}{4} + 3$ It is appropriate to approximate: 3.0 or 3.5 ETT for a child younger than 1 year old 3.5 or 4.0 ETT for a child 1–2 years old For a child 2–10 years old $\frac{\text{(age in years)}}{4} + 3.5$

Procedure 12: Confirmation of Endotracheal Tube Placement

Introduction

Performing pediatric endotracheal intubation in the out-of-hospital setting may be difficult or impossible even for experienced prehospital professionals. Confirming position of the endotracheal tube (ETT) in the trachea is a major challenge because esophageal intubation is a common and dangerous complication of endotracheal intubation. Intubation is often not necessary in the field if there is effective bag-mask ventilation with appropriate chest rise. Furthermore, portable quantitative capnography does not require intubation and may be used in line with bag-mask ventilation as long as there is a good mask seal on the patient's face. Currently there are four methods to confirm placement of the ETT:

1. Clinical assessment
2. Use of exhaled carbon dioxide detection device
3. Use of digital capnometry (quantitative end-tidal CO_2)
4. Use of esophageal aspiration bulb or syringe

Indications

Endotracheal intubation

Contraindications

An adult carbon dioxide detector device cannot be left in place in a child weighing less than 15 kg

Equipment

Stethoscope

Esophageal detector bulb or syringe OR

Colorimetric end-tidal carbon dioxide detector device OR

Quantitative end-tidal CO_2 device, if available

Rationale

A properly positioned ETT makes it possible to effectively oxygenate and ventilate children with critical illnesses or injuries. Esophageal placement of ETT, however, is usually harmful or fatal. Moreover, if the child is moved, a correctly placed ETT may easily dislodge from the trachea to the oropharynx or esophagus. Delayed detection may result in hypoxia. Clinical assessment of placement of the ETT can be inaccurate, especially in infants and small children. Often, there is a lot of noise in the surrounding area (family members or traffic) that may make it hard to hear breath sounds. Also, breath sounds may be transmitted from the esophagus or stomach throughout the chest of a child and mislead the listener. Fortunately, several mechanical adjuncts are available to supplement clinical assessment and help confirm correct ETT placement in the trachea.

Preparation

1. Intubate the infant or child with a correctly sized ETT (see Procedure 11, Endotracheal Intubation).
2. Determine the weight of the patient.
3. Suction any fluid from the ETT.

Esophageal Detector (Aspiration) Bulb or Syringe

1. Remove esophageal detector bulb or syringe from packaging.
   - Use only in children who weigh ≥20 kg.

Colorimetric Exhaled Carbon Dioxide Detector

1. Determine correct size of the carbon dioxide detector.
   - Use a pediatric device if the child weighs less than 15 kg.

- Use an adult device if the child weighs 15 kg or more.
- If an adult device is used on a small child, remove after six breaths (initial confirmation of placement).

2. Check the expiration date on the carbon dioxide detector package.
3. Remove the carbon dioxide detector from its packaging.
4. Inspect the carbon dioxide detector before use for bright purple color and dryness.

Digital Capnometry

1. Place sensor as indicated by manufacturer.
2. Attach sensor probe to monitoring cable.
3. Observe for square waveform that indicates correct ETT placement.
4. Absence of square waveform indicates improperly placed ETT or low exhaled CO_2.

Procedure 12-1

Clinical Assessment

1. Look for bilateral rise and fall of the chest. Remove ETT if there is no chest rise with assisted ventilation. Listen for breath sounds over the stomach. If gurgling is present (like a straw in milk), the ETT is in the esophagus. If breath sounds only are present in the stomach, continue assessment and do not remove the tube unless there is desaturations or bradycardia, as they may be transmitted from the lungs.

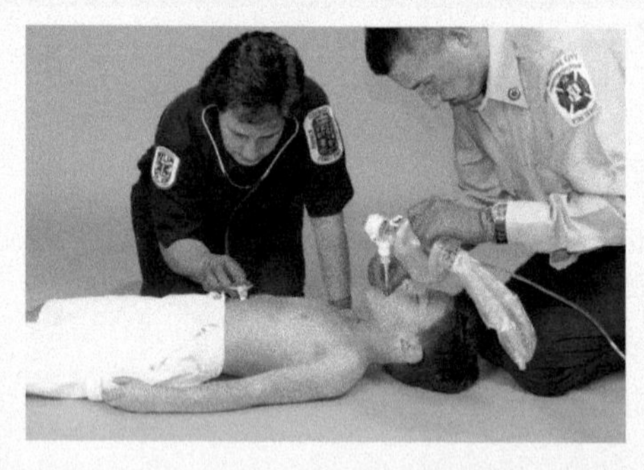

2. Listen for breath sounds in the right midaxillary line, then in the left midaxillary line. If breath sounds are equal, secure the tube. If breath sounds are greater on the right side than on the left side, then the tube may be in the right mainstem bronchus. Slowly pull back the ETT until breath sounds are equal.

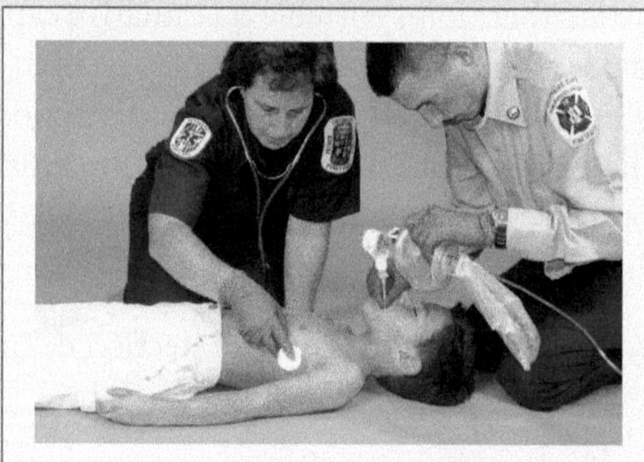

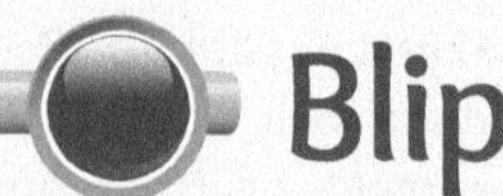

Do not remove the ETT just because breath sounds are heard in the stomach. They may be transmitted sounds from the lungs. If the patient has continued desaturations or bradycardia, perform a direct laryngoscopy to ensure the ETT is through the vocal cords. If it is not, or you are unsure, and the patient has continued desaturations despite giving effective breaths with positive end-expiratory pressure (PEEP), then removing the ETT is appropriate to deliver oxygen with bag-mask ventilation.

Procedure 12-2

Esophageal Detector Bulb or Syringe

1. Attach the device to the end of the ETT right after intubation and before breaths are given.

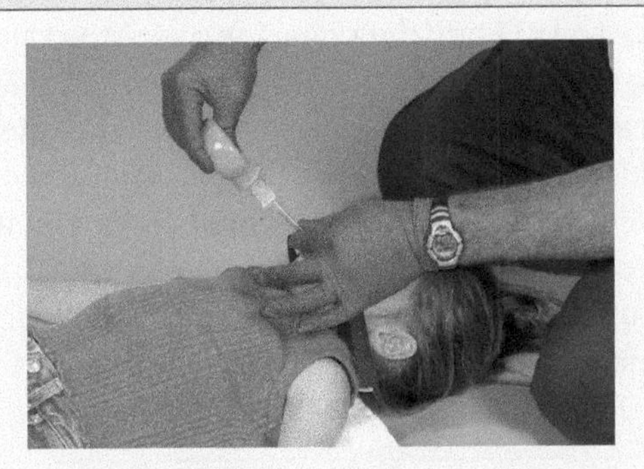

2. Aspirate slowly over 3–5 seconds. If resistance is felt, then the ETT is in the esophagus. Remove it. If air is aspirated, the ETT is in the trachea. Secure it.

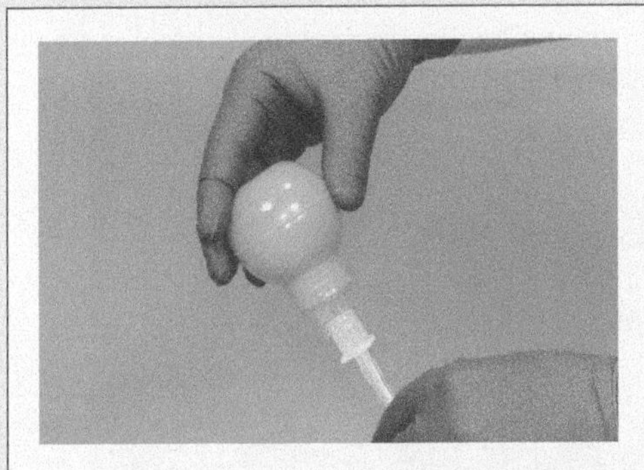

Possible Complications

A faulty device or misinterpretation of results of a carbon dioxide detector or esophageal detector device may result in incorrect ETT placement or incorrectly removing an ETT that was correctly placed.

Rebreathing carbon dioxide may cause hypercarbia in an infant weighing less than 15 kg if an adult-sized detector is left in line. If the child weighs less than 15 kg, use a pediatric device. If the child weighs 15 kg or more, use an adult device.

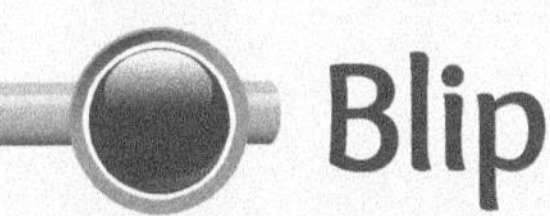

Blip

Do not use an esophageal detector bulb or syringe if the child weighs less than 20 kg.

Procedure 12-3

Colorimetric Carbon Dioxide Detector Device

1. Attach the device to the end of the ETT and attach the other end to the bag-mask device.

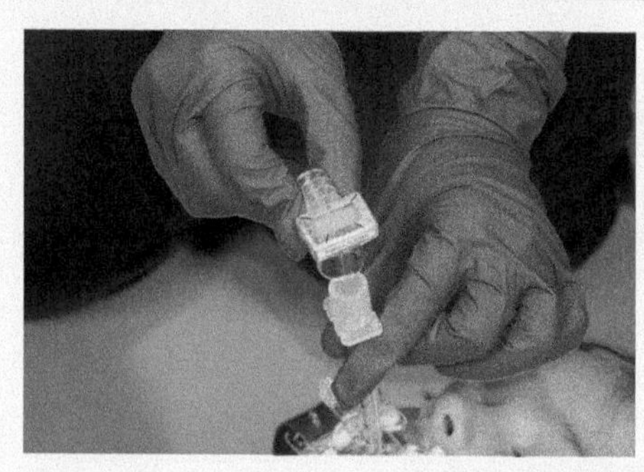

2. Begin ventilation.

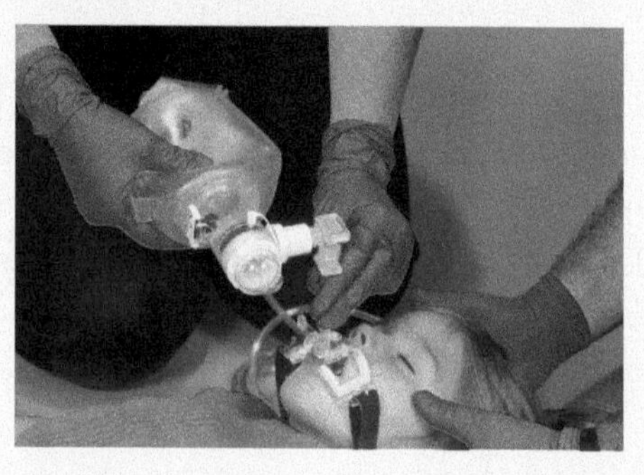

3. Observe the carbon dioxide detector for color change during exhalation. Read only after a total of six breaths. Check the color and act accordingly (**Table P12-1**). Regardless of whether the ETT is in the trachea, the carbon dioxide detector will change to a purple color when 100% oxygen is squeezed through the bag device and ETT into the lungs. The color on exhalation is the one to pay attention to because the color in the expiratory phase of breathing reflects carbon dioxide production. However, do not leave an adult carbon dioxide detector in place after initial confirmation of tube position on a patient weighing less than 15 kg because the adult device has too much dead space and an infant can rebreathe carbon dioxide if it is left in line. Document observations and interventions.

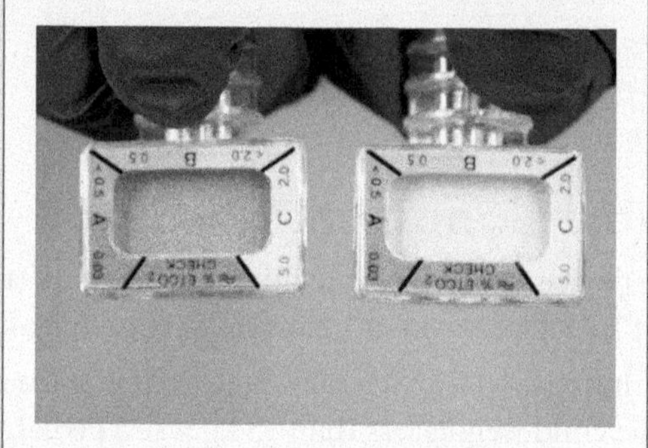

Table P12-1 Use of Colorimetric Exhaled Carbon Dioxide Detector in ETT Placement

Color	Patient With Pulse	Patient Without Pulse
Yellow	Yes—tube correctly placed Leave tube in place and secure it	Yes—tube correctly placed Leave tube in place and secure it
Tan	Think about it Ventilate six more times (while reassessing tube placement) Reassess detector for color change. If still tan, leave tube in place and secure it Attempt to correct any possible cause of low perfusion or low carbon dioxide	Think about it Ventilate six more times (while reassessing tube placement) Reassess detector for color change. If still tan, leave tube in place and secure it Attempt to correct cause of low perfusion or low carbon dioxide
Purple	Problem—tube incorrectly placed or the child is in cardiac arrest or dead and is not producing measurable amounts of carbon dioxide or delivering it to the lungs. Extubate Ventilate with bag-mask device Reintubate	Problem—tube may be incorrectly placed, or the child is dead and not producing measurable amounts of carbon dioxide Look at vocal cords with laryngoscope If tube is incorrectly placed: Extubate Ventilate with bag-mask device Reintubate If tube is between vocal cords, and vocal cord marker is below vocal cords: Leave tube in place Check adequacy of CPR Proceed with ALS protocol

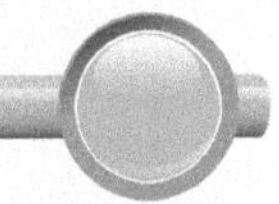

Tip

Remove the carbon dioxide detector from the ETT if endotracheal drugs are given, because a wet detector may not show a correct color change from purple to yellow.

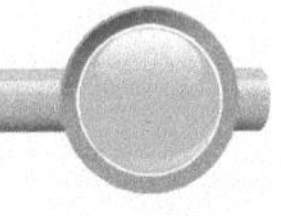

Tip

If the child is in cardiac arrest and not receiving chest compressions, no color change will occur, even if placement is correct, because there is no carbon dioxide being delivered to the lungs.

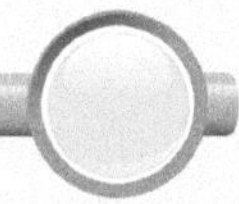

Controversy

An important controversy is whether a carbon dioxide detector or esophageal detector (aspiration) bulb or syringe is better. There is not enough data on efficacy, safety, and feasibility to clearly support one technique alone.

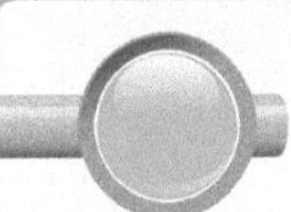

Tip

If the child weighs less than 15 kg, use a pediatric colorimetric exhaled carbon dioxide detector. If the child weighs 15 kg or more, use an adult device.

Procedure 12-4

Quantitative End-Tidal CO_2 ($ETCO_2$)

1. If quantitative $ETCO_2$ is used, a number should register quickly. Accuracy of the $ETCO_2$ number relies on a good mask seal if the patient is not intubated OR minimal leak if an ETT is in correct airway position.

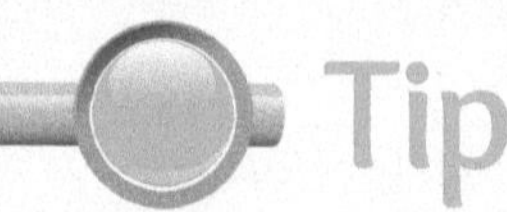

If there is a lot of pulmonary edema or pulmonary hemorrhage, an $ETCO_2$ value may not register.

2. Remember that the number will be low in cardiac arrest and will hopefully improve with high-quality CPR and return of spontaneous circulation (ROSC).

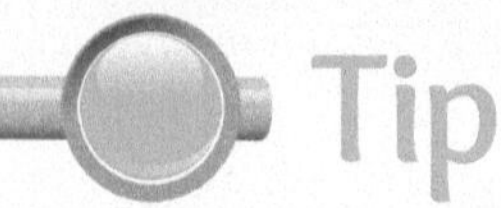

Pulse oximetry requires a pulse and will not register with a cardiac arrest and may be difficult to pick up with delayed capillary refill as may be seen with shock.

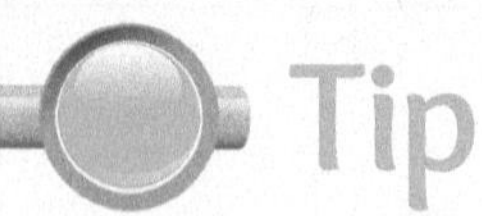

If the child is pulseless and no chest compressions are being performed, there will be a very low (or zero) number on quantitative assessment. Assess quality of CPR (depth, rate, recoil). Patients that have been pulseless for a period of time may not be revivable even with high-quality CPR.

3. Use waveform capnography tracing for quantitative assessment.

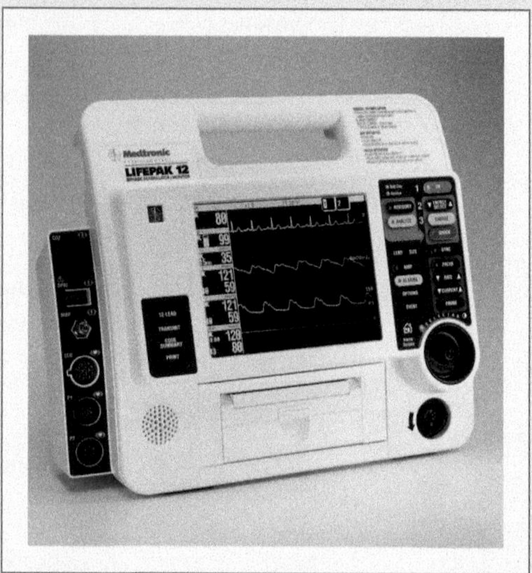

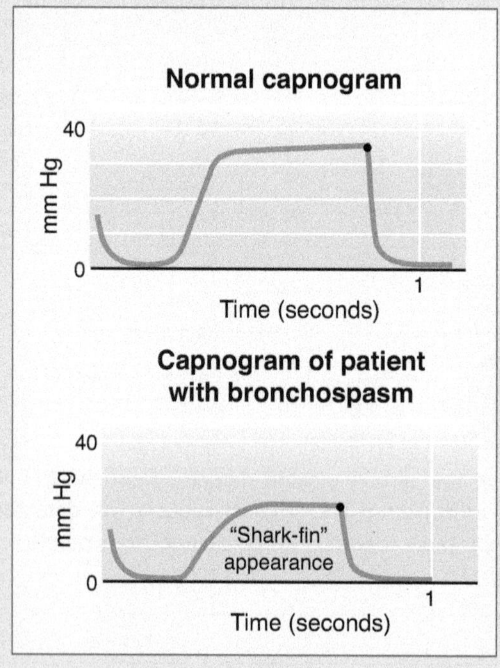

Procedure 13: Advanced Airway Techniques

Introduction

Rarely, standard bag-mask ventilation fails and endotracheal intubation (ETI) is difficult or impossible. Examples of such patients are children with massive head trauma and airway edema or hematomas of the mouth or upper airway, children with multisystem injuries and long transport times, or infants with significant congenital or acquired airway abnormalities that cannot be ventilated. In such dire circumstances, some EMS systems allow prehospital professionals to perform advanced airway techniques. These include use of the laryngeal mask airway (LMA), the gum elastic bougie, the lighted stylet, the King Airway, and rapid sequence intubation (RSI). Needle cricothyrotomy is another option and is explained in detail in this procedure. None of these techniques have been well evaluated in children in the out-of-hospital setting, and each procedure has important benefits, limitations, and contraindications.

Characteristics of children that are red flags for possible problems managing the airway include the following history or physical findings:

History:

1. Past history of difficult intubation or problems with ventilation.
2. Children with congenital anomalies affecting facial bones and oropharyngeal structures including the tongue.
3. History of recurrent stridor or upper airway obstruction.

Physical Findings:

1. Unable to open the mouth widely.
2. Difficulty in fully extending the neck.
3. Presence of a large tongue or dysmorphic facial features.
4. Inability to visualize the entire uvula when depressing the tongue with a tongue blade.
5. Trauma to the face, mouth, tongue, or neck.

Supraglottic Airway Device

Laryngeal Mask Airway (LMA)

The LMA is a device used frequently in EDs and hospitals to ventilate children. It consists of a tube with a distal inflatable mask that is inserted into the mouth. When the mask is inflated, air goes into the trachea. A bag-mask device can then be connected to the tube to provide rescue breathing. There is little out-of-hospital experience with LMAs, and the few reported trials are in adults. Hence, the safety and efficacy of this procedure in children in the out-of-hospital setting are unknown. However, the procedure is simple and fast, the success rates in hospitals are excellent, and the risks are small. EMS systems may soon be introducing the LMA for pediatric rescue breathing, and it may be an easier rescue technique than ETI in children who cannot be effectively ventilated by a bag-mask device. This technique requires special equipment and special training. Also, the epiglottis may flip over and interfere with good positioning of the LMA device.

Indications

A child who requires ventilation

Failed bag-mask ventilation

Failed ETI attempt

Contraindications

Severe upper airway obstruction

An awake patient with intact airway reflexes

Patients requiring high pressures to ventilate (asthma, bronchiolitis)

A relative contraindication is a full stomach, because the LMA does not fully protect against aspiration

Equipment

LMA have eight sizes: 1, 1.5, 2, 2.5, 3, 4, 5, and 6

Water-soluble lubricant

Syringe

Oxygen source

Suction

Ventilation bag

Monitors (pulse oximeter, capnography)

Preparation

1. Select the LMA size for the patient (see **Table P13-1** for sizing).
2. Select an appropriate resuscitator bag: although a small child can be safely and effectively ventilated using an adult bag, a pediatric bag will not work for a large child. Pediatric tidal volume is approximately 8 mL/kg. The bag should have a volume of 450–750 mL. An adult bag (1,200 mL) is acceptable for larger children or adolescents.
3. Connect the oxygen tubing.
4. Once inserted, connect the bag device to the end of the LMA.

Table P13-1 LMA Size/Cuff Volume by Weight

LMA Size	Cuff Volume	Weight of Patient
1	4 mL	<5 kg
1.5	7 mL	5–10 kg
2	10 mL	10–20 kg
2.5	14 mL	20–30 kg
3	20 mL	30–50 kg
4	30 mL	50–70 kg
5	40 mL	>70 kg
6	50 mL	>100 kg

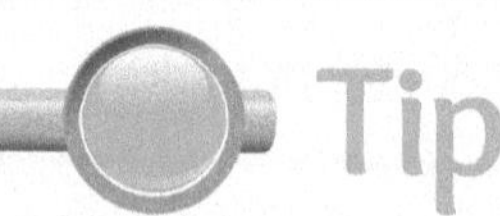

The LMA is a fast and simple device and is widely used for children in the ED and hospital.

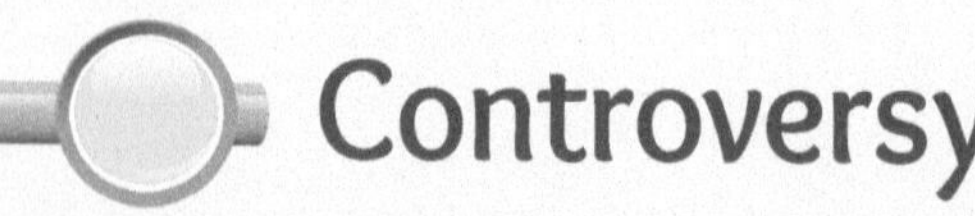

The LMA has not been studied in children in the out-of-hospital setting, and risks and benefits are unknown.

Procedure 13-1

LMA Insertion Methods–Classic

1. Deflate the cuff of the mask.

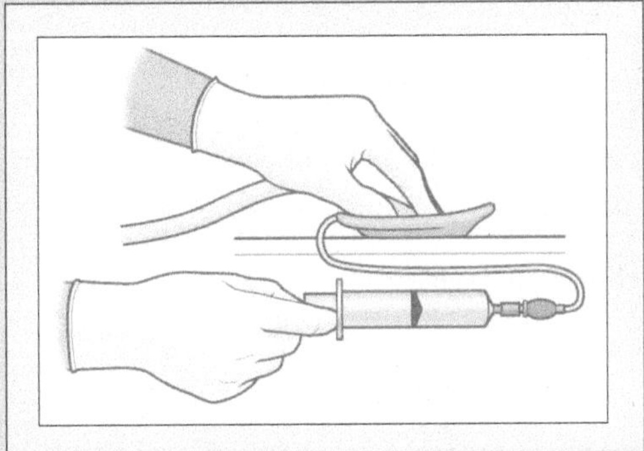

2. Hold the LMA like a pen, with the index finger of the dominant hand at the junction of the mask and the tube.

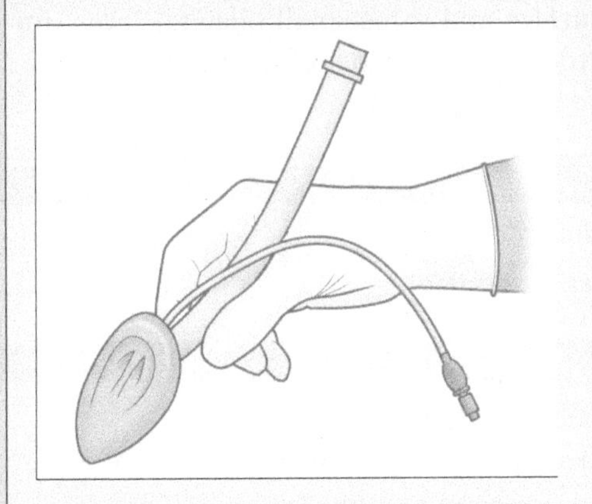

3. Slide the LMA along the hard palate, pushing it back against the palate as it is advanced toward the hypopharynx. This prevents the tip from folding over on itself and reduces interference from the tongue.

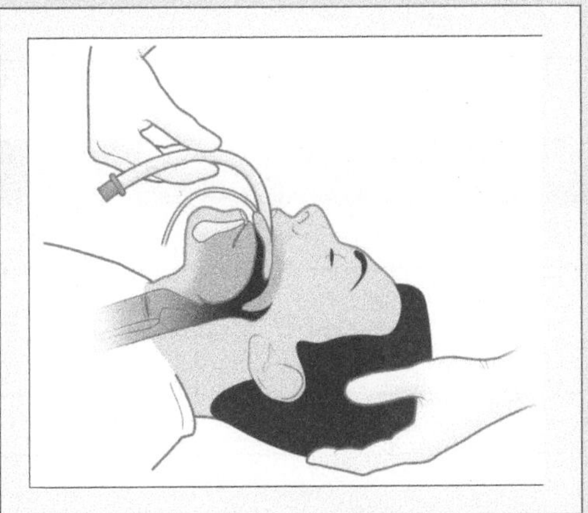

4. Advance with gentle pressure until resistance is met.

5. If necessary, continue pressure on the tube with the nondominant hand to fully advance the LMA to its proper position.

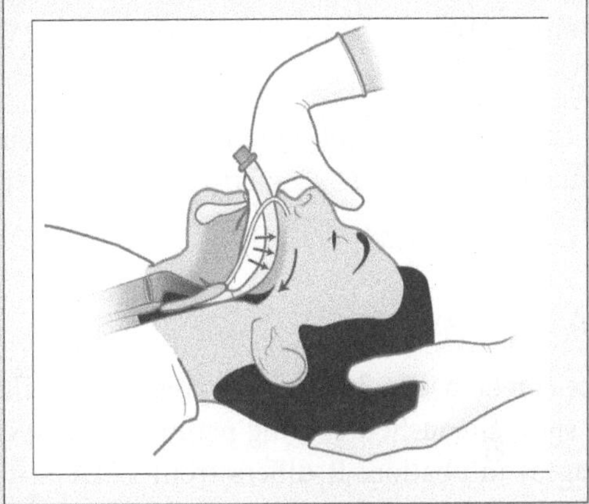

6. Once in place, loosen grip. Then inflate the cuff, allowing it to acquire its natural position.

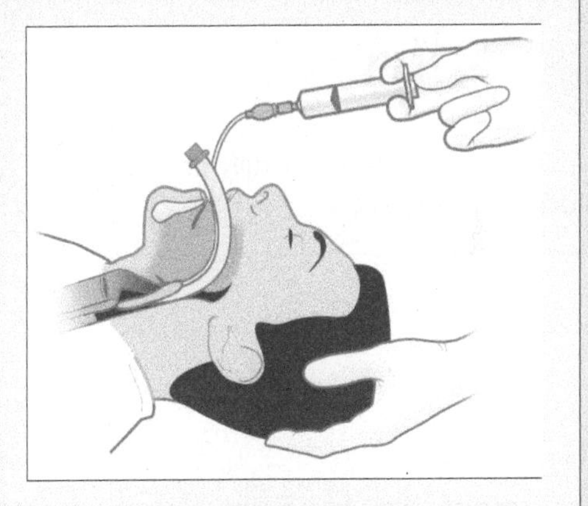

7. Attach to bag device.

Procedure 13-2

LMA Insertion Methods–180° Rotation

1. Invert the deflated mask "inside-out."
2. Then insert the LMA into the mouth in a 180-degree rotated position, with the mask's orifice facing the palate.
3. Push the LMA toward the hypopharynx until it enters the pharynx (detected by a sudden loss of resistance). In contrast to the classic method, do not use the index finger as a guide.
4. Then turn the LMA 180 degrees back to its normal position.
5. Inflate the cuff. Apply a water-soluble lubricant to the posterior surface. Rub the lubricant over the anterior hard palate.
6. Attach to bag device.

King Airway

This device can be used with positive pressure ventilations as well as spontaneously breathing patients. It is designed for esophageal intubation. It differs from LMA in that it has two areas that inflate: the proximal cuff inflates near the base of the tongue and separates the laryngopharynx from the oropharynx and nasopharynx; and the distal cuff inflates in the esophagus, which prevents insufflation of the stomach. A single valve inflates both the proximal and distal cuffs. There are two main ventilation outlets on the anterior surface and three small bilateral "eyes" for additional ventilation on the sides of the tube.

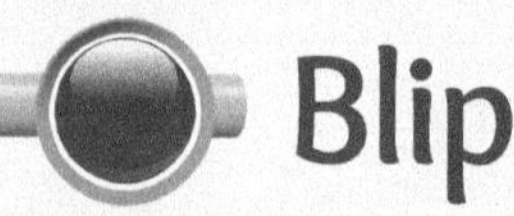

Blip

King Airway and LMA may not fully protect from regurgitation and aspiration.

Indications

Failed ETI attempt

Failed bag-mask ventilation

Contraindications

Responsive patients with an intact gag reflex

Patients with known esophageal disease

Patients who have ingested caustic substances

Preparation

1. Choose correct size based on patient's height (see **Table P13-2** for sizing).
2. Test cuff inflation system for air leak.
3. Apply water-soluble lubricant to distal tip.

Table P13-2 King LT-D Sizing and Information

King LT-D Size	2	2.5	3	4	5
Connector color	Green	Orange	Yellow	Red	Purple
Recommended patient height (weight)	35–45 inches (12–25 kg)	41–51 inches (25–35 kg)	4–5 feet	5–6 feet	>6 feet
Cuff volume	25–30 mL	30–40 mL	45–60 mL	60–80 mL	70–90 mL

Source: http://www.scdhec.gov/health/ems/ResourcesKingLT.pdf

Procedure 13-3

King Airway Insertion

1. Deflate the cuffs and apply water-soluble lubricant to distal tip.
2. Hold the King Airway with your dominant hand. With the nondominant hand, hold the mouth open and apply chin lift.

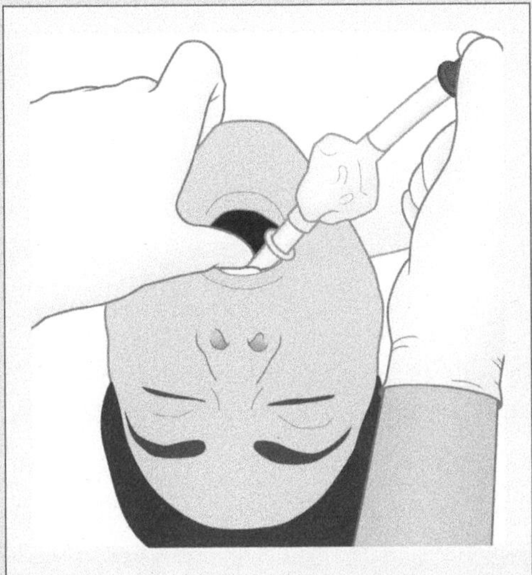

3. Using lateral approach, insert the King Airway into the mouth.

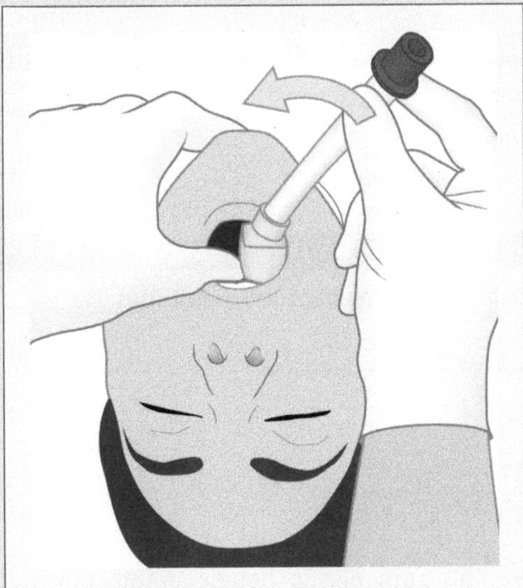

4. Advance the tube behind the base of the tongue while rotating the tube back to midline so that the blue orientation line faces the chin of the patient.
5. Without excessive force, advance the tube so that the base of the connector is aligned with the teeth or gums.

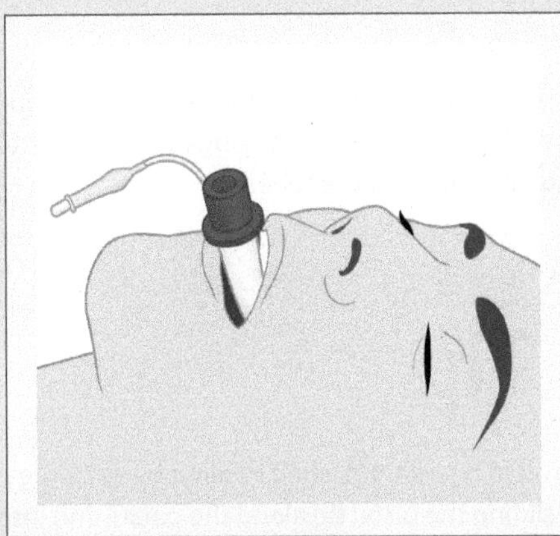

6. Inflate cuffs with appropriate volumes (see Table P13-2).
7. Attach the bag to the connector.

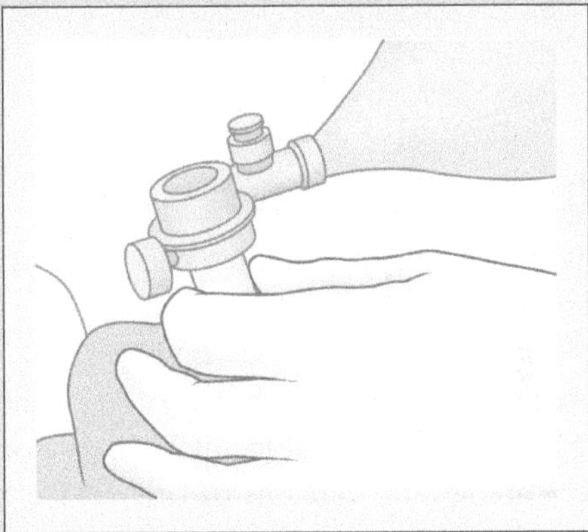

8. While bagging the patient, gently withdraw the tube until ventilation becomes easy.
9. If necessary, adjust cuff inflation to obtain a seal for the airway at the peak ventilation pressure used.

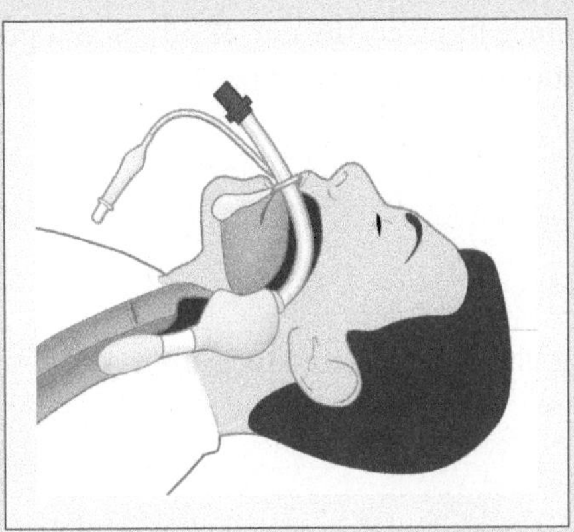

(*continues*)

Procedure 13-3 (continued)

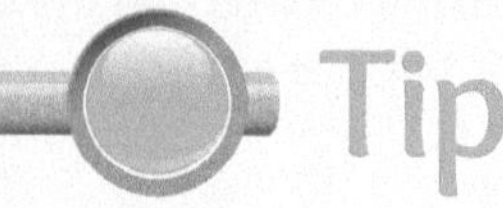

Tip

Instead of the chin lift method, a laryngoscope or tongue depressor can be used to lift the tongue anteriorly to allow easy advancement of the tube.

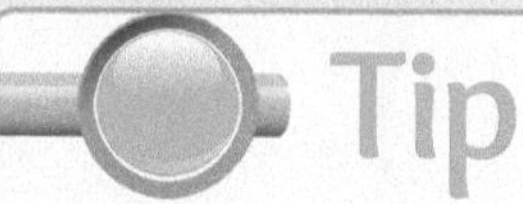

Tip

Insertion can also be accomplished midline by applying a chin lift and sliding the distal tip along the palate and into position in the proximal esophagus. Head extension may also be helpful.

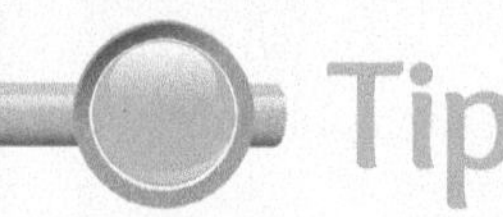

Tip

Initially placing the tube deeper, inflating the cuffs, and then retracting until ventilation becomes easy and free flowing is preferred, because a shallow insertion requires deflation of the cuffs to insert the tube deeper.

Gum Elastic Bougie

Sometimes it is difficult to visualize the vocal cords for ETI. There are many reasons for failure to see the anatomy, especially if the child has muscle tone. The gum elastic bougie or endotracheal tube (ETT) introducer is a long flexible stylet that facilitates insertion of an ETT. There are several versions of this device that are available and may prove useful in facilitating intubation. The cartilaginous rings structure of the trachea allows the operator to feel the gum elastic bougie in the correct location. The semi-rigid tube or rod can be angled to pass into the trachea and as the device brushes against the tracheal rings, the rod can be palpated to be in position. Once in place, the device serves as a guide for placement of the ETT. Airway injury also is a risk.

Indication

An adjunct for the difficult airway when direct visualization of the vocal cords is impossible because of secretions or blood obstructing the view

Contraindications

Major facial trauma

Laryngeal fracture

Severe upper airway obstruction

Equipment

Gum elastic bougie device in pediatric and adult sizes

All equipment described under ETI

Preparation

1. Prepare the child for ETI (see Procedure 11).
2. Ensure the gum elastic bougie points upward in a J-shape configuration.

Procedure 13-4

Gum Elastic Bougie Device

1. Place the lubricated ETT over the straight end of the gum elastic bougie.
2. Visualize the cords with laryngoscopy.
3. Insert the J-shaped end of the gum elastic bougie through the cords, advancing the device until clicks are palpated indicating the presence of tracheal rings.
4. Slide the ETT over the gum elastic bougie into the trachea.
5. Remove the laryngoscope, then the gum elastic bougie.
6. Ensure the ETT is in the trachea by end-tidal CO_2 detection or an esophageal detector device, and that the tube has a correct position at the lips.
7. Secure the ETT.

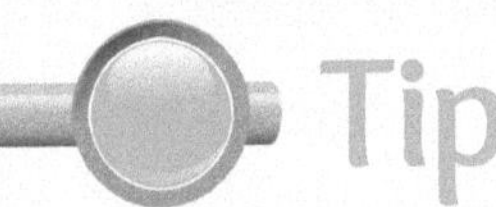

Tip

A gum elastic bougie is particularly helpful when a very anteriorly placed larynx makes visualization of the vocal cords difficult.

Lighted Stylet

The lighted stylet uses a stylet with a fiberoptic tip that is brightly illuminated as the tube is passed into the trachea. It is a blind intubation technique and uses the light's position visualized on the external area of the neck over the trachea to determine positioning. The technique does not require airway visualization. The lighted stylet is particularly useful when copious blood or secretions obstruct direct laryngoscopy.

Indications

An adjunct for the difficult airway when direct visualization of the vocal cords is impossible due to secretions or blood obstructing the view.

Contraindications

Major facial trauma

Laryngeal fracture

Severe upper airway obstruction

Equipment

Lighted stylet of appropriate diameter to fit through ETT

ETI equipment

Preparation

1. Follow ETI procedure (Procedure 11).

Procedure 13-5

Lighted Stylet

1. Select an appropriate size ETT that allows a lighted stylet to fit within the lumen.
2. Apply a water-soluble lubricant to the opening of the ETT to allow easy advancement of the stylet without sticking. Test the light source on the stylet.
3. Insert the lighted stylet so that the light source is at the tip of the ETT.
4. Bend the ETT/stylet assembly to a sharp angle of greater than 90 degrees. Place the bend at the same distance as the distance from the patient's thyroid cartilage to the angle of their mandible.
5. Apply gentle cricoid pressure. Darken the ambulance or treatment room. Place the patient's head in a neutral position; lift the jaw forward to elevate the tongue and epiglottis while inserting the ETT/stylet assembly into the mouth.
6. If the mouth is easily opened, the stylet can be introduced in the midline and advanced over the base of the tongue. If this is difficult, the ETT/stylet assembly can be turned 90 degrees, advanced into the oropharynx, and turned for insertion when the angle of the assembly reaches the base of the tongue.
7. As the assembly is passed into the trachea, observe for a circular "tracheal glow" that can be observed on the skin over the larynx and trachea.

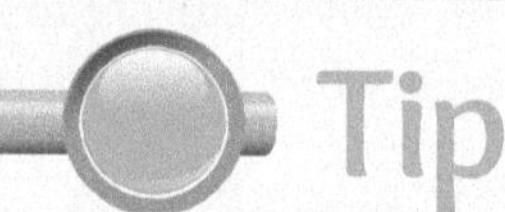

The brightness of the glow that confirms appropriate ETT placement can be assessed by shining the light through the patient's cheek before insertion of the tube.

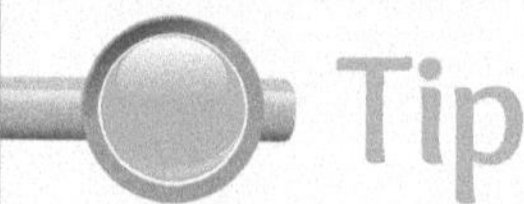

A lighted stylet positioned in the piriform fossa or vallecula will not provide appropriate tracheal glow. A very obese patient may also make it difficult to see the characteristic tracheal glow.

Procedure 14: Intramuscular Injections

Introduction

The intramuscular (IM) route is acceptable for giving several important medications to children. These medications include epinephrine and morphine sulfate. The IM route has limitations, but when inhalation, intravenous (IV), or intraosseous (IO) delivery of medication is not possible, IM administration may be lifesaving.

Indication

Administration of medications when vascular access is not possible or practical

Contraindications

Poor perfusion

Availability of alternative effective routes: oral, inhalation, IV, IN, or IO

Equipment

Tuberculin or 3-mL syringe

22- or 25-gauge needle (5/8- to 1½-inch for IM injection)

Rationale

IM administration allows the medication to absorb slowly but steadily. The advantages of the IM technique is easy delivery and high safety. The disadvantages are poor patient acceptance and delayed effect. Avoid IM medications in patients with low perfusion because absorption is unpredictable. Sometimes, in situations involving a child with low venous pressures, such as in anaphylaxis, IM is an excellent first choice for delivery while vascular access is attempted.

The IM route may result in nerve damage, particularly if the injection is in the buttocks of an infant or small child.

Preparation

1. Explain the procedure using developmentally appropriate terminology. Avoid using the word "shot" because the child may associate this with being shot by a gun. Be honest and tell the child it will hurt but be over as quickly as possible. Describe the needle stick as a pinch or a bee sting.
2. Select the medication. Confirm that the child is not allergic to any medications.
3. Select the appropriate syringe and needle. Keep needles out of the child's sight.

   Needle Length for IM Injection
   - For the ventrogluteal or dorsogluteal sites, use a needle slightly longer than one half of the distance between the thumb and finger when the skin at the injection site is grasped.
   - For the deltoid and vastus lateralis sites, use a 1-inch needle if the skin is grasped. If the muscle is stretched, use a 5/8-inch needle.
4. Cleanse the top of the medication vial with an alcohol wipe or open the ampule.
5. Withdraw the appropriate volume of medication, based on the child's milligram per kilogram dose. Calculate the dose or obtain from length-based resuscitation tape or resuscitation software (see Procedure 2).
   - The maximum volume IM is:
     - 2 mL in older children
     - 1 mL in small children and older infants
     - 0.5 mL in small infants

6. Select the appropriate injection site (**Table P14-1**). Consider the following factors:
   - The volume of medication
   - The condition of the muscle
   - The type of medication
   - The child's ability to be properly positioned
7. Position and secure the child. Consider letting the caregiver hold the child in one of the following ways:
   - Have the child sit on the caregiver's lap, facing to the side. Put one of the child's arms around the caregiver's waist and have the caregiver hold the child close to his or her chest. The caregiver can hold the child's arms or legs.
   - Position the child straddling the caregiver's lap, sitting chest to chest. Tell the caregiver to hug the child. The caregiver can help to hold an arm or leg.

Possible Complications

Abscess

Cellulitis

Damage to blood vessel, nerve, or tendon

Redness or swelling at the site

Adverse reaction to the medication

Pain at site

Table P14-1 Appropriate Sites for IM Injections

Site	Indications	Landmarks	Considerations	Disadvantages
Vastus lateralis muscle: Largest muscle group in children under 3 years of age	Use in infants and small children Preferred site for all ages	Palpate the greater trochanter and the knee joint; divide the distance into thirds Use middle third for injection site	Can be used for IM injections in young children	Possible thrombosis of the femoral artery More painful than deltoid or gluteal sites.
Ventrogluteal muscle: Large muscle with few nerves and blood vessels	Use in children over 3 years of age	Have the child lie on his side and bend the upper leg forward in front of the lower leg Palpate greater trochanter and anterior and posterior iliac crests Place palm over greater trochanter with fingers open in a V shape pointing towards iliac crests Inject into center of the V shape	Well-defined landmarks to identify the site	None
Dorsogluteal site	Use in children over 3 years of age	Have the child lie on his stomach and rotate his legs and toes inward Palpate greater trochanter and posterior iliac spine; draw an imaginary line between these two points Inject lateral and above the imaginary line	In an older child, larger volumes of medication (2 mL) can be injected because the muscle mass is larger.	Contraindicated in children under 3 years of age and those who have not been walking for at least 1 year Medication may inadvertently be given into fat in older child with a large fat mass May damage the sciatic nerve, which tracks out from the lower lumbar spine and goes underneath the gluteal muscles
Deltoid	Use for small volumes of medication. Used in children 18 months of age and older	Palpate the shoulder and go two fingerbreadths below Give the injection in the upper third of the muscle	Faster absorption rate than gluteal site Fewer side effects from the injection and less painful site	May damage the radial nerve in young children Because of the limited muscle mass, only small volumes of medication can be injected

Procedure 14-1

IM Injection

1. The vastus lateralis site is preferable. Use the ventrogluteal or dorsogluteal sites if the thigh muscle is not accessible in children older than 3 years.
2. Stretch the skin and insert the needle at a 90-degree angle.
3. If the patient's muscle mass is small, grasp the body of the muscle between the thumb and forefingers.
4. Release the skin and pull back on the plunger to aspirate for blood.
5. If no blood appears, inject the medication. If blood appears, remove the syringe and start the procedure again.
6. Apply gentle pressure to the site with a gauze pad. Do not massage the site.

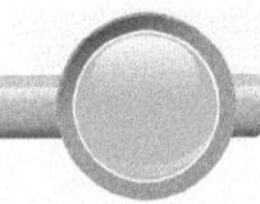

Tip

Select the injection site based on age, anatomic considerations, and volume of medication to be given.

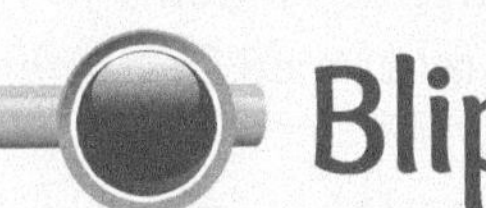

Blip

Avoid injecting close to a major nerve because it may cause nerve damage.

Procedure 14-2

After the Injection

1. Praise the child. Apply an adhesive bandage to the site.

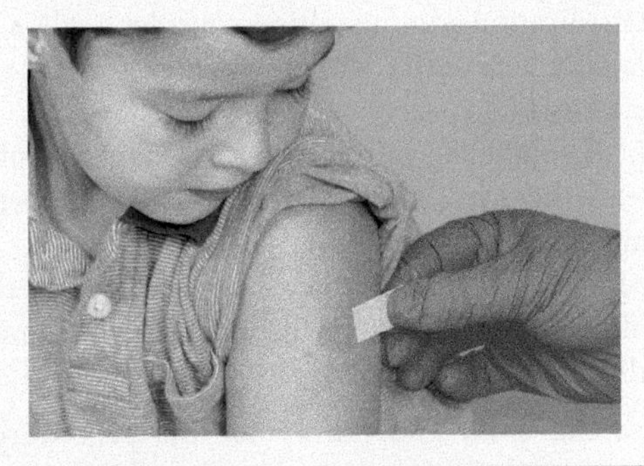

2. Dispose of the syringe in a sharps container.

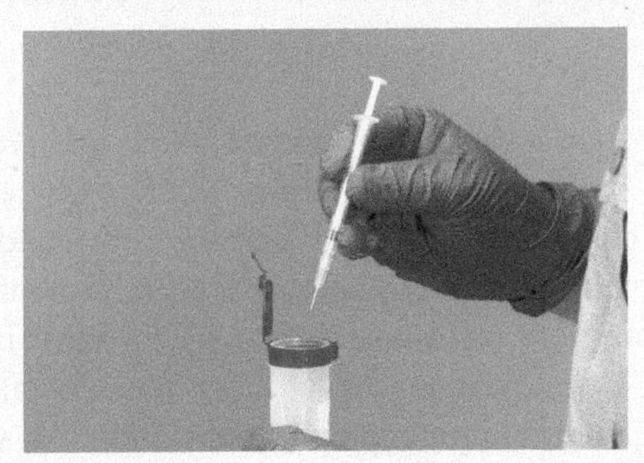

3. Write down the name of the medication, dosage, route, time, and any effects.

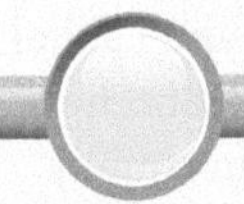

Controversy

Some experts believe that the dorsogluteal site should not be used until the child has been walking for at least 1 year.

Procedure 15: Intravenous Access

Introduction

Establishing intravenous (IV) access is a time-honored method of fluid and drug administration. However, unlike the situation with an adult, securing IV access in a pediatric patient is often difficult or impossible in the out-of-hospital setting. Fortunately, the majority of pediatric patients do not require IV access before emergency department (ED) arrival, and many out-of-hospital medications do not require an IV route for administration.

Indications

Cardiopulmonary arrest

Shock

Cardiac dysrhythmia

Illness or injury possibly requiring immediate IV drug or fluid administration

Contraindications

Availability of another reliable administration route

Brief transport time

Consider vascular access on the way to the ED in the following situations:

- Multisystem injury
- Shock

Equipment

IV catheters, 14- to 24-gauge

IV tubing (macrodrip or microdrip)

Extension connector

IV solution

Rubber band or elastic band tourniquet

Adhesive tape or occlusive dressing

Gauze pad

Pediatric arm board

Rationale

IV access makes it easier to give medications and provides a route for fluid therapy in illness or injuries where there is possible blood or fluid loss. IV delivery is the gold standard for giving medications because it permits predictable delivery and more rapid onset of action for most important drugs. The indications for IV access must be carefully weighed against common complications and risks associated with the procedure. These include diversion from airway and breathing management, possible delays to ED care, and pain to the child. Also, there is a risk to the prehospital professional from exposure to bloodborne pathogens. However, in certain children, such as the critically ill child with shock, IV therapy in the field can be life saving.

Preparation

1. Assemble the equipment. Select the appropriate IV solution and tubing.
   - Inspect the solution for cloudiness, expiration date, leakage, or contamination.
   - Use microdrip IV tubing for giving medication.
   - For fluid administration, use a macrodrip.
   - For medication administration consider a saline lock: male Luer lock device with injection port and normal saline flush.
   - Spike the fluid bag with the tubing, clamp the tubing, squeeze the drip chamber until it is half full, open the clamp, and flush the tubing.
   - Select the appropriate catheter, depending on need for fluid volume. Use a smaller catheter when only medications are indicated.
2. Prepare the child and family for the procedure. Use developmentally appropriate language to explain the procedure.
3. Select the site.
   - The scalp is a potential site in newly borns.
   - The best sites in the infant are the hands, antecubital fossa, and saphenous vein at the ankle or feet. The dorsum (back) of the hand is a good site in chubby infants. To access that site, grasp the child's hand with the fingers closed and flex the wrist downward.

- In toddlers and older children, potential sites are the hands and antecubital areas. Use the child's nondominant extremity if possible.
- Ideally, avoid inserting the catheter over a joint.
- Consider the antecubital fossa when fluid boluses are required because veins that are more distal in the forearm or hand are usually smaller.
- Hand veins are often mobile under the skin and may move with contact with the catheter.

4. Position the patient supine, or in the caregiver's lap if the child is under school age. Secure the child's legs to avoid kicking. The caregiver can help hold the child and immobilize the insertion site.
5. Apply the rubber band or tourniquet proximal to the entry site. Do not make it too tight. The tourniquet should not block arterial flow. If it is necessary to make the vein more visible, do the following:
   - Place the extremity in a dependent position.
   - Tap or massage the site.
   - Ask the older child to clench and unclench their fist.
6. Cleanse the site with antiseptic solution.

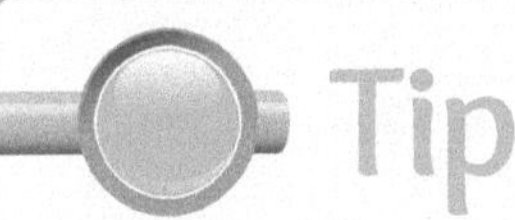

If IV access is for giving medication only, use microdrip tubing. For giving fluid, use macrodrip tubing.

Troubleshooting

1. If the fluid is not infusing properly, assess the following:
   - Make sure the tourniquet has been released.
   - Make sure the child's arm is not bent.
   - Make sure the tape is not too tight.
   - Make sure the tubing is not kinked.
   - Make sure the clamp is open.
   - Lower the fluid bag below the extremity and assess for a backflow of blood into the tubing.
   - Raise the fluid bag higher if possible.
2. If none of the above measures are effective, discontinue the IV and restart in another site.

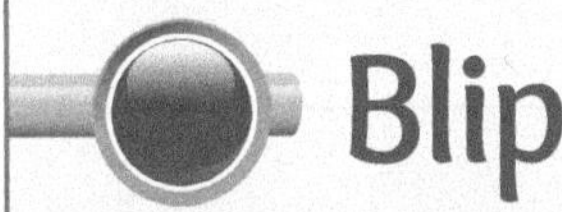

Never delay transport in any critically injured infant or child; consider IV attempts on the way to the hospital.

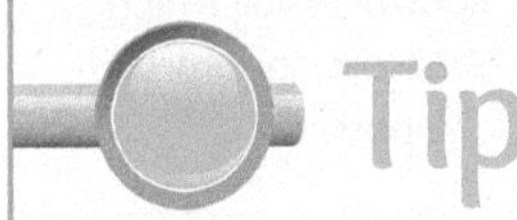

Reward and comfort the child after the procedure.

Procedure 15-1

Intravenous Access

1. Insert the needle. Stabilize the vein by pulling the skin taut distally from the insertion site. Insert the catheter through the skin with the bevel up, at a 30-degree angle. Insert the catheter slowly; blood return may be delayed for a few seconds. When there is a flashback of blood, advance the needle and catheter into the vein and then remove the needle. Never pull the catheter back over the needle because this may cause shearing of the catheter tip. Release the tourniquet. Compress the vein proximal to the site to prevent blood loss through the catheter while connecting the tubing. It is also helpful to position a gauze pad under the catheter at this time. Connect the tubing or male Luer lock to the catheter. If a saline lock (male Luer lock with injection port) is used, a 2- to 5-mL saline flush should be used to maintain patency.
2. Stabilize the catheter with tape or occlusive dressing. Avoid placing an excess amount of tape or gauze over the site because it obstructs the view of the site. Use a clear medicine cup or other device to protect the site while allowing access and visualization.
3. Immobilize the extremity. Be careful not to apply the tape too tightly, because this blocks the flow of blood through the vein.
4. Monitor the solution drip rate to avoid giving too much or too little fluid.
5. Dispose of the needle.

Possible Complications

Pain

Infiltration (look for pain or edema at the site, inability to infuse fluids, or lack of blood return; discontinue IV and insert at another site)

Hypothermia from giving too much room-temperature fluid to an infant

Skin infection

Thrombophlebitis

Inadvertent fluid overload

Catheter shear

Inadvertent arterial puncture

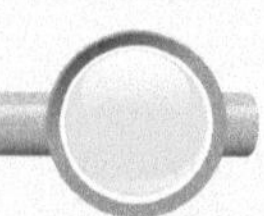

Controversy

Few children require IV access in the field or on the way to the ED. Injured children must always be transported before attempting IV access. For ill children, especially if there is a short transport time, it is controversial which ones need IV access, and whether IV access should be attempted on scene or on the way to the hospital.

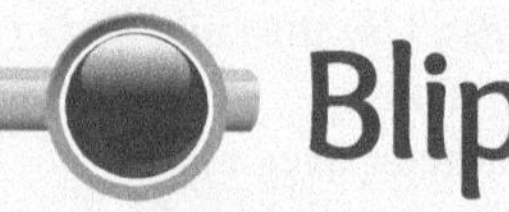

Blip

Do not use words like "stick" or "needle" when describing the procedure to the child. Instead, consider an explanation such as, "I will be putting a soft tube into your arm to give your veins a drink."

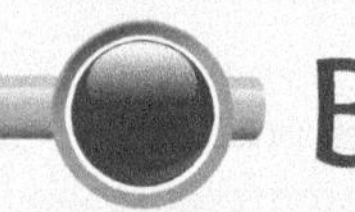

Blip

Be careful not to secure the tape too tightly to immobilize the extremity, because this blocks blood flow in the vein.

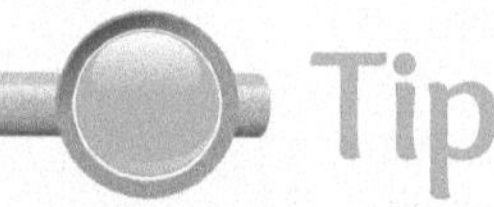

Tip

Position the child and secure the site before beginning the procedure.

Procedure 16: Intraosseous Needle Insertion

Introduction

Establishing vascular access is often difficult or impossible during life-threatening emergencies in infants and young children. The intraosseous (IO), intramedullary, or marrow route for the delivery of resuscitation fluids and medications has been used for more than 50 years in children and adults. Many studies have confirmed that the IO space is an excellent route for medications and fluids. The primary technical problem is successfully piercing the bony cortex (outer layer of the bone) in older children. The bones of neonates and infants are usually soft and the IO space is relatively large, so needle insertion is easier in children of these younger age groups. Good equipment, preparation, and effective technique are especially important for success.

Indication

Severe illness or injury requiring immediate drugs or fluids, when intravenous (IV) access is impossible or unlikely to be successful

Contraindications

Available secure IV line

Fracture or prior failed IO attempt

Equipment

IO needles

Skin cleansing solution

Normal saline and IV tubing

10-mL syringe

Extension connector and stopcock (optional)

Rationale

Using an IO needle to give drugs or fluids is an excellent alternative to cannulating peripheral veins in critically ill or injured children. The IO space is highly vascular and functions as a noncollapsible vein. Needle insertion into this space is a rapid, safe, effective, and acceptable route. In the setting of cardiac arrest, unnecessary time should not be wasted attempting intravenous access. There are several possible sites, but the easiest location is the proximal tibia. The IO space is suitable for infusion of all parenteral medications, crystalloid fluids, or blood products—which quickly traverse the small veins of the bone and eventually enter into the central circulation. Complications are usually minor and infrequent.

Preparation

Tibia and Femur Sites

1. Place the patient in the supine position.
2. Put a small towel roll under the knee.
3. Prepare the skin over the insertion site.

Possible Complications

Compartment syndrome

Failed infusion

Growth plate injury

Bone infection

Skin infection

Bone fracture

Procedure 16-1

Proximal Tibia Site

1. Use the flat surface of the proximal medial tibia, just below and medial to the tibial tuberosity on the flat side of the bone.
2. Introduce the traditional IO needle in the skin, directed away from the growth plate or pointing toward the foot.

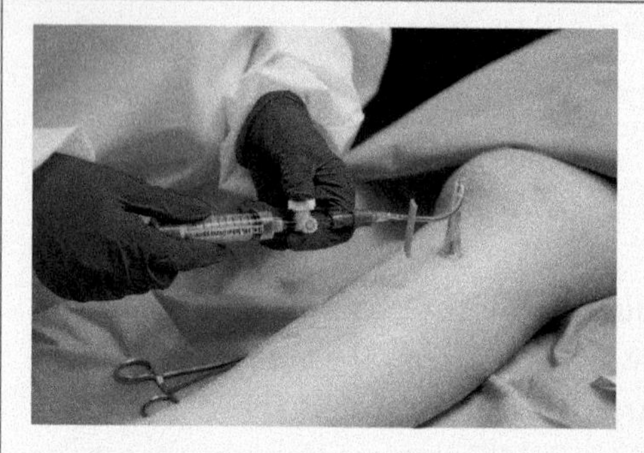

Procedure 16-2

Distal Tibia Site

1. Use the flat surface of the medial distal tibia above the medial malleolus.
2. Introduce the traditional IO needle in the skin directed away from the growth plate or toward the knee.

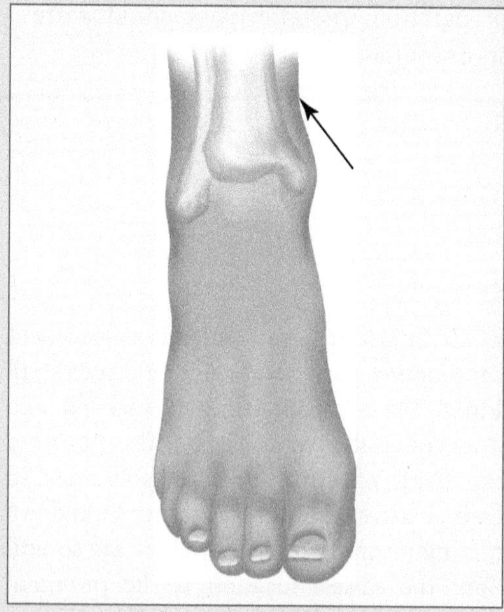

Procedure 16-3

Distal Femur Site

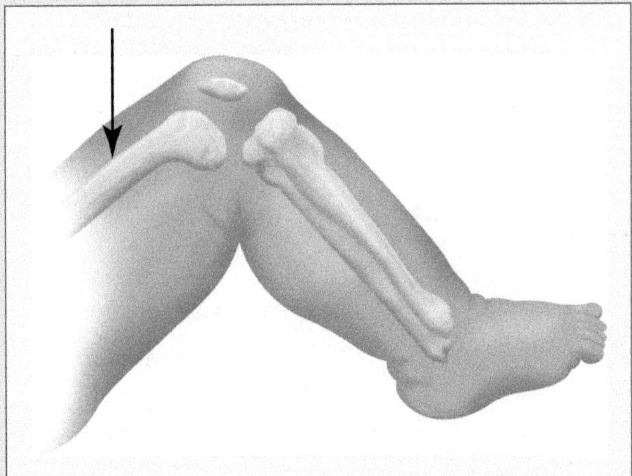

1. Use the distal third of the femur, estimate distance through soft tissue to reach bony surface of femur, and ensure that IO needle has been adjusted to a length that allows bony penetration.

2. Introduce the traditional IO needle in the skin, directed away from the growth plate or pointing toward the trunk.

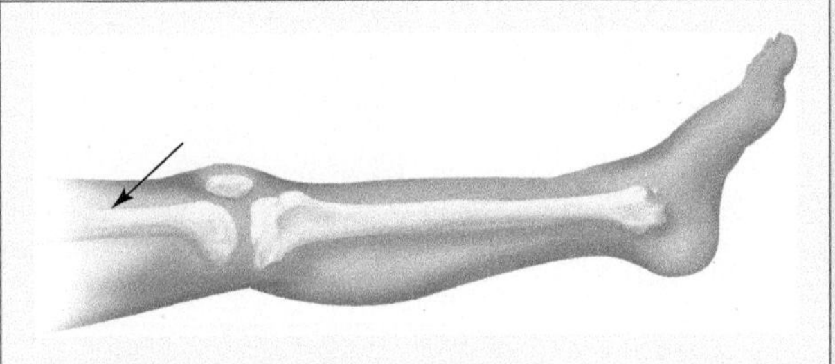

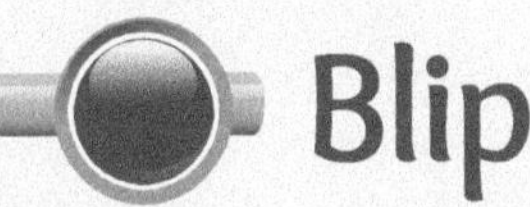

Blip

Although IO access is easy, quick, and safe, it is painful in a conscious child and therefore is only practical in a critically ill or injured child.

Procedure 16-4

Proximal Humerus Site

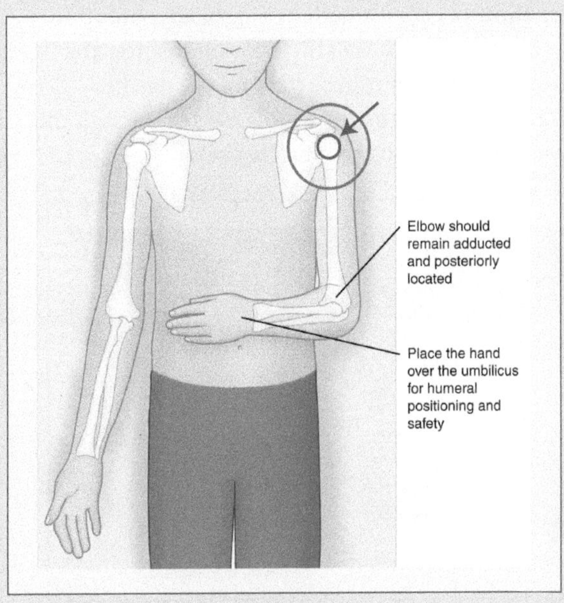
Elbow should remain adducted and posteriorly located
Place the hand over the umbilicus for humeral positioning and safety

1. With the child's hand resting on the abdomen and elbow held close to the body, palpate up the length of the humerus until a "notch" or "groove" followed by a protrusion is felt. This groove represents the surgical neck of the humerus.

2. The insertion point for the IO needle is located approximately 1 cm above the surgical neck.

(continues)

Procedure 16-4 *(continued)*

3. Secure the arm in place to prevent accidental dislodgement of the IO catheter.

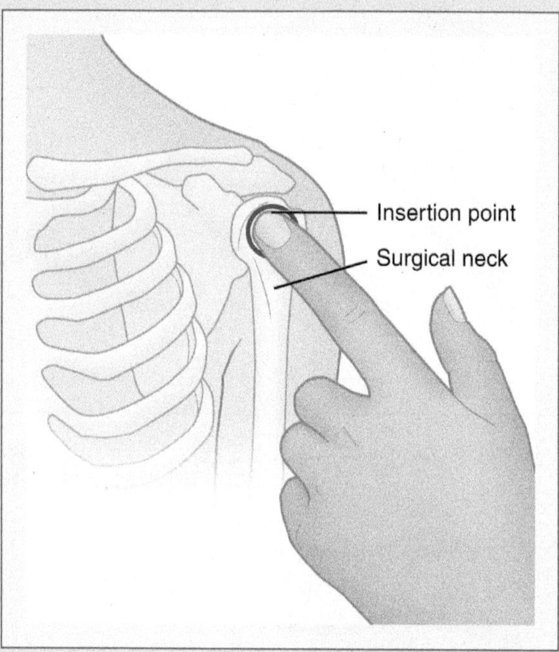

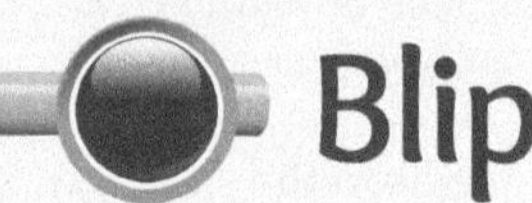

Blip

The proximal humerus should only be utilized in children whose appropriate anatomical landmarks can be identified.

Procedure 16-5

Traditional IO Insertion

1. Pierce the bony cortex with a firm, twisting motion. Use a back-and-forth twisting motion to enter the marrow space. Do not push hard on the needle. A "pop" may be felt as the needle passes through the bony cortex and into the marrow cavity.

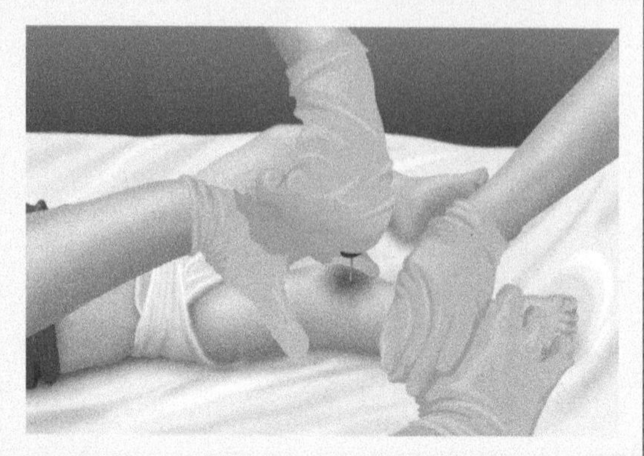

2. Remove the stylet. Any bone marrow aspirated may be used for a glucose check or other testing. However, sometimes marrow cannot be aspirated. Confirm correct placement by infusing 10 mL of normal saline without resistance or swelling around the site due to leakage of fluid.

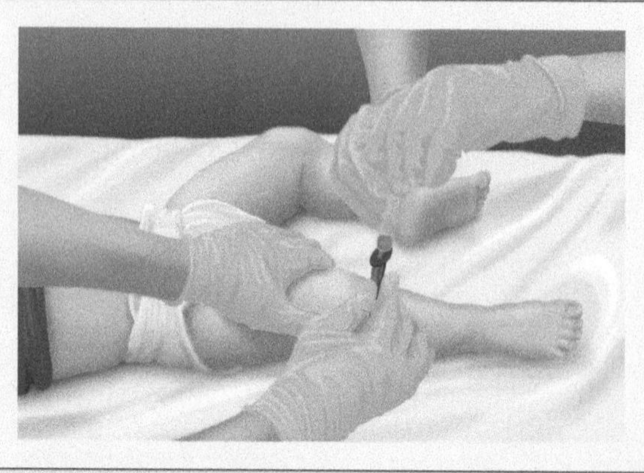

(continues)

Procedure 16-5 *(continued)*

3. Attach IV line to the hub, or to an extension connector and stopcock, and infuse fluids or drugs directly into IO space.

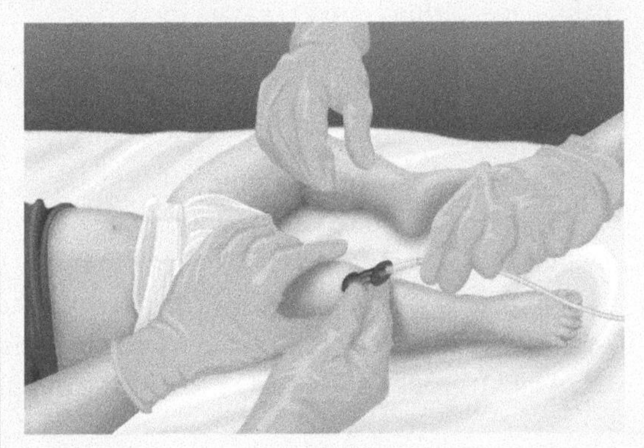

4. Secure the needle to the overlying skin with tape. Monitor the calf to ensure that there is no swelling to indicate leakage of fluid.

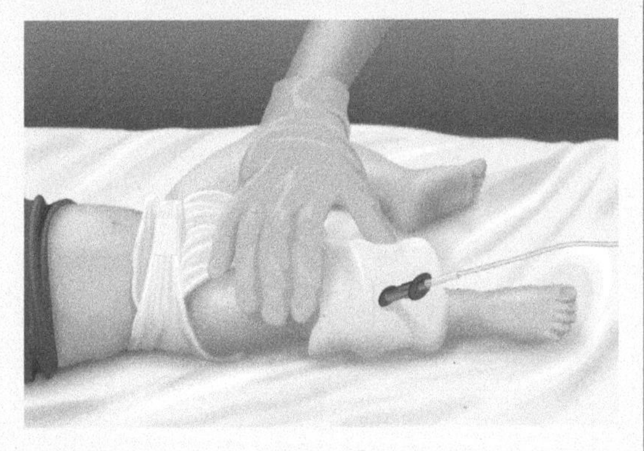

5. Continuously infuse fluids to maintain patency of IO line.

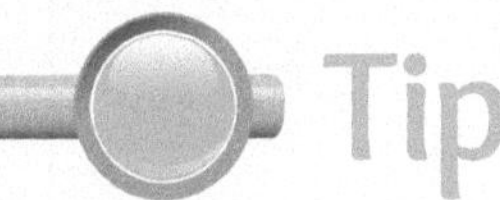

When placing a traditional IO needle, use firm pressure and a twisting motion.

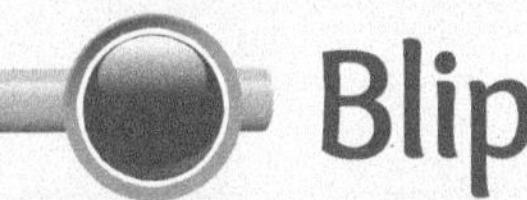

Insert the IO needle gently. Too much force may push the needle all the way through the bone and into the soft tissues.

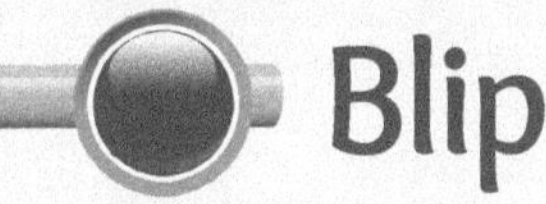

Avoid placing your hand on the calf to prevent possible injury from through-and-through IO needle penetration.

Procedure 16-6

EZ-IO Insertion

An alternate to the traditional manual IO is the EZ-IO (**Figure P16-1**). This device is approved for IO access in the anterior tibia and proximal tibia in children.

1. Select the appropriate needle for the patient's age. The adult set (for patients ≥40 kg) is 25 mm in length and red. The pediatric set (for children 3–39 kg) is 15 mm in length and blue. There is also a larger adult needle (for those ≥40 kg with excessive tissue at the insertion site), which is 45 mm in length and yellow.
2. Attach the needle to the EZ-IO drill.

(continues)

Procedure 16-6 *(continued)*

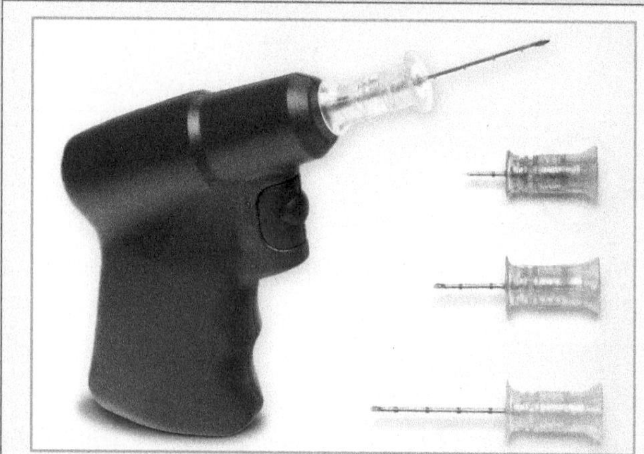

Figure P16-1 EZ-IO tool.

3 Position the needle and EZ-IO drill at 90 degrees to the bone. Press the trigger on the drill handle and apply moderate pressure, while letting the drill do the work for you. When you feel the "pop," you're in. (The pain from the EZ-IO insertion is generally similar to that of peripheral IV insertion.) As with traditional IO insertion, refrain from placing your other hand on the popliteal fossa and adjacent calf to prevent possible palm penetration from excessive force.

4 Disconnect the EZ-IO drill while leaving the needle in place.

5 Withdraw the needle stylet and confirm placement by aspiration of blood with the syringe; however, the inability to aspirate blood does not necessarily indicate improper placement. Confirm correct placement by infusing 10 mL of normal saline without resistance or swelling around the site due to leakage of fluid.

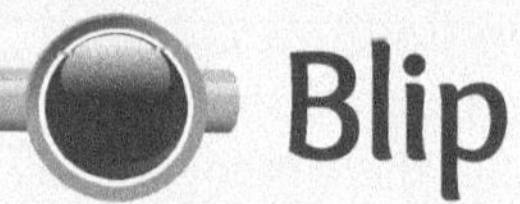

Blip

If the drill stops, you are pushing too hard.

Procedure 17: Cardiopulmonary Resuscitation

Introduction

Cardiopulmonary arrest (CPA) occurs when a patient's heart and lungs stop functioning. In children, CPA usually begins as a primary respiratory arrest. This is in contrast to adults, in whom CPA or "sudden death" is almost always a primary cardiac event that occurs with onset of ventricular fibrillation (VF) and an abrupt change in the heart's electrical activity. Because cessation of effective breathing is often the precipitating factor in pediatric CPA, airway management and ventilation are to children in CPA what defibrillation is to adults. Cardiopulmonary resuscitation (CPR) refers to basic airway management, artificial ventilation, and chest compressions to provide oxygen and circulation to core organs: the heart, brain, and lungs. In children, CPR has been shown to improve survival from drowning, and it may also benefit patients in CPA from other causes. Asphyxial cardiac arrest is more common than VF cardiac arrest in infants and children, and ventilations are extremely important in pediatric resuscitation.

Indications

Newly born, neonate, infant, or child of any age who is apneic and pulseless

Newly born with a heart rate less than 60 beats/min and not improving after standard newborn care

Neonate, infants, and children with a heart rate less than 60 beats/min and poor perfusion

Contraindication

Newly born, infant, or child with effective perfusion (palpable central or peripheral pulse)

Equipment

Mouth-to-mask device

Bag-mask device, infant or child

Airway adjuncts

Appropriate mask sizes

Rationale

CPR encompasses the basic procedures for sustaining critical oxygenation, ventilation, and perfusion recommended by the American Heart Association. The pediatric techniques are slightly modified from the adult techniques to reflect the known differences in CPA between age groups. Furthermore, there are specific differences between infants and children, including number of rescuers, placement of hands and fingers, rates of ventilation, and rates and depth of chest compressions.

Preparation

1. Position a child on a hard surface. Position a neonate or infant on a hard surface or on the forearm of the rescuer with the hand supporting the head.

Pediatric Assessment

1. ABC assessment if patient is awake and moving.
2. CAB assessment—if patient is unresponsive and not breathing (gasps do not count as breathing), check pulse.
3. If no pulse detected in 10 seconds, start chest compressions (see ratios in **Table P17-1**).
4. If definite pulse greater than 60 per minute, then administer one breath every 3 to 5 seconds.
   - Infant BLS guidelines apply to infants less than 1 year of age.
   - Child BLS guidelines apply to children 1 year of age until puberty. For teaching purposes, puberty is defined as breast development in girls and the presence of axillary hair in boys.
   - Adult BLS guidelines apply at and beyond puberty.

High-Quality CPR

High-quality CPR is defined by:

1. Chest compressions of appropriate rate and depth.
2. Push fast: push at a rate of 100–120 compressions per minute.
3. Push hard: push with sufficient force to depress at least one-third the anteroposterior (AP) diameter of the chest or approximately 1.5 in (4 cm) in infants and 2 in (5 cm) in children.
4. Allow complete chest recoil after each compression to allow the heart to refill with blood. Incomplete recoil during CPR is associated with higher intrathoracic pressures and significantly decreased venous return, coronary perfusion, blood flow, and cerebral perfusion.
5. Minimize interruptions of chest compressions.
6. Avoid excessive ventilation.
7. See ratios in **Table P17-1** for ratio of chest compressions to ventilation.
8. Rescuers should rotate the compressor role every 2 minutes to avoid fatigue.
9. Ratios do not apply if patient is intubated. Deliver breaths at a rate of 8–10 per minute and continuous chest compressions (one breath approximately every 6 seconds)
10. If the patient has return of spontaneous circulation (ROSC) with a perfusing rhythm and pulse, then breaths can be delivered at a rate of approximately 20 per minute (one breath every 3 seconds).

Table P17-1 Chest Compressions to Ventilation Ratios

Age	Compressions (min)/Ratios	Depth (inches)	Hand Placement
Newly born	3:1 ratio of compressions to ventilations (90 compressions to 30 breaths every minute); consider 15:2 if cardiac in origin	Compress approximately one-third of AP chest diameter	Two thumbs encircling the chest and supporting back (may prefer higher coronary perfusion pressure than two-finger technique)
Infant	100–120/min; 30:2 ratio of compressions to breaths for lone rescuer; 15:2 if two rescuers	Compress at least one-third the depth of the chest or about 4 cm (1.5 in)	Lone rescuers (whether lay rescuers or health care providers) should compress the sternum with two fingers placed just below the intermammary line; do not compress over the xiphoid or ribs
Child	100–120/min; 30:2 ratio of compressions to breaths for lone rescuer; 15:2 if two rescuers	Compress at least one-third of the AP dimension of the chest or approximately 5 cm (2 in)	Lone rescuers (whether lay rescuers or health care providers) should compress the lower half of sternum with heel of one or two hands
Adolescent	100–120/min; 30:2 ratio of compressions to breaths	Compress at least one-third of the AP dimension of the chest or approximately 5 cm (2 in)	Place the heel of one hand on the center of the chest (lower half of the sternum). Place the heel of your other hand over the first hand.

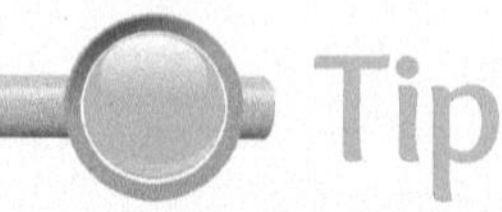

Tip

Manipulation of the head to keep the airway in a neutral position is essential for effective ventilation. A towel roll under the shoulders of the infant or small child may help maintain neutral head position.

Procedure 17-1

Performing CPR on an Infant

1. Position the infant on a firm surface. Place two fingers in the middle of the sternum just below a line between the nipples. Use two fingers to compress the chest at least one-third the AP diameter of the chest or about 4 cm (1.5 inches) at a rate of 100–120 per minute. Allow the sternum to return to its normal position between compressions.

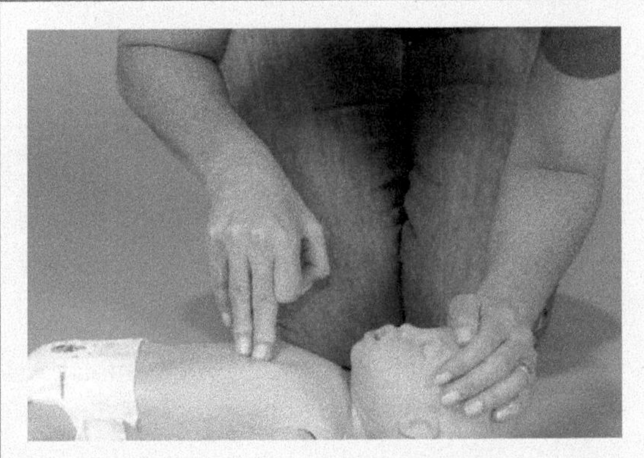

2. Coordinate compressions with ventilations in a 30:2 ratio (one rescuer) or 15:2 (two rescuers), pausing for two ventilations at the end of each cycle. Continue cycles of compressions and ventilations until an automated external defibrillator (AED) becomes available or the infant shows signs of spontaneous breathing.

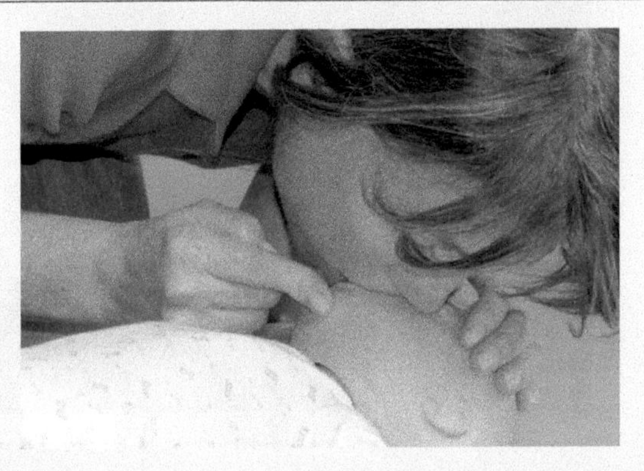

3. If two rescuers are present, compressions can also be performed at a ratio of 15 compressions to two breaths using the two thumb-encircling-hands technique.

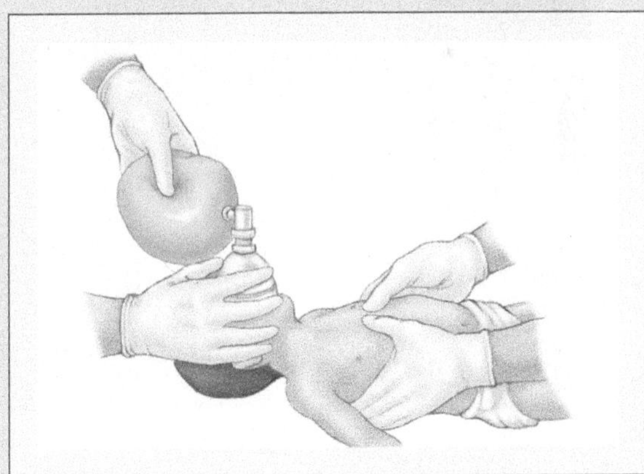

Procedure 17-2

Performing CPR on a Child

1. Place the child on a firm surface. Prepare to place the heel of one or both hands in the center of the chest, in between the nipples, avoiding the xiphoid process.

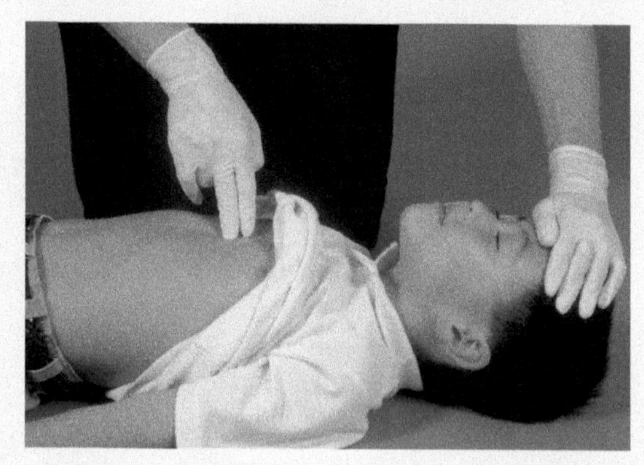

2. Compress the chest at least one-third the AP diameter of the chest or approximately 5 cm (2 inches) at a rate of 100-120 per minute.

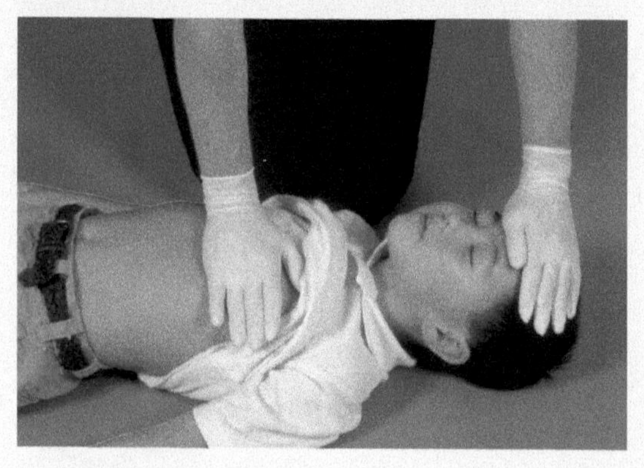

3. Coordinate compressions with ventilations in a 30:2 ratio (one rescuer) or 15:2 (two rescuers). At the end of each cycle, pause for two ventilations. Perform mouth-to-mask ventilation with 100% oxygen. Give two breaths of 1 second each.

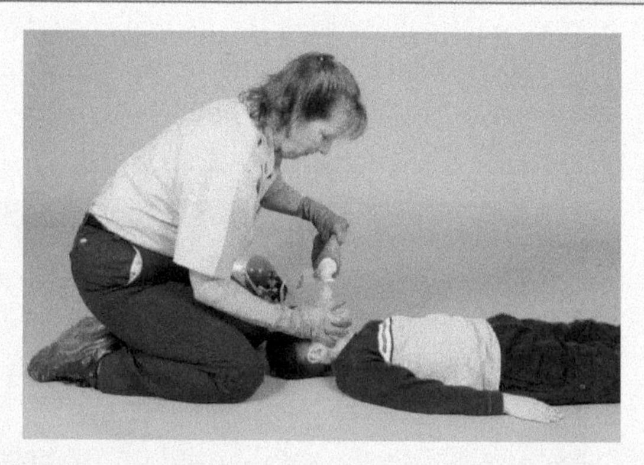

4. Continue cycles of compressions and ventilations until an AED becomes available or the patient shows signs of spontaneous breathing. If the child resumes effective breathing, place him or her in a position that allows for frequent reassessment of the airway and vital signs during transport.

Possible Complications

Coronary vessel injury

Diaphragm injury

Hemopericardium

Hemothorax

Interference with ventilation

Liver injury

Myocardial injury

Pneumothorax

Rib fractures

Spleen injury

Sternal fracture

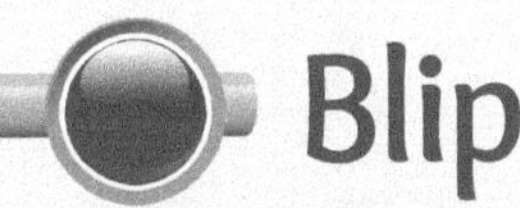

Blip

A common problem in the transition from one-rescuer to two-rescuer child CPR is the lack of coordination between ventilations and compressions.

Use of End-Tidal Carbon Dioxide ($ETCO_2$) for Quality of Compressions

1. Exhaled CO_2 is reflective of cardiac output during a cardiac arrest, because pulmonary blood flow must exist for $ETCO_2$ to register.
2. Quantitative $ETCO_2$ may be used to monitor quality of CPR. Normal $ETCO_2$ with a good mask seal or if the patient is intubated is approximately 35–45 mm Hg. During a cardiac arrest, the $ETCO_2$ value will be much lower and can theoretically reach 0 if the patient has no pulse and is not receiving chest compressions.
3. Potential goals for quantitative $ETCO_2$ during a pulseless arrest are greater than 15 mm Hg.
4. If ROSC is achieved, the $ETCO_2$ will begin to rise, reflecting increasing blood flow for cardiac output.
5. After circulation (ROSC) is restored, monitor systemic oxygen saturation. It may be reasonable, when appropriate equipment is available, to titrate oxygen administration to maintain the oxyhemoglobin saturation greater than or equal to 94%.

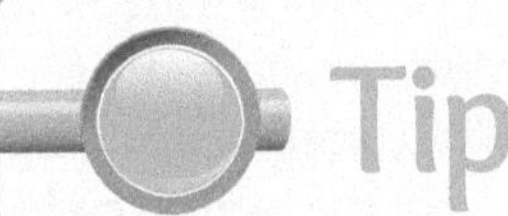

Tip

CO_2 may be lowered through prolonged O_2 administration above what is necessary due to lowering of systemic vascular resistance.

Procedure 18: AED and Defibrillation

Introduction

Synchronized cardioversion for tachydysrhythmias has long been part of adult emergency care. However, ventricular dysrhythmias are rare in children, especially in infants, and pediatric supraventricular tachycardia (SVT) is usually treatable with medical therapy. All providers should be prepared to provide synchronized cardioversion or defibrillation in appropriate situations. Ventricular fibrillation (VF) is observed in 5%–15% of pediatric and adolescent arrest. However, when a child develops VF or pulseless ventricular tachycardia, defibrillation (unsynchronized cardioversion) may be lifesaving. Synchronized cardioversion may resuscitate a child in shock with SVT. Synchronized cardioversion provides a shock that is timed (synchronized) with the QRS complex, avoiding delivery during the refractory period of the cardiac cycle, when a shock could produce VF. Use the synchronized mode for selected cases of SVT or ventricular tachycardia with a pulse, and the asynchronized (defibrillation) mode for VF or ventricular tachycardia without a pulse.

Indications

Ventricular fibrillation

Pulseless ventricular tachycardia

SVT with shock and no vascular access rapidly available (synchronized)

Ventricular tachycardia with shock and unresponsiveness with pulse

Atrial fibrillation or atrial flutter with shock

Contraindications

Conscious patient with good perfusion

Equipment

Automatic external defibrillator with pads appropriate for age

Standard defibrillator with paddles or pads appropriate for age

Rationale

When a child's heart rhythm deteriorates into ventricular tachycardia or fibrillation, there is usually a severe systemic insult, such as profound hypoxia, ischemia, electrolyte abnormalities, electrocution, or myocarditis. Death may result if treatment is delayed. SVT, in contrast, is usually a more stable cardiac rhythm. When the child is pulseless and has VF or ventricular tachycardia, perform defibrillation as quickly as possible with the appropriate technique. If a child has SVT or ventricular tachycardia with a pulse and shock, use synchronized cardioversion.

Do not attempt to perform synchronized cardioversion on a child with SVT who is well perfused.

Preparation

1. Open airway and ventilate with bag-mask device with 100% oxygen if indicated, while assembling equipment for cardioversion or defibrillation.
2. If child is pulseless, begin closed-chest compressions, until an automated external defibrillator (AED) or conventional defibrillator is available.

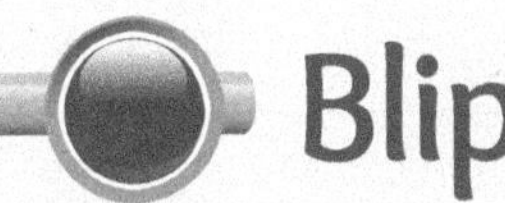

Blip

Do not deliver synchronized cardioversion to a conscious child with SVT or ventricular tachycardia unless the child is in shock and has no intravenous (IV) or intraosseous (IO) access rapidly available for medical treatment.

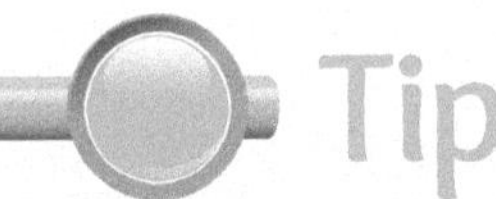

Tip

For a child with ventricular fibrillation or pulseless ventricular tachycardia, use the asynchronized (defibrillation) mode.

Procedure 18-1

Conventional Defibrillator Use

1. Apply the paddles or pads directly to the skin. Place one paddle or pad on the anterior chest wall on the right side of the sternum inferior to the clavicle and the other paddle or pad on the left midclavicular line at the level of the xiphoid process. As another option, use the anterior-posterior position.

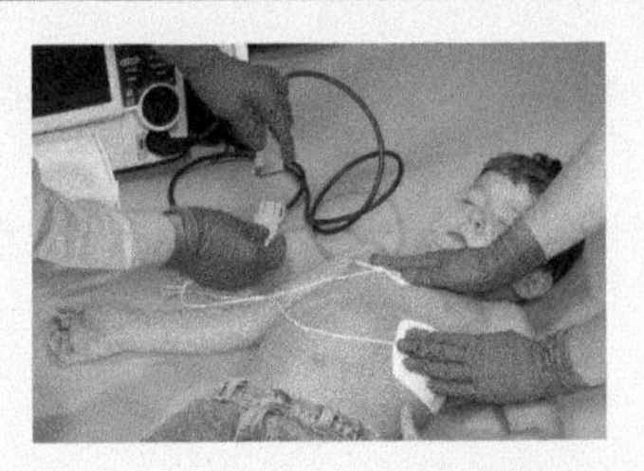

2. Clear the nearby area to avoid shocking someone. Announce, "I am going to shock on three. One, I am clear. Two, you are clear. Three, everybody is clear."

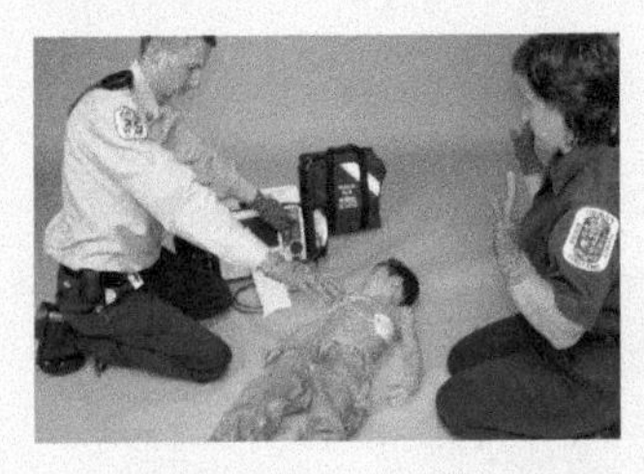

3. Begin recording rhythm. Deliver the electrical countershock with firm pressure.

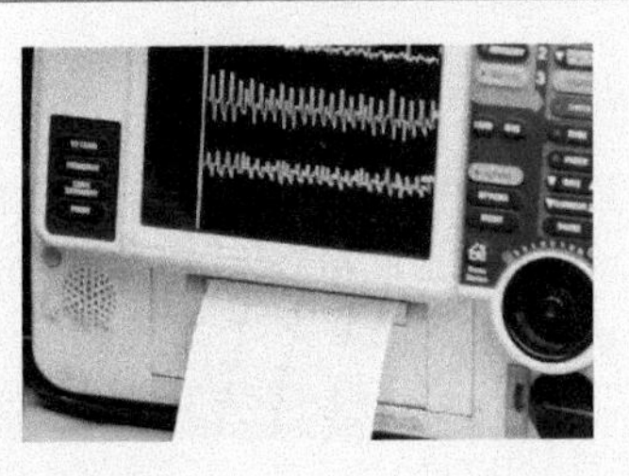

4. If CPR was being performed prior to shock, resume CPR for 2 minutes. Then check monitor for a change in rhythm, and check pulse.

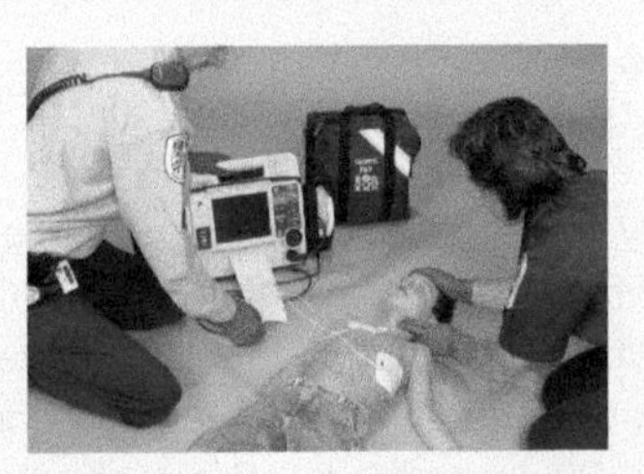

5. If the first electrical shock is unsuccessful, resume CPR, then reanalyze the rhythm after 2 minutes (five cycles) of CPR. Give specific dysrhythmia treatment with epinephrine or other drugs, as per EMS protocol. Treat bradycardia or other dysrhythmias.

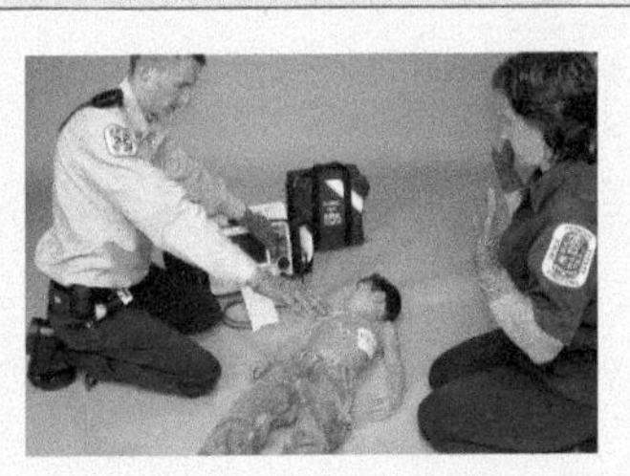

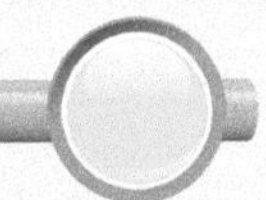

Controversy

The preferred paddle location in children is controversial and no study in humans has compared the two techniques. Anterior chest wall placement has the advantage of a supine child and easier airway management. Anterior-posterior placement may allow larger paddles and more effective delivery of the charge.

Preparation

Conventional Defibrillator Use

1. Select the proper paddle or pad size. Use the 8-cm adult paddles if these will fit on the chest wall; otherwise, use the 4.5-cm pediatric paddles (**Table P18-1**).
2. Prepare paddles or skin electrodes with electrode jelly, paste, or saline-soaked gauze pads, or use self-adhesive defibrillator pads. Do not let jelly or paste from one site touch the other and form an "electrical bridge" between sites, which could result in ineffective defibrillation or skin burns.
3. Establish appropriate electrical charge (**Table P18-2**).
4. Select synchronized or asynchronized mode.
5. Properly charge pack and stop chest compressions.

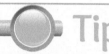

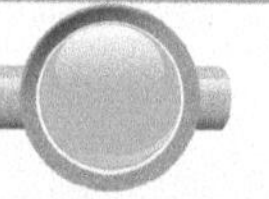

Tip

Maintain high-quality chest compressions until defibrillator is charged when you are analyzing rhythm OR as long as possible when using AED mode. Immediately resume compressions once rhythm is analyzed and does not suggest a shock OR immediately after a shock is delivered.

Table P18-1 Paddle Size

Paddle Size
• 8-cm Adult paddles (use in children older than 12 months of age or weighing more than 10 kg) On anterior chest wall, OR Anterior-posterior
• 4.5-cm Pediatric paddles (use in infants up to 12 months of age or weighing less than 10 kg) on the anterior chest wall

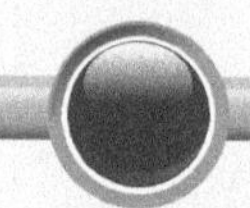

Blip

Failure to firmly apply paddles to the chest wall decreases effective delivery of charge.

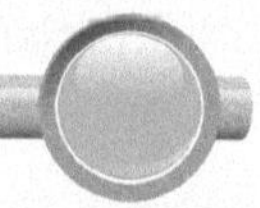

Tip

Consider giving a benzodiazepine before cardioversion if patient is awake.

Procedure 18-2

One Rescuer with an AED

For children younger than 8 years of age, use a child-pad cable system if available.

1. Verify unresponsiveness.
2. Look for no breathing or only gasping and check pulse.

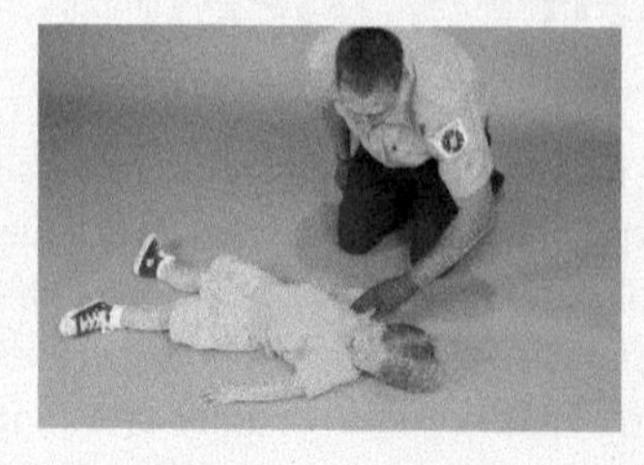

3. If not breathing but with a pulse, begin bag-mask ventilations.
4. If no pulse, begin CPR with 30 compressions and 2 breaths.

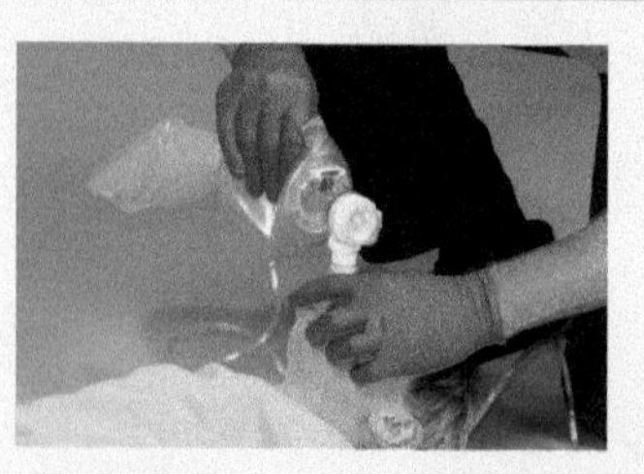

5. Apply AED as soon as it is available.
6. POWER ON the AED and follow voice prompts. Some devices will turn on when the AED lid or carrying case is opened.

(continues)

Procedure 18-2 *(continued)*

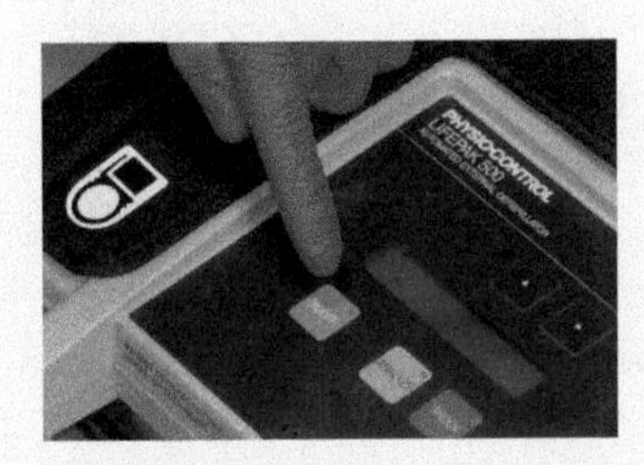

7 ATTACH the AED. Select the correct pads for victim's size and age (adult versus child). Peel the backing from the pads. Attach the adhesive pads to the victim as shown on the pads. (If only adult pads are available, and they overlap when placed on the chest, use an anterior [chest] and posterior [back] placement.) Attach the electrode cable to the AED (if not preconnected).

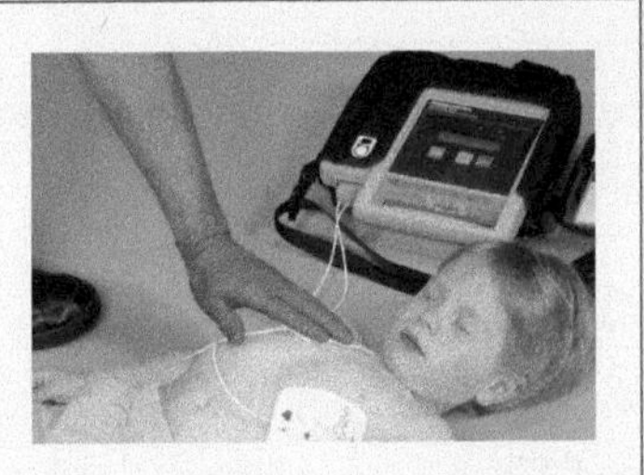

8 Allow the AED to ANALYZE the victim's rhythm ("clear" victim during analysis). Deliver a SHOCK if needed ("clear" victim before shock).

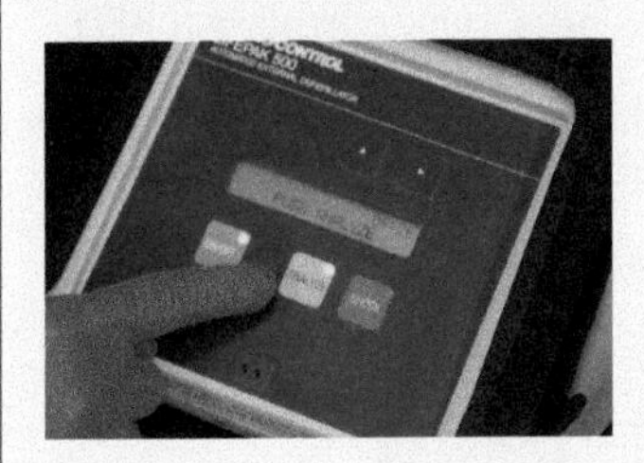

Reasonable variations in this sequence are acceptable.

9 Resume CPR.

Table P18-2 Appropriate Electrical Charge for Countershock

Dysrhythmia	Mode	Charge
Ventricular fibrillation Ventricular tachycardia without a pulse	Defibrillation (asynchronized)	2 J/kg, then 4 J/kg, then 4 J/kg, as needed. Then 4 J/kg after CPR and each dose of medication. More than 4 J/kg may be delivered, but do not deliver more than 10 J/kg.
Ventricular tachycardia with pulse, SVT	Synchronized cardioversion	0.5–1.0 J/kg. Repeat as needed.
Atrial fibrillation and atrial flutter with shock	Synchronized cardioversion	If no result with 0.5–1.0 J/kg, may use up to 2 J/kg

Possible Complications

Ineffective delivery of countershock because of failure to charge, improper positioning on the chest, incorrect paddle size, or improper conduction medium

Burns on the chest wall

Failure to "clear" before voltage discharge, leading to electrical shock of a team member or bystander

Tachydysrhythmia

Bradycardia

Myocardial damage or necrosis

Cardiogenic shock

Embolic phenomena

Procedure 18-3

Two Rescuer AED Sequence of Action

1. Verify unresponsiveness. Have partner get AED.
2. Look for no breathing or only gasping and check pulse.

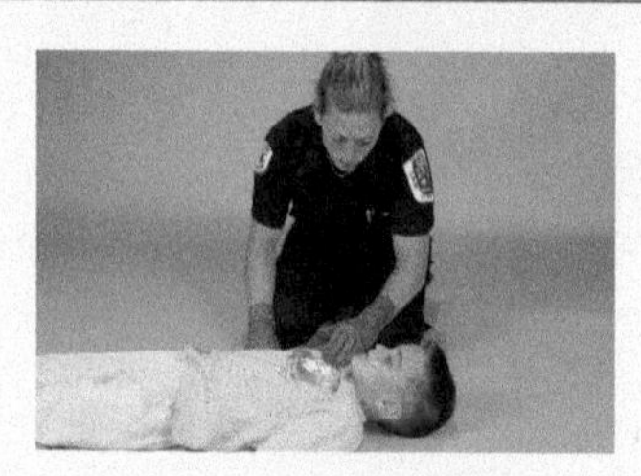

3. If no pulse, start CPR. If not breathing but with a pulse, begin bag-mask ventilations.
4. Apply AED as soon as it is available.
5. Attempt defibrillation with the AED if no signs of circulation are present. Place the AED near the rescuer who will be operating it. The AED is usually placed on the side of the victim opposite the rescuer who is performing CPR. The rescuer begins performing CPR while the rescuer who was performing CPR prepares to operate the AED. (It is acceptable to reverse these roles.)

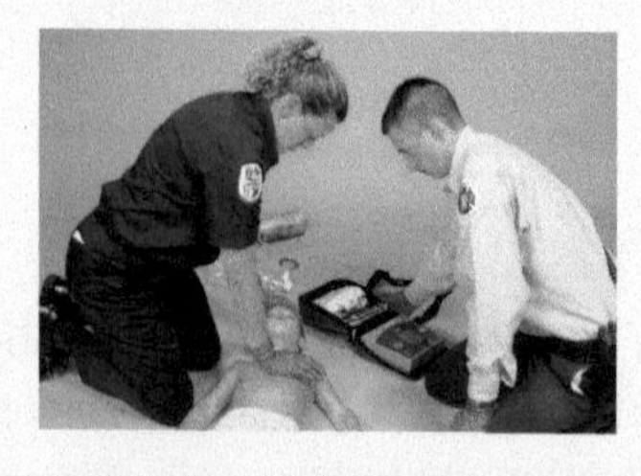

6. The AED operator takes the following actions. POWER ON the AED first (some devices will turn on automatically when the AED lid or carrying case is opened).

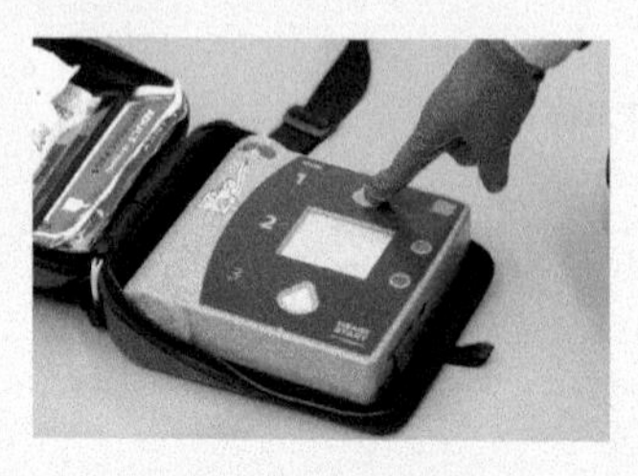

7. ATTACH the AED to the victim. Select correct pads for the victim's size and age. Peel the backing from the pads. Ask the rescuer performing CPR to stop chest compressions. Attach the adhesive pads to the victim as shown on the pads. (If only adult pads are available, and they overlap when placed on the chest, use an anterior [chest] and posterior [back] placement.) Attach the AED connecting cables to the AED (if not preconnected). ANALYZE rhythm. Clear the victim before and during analysis. Check that no one is touching the victim. Press the ANALYZE button to start rhythm analysis (some brands of AEDs do not require this step).

   "Shock Indicated" message. Resume CPR until AED is charged and ready to deliver shock. Clear the victim once more before pushing the SHOCK button ("I'm clear, you're clear, everybody's clear"). Check that no one is touching the victim. Press the SHOCK button (victim may display muscle contractions).

   "No Shock Indicated" message. Resume CPR immediately after the shock is given.

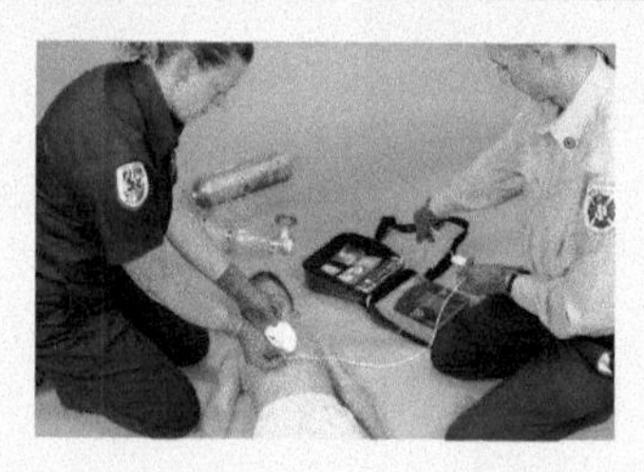

8. After about two minutes of CPR (or when prompted by the AED), analyze rhythm, then follow the "shock indicated" or "no shock indicated" steps as appropriate.

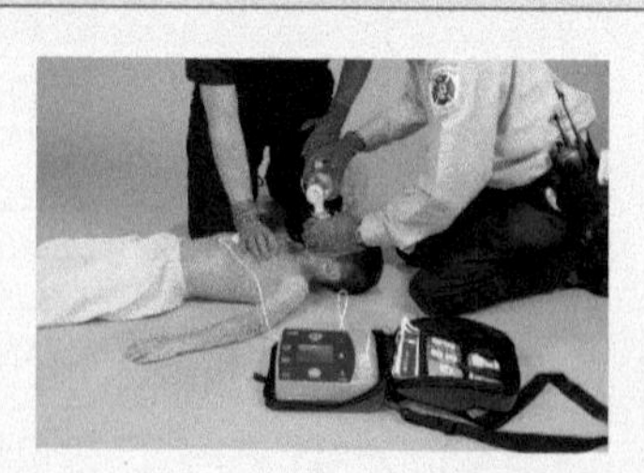

Procedure 19: Endotracheal Tube Drug Instillation

Introduction

The ability of the airways of the lungs to absorb medicines has been recognized for more than a century. Giving medication through an endotracheal (ET) tube is an alternative to intravenous (IV) or intraosseous (IO) drug delivery in a cardiopulmonary resuscitation, when necessary. The airways are well vascularized and can absorb certain emergency medications. Drug dosages and dilutions in ET delivery are different from IV or IO administration. ET drug delivery has been deemphasized; while this route of administration is better than no drug delivery, it is less effective than IV or IO. Once vascular access has been achieved, consideration should be given to repeating drugs if there has been no response to the ET drug delivery.

Indications

Cardiopulmonary resuscitation

Lack of IV or IO access

Contraindication

Functioning IV or IO access

Equipment

ET tube

Long catheter (feeding tube, suction catheter, nasogastric [NG] tube, or umbilical catheter)

Catheter size (in French units): approximately two times ET tube size (in mm) (**Table P19-1**)

Desired drug/diluent mixture

Normal saline

Self-inflating ventilation device

Use 1–3 mL of diluent in infants, and 5–10 mL maximum in older children.

Table P19-1 Suggested Catheter Size per Tracheal Tube

Endotracheal Tube Size (mm)	Catheter Size (Fr)
2.5	5
3.0	6
3.5–4.5	8
5.0–6.5	10
7.0	12

Rationale

If neither IV nor IO access is available for giving drugs during cardiopulmonary resuscitation, the ET route is a good alternative for pediatric drugs (atropine, naloxone, lidocaine, and epinephrine). The absorption, blood levels, onset, and duration of action are different with each drug. ET doses are unique for each agent, and are higher than IV or IO doses because absorption is not as good. While ET drugs are probably not as effective as IV or IO drugs, they can help improve the chances of successful resuscitation while IV or IO access is established.

Preparation

1. Intubate the patient.
2. Stabilize and secure the ET tube.
3. Preoxygenate and ventilate.

Possible Complications

Hypoxia

Hypercarbia

Pneumonitis

Tracheal injury

Adverse side effects of drug itself

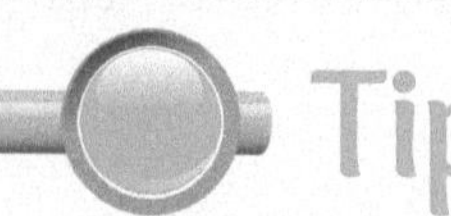

ET drug administration is a potential route for medications during early phases of resuscitation.

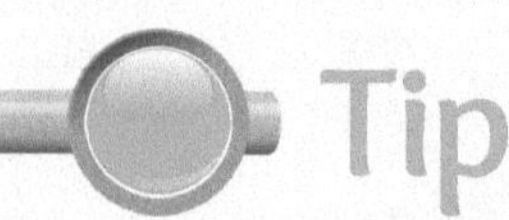

IV and IO are better routes of drug administration than the ET route.

Procedure 19-1

Endotracheal Drug Delivery

1. Draw the calculated drug dose into a syringe.
2. Dilute the medication with normal saline.
3. Insert tip of small feeding tube or catheter past distal tip of ET tube.
4. Instill solution directly into the trachea.
5. Follow with positive-pressure breaths.
6. Ventilate three times with self-inflating ventilation device to disperse the solution into the entire lung. Repeat medications if indicated.

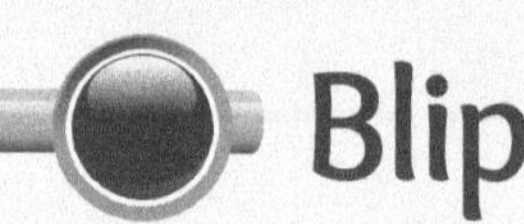

Never give sodium bicarbonate by the ET tube.

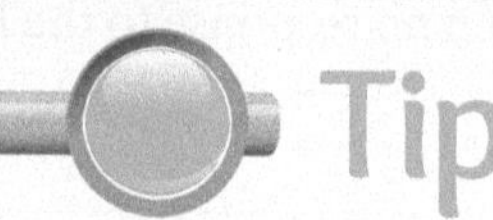

Drugs approved for ET installation: lidocaine, epinephrine, atropine, and naloxone.

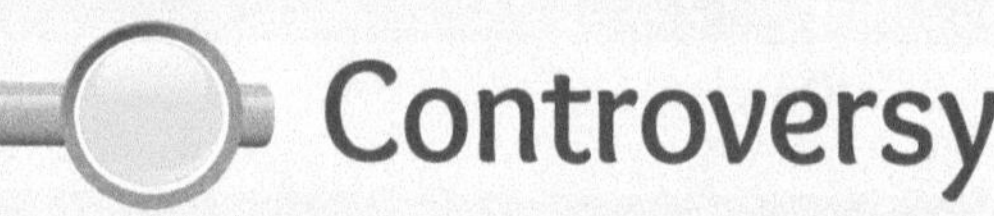

The absorption and extent of central delivery of drugs given by ET tube is not known and dose recommendations have not been validated by scientific studies on children.

Procedure 20: Rectal Administration of Benzodiazepines

Introduction

Rectal drug administration is a well-known delivery technique in children and is useful for many medications, including antipyretics and anticonvulsants. The only rectal medication approved in most EMS systems is diazepam for pediatric status epilepticus. Status epilepticus is a major pediatric medical emergency that may benefit from quick treatment. Although the first priority is airway and breathing, additional therapy may include medication to terminate the seizure. There remains significant controversy regarding the administration of rectal drugs from a safety and effectiveness stance. Rectal diazepam is an effective route with few added complications when other routes of administration are not immediately available. It is important to ask if the parents have administered a rectal gel form of diazepam prior to EMS arrival.

Indication

Status epilepticus

Contraindications

Newborn age (a month or less) (relative)

Recent rectal surgery (e.g., for Hirschsprung disease, imperforate anus) (relative)

Equipment

Lubricant

Tuberculin syringe, or 14- to 20-gauge over-the-needle catheter with 3- to 5-mL syringe

Intravenous (IV) solution of diazepam

Tape (optional)

Rationale

Establishing IV or intraosseous (IO) access is often time consuming and may delay delivery of essential advanced life support (ALS) drugs, especially in infants and toddlers. The rectum is an effective alternative route for emergency drug administration. The rectum is highly vascularized, and certain drugs are quickly absorbed through the lining or mucosa. Diazepam is a lipid-soluble benzodiazepine that is reliably absorbed through the rectum and terminates most seizures without further treatment. It takes a few minutes longer to stop the seizure after rectal administration of diazepam as compared to IV diazepam. Occasionally, as with the IV diazepam preparation, more than one dose of rectal diazepam is necessary. One reason is because of the drug's short duration of action and recurrence of seizure activity.

Rectal lorazepam also has been used in the treatment of status epilepticus. This is less frequently encountered in the out-of-hospital setting because of the manufacturer's recommendations to keep this drug refrigerated. Lorazepam may be stored for up to 30 days unrefrigerated at room temperature.

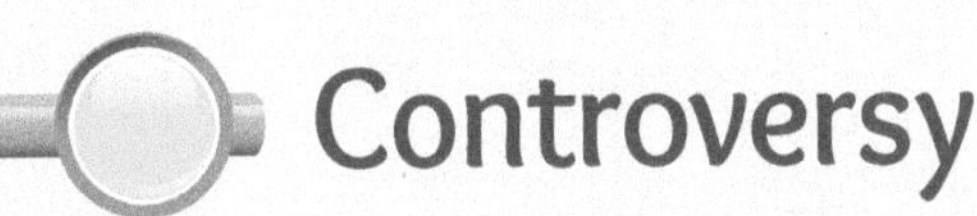

The optimal non-IV route and which drug to use are not known.

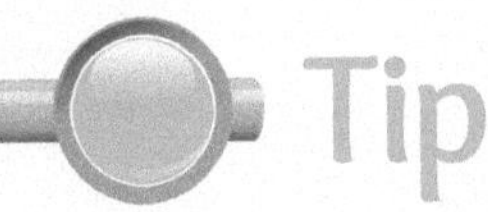

The most serious potential complication of rectal diazepam is respiratory depression, which is usually from the drug, but may be from the prolonged seizure or the underlying cause of the seizure.

Preparation

1. Use the pediatric resuscitation tape or resuscitation software to determine the weight of the child (see Procedure 2), or establish the patient's weight from information provided by the caregiver.
2. Draw up the calculated dose of IV medication into a disposable tuberculin syringe or 3- to 5-mL syringe.
3. Lubricate the syringe or catheter:
    - If using the tuberculin syringe as the administration device, remove needle and apply lubricant to the tip of the syringe.
    - If using a 3- to 5-mL syringe (or tuberculin syringe, to draw up medication only), remove needle, attach over-the-needle catheter (plastic portion only), and lubricate catheter.

Possible Complications

Respiratory depression

Administration that is too high in the rectum with inadequate serum level

Rectal tearing

Procedure 20-1

Rectal Administration of Benzodiazepines

1 Position the patient in the decubitus position, knee-chest position, or supine position with a second prehospital professional or the caregiver holding the legs apart.

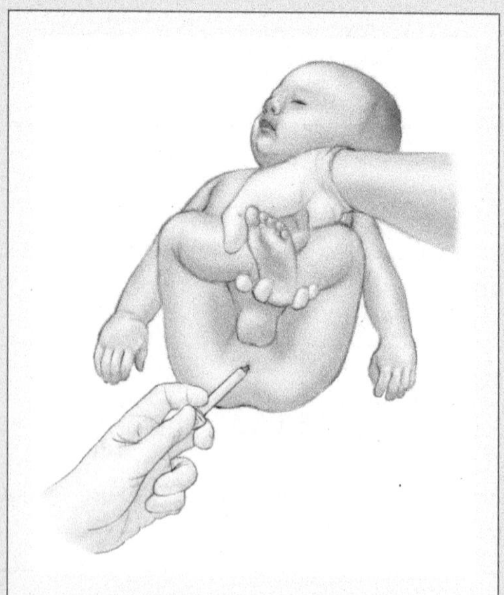

2 Carefully introduce the syringe or over-the-needle catheter approximately 5 cm (2 in) into the rectum. Inject the solution into the rectum. Remove the syringe. Hold buttocks closed for 10 seconds. Tape buttocks closed (optional).

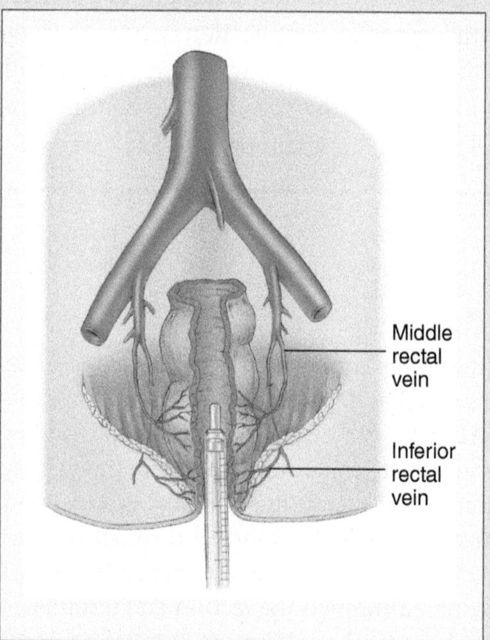

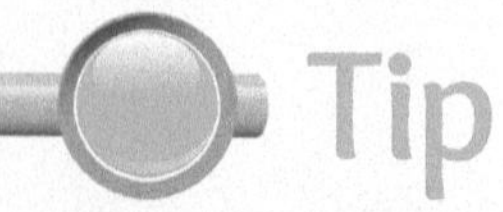

The rectal dose of diazepam is 0.5 mg/kg, to a maximum dose of 20 mg. Onset of action for rectal diazepam is slower than IV dose.

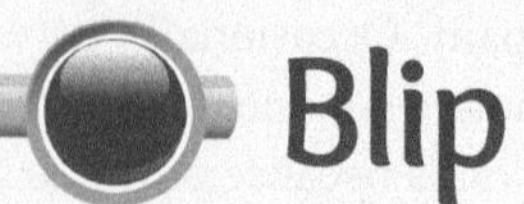

Administration of diazepam too high into the rectum may decrease its anticonvulsant effect, because the drug may be absorbed differently and broken down more quickly in the liver.

Procedure 21: Spinal Motion Restriction

Introduction

Spinal injury may be subtle or difficult to recognize because of altered mental state, distracting injuries, or lack of obvious signs. Failure to recognize potential spinal injury can lead to death or permanent disability. Spinal motion restriction is therefore essential for every child who sustains a suspicious mechanism of injury (where the head, neck, or spine may be involved), who has pain or tenderness of the spine, or who has signs or symptoms of weakness or loss of sensation.

Indications

Any significant mechanism of injury above the clavicles, including the head, face, or neck to the axial spine

Acute weakness or loss of sensation after a potential spinal injury

Pain or tenderness to the neck or spine

Deformity to the neck or spine

Altered mental state after an injury

Contraindications

The combative child is a relative contraindication because forceful restraint of a combative child with spinal or head injury can worsen the injury.

If the risks of agitation and increased spinal movement from full spinal stabilization are greater than the benefits, consider more acceptable but less definitive stabilization options, and document the circumstances clearly.

Equipment

Long spine board

Padding materials (blankets, towels)

Rigid cervical collars in pediatric sizes

Straps with fastening device

Wide tape (2 or 3 in)

Optional equipment:

Head cushions from a cervical spine stabilization device (CID)

Rationale

The spinal column is made of 33 articulating bones, and its structure changes significantly during childhood growth. The age of the child and the physical state of spinal growth are important factors in the incidence and types of pediatric spinal injuries. Whenever the mechanism of injury, signs, or symptoms suggests possible spinal injury, the entire spine must be stabilized. Maintain the anatomic stability of the entire spinal column as carefully as possible, and use age-specific considerations in approaching the child to minimize spinal movement.

Preparation

1. If the child is unstable or the environment is unsafe, quickly remove the patient onto the stretcher or the long spine board using manual spinal stabilization techniques.
2. Spinal boards or extrication devices can be used to move the child onto the stretcher.
3. Anatomic differences, specifically the large size of an infant or child's head, require modification of stabilization procedures. For example, place a thin (1 inch) layer of padding beneath the child's body from the shoulder to the hips.
4. Prepare the child and caregiver for the procedure by explaining actions. Make a game of it for an alert, cooperative child.

Possible Complications

Airway obstruction

Impairment of ventilation

Obscuring hemorrhage or other injuries

Spinal injury from improper technique

Back pain

Procedure 21-1

Initial Manual Spinal Stabilization

1. Gently align the head and neck into a neutral position similar to the "sniffing position." Do not force neutral position if there is resistance to movement, crepitus, or increased spinal pain.

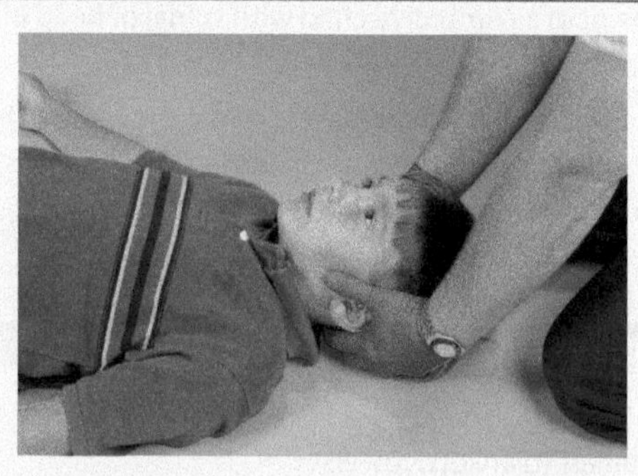

2. Have an additional rescuer(s) restrain other body parts as needed to reduce motion.

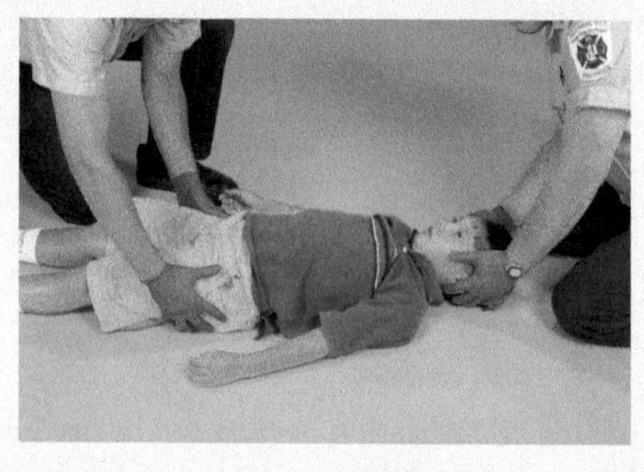

3. Have a second rescuer apply a size-appropriate rigid cervical collar. Evaluate the neck area that will be covered by the cervical collar. Determine the appropriate size with the manufacturer's recommendations. If a correctly sized cervical collar is unavailable, move on to the next step.

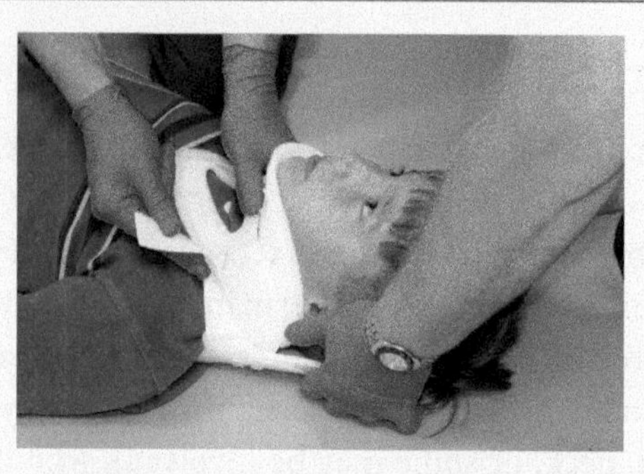

4. Transfer the patient as a unit onto a stretcher or spine board, or alternate stabilization device that is long enough to support the patient's full length. A board or other extrication device can be used to facilitate movement onto the stretcher. Perform the clinical assessment of the patient's back, buttocks, and breath sounds during the log roll or lift and slide process. Be prepared to treat injuries. After placing the child on the stretcher or board, pad all open spaces under the patient before securing the patient.

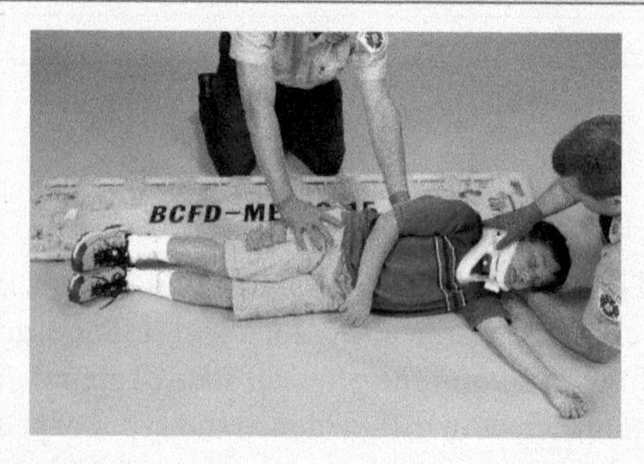

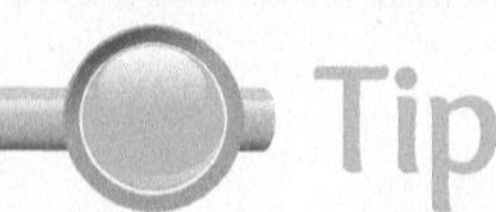

Reassure nervous children that the spinal stabilization is only temporary, but it is necessary. Try distraction.

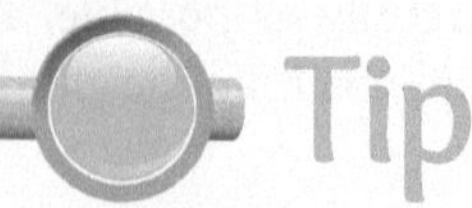

Assign one rescuer to in-line neck stabilization of a combative child.

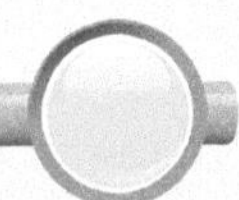

Controversy

The indications for spinal stabilization of infants and toddlers are unknown. Infants and young children cannot verbally communicate symptoms, such as weakness, numbness, or pain, so the threshold for spinal stabilization must be lower than for the older child. However, restraining a conscious child on a spine board or backboard can cause pain and agitation, and is not necessary.

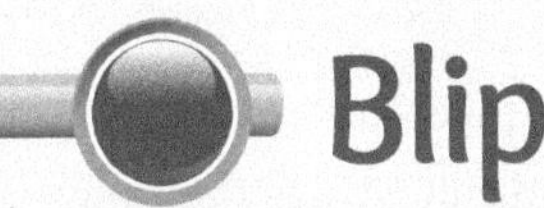

Blip

Do not accept the labeled sizes for cervical collars ("pediatric" or "infant"). Measure each patient individually.

Procedure 21-2

Securing a Patient to a Stretcher or Spinal Stabilization Device

1. Secure the patient's body to the stretcher or board while manually maintaining the neutral alignment of the head and neck. To secure against lateral movement, pad along the patient's sides, especially along the pelvis and legs.

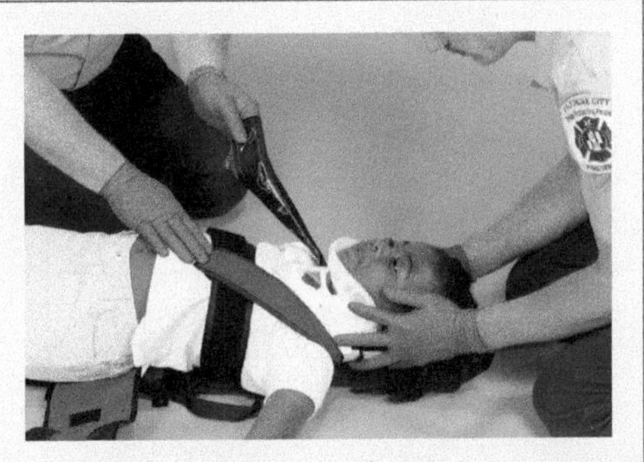

2. Stabilize the cervical spine by using blanket rolls, or blocks from the CID, to restrict lateral head motion and rotation and to prevent upward motion of the shoulders. Do not pad under the young child's head because the large occiput will flex the neck and bends the airway out of neutral position. Secure against axial shifts if the stretcher or board needs to be tilted (going down stairs, fitting into a small elevator, or for elevating the head in cases of head injury).

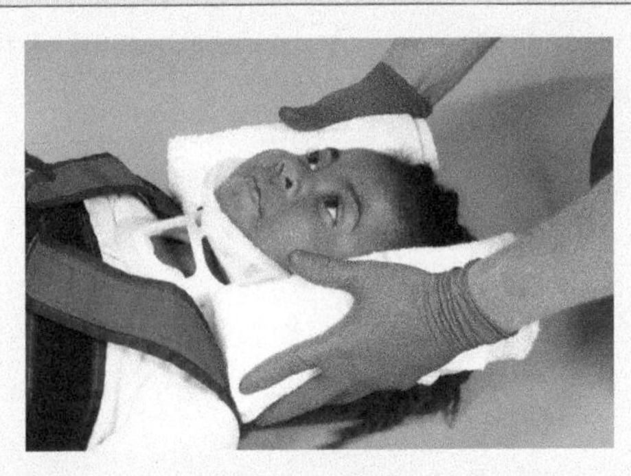

3. Place straps across the patient at the level of the axilla, pelvis, and legs. Do not place straps over the abdomen or use straps to impair movement of the diaphragm.

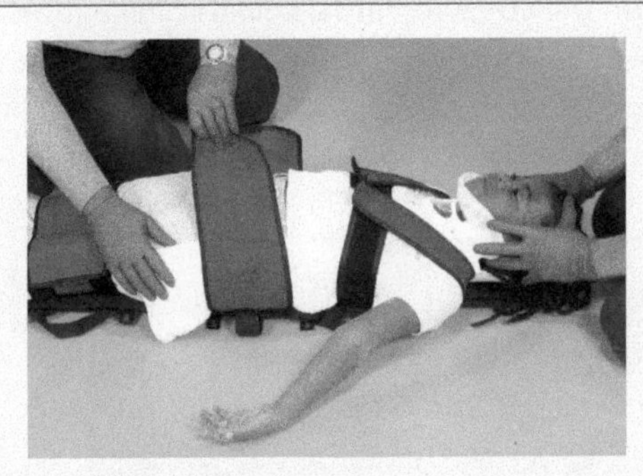

(continues)

Procedure 21-2 *(continued)*

4. Further secure the head with tape directly above the patient's eyebrows. Avoid chin straps that may complicate airway maintenance in case of emesis.

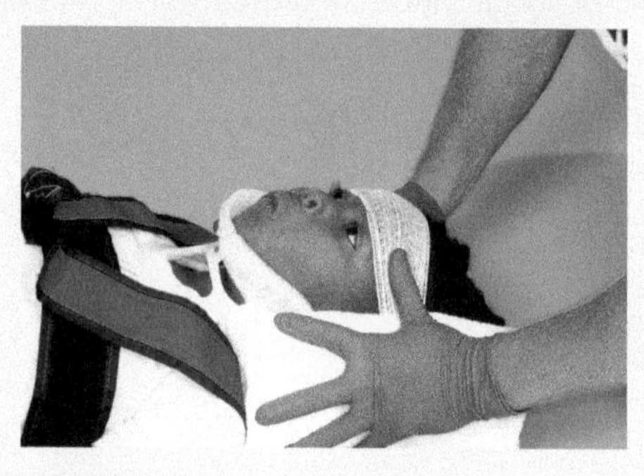

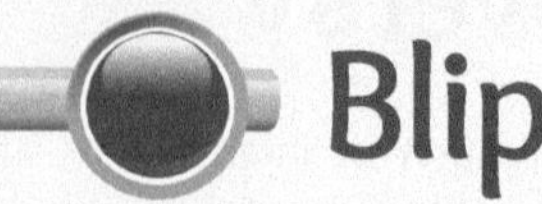

Blip

Never place tape across the child's neck, because this may obstruct the airway.

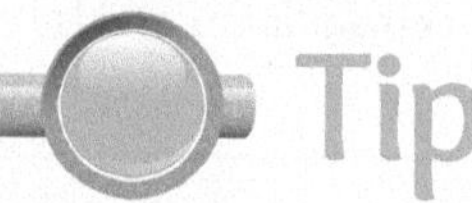

Tip

When using tape, use the longest strips possible to maximize adhesive surface and security.

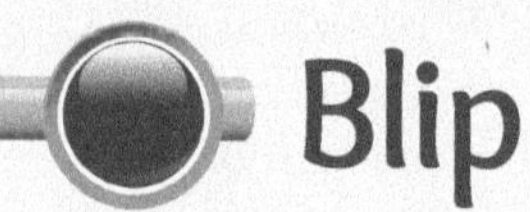

Blip

Do not use sandbags or weighted material because of the risk of injury in the event of movement.

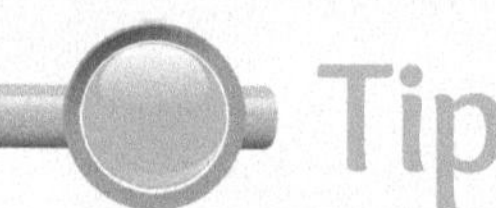

Tip

Spinal boards have been associated with adverse effects in some patients and are not always necessary for maintenance of spinal stabilization.

Procedure 21-3

Pediatric Spinal Stabilization Using a Vest-Type Stabilization Device

1. Perform the steps for initial spinal stabilization. Remove the vest device from its case. Open the head and body flaps. If the child's legs are longer than the device, place the device on a long spine board.

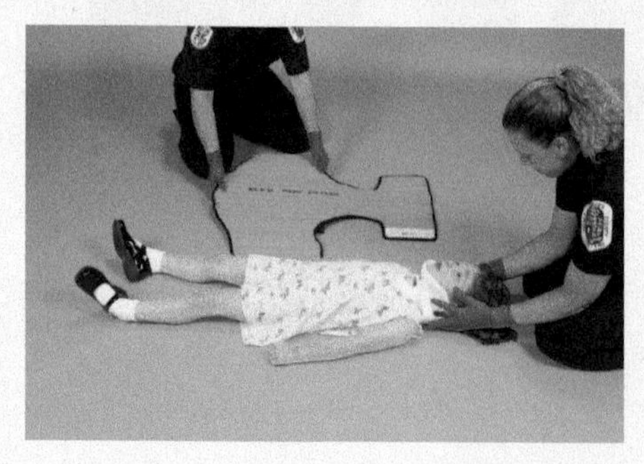

2. If padding is required to keep the child in neutral position, place it on the device.

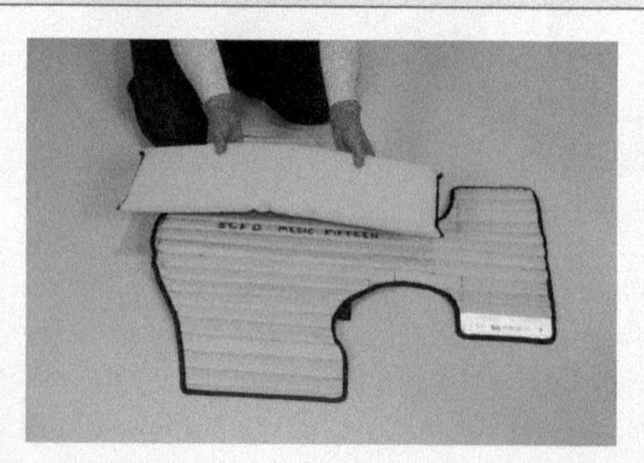

(continues)

Procedure 21-3 *(continued)*

3. Using standard techniques (log roll, or lift and slide), move the patient as a unit onto the device.

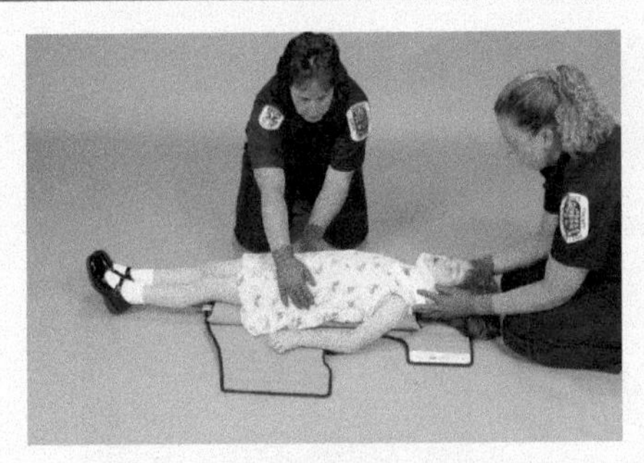

4. Lift the body flaps up and fold them inward on themselves along the lateral sides of the patient. This ensures that the abdomen and chest are not restricted.

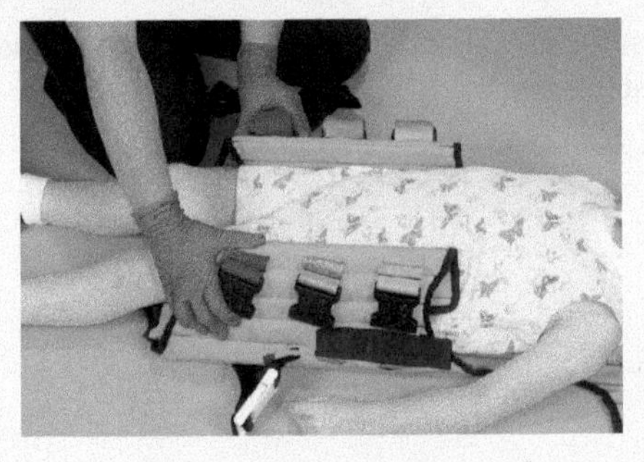

5. Secure the body flaps across the patient's trunk with tape or the attached straps. Make sure not to restrict the child's diaphragm or breathing.

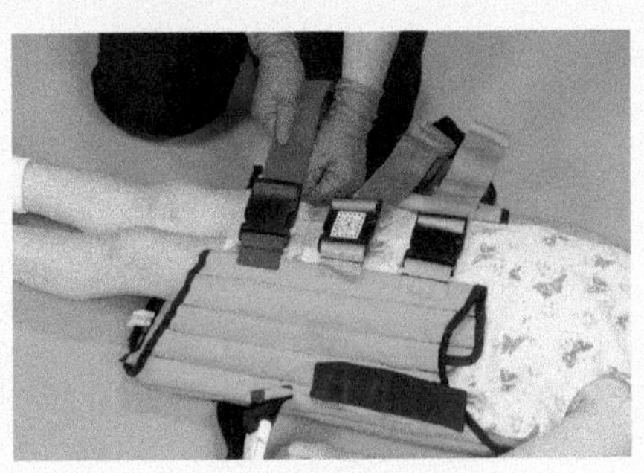

6. Lift the head flaps up along the child's head, and then fold the flaps down to the side so that the top edges are even with the child's forehead.

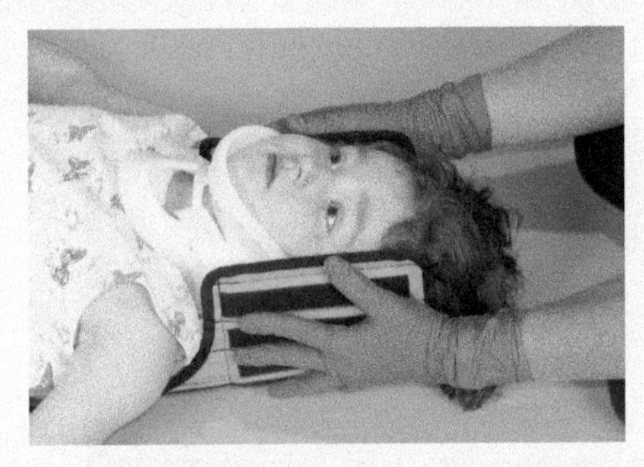

7. Place a strap across the child's forehead, connecting it across both sides of the head flaps. Secure the stabilized child to a long spine board or stretcher.

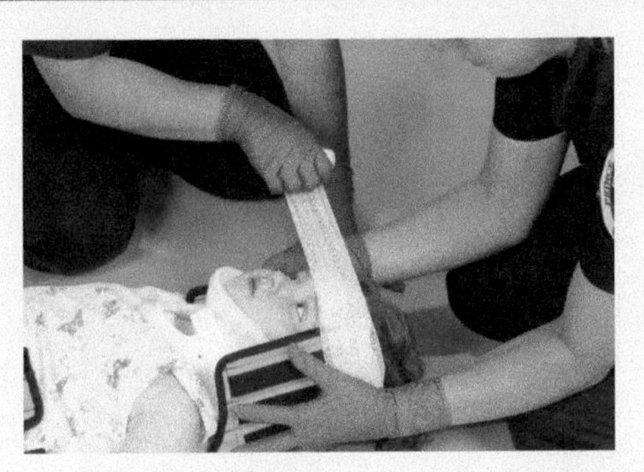

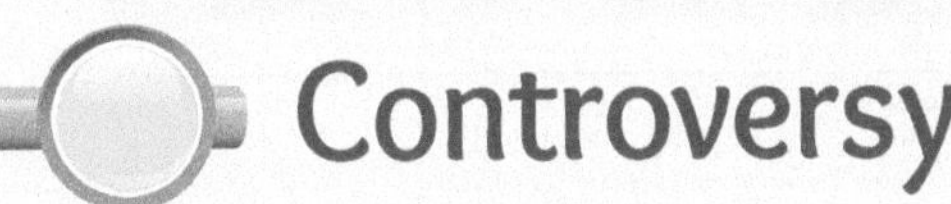

Controversy

The effectiveness and safety of the vest-type spinal stabilization device is controversial. The device is supposed to provide added restraint to a long spine board, but risks and benefits are not established.

Procedure 21-4

Releasing and Monitoring Spinal Stabilization

1. Do not release manual head and neck stabilization until the entire spine is properly stabilized.

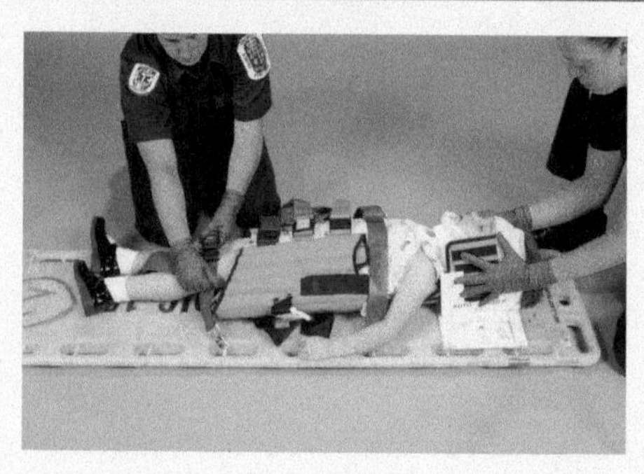

2. Reassess airway, breathing, and circulation for possible compromise caused by spinal stabilization technique.

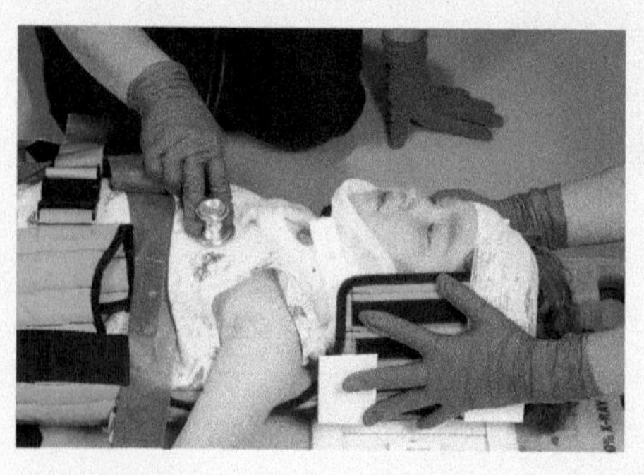

3. Assess the patient's distal neurologic status before and after spinal stabilization.

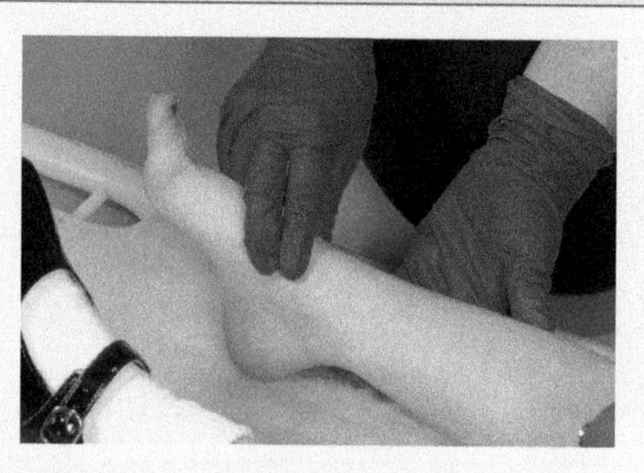

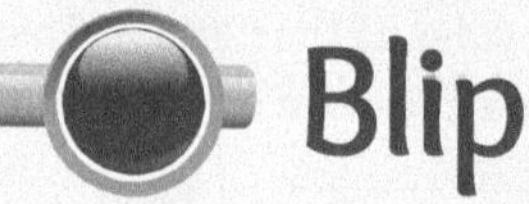

Blip

Never release manual neck stabilization until the spine is properly stabilized.

Procedure 22: Needle Thoracostomy

Introduction

A pneumothorax occurs when air gets between the two pleural membranes of the lung, a potential space that is virtually empty under normal breathing conditions. Tension pneumothorax develops when the air in the pleural space has enough pressure to shift the internal contents of the chest and impair the function of the lungs, heart, and great vessels. Reduction in blood return to the heart and diminished cardiopulmonary function results in shock and cardiopulmonary arrest if the tension pneumothorax is untreated. The child with tension pneumothorax has usually had positive-pressure ventilation in the field and has physiologic abnormalities on assessment, with evidence of increased work of breathing and hypoxia. Classical adult physical findings, such as a shifted trachea or diminished breath sounds on the affected side, may not be detectable in an infant or child. If cardiac output is severely impaired by the tension pneumothorax, the child also exhibits shock.

Indications

Penetrating chest wall injury in a child with poor perfusion accompanied by respiratory distress and hypoxia

Blunt chest wall injury in a child with respiratory distress and hypoxia that worsens with assisted ventilation

Contraindication

History of a severe bleeding disorder, such as hemophilia (relative)

Equipment

14- or 16-gauge over-the-needle catheter

30-mL syringe

Skin cleansing solution

Rationale

When the mechanism of injury, signs, and symptoms suggest tension pneumothorax in a child, create an opening between the pleural space and the atmosphere to immediately reduce elevated intrapleural pressure. This helps reexpand the lung, improve venous return, and restore cardiopulmonary function. The easiest method for creating a communication between the pleural space and the outside atmosphere is by producing an open pneumothorax. The technique requires inserting a large-bore needle into the pleural space and leaving it open to the air.

Preparation

1. Position the child supine.
2. Raise the arm above the head on the affected side, and have the caregiver or second rescuer hold it.
3. Select the site:
   - Second intercostal space at the midclavicular line OR
   - Fourth intercostal space at the anterior axillary line
4. Before preparing the site, count the ribs twice to ensure proper site location. The nipple is usually at the fourth intercostal space.
5. Prepare the site with skin cleansing solution.

Possible Complications

Open pneumothorax

Hemothorax

Diaphragm penetration

Bowel penetration

Hemopericardium

Intercostal nerve or vessel or other intrathoracic vessel injury

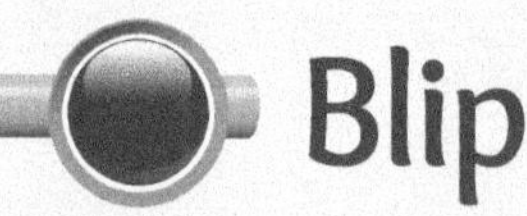

Blip

Do not insert the needle under the rib margin, because the vessels and nerves there are easily injured. Insert ***above*** the rib.

Procedure 22-1

Needle Thoracostomy

1. Attach the needle, with catheter in place, to the syringe.
2. Insert the needle through the skin at 90 degrees and advance until the tip hits a rib.

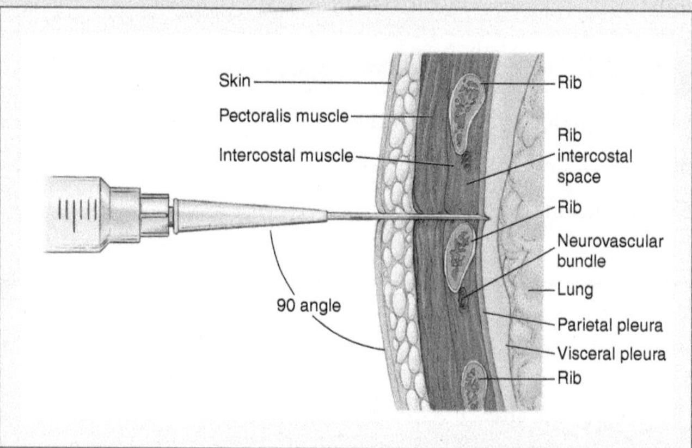

3. Advance the needle over the top of the rib margin.
4. Push the needle tip into the pleural space. A slight "pop" is usually felt when the needle pierces the outside pleural membrane, or parietal pleura.
5. Pull back the plunger of the needle to aspirate air.
6. Remove the syringe and needle and leave the catheter in the pleural space, anchored in the chest wall.
7. Monitor work of breathing, circulation to skin, heart rate, respiratory rate, and blood pressure. Consider doing contralateral needle thoracostomy if the child does not improve.

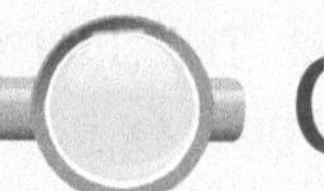

Controversy

The frequency of tension pneumothorax after blunt chest-wall injury is not known, and the indications for needle thoracostomy in this out-of-hospital situation are controversial.

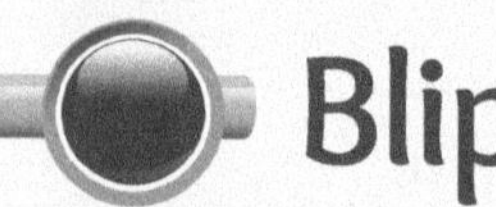

Blip

A shifted trachea or diminished breath sounds may not be detectable in an infant or young child with a tension pneumothorax.

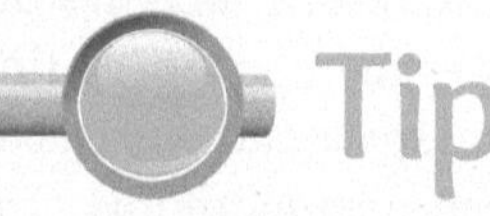

Tip

Suspect a tension pneumothorax when a child with chest injury worsens with assisted ventilation.

Procedure 23: Removing and Replacing a Tracheostomy Tube

Introduction

Children with tracheostomy tubes are increasingly common in the out-of-hospital setting. Most of these children live at home and have trained caregivers. Rarely, a tracheostomy tube problem occurs with a technology-assisted child (TAC) and 9-1-1 is activated.

Indications

Decannulation

Obstruction

Contraindications

Inadequately sized tract or stoma for insertion of a new tracheostomy tube; in this case, insert an endotracheal tube

Lack of a replacement tracheostomy tube or appropriately sized endotracheal tube

New tract and breathing adequately

Equipment

Suction device

Sterile suction catheters

Oxygen

Bag-mask device, standard pediatric and adult mask sizes

Tracheostomy cannulas, appropriately sized for patient

Endotracheal tubes, standard pediatric and adult sizes

Laryngoscope handle with blades

Tape or tracheostomy ties

Gauze pads

5- or 10-mL syringe

Water-soluble lubricant

Scissors

Sterile saline

Stethoscope

Rationale

Treatment of a tracheostomy tube problem usually requires simple techniques, such as suctioning or removal of the old tube and replacement with a new tube. Partial airway obstruction from clogging of the old tube may not be relieved by suctioning alone, or it may be impossible to ventilate a child through an existing tracheostomy tube because of decannulation or severe obstruction. Under these conditions, the prehospital professional may need to place a new tracheostomy tube to save the child's life.

Preparation

1. Ask the caregiver if there are any special problems with the child's trachea or special requirements involving the child's tracheostomy.
2. Ask the caregiver if a replacement tracheostomy tube is available.
3. Speak directly to the child about what to expect and attempt to enlist her cooperation.

Possible Complications

Creation of a false lumen

Subcutaneous air

Pneumomediastinum

Pneumothorax

Bleeding at insertion site

Bleeding through tube

Mainstem intubation with endotracheal tube (usually right mainstem)

Procedure 23-1

Removing an Old Tracheostomy Tube

1. Position the child with the head and neck hyperextended to expose the tracheostomy site.
2. Apply oxygen over the mouth and nose.
3. If the existing tube has a cuff, deflate it. Connect a 5- to 10-mL syringe to the valve on the pilot balloon. Draw air out until the balloon collapses. Cutting the balloon will not deflate the cuff.
4. Cut or untie the cloth ties that hold the tracheostomy tube in place.
5. Withdraw the tracheostomy tube using a slow, steady, outward and downward motion.
6. Assess airway for patency and adequate ventilation.
7. Provide oxygen and ventilation as needed (through the stoma if necessary).

Procedure 23-2

Replacing the Tracheostomy Tube

Insert a tracheostomy tube of the same size and model whenever possible. If this is not available, use a smaller tube or an endotracheal tube of the same inner diameter as the tracheostomy tube.

1. If the tube uses an insertion obturator, place this in the tube. If the tube has an inner and outer cannula, use the outer cannula and obturator for insertion.
2. Moisten or lubricate the tip of the tube (and obturator) with water, sterile saline, or a water-soluble lubricant.
3. Hold the device by the flange (wings) or hold the actual tube like a pencil.
4. Gently insert the tube with an arching motion (follow the curvature of the tube) posteriorly and then downward. Slight traction on the skin above or below the stoma may help.

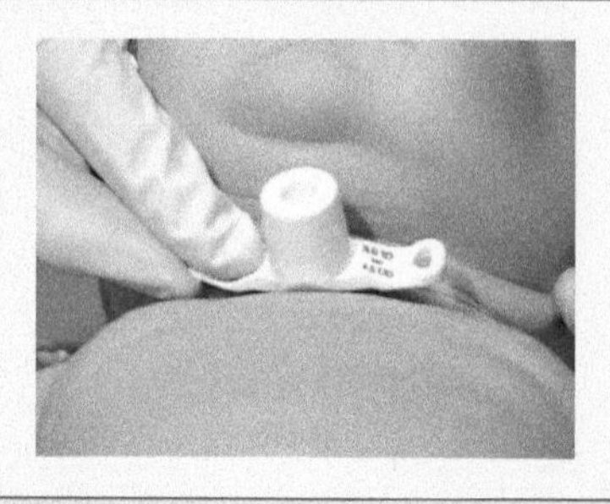

5. Once the tube is in place, remove the obturator, attach the bag-mask device, and attempt to ventilate. If the tube uses an inner cannula, insert to allow mechanical ventilation with a bag-mask device.
6. Check for proper placement by watching for bilateral chest rise, listening for equal breath sounds, and observing the patient. Signs of improper placement include lack of chest rise, unusual resistance to assisted ventilation, air in the surrounding tissues, and lack of patient improvement.
7. If the tube cannot be inserted, withdraw the tube, administer oxygen, and ventilate as needed.
8. Use a smaller-size tracheostomy tube for the second attempt. If still unsuccessful with a smaller tracheostomy tube, insert an endotracheal tube through the stoma. Check the length of the original tracheostomy tube, note the markings on the endotracheal tube, and advance it to the same depth as the original tube. The inserted portion of the endotracheal tube will be approximately half the distance needed for oral insertion. Do not advance the tube too far, or it may go into a mainstem bronchus (usually the right).
9. If still unsuccessful, use a suction catheter as a guide. Insert a small, sterile suction catheter through the tracheostomy tube. Without applying suction, insert the suction catheter into the stoma. Slide the

(continues)

Procedure 23-2 *(continued)*

tracheostomy tube along the suction catheter and into the stoma, until it is in the proper position. Remove the suction catheter. Assess ventilation through the tracheostomy tube.

10. If still unsuccessful, consider orotracheal intubation or transport the patient with ventilation through the stoma using a stoma mask or newborn mask, or through bag-mask device over the nose and mouth while covering the stoma with a sterile gauze.

11. After proper placement, cut the ends of the tracheostomy ties or tape diagonally (allows for easy insertion); pass through eyelets (openings) on the flanges; and tie around the patient's neck, so that only a little finger can pass between the ties and the neck.

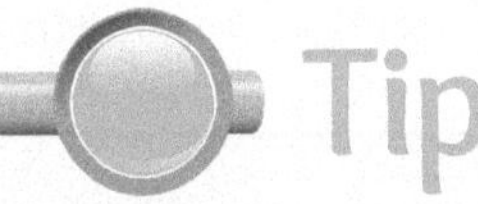

Talk to the caregiver about the size and type of tracheostomy tube and about known problems with the stoma or tube.

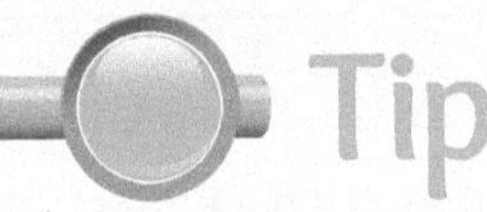

If unable to reinsert a tracheostomy tube, use a similarly sized or smaller endotracheal tube.

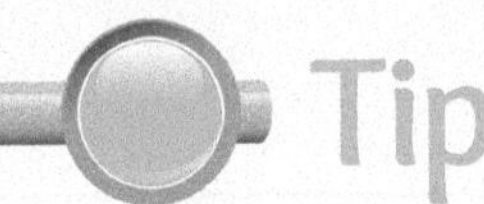

Keep the suction catheter close at hand.

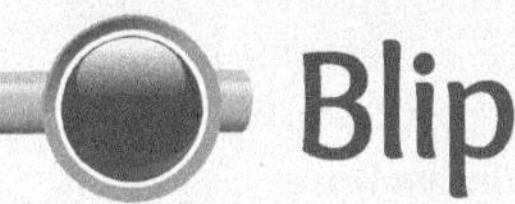

Do not force a tracheostomy tube, especially through a new stoma site. Consider inserting a smaller-size tracheostomy or endotracheal tube.

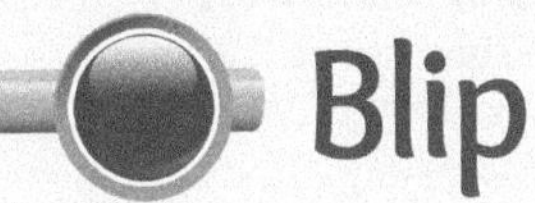

Do not advance an endotracheal tube too far through the stoma.

Note: The following drugs may be used for pediatric prehospital care. Certain drugs may not be available in some EMS systems per local policy. The drugs in tables designated by a green bar are core drugs commonly used in EMS systems. The drugs designated by a yellow bar are optional drugs that are sometimes used for children in EMS systems.

Acetaminophen, APAP, Paracetamol		
Use: Analgesic, Antipyretic	**Recommended Dose** 10–15 mg/kg **Maximum Dose** 1 g	**Precaution:** Ensure proper concentration. Use with caution in patients with liver disease. **Adverse Reactions:** Nausea, vomiting

Activated Charcoal		
Use: Gastric decontamination	**Recommended Dose** Initial dose: < *12 years*: 1–2 g/kg **Maximum Dose** 100 g	**Precaution:** Based on local EMS policy, the prehospital professional should consult either medical oversight or poison control (1-800-222-1222). Iron, lithium, alcohols, ethylene glycol, alkalis, fluoride, mineral acids, and potassium do not bind to activated charcoal. Avoid aspiration. If airway reflexes are impaired, the risk of administering activated charcoal may outweigh the benefits. Commercially available preparations of activated charcoal often contain sorbitol as a cathartic. Fatal hypernatremic dehydration has been reported after repeated doses of charcoal with sorbitol. **Adverse Reactions:** Constipation, obstruction, intestinal bezoar, diarrhea, dehydration, pulmonary aspiration

Adenosine		
Use: Supraventricular tachycardia (SVT)	**Recommended Dose** 0.1 mg/kg rapid IV or IO bolus over 1–2 seconds. Repeat at 0.2 mg/kg. **Maximum Dose** First Dose: 6 mg Second Dose: 12 mg	**Precaution**: Use continuous cardiac monitoring. Avoid use in second or third degree AV block, sick sinus syndrome. **Adverse Reactions:** Nausea, hypotension, dyspnea, bronchospasm, chest pain/pressure, tingling, heart block, dysrhythmias, facial flushing, metallic taste. Bronchoconstriction may occur in asthmatics.

Albuterol (Salbutamol)		
Use: Prevention and acute relief of bronchospasm, Prophylaxis for exercise-induced bronchospasm.	**Recommended Dose** Nebulizer solution (1.25 mg/3 mL, 2.5 mg/3 mL, 5 mg/mL) 2.5-5 mg every 20 minutes for 3 doses. Repeat dose every 1–4 hours as needed. If not already prediluted, dilute in minimum of 2–3 mL of saline for adequate nebulization. May use continuously for status asthmaticus. MDI: 4–8 puffs (90 mcg/puff) every 15–20 minutes for 3 doses. Repeat every 1–4 hours as needed. **Maximum Dose** Not established for status asthmaticus	**Precaution:** Tremors common **Adverse Reactions:** Nausea, palpitations, headache, dizziness, tremor, tachycardia

Amiodarone

Use: Life-threatening ventricular arrhythmias: ventricular fibrillation or tachycardia

Recommended Dose

5 mg/kg IV or IO push for ventricular fibrillation or pulseless ventricular tachycardia.
5 mg/kg IV or IO infusion over 20–60 minutes for wide complex tachycardia.

Maximum Dose

15 mg/kg/day

Precaution: Must dilute with 20 mL of 5% dextrose prior to administration to avoid thrombophlebitis. May cause hypotension and prolonged Q-T interval. Should not use in combination with procainamide. Contraindicated in severe sinus node dysfunction, marked sinus bradycardia, second and third degree AV block.

Adverse Reactions: Hypotension, bradycardia, dysrhythmias, vomiting

Aspirin

Use: Analgesic, Antipyretic

Recommended Dose

10–15 mg/kg

Maximum Dose

1 g

Precaution: Avoid use in children < 16 years with chickenpox or viral illness due to association with Reye's Syndrome.

Adverse Reactions: Nausea, vomiting, abdominal pain, ulcers, rash, urticaria, bronchospasm

Atropine

Use: Sinus bradycardia, Chemical nerve gas and organophosphate pesticide poisoning

Recommended Dose

0.02 mg/kg IV or IO

Minimum single dose of 0.1 mg.

May repeat dose every 5 minutes to maximum total dose of
1 mg for a child and 2 mg for an adolescent or adult.

Maximum Dose

Single Dose: 0.5 mg for a child, 1 mg for an adolescent.

Precaution: Atropine sulfate comes in different concentrations, calculate dosage accordingly. Avoid in tachydysrhythmias. Caution in children with brain damage or spastic paralysis. Anticholinesterase poisonings may require large doses of atropine (nerve gas 0.05–0.1 mg/kg, organophosphate poisoning 0.02–0.05 mg/kg, so maximum dose does not apply.) (Pralidoxime will also be needed.)

Adverse Reactions: Dry mouth, blurred vision, tachycardia, constipation, urinary retention

Calcium Chloride

Use: Ionized hypocalcemia, Hyperkalemia, Hypermagnesemia, Calcium channel blocker toxicity.

Recommended for cardiac resuscitation only in cases of documented hyperkalemia, hypocalcemia, or calcium channel blocker toxicity.

Recommended Dose

20 mg/kg IV or IO slowly (if using 10% CaCl, dose is 0.2 mL/kg).

Inject slowly while monitoring heart rate.

Repeat dose as necessary for desired clinical effects.

Maximum Dose

1000 mg is usual maximum

Precaution: Stop injection if symptomatic bradycardia occurs. Calcium chloride administration results in a more rapid increase in ionized calcium concentrations than calcium gluconate and is preferred for the critically ill child.

Extravascular administration can result in severe skin injury. Highly irritating to tissues. Avoid scalp vein, small hand or foot veins for IV administration.

Adverse Reactions: Tissue extravasation and necrosis; May exacerbate metabolic acidosis. Hypotension, bradycardia, arrhythmias, ventricular fibrillation

Calcium Gluconate (preferred in neonates)

Use: Ionized hypocalcemia, Hyperkalemia, Hypermagnesemia, Calcium channel blocker toxicity.

Recommended for cardiac resuscitation only in cases of documented hyperkalemia, hypocalcemia, or calcium channel blocker toxicity.

Recommended Dose

60 mg/kg IV or IO slowly (if using 10% calcium gluconate, dose is 0.6 mL/kg). Inject slowly while monitoring heart rate.

Repeat dose as necessary for desired clinical effects.

Maximum Dose

1000 mg is usual maximum

Precaution: Stop injection if symptomatic bradycardia occurs. Calcium chloride administration results in a more rapid increase in ionized calcium concentrations than calcium gluconate and is preferred for the critically ill child. Extravascular administration can result in severe skin injury. Highly irritating to tissues. Avoid scalp vein, small hand or foot veins for IV administration.

Adverse Reactions: Tissue extravasation and necrosis, hypotension, bradycardia, arrhythmias, ventricular fibrillation

Dexamethasone

Use: Croup, Asthma

Recommended Dose

Croup:
0.15–0.6 mg/kg IV, IM, or PO

Asthma:
0.6–1.0 mg/kg IV or IM

Maximum Dose

16 mg/day

Precaution: Long acting glucocorticoid

Adverse Reactions: Sodium and fluid retention, hyperglycemia

Diazepam

Use: Seizures, Agitation

Recommended Dose

IV: 0.1 mg/kg every 5–10 minutes. Administer over approximately 2 minutes to avoid pain at intravenous site.

PR: 0.5 mg/kg up to 20 mg

Maximum Dose

IV: 5 mg/dose

PR: 20 mg

Precaution: There is an increased incidence of apnea when combined with other sedative agents or when given rapidly. Be prepared to provide respiratory support. Monitor oxygen saturation. Avoid extravasation to prevent venous thrombosis or phlebitis. Avoid rapid administration to prevent hypotension or respiratory arrest. Avoid prolonged use of parenteral diazepam because it contains 40% propylene glycol as a diluent.

Adverse Reactions: Respiratory depression, drowsiness, bradycardia, hypotension, apnea, pain at injection site

Diphenhydramine

Use: Anaphylaxis, Antihistamine

Recommended Dose

1 mg/kg IV or IO slow push

Maximum Dose

IV: 50 mg

Precaution: May case sedation and respiratory suppression especially if using other sedative agents. May cause hypotension. Overdosage may cause hallucinations and seizures. Rapid IV administration may precipitate seizures. All doses may cause paradoxical excitement or agitation.

Adverse Reactions: Drowsiness, dry mouth, constipation, urinary retention

Dopamine

Use: Hypotension, Shock

Recommended Dose

Neonate: 2–10 mcg/kg/min IV or IO infusion

Children: 2–20 mcg/kg/min IV or IO infusion

Titrate up to desired effect:

5 mcg/kg/min = low dose
10 mcg/kg/min = moderate dose
20 mcg/kg/min = high dose

Maximum Dose

20 mcg/kg/min

Precaution: Infusion rates greater than 20 mcg/kg/minute may produce extreme peripheral vasoconstriction and ischemia. Mix with great caution. Extravascular administration can result in severe skin injury. Avoid small veins. Dopamine is inactivated in an alkaline solution. Correct hypovolemia prior to use.

Adverse Reactions: Ectopic beats, tachycardia, palpitations, vasoconstriction, dyspnea, vomiting

Epinephrine

Use: Croup, Anaphylaxis, Acute asthma, Cardiac arrest, Shock

Recommended Dose

Anaphylaxis: IM, 0.01 mg/kg/dose = 0.01 mL/kg/dose of 1 mg/mL concentration (max 0.3 mg = 0.3 mL). Repeat dose every 5–20 minutes.

Anaphylactic shock: IV 0.01 mg/kg of 0.1 mg/mL concentration Max 0.5 mg

Croup: 0.25–0.5 mg/kg of 1 mg/mL concentration in 3 mL of NS by inhalation (max 5 mL/dose)

Shock: 0.10-1 mcg/kg/min of 0.1 mg/mL concentration

Racemic epinephrine (2.25%) for croup: 0.1 mL/kg by inhalation (maximum 0.5 mL) in 3 mL of NS.

Precaution: Use length-based resuscitation tape or computerized software to verify correct dose. Read concentration on label carefully. Incompatible with alkaline solutions. Extravascular administration can result in severe skin injury.

Anaphylaxis: Some anaphylactic reactions require large doses of epinephrine that may be administered IV.

Cardiac Arrest: If administered through an endotracheal tube, follow the dose with saline flush or dilute in isotonic saline flush (1 to 5 mL) based on patient length/weight.

Adverse Reactions: Tachycardia, palpitations, cardiac dysrhythmias, diaphoresis, vomiting, headache, dizziness

Fentanyl

Use: Analgesic, Anesthetic for intubation and maintenance

Recommended Dose

IV: 1 mcg/kg/dose every 30–60 minutes

IN: 1–2 mcg/kg

Maximum Dose

100 mcg

Titrate to effect

Precaution: There is an increased incidence of apnea when combined with other sedative agents, particularly benzodiazepines. Avoid rapid IV infusion; inject slowly over several minutes. If given rapidly, may cause chest wall or glottic rigidity, which may be reversed with a muscle relaxant.

Adverse Reactions: Apnea, bradycardia, nausea, vomiting

Flumazenil

Use: Reverse sedative effects of benzodiazepines

Recommended Dose

IV: 0.01–0.02 mg/kg over 15 seconds; repeat every 1 min prn. When IV access is unavailable, may be given IM.

Maximum Dose

0.2 mg/dose and to cumulative total dose of 0.05 mg/kg or 1 mg

Precaution: May precipitate acute withdrawal in dependent patients. May precipitate seizures in high risk patients on chronic benzodiazepine, sedative/hypnotics or other coingestants in an overdose. Observe for resedation. Avoid single bolus injection.

Adverse Reactions: Rebound sedation or respiratory depression due to its short duration of action.

Furosemide

Use: Fluid overload, Congestive heart failure, Diuresis, Edema, Pulmonary Edema, Hypertension	**Recommended Dose** *Children*: 1–2 mg/kg IV, IO, or IM **Maximum Dose** 40 mg	**Precaution:** Do not give to child with hypovolemia. Contraindicated in anuria. **Adverse Reactions:** Hypotension, electrolyte depletion, alkalosis, tinnitus, ototoxic

Glucagon

Use: Beta-blocker or Calcium channel blocker overdose, Hypoglycemia	**Recommended Dose** Hypoglycemia due to insulin excess: *Children*: 0.02–0.03 mg/kg for those < 20 kg, for those > 20 kg 1 mg IV, IO, IM; repeat every 20 minutes if needed for clinical effect. Total 3 doses. Beta-blocker or calcium channel blocker overdose: IV: 0.05–0.15 mg/kg followed by 0.07 mg/kg/h (maximum of 5 mg/h) infusion. **Maximum Dose** Pediatric: 1 mg	**Precaution:** Use immediately after reconstitution. Caution in patients with pheochromocytoma. **Adverse Reactions:** Nausea, vomiting

Glucose (Dextrose)

Use: Hypoglycemia	**Recommended Dose** *Newborn*: 2 mL/kg 10% dextrose IV or IO push *Neonate*: 5 mL/kg 10% dextrose IV or IO push *< 2 years*: 2 mL/kg 25% dextrose IV or IO push *> 2 years*: 1 mL/kg 50% dextrose IV or IO push **Maximum Dose** Doses guided by repeated serum glucose level determinations	**Precaution:** Depending on situation hypoglycemia may re-occur. **Adverse Reactions:** Hyperglycemia

Hydrocortisone

Use: Acute adrenal insufficiency/adrenal crisis, Septic shock	**Recommended Dose** 1–2 mg/kg IV, IO, IM **Maximum Dose** 100 mg	**Precaution:** Do not use for head injury. Use with caution in patients with hypertension, heart failure, renal or hepatic impairment. **Adverse Reactions:** Arrhythmias, hypertension, adrenal suppression

Ibuprofen

Use: Analgesic, Antipyretic	**Recommended Dose** 5–10 mg/kg/dose PO **Maximum Dose** 800 mg	**Precaution:** Cross reacts with aspirin allergy, gastrointestinal bleeding. Liquid products may contain alcohol. Do not use in patients with kidney disease. Do not use in infants <6 months. **Adverse Reactions:** Vomiting, gastritis, ulcer formation, rash

Ipratropium

Use: Asthma

Recommended Dose

Nebulized solution (0.5 mg/2.5 mL)

Children < 12 years: 0.25 mg nebulized every 20 minutes for 3 doses

Children > 12 years: 0.5 mg nebulized every 20 minutes for 3 doses

Maximum Dose

0.5 mg

Precaution: Use with albuterol every 20 min x 3.

Adverse Reactions: Tachycardia, dry mouth, headache, cough, hoarseness, blurred vision

Ketamine

Use: Anesthesia for intubation, analgesia for painful procedures

Recommended Dose

IV: 1–2 mg/kg

IM: 3–5 mg/kg

Maximum Dose

100 mg

Precaution: Emergence reactions may occur up to 24 hours postoperatively: delirium, hallucinations, vivid dreams. Avoid use in patients with increased ICP, increased intraocular pressure, or bowel obstruction.

Adverse Reactions: Hallucinations, tonic-clonic movements, nausea, vomiting, decreased cough reflex, nystagmus, tachycardia, bronchospasm, hypertension, bradycardia, hypotension, apnea. May cause purposeless movements.

Lidocaine (Lignocaine)

Use: Ventricular tachycardia, Ventricular fibrillation, Wide-complex SVT

Recommended Dose

Children: IV/IO/ET Loading Dose = 1 mg/kg; repeat in 10–15 minutes for 2 doses if needed; IV continuous infusion after loading dose: 20–50 mcg/kg/min

ET: 2–2.5 times the IV dose

Maximum Dose

IV: 3 mg/kg

Precaution: Contraindicated in complete heart block and wide complex tachycardia due to accessory conduction pathways. Excessive dosage may result in myocardial depression, hypotension, agitation, or seizures. Hypersensitivity to amide anesthetics. If administered through an endotracheal tube, follow the dose with saline flush or dilute in isotonic saline flush (1 to 5 mL) based on patient size.

Adverse Reactions: Arrhythmias, seizures, respiratory depression or arrest

Lorazepam

Use: Anticonvulsant, Anxiety, Sedation

Recommended Dose

Status epilepticus:

Neonates: 0.05 mg/kg IV or IO over 2–5 minutes

Infants and Children: 0.05–0.1 mg/kg IV or IO over 2–5 minutes; max: 4 mg/dose; repeat 0.05 mg/kg second dose in 10–15 minutes if needed

Maximum Dose

4 mg/dose

Precaution: Beware of respiratory depression. There is an increased incidence of apnea when combined with other sedative agents. Monitor oxygen saturation and be prepared to provide respiratory support. May be reversed with flumazenil.

Adverse Reactions: Bradycardia, hypotension, apnea, confusion, hallucinations, myoclonic jerking in preterm infants

Mannitol

Use: Diuresis, Reduces intracranial pressure	**Recommended Dose** IV: 0.25–1 g/kg **Maximum Dose** 1 g/kg body weight	**Precaution:** Inspect vials for crystals. Use 5 micron filter for 20% solutions or greater. Avoid excessive fluid loss with diuresis to prevent dehydration and electrolyte imbalance. **Adverse Reactions:** Dehydration, fluid and electrolyte imbalance, headache, hypovolemia, seizures, water intoxication

Methylprednisolone

Use: Asthma, Croup	**Recommended Dose** Status asthmaticus: 1–2 mg/kg/dose IV or IO **Maximum Dose** 60 mg	**Precaution:** Rapid IV push of high doses in < 20 minutes may cause hypotension, arrhythmias, and sudden death. **Adverse Reactions:** Edema, pituitary-adrenal suppression, hypokalemia, peptic ulcer, nausea, vomiting

Midazolam

Use: Anxiety, Seizures	**Recommended Dose** Status epilepticus: IV, or IO: 0.1 mg/kg; IN 0.2 mg/kg Sedation/anxiolysis IV, IO, or IM: 0.05–0.1 mg/kg IN 0.2 mgHg **Maximum Dose** *6 months–5 years*: 6 mg *> 6 years*: 10 mg	**Precaution:** Avoid rapid IV administration which may produce respiratory arrest and seizures. There is an increased incidence of apnea when combined with other sedative agents, particularly benzodiazepines. Be prepared to provide respiratory support, regardless of route of administration. Monitor oxygen saturation. May be reversed with flumazenil. Myoclonus may occur in premature infants. Paradoxical excitation may occur in children. May be reversed with flumazenil. **Adverse Reactions:** Bradycardia, hypotension, cardiac arrest, apnea, respiratory depression

Morphine

Use: Severe acute and chronic pain, Pulmonary edema, tet spells	**Recommended Dose** *Neonates*: 0.05 mg/kg IM, IV, IO, SQ *Infants and Children*: 0.05–0.1 mg/kg IM, IV, IO, SQ *Adolescents*: 3–4 mg IV or IO, repeat in 5 minutes as needed **Maximum Dose** *Neonates*: 0.1 mg/kg *Infants, children, and adolescents*: 10 mg	**Precaution:** Pediatric patients are more sensitive to the effects of opiates. Hypersensitivity to similar opiates. Some products may contain sulfites. There is an increased incidence of apnea when combined with other sedative agents, particularly benzodiazepines. Be prepared to provide respiratory support, regardless of route of administration. Monitor oxygen saturation. May be reversed with naloxone. **Adverse Reactions:** Respiratory depression, hypotension, rash

Naloxone

Use: Opiate intoxication	**Recommended Dose** *Pediatric*: 0.1 mg/kg/dose IV, IO, IM, ET **Maximum Dose** 2 mg	**Precaution:** Dilute to 1–2 mL with normal saline for ET use. May induce acute withdrawal in opioid dependency. Patients who receive naloxone should be continuously observed for renarcotization for at least 2 hours after last dose of naloxone. Doses may be repeated as needed to maintain opiate reversal. IM absorption may be erratic. Do not administer naloxone to a newborn whose mother is suspected of recently abusing drugs due to risk of acute withdrawal in the infant.

Nitrous oxide, Dinitrogen oxide, N_2O, Laughing gas

Use: Analgesia, Sedation

Recommended Dose
25–50% with oxygen 50:50
Maximum Dose
70–80%

Precaution: Asphyxiation may occur
Adverse Reactions: Malignant hyperthermia, cardiac dysrhythmias, nausea, vomiting, delirium

Norepinephrine

Use: Distributive shock

Recommended Dose
0.05–0.1 mcg/kg/min IV, titrate to desired response
Maximum Dose
1–2 mcg/kg/min

Precaution: Double check concentration and infusion rate. Avoid scalp veins.
Adverse Reactions: Bradycardia, hypertension, arrhythmias, palpitations, pallor, ischemic necrosis, organ ischemia

Phenobarbital, Phenobarbitone

Use: Status epilepticus

Recommended Dose
20 mg/kg IV or IO over 20 min (1 mg/kg/min); not to exceed 50 mg/min
Maximum Dose
1000 mg

Precaution: There is an increased incidence of apnea when combined with other sedative agents. Be prepared to provide respiratory support. Monitor oxygen saturation. Avoid extravasation because parenteral solutions are very alkaline. Be prepared to support respirations.
Adverse Reactions: Drowsiness, hypotension, apnea, paradoxical excitation

Phenytoin, Sodium Diphenylhydantoin (DPH)

Use: Status epilepticus

Recommended Dose
Neonate: 10 mg/kg
Children: 20 mg/kg IV or IO over 20 min (1 mg/kg/min); not to exceed 50 mg/min
Maximum Dose
1000 mg

Precaution: Incompatible with glucose solutions. Monitor heart rate and reduce infusion if rate decreases by 10 beats/min. Rapid IV administration may trigger ventricular fibrillation and cardiac arrest. Avoid extravasation. Injections may contain propylene glycol and benzyl alcohol.
Adverse Reactions: Bradycardia, hypotension, arrhythmias, cardiovascular collapse, nystagmus, drowsiness

Pralidoxime Chloride, 2-PAM, 2-Pyridine Aldoxime Methochloride

Use: Organophosphate poisoning, Carbamate insecticide poisoning with nicotinic symptoms, Anticholinesterase poisoning

Recommended Dose
25–50 mg/kg, up to 2 g, IV over 5–30 minutes, then 10 mg/kg/hr or repeat load every 1–2 hours.
IM: 15 mg/kg (up to 600 mg), repeat as needed every 15 minutes to a maximum of 45 mg/kg
Maximum Dose
2 g/dose
Large total amounts may be required in a severe poisoning.

Precaution: Rapid IV administration may cause tachycardia, laryngospasm, muscle rigidity and transient neuromuscular blockade. IV route preferred, but may be given IM or SC when IV route is not immediately accessible.
Adverse Reactions: Nausea, headache, dizziness, diplopia, hyperventilation

Rocuronium Bromide

Use: Adjunct to general anesthesia to facilitate tracheal intubation and provide skeletal muscle relaxation during mechanical ventilation.	**Recommended Dose** IV: 1 mg/kg **Maximum Dose** 1.2 mg/kg	**Precaution:** Ventilatory support is necessary. Prepare to respond with airway management. Do not mix with alkaline solutions. May interact with certain antibiotics that have neuromuscular blocking actions (e.g., aminoglycosides) and enhance neuromuscular blockade. Toxicity may be increased in patients with pulmonary disease. **Adverse Reactions:** Muscle weakness, hypotension or hypertension, arrhythmias, tachycardia, bronchospasm, hiccoughs

Sodium Bicarbonate

Use: Cyclic antidepressant overdose, Hyperkalemia	**Recommended Dose** *Pediatric*: 1 mEq/kg IV or IO slowly **Maximum Dose** 50 mEq/dose	**Precaution:** Do not mix with calcium, dopamine, epinephrine. May cause tissue necrosis from IV extravasation. Caution with renal impairment. No more than 0.5 mEq/mL for neonatal use. **Adverse Reactions:** Cerebral hemorrhage, edema, hypernatremia, hypokalemia, hypocalcemia, metabolic alkalosis

Succinylcholine, Suxamethonium

Use: Adjunct to general anesthesia, Endotracheal intubation, Mechanical ventilation	**Recommended Dose** IV, IO, or IM: 1–2 mg/kg/dose	**Precaution:** Contraindicated in conditions associated with increased ICP, severe burns, spinal cord injury, neuromuscular disease, myopathy, or malignant hyperthermia. When these contraindications exist, use a nondepolarizing muscle relaxant such as rocuronium. Ventilatory support is necessary. If cardiac arrest occurs immediately after administration of succinylcholine, hyperkalemia must be suspected (particularly in males under 9 years of age). Toxicity is increased in patients with muscle injury, muscle myopathies, rhabdomyolysis, or low pseudocholinesterase levels. Children are more susceptible to developing bradycardia, cardiac arrest, and myoglobinemia. Atropine is recommended prior to the administration of succinylcholine in children. **Adverse Reactions:** Bradycardia, hypotension, arrhythmias, apnea, cardiac arrest, hyperkalemia, malignant hyperthermia

Glossary

abdomen the anatomic portion of the anterior trunk below the ribs and above the pelvis; it contains the stomach, lower part of the esophagus, small and large intestines, liver, gall bladder, spleen, pancreas, and bladder.

abdominal excursions the work of abdominal muscles in infants during the breathing cycle.

abrasion a portion of skin or of a mucous membrane scraped away as a result of injury.

absorb to take in or suck up.

abusive head trauma seen in abused infants and children. The patient has been subjected to violent, whiplash-type shaking injuries inflicted by the abusing individual. This may cause coma, convulsions, and increased intracranial pressure due to tearing of the cerebral veins with consequent bleeding into the brain. (Old term: shaken baby/infant syndrome.)

acceleration-deceleration event a type of injury caused when a moving body part, such as the head, stops its forward motion suddenly.

acid a corrosive substance with low pH.

acidosis excessive acidity of body fluids due to an accumulation of acids (as in diabetic acidosis or renal disease) or an excessive loss of bicarbonate (as in renal disease).

acrocyanosis cyanosis of the extremities; acrocyanosis of the hands and feet may be normal in the infant within the first hour after birth.

activation phase first of three phases in disaster response. This is the notification and initial response phase which includes establishment of the Incident Command System organization and scene assessment.

acute characterized by sharpness or severity, or having a sudden onset, sharp rise, and short course.

adenoidal lymphoid tissue in the back of the mouth and oropharynx.

adrenaline synonym for epinephrine. A hormone produced by the body that increases pulse rate and blood pressure; mediates the "fight-or-flight" response of the sympathetic nervous system when the body is under stress.

adrenergic agents drugs that mimic the effects of epinephrine (adrenaline) and norepinephrine.

adsorb to take up and hold by adsorption.

afebrile seizures a seizure not accompanied by a fever.

agent something that causes an effect; thus, bacteria that cause a disease are said to be agents of the specific disease. An injury agent is the energy causing the damage, such as thermal energy from a burn. A drug is a pharmacologic agent.

agonist a substance that stimulates or activates a specialized receptor on a cell.

airway adjunct an artificial device to maintain an open airway.

alkali a strong base with a high pH, usually corrosive to tissues.

alveoli the air sacs of the lungs in which the exchange of oxygen and carbon dioxide takes place.

amniotic fluid the liquid contained in the amnion, inside the uterus. This fluid is sterile, transparent, and almost colorless. The liquid surrounds and protects the fetus from injury and helps maintain an even temperature.

analgesia, analgesic a drug that relieves pain.

anaphylactic reaction an extreme, life-threatening systemic allergic reaction that may include shock and respiratory failure.

anaphylaxis a severe form of hypersensitivity reaction that produces dangerous physiologic changes, such as bronchospasm, shock, and airway edema.

anatomic relating to the anatomy or structure of an organism.

ancillary something that assists another action or effect but is not essential to the accomplishment of the action.

antecubital fossa the triangular area lying anterior to and below the elbow, bounded medially by the pronator teres muscle and laterally by the brachioradialis muscles.

anthrax a deadly bacteria (*Bacillus anthracis*) that lies dormant in a spore (protective shell); the germ is released from the spore when exposed to the optimal temperature and moisture. The route of entry is inhalation, cutaneous, or gastrointestinal (from consuming food that contains spores).

antibiotic any of a variety of natural or synthetic substances that inhibit growth of, or destroy, bacteria that are responsible for infectious diseases.

anticonvulsant agent that prevents or stops convulsions.

antigen protein recognized by the immune system which causes an allergic reaction.

antipyretic an agent that reduces fever.

antivenin a serum that counteracts the effect of venom from an animal or insect.

anxiolysis reduction of anxiety, agitation, or tension.

apnea a temporary cessation of breathing.

apneic characterized by absence of breathing.

apparent life-threatening event (ALTE) an unexplained sudden episode of color change (cyanosis or pallor), tone change (limpness, stiffness), or apnea that required mouth-to-mouth resuscitation or vigorous stimulation.

asphyxia a condition caused by insufficient oxygen.

assessment evaluation.

assisted ventilation to provide ventilation mechanically.

asthma a disease caused by increased responsiveness of the tracheobronchial tree to various stimuli. The result is paroxysmal constriction of the bronchial airways. Clinically, there is severe dyspnea accompanied by wheezing.

asymmetric without symmetry.

asystole cardiac standstill; absence of contractions of the heart.

ataxia an abnormal gait.

atrioventricular heart block blockage of the electrical impulse from the atrium of the heart to the ventricle.

atrium one of two (right and left) upper chambers of the heart. The right atrium receives blood from the vena cava and delivers it to the right ventricle, which, in turn, pumps blood into the blood vessels of the lungs. The left atrium receives blood from pulmonary veins and delivers it to the left ventricle, which, in turn, pumps blood into the body.

auscultate to listen, as with a stethoscope.

auscultation the process of listening for sounds within the body with a stethoscope.

automatic implantable cardioverter-defibrillator (AICD) an implantable electronic device designed to monitor heart rhythm and determine if it is abnormal and needs to be corrected.

AVPU (alert, verbal, painful, unresponsive) scale the components of the AVPU scale are used to assess the level of consciousness: Alert, Voice, Painful, Unresponsive.

avulsion a tearing away of a part or structure.

axial loading vertical pressure on the spine.

axillary temperature the temperature taken in the armpit.

axonal shearing a tearing of axons or nerve sheaths, caused by sudden movement, to produce severe brain injury.

baseline a known or initial value with which subsequent observations can be compared.

basilar skull fracture a fracture into the base of the skull, sometimes associated with brain hemorrhage or brain injury.

Battle sign bruising behind the ear; an indication of basilar skull fracture.

benzodiazepines a family of sedative-hypnotic drugs useful for treatment of seizures and agitation.

bezoar a hard mass of entangled material sometimes found in the stomach and intestines.

bilateral pertaining to, affecting, or relating to two sides.

biological agents organisms that cause disease, including viruses, bacteria, and toxins.

biological pathogens a microorganism that can cause disease in a host.

blood pressure the perfusing pressure of blood.

brachial pertaining to a main artery and vein of the arm.

bradycardia a slow heartbeat.

brain death cessation of brain function.

brain perfusion blood circulation in the brain.

brainstem the stemlike part of the brain that connects the cerebral hemispheres with the spinal cord.

brainstem functions bodily functions controlled by the brain stem that are necessary for life, such as breathing.

brainstem herniation bulging and compression of brain tissue; causes breathing to stop and death of the patient.

bronchiolitis inflammation of the bronchioles by a virus.

bronchoconstriction narrowing of the bronchial tubes.

bronchodilator a drug that helps open the airways to improve air movement and reduce wheezing.

bronchopulmonary dysplasia (BPD) iatrogenic chronic lung disease that develops in premature infants following a period of oxygen therapy.

bronchovesicular pertaining to the tree of pulmonary passages.

buccal between the teeth and mucosa of the mouth.

buckle fracture a minor fracture only partially through the bone, in which the top layer of bone on one side is compressed, forming a slight angle or "buckle" in the surface.

bulging fontanelle an elevation of the immature opening of bone in the front of the skull; this sign may suggest increased intracranial pressure.

calcium channel blockers a family of drugs that helps reduce the speed of conduction through the heart and the overall work of the heart.

cannulating to introduce a catheter through a vein or passageway.

capillary refill time (CRT) a test that evaluates distal circulatory system function performed by pushing on an area such as a nail bed and watching the speed of its return of pinkness after releasing the pressure.

capnometry the use of a capnometer, a device that measures the amount of expired carbon dioxide.

cardiac arrest the cessation of cardiac mechanical activity, determined by the inability to palpate a central pulse, unresponsiveness, and apnea.

cardiac dysrhythmia an abnormal cardiac rhythm.

cardiac medication various medications used to treat for heart disease and cardiovascular conditions.

cardiogenic shock a reduced cardiac output secondary to abnormal cardiac function.

cardiomyopathy disease of the myocardium, especially due to primary disease of the heart muscle.

cartilage a specialized type of dense connective tissue, softer than bone, that is common in the skeletons of children.

cartilaginous growth plates the horizontal part of the bone which grows as the human body matures.

cathartic a purgative agent for the bowel.

caustic corrosive and burning; destructive to living tissue.

CBRNE chemical, biologic, radiation, nuclear, and explosive.

central cyanosis slightly bluish, grayish, or dark purple discoloration of the skin (on the trunk and face) due to presence of hypoxia.

central nervous system (CNS) CNS consists of the brain and spinal cord; it controls vital body functions.

central venous catheter catheter inserted into the vena cava to permit intermittent or continuous monitoring of central venous pressure and to facilitate obtaining blood samples for analysis.

cerebral cortex the higher brain; the source of the senses, thinking, feeling, and voluntary movement.

cerebral edema swelling of the brain.

cerebral spinal fluid (CSF) shunt tube that allows fluid manufactured in the ventricles of the brain from the subarachnoid space to drain in another part of the anatomy outside of the brain, such as the peritoneum. This can lower pressure in the brain.

cervical of, pertaining to, or in the region of the upper spine.

chest wall the musculoskeletal framework of the chest.

child maltreatment a general term applying to all forms of child abuse and neglect.

child neglect failure by those responsible for caring for a child to provide for the child's nutritional, emotional, and physical needs.

child protective services (CPS) this agency is the community legal organization responsible for protection, rehabilitation, and prevention of child maltreatment and neglect. CPS has the legal authority temporarily to remove from home children at risk for injury or neglect and to secure foster placement.

children with special health care needs (CSHCN) those who have or are at increased risk for a chronic, physical, developmental, behavioral, or emotional condition and who also require health and related services of a type or amount beyond that required by children generally.

choanal atresia a narrowing or blockage of the nasal airway by membranous or bony tissue; a congenital condition (present at birth).

cholinergic crisis a crisis involving cholinergic drugs, pesticides or "nerve gases" designed for chemical warfare. Cholinergic agents overstimulate normal body functions that are controlled by the parasympathetic nerves.

cholinergic impulses description of a neuron that secretes the neurotransmitter acetylcholine.

circadian rhythm the regular recurrence, in cycles of about 24 hours, of biological processes or activities, such as sensitivity to drugs and stimuli, hormone secretion, sleeping, feeding, etc. This rhythm seems to be set by a biological clock that seems to be set by recurring daylight and darkness.

clavicles the collarbone; a bone, curved like the letter f, that articulates with the sternum and scapula.

coin rubbing cultural ritual intended to treat an illness by rubbing hot coins, often on the back, which produces rounded and oblong red, patch, flat skin lesions.

colostomy the surgical establishment of an opening between the colon and the surface of the body for the purpose of providing drainage of the bowel.

commotio cordis sudden cardiac arrest from a blunt, nonpenetrating blow to the chest. The basis of the cardiac arrest is ventricular fibrillation (a chaotically abnormal heart rhythm) triggered by chest wall impact immediately over the anatomic position of the heart.

compensated shock a clinical state in which there are clinical signs of inadequate tissue perfusion, but the patient's blood pressure is in the normal range.

compensatory mechanisms physiologic responses, initiated to help return the body's vital functions to normal after a severe insult to breathing, perfusion, or metabolic function.

complex febrile seizure a self-limited seizure in a previously healthy child between the ages of 6 months and 6 years that is associated with an elevated fever, which lasts longer than 15 minutes, and may have focal motor activity.

complex partial seizure characterized by alteration of consciousness with or without complex focal motor activity.

compression a squeezing together; state of being pressed together.

concussion a brain injury causing any type of altered state of consciousness.

congenital present at birth.

congenital anomalies an anatomic structure that is unusual or different at birth.

congenital diaphragmatic hernia a developmental defect of the diaphragm in which the abdominal organs herniate into the chest.

congenital heart disease heart disease that is present from birth.

congestive heart failure a disorder in which the heart loses part of its ability to effectively pump blood, usually as a result of damage to the heart muscle and usually resulting in a backup of fluid into the lungs.

consent for care permission to render care.

constipation infrequent defecation with passage of unduly hard and dry fecal material.

contact burn a thermal burn from direct contact with a hot object, fluid, or gas.

contraindication a condition indicating that a treatment is inappropriate.

core perfusion blood circulation in the core of the human body.

corrosive producing corrosion or destruction of tissue.

cortical pertaining to or of the outer layer of the brain.

crackles rales; lung sounds that suggest fluid in alveoli.

cranium the area of the head above the ears and eyes; the skull. The cranium contains the brain.

crepitus the noise or feel of gas in soft tissues.

critical incident stress management (CISM) a process that confronts the responses to critical incidents and defuses them, directing the emergency service personnel toward physical and emotional equilibrium.

crowning stage in delivery when the fetal head presents at the vaginal opening.

cupping the cultural practice of placing warm cups on the skin to pull out illness from the body. This results in red, flat, rounded skin lesions which are often more intensely red at the borders.

Cushing triad the combination of hypertension, bradycardia and irregular respirations that occurs with increased intracranial pressure.

cyanide a colorless gas that has an odor similar to almonds, and which is a chemical asphyxiant used in many industrial processes; exposure can occur from by-products of combustion at structure fires.

cyanosis slightly bluish, grayish, slatelike, or dark purple discoloration of the skin due to presence of hypoxia.

cyanotic heart disease a type of congenital heart disease with a right to left shunt resulting in partially oxygenated blood in the systemic circulation.

cyclic antidepressants a type of antidepressant drug that may cause coma, seizures, and conduction disturbances if taken in an overdose.

decerebrate a posture characterized by rigid extension of the arms and legs; indicates pressure on the brain stem at the level of the pons and may appear in patients with severe brain swelling.

decompensated shock a shock state characterized by low blood pressure, which will rapidly progress to cardiac arrest if not rapidly corrected.

decontamination the process of removing a poison.

decorticate a posture characterized by flexion of the arms and extension of the legs; indicates pressure on the cerebral cortex and subcortical white matter with preservation of brainstem function and may appear in patients with severe brain trauma.

defibrillator an electrical device that shocks the heart; it may be used externally or in the form of an automatic implanted defibrillator.

demarcated a defined area in a boundary.

dendrite a projection from a neuron that makes connections with an adjacent cell.

dextrose a form of glucose (or sugar) found naturally in animal and plant tissue and derived synthetically from starch.

diabetes mellitus a metabolic disorder in which the ability to metabolize sugar is impaired, usually because of a lack of insulin.

diabetic ketoacidosis a form of acidosis in diabetes in which certain acids accumulate when insulin is not available.

diagnostic testing tests used to determine the cause of an illness or disorder.

diaphoretic a state of excessive perspiration because of high physiologic stress.

diaphragm the muscle separating the chest from the abdominal cavity, which allows breathing.

diaphysis the shaft of a long bone.

diastolic pressure the pressure that remains in the arteries during the relaxing phase of the heart's cycle (diastole) when the left ventricle is at rest.

diffuse axonal injury an injury to the brain, resulting in diffuse brain swelling

dilated widened.

direct medical control physician instructions that are given directly by phone or radio.

dirty bomb name given to a bomb that is used as a radiological dispersal device (RDD).

disaster a widespread event that disrupts community resources and functions, in turn threatening public safety, citizens' lives, and property.

distal farthest from the center.

distal extremities structures that are farther from the trunk or nearer to the free end of the extremity.

distention inflation, enlargement.

distributive shock a clinical state characterized by maldistribution of blood volume and vascular tone.

diving reflex submersion of the face and nose in water to produce a vagal reaction; used to terminate an important dysrhythmia of childhood called supraventricular tachycardia.

Do Not Resuscitate (DNR) written documentation giving permission to medical personnel not to attempt resuscitation in the event of cardiac arrest.

Down syndrome a congenital disorder in which a person is born with three copies of chromosome 21 (trisomy 21). Clinical features include mental retardation, slanting eyes, a broad short skull, broad hands and short fingers. Other congenital abnormalities include heart defects and esophageal atresia.

dressings protective covering for diseased or injured parts.

dysphagia inability to swallow or difficulty in swallowing.

dysrhythmias abnormal, disordered rhythm.

edema a local or generalized collection of tissue fluid.

effortless tachypnea tachypnea, without the signs of increased work of breathing; this represents the child's attempt to blow off extra carbon dioxide to correct the acidosis generated by poor perfusion.

electrocardiogram (ECG) a 12-lead electrocardiographic recording used to evaluate the heart and its rhythm.

emancipated minor person legally under age but recognized by the state as having the legal capacity to consent for self (usually over 14 years of age).

emergency exception rule see doctrine of implied consent.

emesis vomiting.

emotional abuse the intentional infliction of emotional harm to a child.

emotional neglect the intentional omission of emotional support to a child.

empathy the awareness of and insight into the feelings, emotions, and behavior of another person.

EMS-EMSC Continuum the linked community services set up to prevent and treat childhood emergencies. The continuum includes prevention, the primary physician, out-of-hospital care, ED care, hospital care, and rehabilitation.

encephalitis inflammation of the brain.

endotracheal intubation a method of intubation in which an endotracheal tube (ETT) is placed through a patient's mouth, directly through the larynx between the vocal cords, and into the trachea, to open and maintain an airway.

enterovirus species of virus that causes gastrointestinal or respiratory disease in children.

envenomation the act of injecting venom, such as by a snake or insect.

environment the surroundings, conditions, or influences that affect an organism or an injury.

environmental assessment evaluation of the scene to draw clues about what is wrong and the best route to take for treatment. Gathering information by observing things like damage to a vehicle or medication bottles in the patient's home.

epiglottis a leaf or omega-shaped structure located immediately posterior to the root of the tongue that prevents food and secretions from entering the trachea.

epiglottitis inflammation of the epiglottis.

epilepsy a condition of recurrent seizures.

epinephrine a substance produced by the body (commonly called adrenaline) and that has a vital role in the function of the sympathetic nervous system; also a drug produced by pharmaceutical companies that increases blood pressure and causes bronchodilation; the drug of choice for an anaphylactic reaction.

epiphysis the ends of the bone that are the secondary ossification centers.

esophagus a muscular canal that carries food from the pharynx to the stomach.

etiology cause and origin of disease.

evaporation change from liquid to vapor.

exhalation the process of breathing out.

extensor posturing see decerebrate.

extraocular movement of the eyes in various directions.

feeding tube a tube placed into the stomach through the mouth, nose, or skin.

fetal-placental transfusion the transfusion of blood from the baby to the placenta, leading to a decrease in the infant's blood volume. This can occur if the baby is held higher than the uterus or womb prior to clamping the cord.

fetus a human or mammal in an early form of intrauterine development.

flaccidity weak, lax, and soft.

flail chest an unstable condition of the chest wall due to two or more fractures of the ribs resulting in ineffective breathing.

flexion the act of bending.

flexural creases the creases behind the knees or inside the elbows.

focal limited to a part of the body.

fontanelle a soft spot of undeveloped bone lying between the cranial bones of the skull of a fetus or infant.

fulminant pneumonia sudden and intense inflammation of the lungs with infection.

gag reflex the protective reflex that keeps food, fluid, or secretions from getting into the trachea.

gastric decompression the removal of air and other contents from the stomach.

gastric feeding tube a tube that provides a channel directly into a patient's stomach, allowing removal of gas, blood, and toxins, or insertion medications and nutrition.

gastroenteritis inflammation of the stomach and intestinal tract.

gastroesophageal reflux a condition in which the liquid content of the stomach regurgitates (backs up, or refluxes) into the esophagus.

gastrointestinal (GI) decontamination the removal of poison from the stomach.

gastrostomy tube (G-tube) a feeding tube placed directly through the wall of the abdomen.

generalized seizure characterized by movements (often tonic-clonic) that indicate involvement of both cerebral hemispheres.

gestation the length of time from conception to birth.

glial cells specialized cells that surround neurons, providing mechanical and physical support and electrical insulation between neurons.

glottis the sound-producing apparatus of the larynx, consisting of two vocal folds.

glucagon a hormone that has the property of increasing the concentration of sugar in the blood.

greenstick fracture a fracture involving only part of the outer layer or cortex of a bone.

grunting a short, low-pitched sound at the end of exhalation, present in children with moderate to severe hypoxia; it reflects poor gas exchange because of fluid in the lower airways and air sacs.

hazardous materials (HazMat) any substance that is toxic, poisonous, radioactive, flammable, or explosive and causes injury or death with exposure.

head bobbing the head lifts and tilts back during inspiration, then moves forward during expiration; a sign of increased work of breathing.

health information exchanges (HIEs) the sharing of healthcare information electronically across organizations within a region, community, or hospital system.

hematocrit a measure of red blood cell mass in the serum. An average figure for humans is 45 percent.

hematoma a swelling or mass of blood confined to a organ, tissue, or space and caused by a break in a blood vessel.

hemodialysis a form of dialysis in which the blood is removed from the patient through a catheter or fistula, and then returns to the body through another needle, removing various toxins, electrolytes, and fluid in the process.

hemodynamically stable not changing or fluctuating in relation to the mechanics of blood circulation.

hemopericardium accumulation of blood around the heart muscle in the pericardial sac.

hemophilia a congenital condition in which the patient lacks one or more of the blood's normal clotting factors.

hemostat instrument clamp; in its closed position it squeezes tissues or vessels and arrests the flow of blood.

hepatomegaly enlargement of the liver.

hives wheals; an itchy rash caused by contact with or ingestion of an allergic substance or food.

homeostasis the maintenance of a relatively stable internal physiologic environment.

host the organism acted upon in an injury or illness process.

hydrocarbon a basic organic compound made up only of hydrogen and carbon.

hydrocephalus the increased accumulation of cerebrospinal fluid within the ventricles of the brain.

hydrochloric acid a powerful and corrosive aqueous solution of hydrogen chloride (HCl).

hymenoptera insects such as bees, ants, and wasps.

hyperalimentation the administration of nutrients by intravenous feeding.

hyperoxia increased oxygen in the blood.

hyperthermia unusually elevated body temperature.

hypertrophic cardiomyopathy (HCM) a condition in which the heart muscle is unusually thick, which means that the heart has to pump harder to get blood to leave.

hypnotic drug pertaining to sleep or sedation.

hypocarbia decreased carbon dioxide in the blood, usually from an excess rate of ventilation.

hypoglycemia low blood sugar.

hypoperfusion inadequate circulation.

hypotension decrease of systolic and diastolic blood pressure below normal for age, representing decompensated shock.

hypotensive (decompensated) shock a shock state characterized by low blood pressure, which will rapidly progress to cardiac arrest if not rapidly corrected.

hypothermia having a body temperature below normal range.

hypotonia reduced muscular tension.

hypovolemia diminished blood volume.

hypovolemic shock a clinical state of reduced intravascular volume.

hypoxemia a decreased oxygen saturation in blood detected by pulse oximetry or direct measurement of oxygen saturation in an arterial blood gas sample.

hypoxia a pathological condition in which the body as a whole (generalized hypoxia) or region of the body (tissue hypoxia) is deprived of an adequate oxygen supply.

hypoxic stress a subnormal concentration of oxygen.

ileostomy the surgical establishment of an opening between the small bowel and the surface of the body for the purpose of providing drainage of the bowel.

impending brainstem herniation when brain tissue, cerebrospinal fluid, and blood vessels are moved or pressed away from their usual position inside the skull.

impending herniation syndrome clinical state in which there is severely abnormal brain pressure, just before the moment of tissue herniation and compression of brain tissue

implementation phase second of the three phases in disaster response. Activities during this phase include: search and rescue, victim triage, initial stabilization and transport, and definitive management of scene hazards and victims.

implied consent a type of consent in which a patient who is unable to give consent is given treatment under the legal assumption that he or she would want treatment if thinking in a normal way.

in utero within the uterus.

indirect medical control existing or standing orders, written policies, procedures, and protocols.

indwelling central venous catheter small, flexible plastic tube inserted into a large vein above the heart, usually the subclavian vein, through which access to the blood stream can be made. This catheter is left in place and allows drugs and blood products to be given and blood samples withdrawn painlessly.

informed consent permission for treatment given by a competent patient after the potential risks, benefits, and alternatives to treatment have been explained.

infusion a liquid substance introduced into the body for therapeutic or diagnostic purposes.

inspiratory the process of moving air into the lungs.

insulin a hormone produced by the islet of Langerhans (an exocrine gland in the pancreas) that enables sugar in the blood to enter the cells of the body; used in synthetic form to treat and control diabetes mellitus.

intercostal between the ribs.

intercurrent intervening.

intra-abdominal within the abdomen.

intracranial within the cranium or skull.

intracranial hypertension increased pressure of the cerebrospinal fluid that impairs brain function.

intramuscular medications injections into a muscle; a medication delivery route.

intranasal within the nasal cavity; a medication delivery route.

intraosseous within the marrow cavity of a bone; intramedullary; a medication delivery route.

intravascular volume the water portion of the circulatory system surrounding the blood cells.

ipecac an oral medicine to induce vomiting; this medicine is no longer recommended for use by prehospital professionals.

ischemia deficiency of blood supply.

jaundice a condition characterized by yellowness of skin, whites of eyes, mucous membranes, and body fluids due to deposition of excess bilirubin in the blood (hyperbilirubinemia).

jugular venous distension a prominence of the jugular veins as they fill with blood; if patient is not supine, indication that the blood may be having difficulty flowing back into the right side of the heart. This can be caused by pericardial tamponade, tension pneumothorax, or right-sided heart failure.

lactic acidosis the metabolic acidotic state resulting from the accumulation of lactic acid secondary to anaerobic cellular metabolism.

laryngoscope an instrument for examining the larynx.

laryngoscopy an examination of the interior of the larynx.

larynx the enlarged upper end of the trachea, below the root of the tongue, that contains the vocal cords.

lateral pertaining to the side.

lateral decubitus position the position with the patient on his or her side.

legal authority the ability to make medical decisions under the law.

lethargy listlessness; weakness.

leukemia a cancerous condition in which certain cell lines begin to grow abnormally fast.

localizes when a patient is able to respond to the site of a specific noxious or painful stimulus (e.g., when a patient reaches for and pushes away the hand that is pinching them during a neurologic exam).

long QT syndrome a condition characterized by a QT interval exceeding approximately 450 ms.

lordosis forward curve of the lumbar spine.

lye corrosive, alkaline cleaning liquid.

malaise discomfort, uneasiness, or generalized ill feeling, often indicative of infection.

malposition when something is in an incorrect or abnormal position.

mandible the horseshoe-shaped bone forming the lower jaw.

mass-casualty incident (MCI) an emergency situation involving more than one patient, and which can place such great demand on equipment or personnel that the system is stretched to its limit or beyond.

mature minor a person without the formal legal status of an emancipated minor, but having similar characteristics: married, pregnant, on active-duty status in the armed service, or 15 years or older and living separate and apart from his or her guardians. This person has the legal right to give consent for treatment as well as the legal right to refuse.

meconium the bowel contents of a fetus. The presence of meconium in amniotic fluid means the fetus may have suffered some type of stress, such as hypoxia, and may be depressed and need to be resuscitated.

mediastinum the space between the lungs, in the center of the chest, that contains the heart, trachea, mainstem bronchi, part of the esophagus, and large blood vessels.

medical control physician instructions that are given directly by radio (online or direct) or indirectly by protocols or guidelines (off-line or indirect), as authorized by the medical director of the service program.

medical home an approach to providing health care services in a high quality and cost-effective manner. Children and their families who have a medical home receive the care that they need from a pediatrician or family physician that they know and trust. The pediatric health care professional and parents act as partners in a medical home to identify and access all the medical and nonmedical services needed to help children and their families achieve their maximum potential.

medical responsibility the moral and legal duty to provide medical care in an emergency.

medicolegal related to medical jurisprudence or forensic medicine.

mediport a central catheter that is implanted under the skin.

meninges a set of three tough membranes, the dura mater, arachnoid, and pia mater, that encloses the entire brain and spinal cord.

meningitis inflammation of the membranes of the spinal cord or brain.

meningococcal sepsis blood-borne infection with the bacteria *Neisseria meningitidis* leading to sepsis (fever or hypothermia, shock, and hypotension).

meningococcemia infection of the blood stream by the bacteria *Neisseria meningitidis*. This is usually a severe infection characterized by fever, shock and a characteristic purpuric rash (bruising of the skin) with or without meningitis.

metabolic acidosis a metabolic state of acidosis resulting from retention of hydrogen or other positively charged ions not related to respiratory compromise.

midaxillary (line) imaginary vertical line drawn through the middle of the axilla (armpit), parallel to the midline.

military anti-shock trousers (MAST) a garment designed to put pressure on the lower extremities and abdomen in order to squeeze blood from the peripheral vessels so as to increase core organ circulation. This is no longer recommended in children.

minor a person not of legal age and thus requiring consent from a legal guardian for medical or surgical care.

minute ventilation the volume of air exchanged per minute [minute ventilation =tidal volume × respiratory rate].

miosis abnormal contraction of pupils.

Mongolian spots blue-gray areas of discoloration of the skin caused by abnormal pigment, not by trauma or bruising.

mortality death.

motor activity muscle use.

mottling a condition of abnormal skin circulation, caused by vasoconstriction or inadequate circulation.

multisystem trauma injury involving more than one organ system, such as combined injury to the chest, abdomen, and brain.

myocardial depression when the heart muscle is not working adequately.

myocardial function a measure of how well the heart is working.

myocardial infarction the death of part of the heart muscle caused by partial or complete occlusion of one or more of the coronary arteries.

myocarditis inflammation of the myocardium.

narcotic an opiate drug that produces analgesia and sedation, as well as euphoria when used for recreational purposes.

nasal cannula an oxygen-delivery device in which oxygen flows through two small, tubelike prongs that fit into the patient's nostrils.

nasal flaring flaring out of the nostrils, indicating increased work of breathing and hypoxia.

nasopharyngeal airway (NPA) airway adjunct inserted into the nostril of a conscious patient who is not able to maintain a natural airway.

needle decompression the removal of air from a closed space, such as from the pleura.

neonatal seizures seizures that occur in neonates.

nerve agents a class of chemicals including organophosphates; they function by blocking an essential enzyme in the nervous system, which causes the body's organs to become overstimulated.

neurogenic shock shock caused by paralysis of the nerves that control the size of the blood vessels, leading to widespread dilation and pooling of blood in the peripheral vessels to the extent that adequate perfusion cannot be maintained; seen in patients with spinal cord injuries.

neurovascular concerning both the nervous and vascular systems.

nonpulsatile fontanelle when the fontanelle or "soft spot" on an infant's head is full, usually tense and does not seem to beat or pulse with each beat of the heart.

nuclear bomb a bomb which is extremely powerful due to its use of atomic energy as a source of its explosive nature. In addition to the actual explosive force of the bomb, injury is caused in a wider area by the radiation released by the explosion.

obstetric having to do with pregnancy, delivery of a baby.

obstructive shock shock or inadequate tissue perfusion that is caused by a restriction to blood flow out from the heart (e.g., shock due to a critical coarctation or severe narrowing of the aorta, tension pneumothorax, or cardiac tamponade).

obturator an inner stabilizing structure that gives stiffness to a hollow tube, to allow insertion or clearing of an obstruction.

occlusion the closure of a passage.

occlusive dressing a dressing that covers completely.

occult illness an illness that is not immediately obvious or is "hidden." An illness that does not have obvious symptoms.

operations administrative processes.

opiates see narcotics.

oral glucose a simple sugar that is readily absorbed by the bloodstream; it is carried on the EMS unit.

organophosphate insecticide a type of poison with cholinergic properties, used as an insecticide.

oropharyngeal airway (OPA) an airway adjunct inserted into the mouth to keep the tongue from blocking the upper airway and to make suctioning the airway easier.

oropharynx the part of the pharynx lying between the soft palate and upper portion of the epiglottis.

ossification the formation of bone. An ossification center is an area where cartilage is transformed through calcification into a new area of bone.

osteogenesis imperfecta a genetic disorder in which the bones are brittle, and results in fractures.

ostomies a surgical opening made in the skin as a way for waste products to leave the body.

otorrhea any flow or discharge from the ear.

pallor lack of color; paleness.

palpation physical touching for the purpose of obtaining information.

paradoxical irritability a marker for possible serious pediatric illness, consisting of a particular type of irritability where attempts to console further distress the child.

pathology the study and diagnosis of disease.

pathophysiology the study of how disease or injury affects the body.

pedal related to the foot (e.g., pedal pulses are pulses found in the foot).

pedal relating to the foot or feet.

pediatric assessment triangle (PAT) assessment tool that allows rapid formation of a general impression of the type and level of illness or injury in an infant or child without touching him or her; consists of assessing appearance, work of breathing, and circulation to the skin.

pediatric critical care center a type of specialized center for children with advanced resources (such as a pediatric intensive care unit) for care of the critically ill.

pediatric trauma center a type of specialized center for children with advanced resources for care of critically injured children.

pelvic fractures breaks through one or more bones of the pelvis (the hip bones and the sacrum and coccyx or lower parts of the spine).

percutaneous endoscopic gastrostomy (PEG) a procedure that places a tube through the abdominal wall and into the stomach.

perfusion blood circulation.

pericardial tamponade compression of the heart due to a buildup of blood or other fluid in the pericardial sac.

periosteum the membrane, made up of a double layer of connective tissue, that covers all bones, except the articular surfaces.

peripheral cyanosis slightly bluish or dark purple discoloration of the skin (on the hands and feet only).

peripheral vasoconstriction when the blood vessels in the outer extremities (hands and feet especially) constrict (get smaller in size through the contraction of the smooth muscle in the blood vessel walls) and therefore lead to a decrease in blood flow to those areas. This may produce peripheral cyanosis (bluish discoloration of the hands and feet) and prolonged capillary refill time.

peripherally implanted central catheter (PICC) an indwelling line that is partially implanted under the skin and partially exposed above the skin.

peritoneal dialysis a type of dialysis in which a special solution is instilled through a catheter into the patient's abdomen, and that draws toxins, electrolytes, and other fluids from the body through the peritoneal membrane.

peritoneum the membrane lining the abdominal cavity (parietal peritoneum) and covering the abdominal organs (visceral peritoneum).

petechiae small, purplish, nonblanching spots on the skin that appear in certain severe fevers and may be indicative of possible sepsis.

petechial related to petechiae, small purplish, nonblanching spots on the skin. Petechiae represent small areas of hemorrhage into the skin and may be seen with infections, especially sepsis.

petechial rash rash which contains petechiae, small areas of hemorrhage into the skin that do not blanch when they are pressed on.

pharynx passageway for air from nasal cavity to larynx and food from mouth to esophagus.

phencyclidine (PCP) a hallucinogen, referred to as PCP or angel dust. Moderate doses cause elevated blood pressure, rapid pulse, increased skeletal muscle tone, and, sometimes, myoclonic jerks.

physeal plate pertaining to growth or to the segment of bone that is concerned with growth.

physical abuse see child maltreatment.

physical neglect see child neglect.

physiologic concerning body function.

Pierre Robin syndrome a condition present at birth marked by a small lower jaw (micrognathia). The tongue tends to fall back and downward (glossoptosis), and there is a cleft soft palate.

placenta the tissue attached to the uterine wall that nourishes the fetus through the umbilical cord.

plague an illness caused by infection with the bacteria *Yersinia pestis*. The disease is characterized by fever and chills followed by a severe illness with pneumonia, headache, and delirium. It is transmitted to humans by the bites of fleas from infected rodents and has a high fatality rate. It is an agent that could possibly be used as a weapon of bioterrorism.

pleura the serous membrane that enfolds both lungs and is reflected upon the walls of the thorax and diaphragm.

pleural space the space between the parietal and visceral layers of the pleura.

pneumomediastinum air or gas in the mediastinal tissues.

pneumonia an inflammation of the lungs caused primarily by bacteria, viruses, and chemical irritants.

pneumothorax a collection of air in the pleural cavity, which if under pressure may cause severe physiologic changes with poor venous return and inadequate cardiac output.

policies medicolegal operational standards to guide prehospital professionals intended to help with decision-making in difficult or legally sensitive field situations.

polypharmacy an ingestion involving more than one drug.

positive-pressure ventilation assisted ventilation.

posteriorly from the back, from behind, or from underneath.

postictal state the confused state of a patient after having a seizure.

postpartum after childbirth.

posturing abnormal body positioning after a brain injury; it may be in response to painful stimuli.

preterm labor labor beginning prior to the 37th week of gestation.

primary brain injury injury resulting from the direct biomechanical effects of the impact forces on the brain which result in direct impact or sudden movement causing shear stress of the brain.

procedure a physical intervention.

prone lying horizontal with face downward.

propylene glycol a solvent in medicines.

protocol a step-by-step process for treatment.

proximal nearest the point of attachment, center of the body, or point of reference; opposite of distal.

pulmonary contusion a bruise of the lung.

pulmonary edema a build-up of fluid in the lungs.

pulmonary intoxicants toxins or poisons which may be absorbed through (e.g., by inhalation) or cause harm to the respiratory system.

pulseless electrical activity (PEA) an organized cardiac rhythm on the cardiac monitor in absence of a palpable pulse.

purpura a rash that looks like bruising of the skin that is usually seen in overwhelming infections (sepsis) or when a patient has an inflammation of the blood vessels (vasculitis).

purpuric pertaining to bruising of the skin.

pus the liquid product of inflammation, generally yellow in color.

QRS complex the electrical shape of a major portion of the heart rhythm on the cardiac monitor, representing ventricular electrical activity.

quadriplegia a condition that causes paralysis of all four extremities (both arms and both legs) usually due to an injury in the upper cervical portion of the spinal cord.

quality assurance (QA) a formalized process of reviewing patient care activities and patient outcomes in an attempt to promote high quality care and insure that the best possible outcomes are achieved while identifying and correcting actions that lead to poor patient care.

quality improvement (QI) a system of internal and external reviews and audits of all aspects of the system.

racemic including all isomers of a drug, such as epinephrine.

radial pertaining to the radius, the larger and more lateral of the two bones in the forearm.

rapid sequence intubation (RSI) a specific set of procedures, combined in rapid succession, to induce sedation and paralysis and intubate a patient quickly.

reactivity the capacity for reacting to a stimulus.

reassessment the part of the assessment process in which problems are reevaluated and responses to treatment are assessed.

recovery phase final of three phases in disaster response. Activities include: scene withdrawal, return to normal operations, and debriefing.

renal dialysis a technique for filtering the blood of its toxic wastes, removing excess fluids, and restoring the normal balance of electrolytes.

respiratory arrest the absence of respirations (i.e., apnea) with detectable cardiac activity.

respiratory depression a condition in which there is a slowing of the respiratory rate and decreased respiratory effort usually due to some effect on the respiratory center in the medulla of the brain. This may be caused by trauma, illness, or the effects of drugs (e.g., morphine or diazepam) or toxins (e.g., ethanol).

respiratory distress a clinical state characterized by increased respiratory rate, effort, and work of breathing.

respiratory failure a clinical state of inadequate oxygenation, ventilation, or both.

respiratory syncytial virus (RSV) a virus that commonly causes bronchiolitis.

retractions physical drawing in of the chest wall between the ribs that occurs with increased work of breathing.

rhinorrhea thin watery discharge from the nose.

ricin neurotoxin derived from mash that is left from the castor bean. When introduced into the body, ricin causes pulmonary edema and respiratory and circulatory failure, leading to death.

salivation the act of secreting saliva.

SALT sort, assess, livesaving interventions, and treatment/transport: a triage system.

saphenous veins two superficial veins, the great and small, passing up the leg.

scald a burn to skin or flesh caused by moist heat and hot vapors, as steam.

scaphoid the wrist bone that is found just beyond the most distal portion of the radius.

scoliosis a lateral curvature of the spine.

scopolamine an anticholinergic agent with action similar to atropine.

secondary assessment a step in the patient assessment process in which a systematic physical examination of the patient is performed. The examination may be a systematic full-body evaluation or an assessment that focuses on a certain area or region of the body, often determined through the chief complaint.

secondary brain injury injury to the brain resulting from factors occurring after the initial biomechanical effects of the primary brain injury (such as hypoxia and hypotension).

secretion the process of producing liquid materials into the blood or body cavities.

sedative an agent that relaxes.

semi-Fowler's position the position of a patient who is lying in a bed in a supine position with the head of the bed at approximately 30 degrees.

sepsis a pathological state, usually in a febrile patient, resulting from the presence of invading microorganisms or their poisonous products in the bloodstream.

septic shock shock from infection, involving hypotension and signs of inadequate organ perfusion.

serial examinations the act of repeatedly examining a patient to carefully watch and document the progression of signs or symptoms in an attempt to develop a diagnosis (e.g., serial examinations of the abdomen to decide if someone with abdominal trauma may have a perforation of the intestine) or to watch for a change in their condition (e.g., serial examinations of a child with a head injury to monitor their neurologic status and watch for signs of increasing intracranial pressure).

serum glucose the level of blood sugar.

sexual abuse rape, sexual assault, or sexual molestation.

shaken baby syndrome/abusive head trauma a syndrome seen in abused infants and children. The patient has been subjected to violent, whiplash-type shaking injuries inflicted by the abusing individual. This may cause coma, convulsions, and increased intracranial pressure due to tearing of the cerebral veins with consequent bleeding into the brain.

shock a clinical syndrome in which the blood flow and oxygen delivery are inadequate for normal organ function.

sickle cell disease a hereditary disease characterized by abnormal clumping together of deformed red blood cells. The patients have painful crises, anemia, infection-risks, strokes, and other serious complications.

simple febrile seizure a brief (less than 15 minutes), self-limited, generalized convulsion in a previously healthy child between the ages of 6 months and 6 years that is associated with an elevated fever. Children with simple febrile seizures have relatively short postictal periods after which they return to their baseline with a nonfocal neurologic examination.

simple partial seizures a focal (localized) seizure which involves a motor or sensory abnormality (e.g., twitching of one hand or a visual disturbance) in a patient who remains conscious. In children, partial seizures are usually motor seizures and frequently will progress to generalized seizures.

Sims position a semi-prone position with the patient on her side, with her opposite knee and thigh drawn well up to facilitate delivery of a baby.

sinus arrhythmia a variation in the resting heart rate often seen in children and adolescents. As the child breathes in the heart rate increases slightly and as they exhale the heart rate decreases. This is a normal variation in children and not truly an arrhythmia. On ECG each QRS complex is preceded by a P wave and there are no missed or skipped beats.

sinus tachycardia rapid heart rate in a child with normal conduction.

slurry a thin, watery mixture.

smallpox a rare, highly contagious viral disease; it is most contagious when blisters begin to form.

sniffing position an upright position in which the patient's head and chin are thrust slightly forward to keep the airway open; the child appears to be sniffing.

soft-tissue injuries injuries to the skin, fat, muscles, ligaments, and tendons.

spasticity increased tone or contractions of muscles causing stiff and awkward movements.

spina bifida a congenital anomaly where the posterior elements of the vertebrae have failed to fuse together. The spinal cord and its associated coverings (meninges) may protrude through this defect in the vertebrae leading to a range of neurologic impairment in the lower extremities depending on the degree and level of the protrusion. When the defect is isolated to the bony structures without spinal cord or meningeal abnormality this is termed spina bifida occulta.

spinal motion restriction the preferred practice of maintaining the spine in anatomic alignment to minimize gross movement, without mandating the use of specific adjuncts. True spinal immobilization is difficult to achieve. The use of a backboard should be judicious, so that the potential benefits outweigh the risks.

spinal protection the preferred term for describing the procedure used by prehospital or hospital-based professionals, with or without the use of adjuncts, to help maintain appropriate alignment of the spine.

spine the vertebral column.

spleen the major abdominal organ involved in the production and destruction of red blood cells and immune cells. It is filled with blood and can hemorrhage after injury.

splinting fixation with a splint.

(START) Simple Triage and Rapid Treatment a triage system.

status epilepticus a state of continuous seizures or multiple seizures without an intervening return to consciousness.

sterile free from living microorganisms.

stress forces that disrupt equilibrium or produce strain.

stridor a harsh sound during inspiration, high-pitched due to partial upper airway obstruction.

subcostal beneath the ribs.

subdural hemorrhage bleeding beneath the dura mater.

subglottic beneath the glottis.

substernal situated beneath the sternum.

sucking chest wound an open or penetrating chest-wall wound through which air passes during inspiration and expiration.

sudden unexpected infant death (SUID) the sudden death of an infant younger than 1 year that cannot be explained because a thorough investigation was not conducted and cause of death could not be determined.

superior vena cava one of the two largest veins in the body that carries blood from the upper extremities, head, neck, and chest into the heart.

supine lying on the back with the face upward.

supraclavicular located above the clavicle.

supraglottic the area above the glottis or true vocal cords.

suprasternal above the sternum.

suprasternal retractions when the muscles and skin above the sternum sink in above the manubrium as the patient attempts to breathe.

supraventricular tachycardia (SVT) an abnormal heart rhythm with a rapid rate and narrow QRS complex.

symmetry correspondence in shape, size, and relative position of parts on opposite sides of a body.

sympathomimetic agents adrenergic drugs; producing effects resembling those resulting from stimulation of the sympathetic nervous system, such as effects following the injection of epinephrine.

symphysis pubis the junction of the pubic bones in the midline on the lower part of the abdomen.

symptomatic ventricular dysrhythmias abnormal ventricular electrical impulses (e.g., ventricular tachycardia) that are associated with symptoms on the part of the patient.

synaptic connections connections between two or more nerves (i.e., synapses).

tachycardia rapid heart rate.

tachypnea rapid respiration.

tamponade compression of tissues.

temporary protective custody when a legal guardian suffers from diminished judgement, law enforcement officers may place a minor in some form of temporary protective custody. While this may allow the prehospital professional to transport a minor to a medical facility for purposes of medical evaluation, it does not give the prehospital professional the right medically to treat a minor.

tension pneumothorax an accumulation of air or gas in the pleural cavity that progressively increases and causes serious hemodynamic changes.

terrorism a violent act dangerous to human life, in violation of the criminal laws of the United States or of any state, to intimidate or coerce a government, the civilian population, or any segment thereof, in furtherance of political or social objectives.

thermoregulation heat regulation.

thoracic pertaining to the chest or thorax.

thoracic excursions the movements of the chest wall (rib cage and muscles) associated with respirations.

thoracostomy opening of the chest wall to allow drainage of the chest cavity.

tidal volume the amount of air that is exchanged with each breath.

titratable the ability to adjust the desired effect of an agent by giving more or less of that agent as needed over time (e.g., using an intravenous catheter to slowly give more analgesic or sedative agents until a patient is just quiet enough to effectively complete a procedure).

tonic-clonic a seizure that features rhythmic back-and-forth motion of an extremity and body stiffness.

totally implanted device a catheter totally implanted and not visible to the eye (mediport).

trachea a cylindrical cartilaginous tube from the larynx to the bronchial tubes. It extends from the 6th cervical to the 5th thoracic vertebra, where it divides at a point called the carina into two bronchi, one leading to each lung.

tracheitis an inflammation of the trachea.

tracheostomy operation of incising the skin over the trachea and making a surgical wound in the trachea in order to permit an airway during tracheal obstruction.

tracheostomy tube a tube inserted into the trachea in children who cannot breathe or maintain a clear airway on their own.

transdermal through the skin.

transient not lasting; of brief duration.

transmucosal to pass across a mucous membrane (e.g., the absorption of a toxin or pharmaceutical agent across the mucous membranes of the mouth).

traumatic brain injury (TBI) the preferred term for head trauma.

tripoding an abnormal position to keep the airway open; it involves leaning forward onto two arms stretched forward.

trismus tonic contraction of the muscles of mastication.

tympanic temperature body temperature measurement made by the use of a device which measures the reflectance of infrared light from the tympanic membrane (ear drum).

umbilical catheterization placing a cannula into the umbilical artery or vein.

umbilical cord the attachment connecting the fetus with the placenta.

universal precautions protective measures that have traditionally been developed by the Centers for Disease Control and Prevention (CDC) for use in dealing with objects, blood, body fluids, or other potential exposure risks of communicable disease.

universal standards for pediatric emergency care standards of care agreed upon and promoted by experts in pediatric emergency care and the organizations they represent for the management of children throughout the emergency medical system.

uterus an organ in the female reproductive system for containing and nourishing the embryo and fetus from the time the fertilized egg is implanted to the time of birth of the fetus.

vagal pertaining to the vagus nerve.

vagal nerve stimulator (VNS) a small device implanted under the skin near the collarbone as a treatment for epilepsy.

vaginal introitus the vaginal opening.

vagus nerve the cranial nerve (X) that provides motor functions to the soft palate, pharynx, and larynx and carries taste bud fibers from the posterior tongue, sensory fibers from the inferior pharynx, larynx, thoracic, and abdominal organs, and parasympathetic fibers to thoracic and abdominal organs.

varicella (chicken pox) an acute viral disease with mild constitutional symptoms (headache, fever, malaise) followed by an eruption appearing in crops and characterized by macules, papules, and vesicles.

vascular tone the amount of constriction in a blood vessel or more generally, the overall amount of constriction in the blood vessels of the body. This is a reflection of the acute cardiovascular health of the patient. Patients in shock often have marked vasoconstriction in an attempt to increase their vascular tone and blood pressure to maximize perfusion to vital organs. When there is a loss of vascular tone (e.g., in sepsis or spinal shock) there is often generalized vasodilatation and severe hypotension.

vasculitis inflammation of the blood vessels which usually is associated with pain, swelling, and often leakage of fluid and blood from the vessels into other organs. When this occurs in the skin a purpuric rash often develops.

vasoconstriction decrease in the caliber of blood vessels.

vasodilatation dilatation of blood vessels.

vasomotor pertaining to the nerves having muscular control of the blood vessel walls.

vasopressor agent a drug that increases vascular tone and increases blood pressure.

ventilation-perfusion mismatch a pathologic state where the oxygen going into the lungs is not mixing appropriately with the blood circulating through the lungs.

ventilator a mechanical device for artificial ventilation of the lungs.

ventricle one of two (right and left) lower chambers of the heart. The left ventricle receives blood from the left atrium (upper chamber) and delivers blood to the aorta. The right ventricle receives blood from the right atrium and pumps it into the pulmonary artery.

ventricular fibrillation (VF) disorganized, ineffective twitching of the ventricles, resulting in no blood flow and a state of cardiac arrest.

ventricular tachycardia (VT) a rapid heart rhythm in which the electrical impulse begins in the ventricle (instead of the atrium), which may result in inadequate blood flow and eventually deteriorate into cardiac arrest.

vertebral bodies the 33 bones that make up the spinal column.

vesicants blister agents; the primary route of entry for vesicants is through the skin.

viral myocarditis a viral infection of the heart which frequently leads to dysrhythmias, especially ventricular dysrhythmias and poor muscle function which produces congestive heart failure.

visual analogue scores (VAS) scales generated by asking a patient or subject to quantify the amount of a sensation they are feeling (usually pain) by pointing to where on a line their sensation is. By measuring how far along the line the patient points one can use this as a measure of that sensation. A frequently used technique for the measurement of pain in research studies.

vital signs the key signs that are used to evaluate the patient's overall condition, including respirations, pulse, blood pressure, level of consciousness, and skin characteristics.

vocal cords two small folds of tissue in the larynx which vibrate as air moves across them to produce sound.

volume resuscitation replenishing the blood volume.

wheezing production of whistling sounds during expiration such as occurs in asthma and bronchiolitis.

womb uterus; female organ for containing, protecting, and nourishing the fetus.

work of breathing an indicator of oxygenation and ventilation. Work of breathing reflects the child's attempt to compensate for hypoxia.

Index

Note: Page numbers followed by f and t denote figures and tables.

A

B

C

D

E

I

J

K

L

N

Q

R

S

T

U

V

W

Y

Additional Credits

Unless otherwise indicated, all photographs and illustrations are under copyright of Jones & Bartlett Learning, courtesy of Maryland Institute for Emergency Medical Services Systems, or have been provided by the author(s).

Cover & Title Page © Getty Images/ Bruce Ayres

Chapter 1

Opener © Mark C. Ide; **FIG 1-4** Courtesy of the Health Resources and Services Administration (HRSA), Maternal and Child Health Bureau (MCHB), Emergency Medical Services for Children (EMSC Program); **FIG 1-3** © Photos.com; **FIG 1-8** © Hemera/ Thinkstock; **FIG 1-12** Courtesy of the Health Resources and Services Administration (HRSA), Maternal and Child Health Bureau (MCHB), Emergency Medical Services for Children (EMSC Program.); **FIG 1-17** From Hockenberry MJ, Wilson D: Wong's essentials of pediatric nursing, ed. 8, St. Louis, 2009, Mosby. Used with permission. Copyright Mosby.

Chapter 2

FIG 2-04 © Photodisc/Getty Images; **FIG 2-10** © Stockbyte/Creatas; **FIG 2-12** © Photos.com

Chapter 3

Opener © PROJEKTOGRAF/ ShutterStock, Inc.

Chapter 4

Opener © Craig Jackson/In the Dark Photography; **FIG 4-4** © FreeBirdPhotos/Shutterstock. **FIG 4-5** Courtesy of Lisa Wise; **FIG 4-7** Courtesy of Susan Fuchs, MD

Chapter 5

Opener © nano/istockphoto.com; **FIG 5-1** From 12-Lead ECG: The Art of Interpretation, courtesy of Tomas B. Garcia, MD.; **FIG 5-7** © Glen Ellman

Chapter 6

Opener © CORBIS/age fotostock; **FIG 6-2** Courtesy of Rhonda Beck; **FIG 6-3** Accu-Chek® Aviva used with permission of Roche Diagnostics; **FIG 6-4** © Stock Connection Distribution/Alamy Images

Chapter 7

Opener © Pears2295/istockphoto.com; **FIG 7-12** Courtesy of the State of North Carolin EMSC.; **FIG 7-17** © Charles Stewart & Associates; **FIG 7-18** Courtesy of Allied Healthcare Products, Inc.

Chapter 8

Opener © Purestock/Thinkstock; **FIG 8-1** © Image Source/age footstock

Chapter 9

Opener © Alexey Stiop/ShutterStock, Inc.; **FIG 9-1** © 2002 Lou Roming, MD, FAAP, FACEP; **FIG 9-2** Chemical Hazards Emergency Medical Management, U.S. Department of Health & Human Services, http://chemm.nlm.nih.gov/chemmimages/salt.png; **FIG 9-3** Courtesy of Dave Saville/FEMA; **FIG 9-4** Courtesy of Harald Richter/National Severe Storms Laboratory (NSSL)/ NOAA; **FIG 9-5** © Shannon Hicks/ Newtown Bee/AP Images; **FIG 9-6** Courtesy of CDC/Dr. John Noble, Jr.

Chapter 10

Opener © Rubberball/Corbis; **TAB 10-7** AAP, The APGAR Score, Pediatrics Vol. 117 No. 4 April 1, 2006, pp. 1444 -1447; **FIG 10-10** © Eddie Lawrence/Science Source. **FIG 10-22** Courtesy of Neotech Products, Inc.

Chapter 11

Opener © Realistic Reflections/ Getty Images; **FIG 11-1** Courtesy of Dr. Hudson/CDC; **FIG 11-2** Courtesy of Cindy Bissell; **FIG 11-11** Courtesy of Cindy Bissell; **FIG 11-13A** © Visuals Unlimited, Inc.; **FIG 11-13B** © Michael English, MD / Custom Medical Stock Photo; **FIG 11-14** © Craig Jackson/In the Dark Photography

Chapter 12

Opener © Glen E. Ellman; **FIG 12-2** © Photos.com; **FIG 12-3** © Glen E. Ellman; **FIG 12-4** © Sean O'Brien/ Custom Medical Stock Photo

Chapter 13

Opener © Pixel Memiors/ ShutterStock, Inc.; **TAB 13-2** Source: Child Welfare Information Gateway. 2012. Child Maltreatment 2010: Summary of Key Findings. http://www.childwelfare.gov/pubs/factsheets/canstats.cfm. Accessed September 11, 2012.

Chapter 14

Opener © Steve Hamblin/Alamy Images

Chapter 15

Opener © VStock LLC/age fotostock; **FIG 15-3** Courtesy, Serenity Safety

Products; **FIG 15-4 & 15-5** Source: National Highway Traffic Safety Administration. Working Group Best-Practice Recommendations for the Safe Transportation of Children in Emergency Ground Ambulances, DOT HS #811 677, Appendix D. Used with permission, Automotive Safety Program, Riley Hospital for Children; **TAB 15-1** National Highway Traffic Safety Administration; **FIG 15-9** Courtesy of IMMI

Chapter 16

Opener © CREATISTA/ShutterStock, Inc.; **FIG 16-1A** © glenda/ShutterStock, Inc.; **FIG 16-1B** © Alexander Raths/ ShutterStock, Inc.; **FIG 16-1D** © AbleStock; **FIG 16-1E** © glenda/ ShutterStock, Inc.; **FIG 16-2** © Libortom/istockphoto.com; FIG **16-4** ©LiquidLibrary; **FIG 16-8** © Dennis MacDonald/PhotoEdit Inc.; **FIG P16-1** Courtesy of VidaCare Corporation.